OXFORD MEDICAL PUBLICATIONS

Oxford Handbook for the Foundation Programme

Naomi Grant

Oxford Handbook for the Foundation Programme

Stephan Sanders

James Dawson

Shreelata Datta

Simon Eccles

OXFORD
UNIVERSITY PRESS

OXFORD
UNIVERSITY PRESS

Great Clarendon Street, Oxford OX2 6DP

Oxford University Press is a department of the University of Oxford.
It furthers the University's objective of excellence in research, scholarship, and education by publishing worldwide in

Oxford New York

Auckland Cape Town Dar es Salaam Hong Kong Karachi
Kuala Lumpur Madrid Melbourne Mexico City Nairobi
New Delhi Shanghai Taipei Toronto

With offices in

Argentina Austria Brazil Chile Czech Republic France Greece
Guatemala Hungary Italy Japan Poland Portugal Singapore
South Korea Switzerland Thailand Turkey Ukraine Vietnam

Oxford is a registered trade mark of Oxford University Press in the UK and in certain other countries

Published in the United States
by Oxford University Press Inc., New York

Reprinted 2006 (with corrections)

Medical Protection Society edition printed 2006

British Library Cataloguing in Publication Data
Data available

Library of Congress Cataloging in Publication Data
Data available

Typeset by Newgen Imaging Systems (P) Ltd., Chennai, India
Printed in China on acid-free paper by Phoenix Offset

ISBN 0–19–920499–3 978–0–19–920499–1

10 9 8 7 6 5 4 3 2 1

Contents

To every doctor who's ever stood there thinking:
'What on earth do I do now?'

Preface

Being a junior doctor can be hard. Really hard.

From the first day you are expected to manage sick patients in an alien environment with minimal experience and even less confidence. The bleep will go off incessantly and often you will not know what to do. The patients will never have the right symptoms or signs, yet will expect you to cure them instantly.

We have written this book to try to make life as a junior doctor a little bit easier; a metaphorical ice axe on a vertical learning curve. We have tried to keep it as simple as possible so that tired minds can make sense of the text. We hope it helps.

No book is perfect; we've done our very best. If you do not agree with what we have written, think we have missed something or have an idea to make it better please let us know. You can fill in the enclosed comments card or email us at the address below. We welcome comments from everyone.

Comments, thoughts, hints, brainwaves or interest in getting involved in future editions to:

ohfp.uk@oup.com

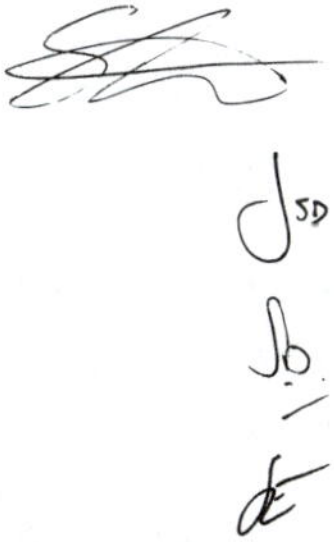

Foreword

Dame Lesley Southgate, Professor of Medical Education, St George's Hospital, University of London

Transitions are marked in our lives by excitement and anticipation, anxiety and anticlimax, and a sense that nothing will ever be the same again. Graduating as a doctor, and taking responsibility for patient care is no exception, and every member of the profession has vivid memories of those times. Including extreme measures to deal with bleeps that go off day and night, patients whose kindness and patience supported faltering clinical confidence, the reality of breaking bad news for real, and the funny side of clinical practice which can only be shared with close colleagues.

Medical education and training are currently undergoing the most significant reforms for many years. The establishment of the foundation programme to replace the PRHO and first SHO years sees the introduction of structure and supervision intended to promote the development of professionalism and clinical competence, particularly directed towards the care of the acutely ill. This at a time of increasing workload and a commitment to patient safety that is stretching the entire NHS workforce and which means that new doctors are entering a rapidly changing scene, where the structure of specialist training is being redefined. The curriculum for the foundation programme, and the assessments that will support it, will direct the trainee's attention to everyday clinical practice, and the knowledge and skills that must underpin those activities that result from the increased responsibility that a doctor, rather than a medical student, has.

In this book, written by doctors who are themselves in training, there is practical guidance which will help the reader to integrate the bewildering range of experiences that they will encounter into a theoretical and structured approach to learning in the workplace. They pay attention to the professional development of the reader, and provide a companion to bring help in tricky situations. And the authenticity of the voices of the authors and their amused but kind tone, itself reflects the spirit that many established clinicians will remember from their own days as a trainee.

May 2005

Acknowledgements

It would not have been possible to write this text without drawing from the wisdom of the other textbooks in the *Oxford Handbook* series. The following *Oxford Handbooks* were essential:

- ***Oxford Handbook of Clinical Medicine*** 6E by Murray Longmore, Ian Wilkinson and Supraj Rajagopalan
- ***Oxford Handbook of Clinical Specialties*** 6E by Judith Collier, Murray Longmore and Peter Scally
- ***Oxford Handbook of Acute Medicine*** 2E by Punit Ramrakha and Kevin Moore
- ***Oxford Handbook of General Practice*** 1E by Chantal Simon, Hazel Everitt, Jon Birtwistle and Brian Stevenson

The authors would like to express their extreme gratitude to these authors for writing such superb texts and allowing us to use them in writing this new one. We hope that it is worthy to sit alongside them.

We would especially like to thank the following wonderful people who have given their time, insight and experience to help us:

Dr Jenny Wright, Miss G Wilson, Dr Adrian Wills, Dr V Weston, Dr John Ward, James Wallace, Will Topping, Dr Kate Thomson, Mr Robert Sutcliffe, Mr Mike Smith, Helen Smith, Dr Gary Smith, Deborah Sanders, Dr TA Roper, Mr Manjeet Riyat, Anne Peppitt, Mr J Oni, Mr David Nunns, Dr Roger Neighbour, Dr Tamanna Moore, Dr Joanne Malkin, Dr Penny Law, Dr J Lamb, Dr William Kinnear, Leofranc Holford-Strevens, Dr Roger Holden, Imogen Hart, Dr David Gray, Dr Chris Gornall, Dr A G Gazis, Dr David Garner, Dr Doug Forrester, Katie Fletcher, Dr J English, Dr Jo Eastwood, David Connor, Gill Comrie, Mr Jaimie Coleman, Dr Lizzie Clark, Mrs S N Chandrasekar, Prof J Birchall, Dr Bryn Baxendale, Dr Helen Barnes, Prof A Aitkenhead, Dr Guru Aithal

We would also like to thank the following institutions for their advice and allowing us to reproduce images: Resuscitation Council UK, National Institute of Clinical Excellence, Complementary Medical Association, Paracetamol Information Centre, British Complementary Medical Association.

A huge thank you to all the staff at Oxford University Press for their support, guidance and humour. In particular:

- Alison Langton
- Michele Marietta
- Ali Bowker
- Kate Martin
- Barry Wheat

Finally we are very grateful to Professor Dame Lesley Southgate, a legend in postgraduate medicine, for her time and wisdom in writing our Foreword.

Abbreviations and symbols

A+E	Accident and emergency
AAA	Abdominal aortic aneurysm
ABG	Arterial blood gas
ABPI	Ankle brachial pressure index
ABx	Antibiotics
ACD	Anaemia of chronic disease
ACEi	Angiotensin-converting enzyme inhibitor
ACS	Acute coronary syndrome
ACTH	Adrenocorticotrophic hormone
ADH	Antidiuretic hormone
ADHD	Attention deficit hyperactivity disorder
ADL	Activities of daily living
AED	Automated external defibrillator
AF	Atrial fibrillation
AFB	Acid-fast bacilli
αFP	α-fetoprotein
AFP	α-fetoprotein
AICU	Adult intensive care unit
AIDS	Acquired immunodeficiency syndrome
ALL	Acute lymphoblastic leukaemia
ALP	Alkaline phosphatase
ALS	Advanced Life Support
ALT	Alanine aminotransferase
AML	Acute myeloid leukaemia
ANA	Antinuclear antibody
ANCA	Antineutrophil cytoplasmic antibody
AO	Arbeitsgemeinschaft für osteosynthesefragen (AO screws)
AP	Anteroposterior
APH	Antepartum haemorrhage
APLS	Advanced Paediatric Life Support
APTT	Activated partial thromboplastin time
APTTr	Activated partial thromboplastin time ratio
AR	Aortic regurgitation
ARDS	Acute respiratory distress syndrome
ARF	Acute renal failure
AS	Aortic stenosis
ASA	American Society of Anesthesiologists
ASAP	As soon as possible
ASD	Atrial septal defect

ASIF	Association for the Study of Internal Fixation
AST	Aspartate transaminase
ATLS	Advance Trauma Life Support
ATN	Acute tubular necrosis
AV	Atrio-ventricular
AVR	Aortic valve replacement
AXR	Abdominal X-ray
B_{12}	Vitamin B_{12}
Ba	Barium
BCG	Bacille Calmette-Guérin (TB vaccination)
bd	Bis die (twice daily)
BE	Base excess/Barium enema
BFG	Big friendly giant
β-HCG	β-human chorionic gonadotrophin
BiC	Bicarbonate
BIH	Benign intracranial hypertension
BiPAP	Biphasic positive airways pressure
BKA	Below knee amputation
BLS	Basic Life Support
BM	Boehringer-Mannhein meter (capillary blood glucose)/Bone marrow
BMA	British Medical Association
BMI	Body mass index
BMJ	British Medical Journal
BNF	British National Formulary
BP	Blood pressure
BPH	Benign prostatic hypertrophy
BX	Biopsy
C+S	Circulation and sensation
Ca^{2+}	Calcium
ca	Carcinoma
CABG	Coronary artery bypass graft
CAH	Congenital adrenal hyperplasia
CBD	Common bile duct
CBT	Cognitive-behavioural therapy
CCF	Congestive cardiac failure
CCST	Certificate of Completion of Specialist Training
CCT	Certificate of Completion of Training
CCU	Coronary care unit
CDH	Congenital dislocation of the hip
CDT	*Clostridium difficile* toxin
CEA	Carcinoembryonic antigen
CEPOD	Confidential Enquiry into Perioperative Deaths
CHD	Coronary heart disease
CI	Contraindication/Cardiac index

CJD	Creutzfeldt-Jakob Disease
CK	Creatine kinase
CK-MB	Heart-specific creatine kinase (MB-isoenzyme)
Cl^-	Chloride
CLL	Chronic lymphocytic leukaemia
CLO	Camplyobacter-like organism
Cm	Centimetres
CML	Chronic myeloid leukaemia
CMV	Cytomegalovirus
CN	Cranial nerves
CNS	Central nervous system
CO	Carbon monoxide
CO_2	Carbon dioxide
COAD	Chronic obstructive airway disease
COC	Combined oral contraceptive
COCP	Combined oral contraceptive pill
COPD	Chronic obstructive pulmonary disease
CPAP	Continuous positive airway pressure
CPK	Creatine phosphokinase
CPN	Community psychiatric nurse
CPR	Cardiopulmonary resuscitation
CRF	Chronic renal failure
CRP	C-reactive protein
CRT	Capillary refill time
CSF	Cerebrospinal fluid
CSOM	Chronic suppurative otitis media
CSU	Catheter specimen of urine
CT	Computer tomography
CTPA	CT pulmonary angiogram
CUS	Catheter urine sample
CV	Curriculum vitae
CVA	Cerebrovascular accident
CVP	Central venous pressure
CVS	Cardiovascular system
CXR	Chest X-ray
d	Days
D+C	Dilatation and curettage
D+V	Diarrhoea and vomiting
DEXA	Dual-energy X-Ray absorptiometry (DXA)
DH	Drug history
DHS	Dynamic hip screw
DI	Diabetes insipidus
DIB	Difficulty in breathing
DIC	Disseminated intravascular coagulation
DKA	Diabetic ketoacidosis

dl	Decilitre
DM	Diabetes mellitus
DNA	Deoxyribonucleic acid/Did not attend
DNR	Do not resuscitate
DoB	Date of birth
DOH	Department of Health
DRE	Digital rectal examination
DTP	Diptheria, tetanus and pertussis
DU	Duodenal ulcer
DVLA	Driver and Vehicle Licensing Agency
DVT	Deep vein thrombosis
d/w	Discuss(ed) with
Dx	Diagnosis
DXA	Dual-energy X-Ray absorptiometry (DEXA)
DXT	Deep radiotherapy
EBM	Evidence-based medicine
EBV	Epstein–Barr virus
ECG	Electrocardiogram
ECHO	Echocardiogram
ECS	Endocervical swab
EEA	European Economic Area
EEG	Electroencephalogram
EMD	Electromechanical dissociation or pulseless electrical activity (PEA)
EMG	Electromyogram
ENT	Ear, nose and throat
EØ	Eosinophil
EPO	Erythropoietin
ERCP	Endoscopic retrograde cholangiopancreatography
ERPC	Evacuation of retained products of conception
ESM	Ejection systolic murmur
ESR	Erythrocyte sedimentation rate
ESRF	End-stage renal failure
ET	Endotracheal
ETOH	Ethanol (alcohol)
EUA	Examination under anaesthetic
EWTD	European Working Time Directive
F1	Foundation year one
F2	Foundation year two
FB	Foreign body
FBC	Full blood count
FDP	Fibrin degradation product
FEV_1	Forced expiratory volume in one second
FFP	Fresh frozen plasma
FH	Family history/Fetal heart

FiO_2	Fractional inspired oxygen content
FOB	Faecal occult blood
FOOSH	Fall on outstretched hand
FP	Foundation Programme
FP1	Foundation Programme, year one
FP2	Foundation Programme, year two
FRC	Functional residual capacity
FSH	Follicle stimulating hormone
FVC	Forced vital capacity
G	Gram
G+S	Group and save
G6PD	Glucose-6-phosphate dehydrogenase
GA	General anaesthetic
GB	Gall bladder
GCS	Glasgow Coma Score
GFR	Glomerular filtration rate
γGT	γ-glutamyl transpeptidase
GGT	γ-glutamyl transpeptidase
GH	Growth hormone
GI	Gastrointestinal
GMC	General Medical Council
GN	Glomerulonephritis
GORD	Gastro-oesophageal reflux disease
GP	General practitioner
GTN	Glyceryl trinitrate
GTT	Glucose tolerance test
GU	Genitourinary
h	Hour
HAV	Hepatitis A virus
Hb	Haemoglobin
HbA_{1c}	Glycosylated haemoglobin
HBV	Hepatitis B virus
HCA	Health care assistant
HCC	Hepatocellular carcinoma
HCG	Human chorionic gonadotrophin
HCO_3^-	Bicarbonate
HCT	Haematocrit
HCV	Hepatitis C virus
HDL	High-density lipoprotein
HDU	High dependency unit
HELLP	Haemolysis, elevated liver enzymes, low platelets (syndrome)
HIV	Human immunodeficiency virus
HLA	Human leucocyte antigen
HOCM	Hypertrophic obstructive cardiomyopathy
HONK	Hyperosmolar non-ketotic (coma)

HR	Heart rate
HRT	Hormone replacement therapy
HSP	Henoch Schönlein purpura
HSV	Herpes simplex virus
HTN	Hypertension
HUS	Haemolytic uraemic syndrome
HVS	High vaginal swab
I+D	Incision and drainage
IBD	Inflammatory bowel disease
IBS	Irritable bowel syndrome
ICP	Intracranial pressure
ICU	Intensive care unit
ID	Identification
IDDM	Insulin-dependent diabetes mellitus
IE	Infective endocarditis
Ig	Immunoglobulin
IgE	Immunoglobulin E
IgG	Immunoglobulin G
IHD	Ischaemic heart disease
ILS	Immediate Life Support
IM/im	Intramuscular
INH	By inhalation
INR	International normalised ratio
ITP	Idiopathic thrombocytopenic purpura
ITU	Intensive care unit
iu	International unit
IUCD	Intrauterine contraceptive device
IUP	Intrauterine pregnancy
IV/iv	Intravenous
IVDU	Intravenous drug user
IVI	Intravenous infusion
IVP	Intravenous pyelogram
IVU	Intravenous urogram
Ix	Investigation(s)
JACCOL	Jaundice, anaemia, clubbing, cyanosis, oedema, lymphadenopathy
JDC	Junior Doctors' Committee
JFDI	Just … do it
JVP	Jugular venous pressure
K^+	Potassium
KCL	Potassium chloride
kg	Kilogram
K-nail	Küntscher nail
kPa	Kilopascal
KUB	Kidneys, ureter, bladder (X-ray)

K-wire	Kirschner wire
l	Litre
LA	Local anaesthetic
LACS	Lacunar circulation stroke
LAD	Left axis deviation/Left anterior descending
LBBB	Left bundle branch block
LDH	Lactate dehydrogenase
LDL	Low-density lipoprotein
LFT	Liver function test
LH	Luteinising hormone
LIF	Left iliac fossa
LMN	Lower motor neurone
LMP	Last menstrual period
LMWH	Low-molecular-weight heparin
LN	Lymph node
LØ	Lymphocyte
LP	Lumbar puncture
LSCS	Lower segment Caesarean section
LUQ	Left upper quadrant
LVF	Left ventricular failure
LVH	Left ventricular hypertrophy
MAOI	Monoamine oxidase inhibitor
mane	In the morning
MAP	Mean arterial pressure
M,C+S	Microscopy, culture and sensitivity
MCTD	Mixed connective tissue disease
MCQ	Multiple choice question
MCV	Mean cell volume
MDDUS	Medical and Dental Defence Union of Scotland
MDU	Medical Defence Union
ME	Myalgic encephalitis
MEWS	Modified Early Warning Score
mg	Milligram
Mg^{2+}	Magnesium
MI	Myocardial infarction
min	Minutes
MMC	Modernising Medical Careers
mmH_2O	Millimetres of water
mmHg	Millimetres of mercury
MMR	Measles, mumps and rubella
MND	Motor neurone disease
MPS	Medical Protection Society
MR	Mitral regurgitation
MRCP	Magnetic resonance cholangiopancreatography
MRI	Magnetic resonance imaging

MRSA	Methicillin-resistant *Staph. aureus*
ms	Milliseconds
MS	Multiple sclerosis/Mitral stenosis
MST	Morphine sulphate
MSU	Mid-stream urine
mth	Months
MVR	Mitral valve replacement
N+V	Nausea and vomiting
N_2O	Nitrous oxide
Na^+	Sodium
NACL	Sodium chloride
NAD	Nothing abnormal detected
NAI	Non-accidental injury
NBM	Nil by mouth
NEB	By nebuliser
NG/ng	Nasogastric
NGO	Non-governmental organisation
NGT	Nasogastric tube
NHS	National Health Service
NICE	National Institute for Clinical Excellence
NICU	Neonatal intensive care unit
NIDDM	Non-insulin dependent diabetes mellitus
NØ	Neutrophil
nocte	At night
NPA	Nasopharyngeal aspirate
NSAID	Non-steroidal anti-inflammatory drug
NSTEMI	Non-ST-elevation myocardial infarction
NTN	National training number
NVD	Normal vaginal delivery
O_2	Oxygen
OA	Osteoarthritis
Obs	Observations
OCP	Oral contraceptive pill/Ova, cysts and parasites
od	Omni die (once daily)
OD	Overdose
OGD	Oesophagogastroduodenoscopy
OHA	Oxford Handbook of Anaesthetics
OHAEM	Oxford Handbook of Accident and Emergency Medicine
OHAM	Oxford Handbook of Acute Medicine
OHCC	Oxford Handbook of Critical Care
OHCLI	Oxford Handbook of Clinical and Laboratory Investigation
OHCM	Oxford Handbook of Clinical Medicine
OHCS	Oxford Handbook of Clinical Specialties
OHGP	Oxford Handbook of General Practice
OHOG	Oxford Handbook of Obstetrics and Gynaecology

OHP	Overhead projector
om	Omni mane (in the morning)
on	Omni nocte (at night)
ORIF	Open reduction and internal fixation
OSCE	Objective structured clinical examination
OT	Occupational therapy
P	Pulse
PA	Posteroanterior
$PaCO_2$	Partial pressure of arterial carbon dioxide
PACS	Partial anterior circulation stroke
PAN	Polyarteritis nodosa
PaO_2	Partial pressure of arterial oxygen
PBC	Primary biliary cirrhosis
PCA	Patient-controlled analgesia
PCO_2	Partial pressure of carbon dioxide
PCOS	Polycystic ovary syndrome
PCR	Polymerase chain reaction
PCT	Primary care trust
PCV	Packed cell volume
PDA	Patent ductus arteriosus/Personal digital assistant
PE	Pulmonary embolism
PEA	Pulseless electrical activity
PEFR	Peak expiratory flow rate
PERLA	Pupils equal and reactive to light and accommodation
PICU	Paediatric intensive care unit
PID	Pelvic inflammatory disease
PMETB	Postgraduate Medical Education and Training Board
PMH	Past medical history
PMT	Pre-menstrual tension
PND	Paroxysmal nocturnal dyspnoea
PNS	Peripheral nervous system
PO_4^{3-}	Phosphate
PO/po	Per os (by mouth)
pO_2	Partial pressure of oxygen
PoC	Products of conception
POCS	Posterior circulation stroke
POP	Plaster of Paris/Progesterone only pill
PPH	Postpartum haemorrhage
PPI	Proton pump inhibitor
PR/pr	Per rectum
PRHO	Pre-registration house officer
PRN	Pro re nata (as required)
PRV	Polycythaemia rubra vera
PSA	Prostate specific antigen
PSH	Past surgical history

PT	Prothrombin time
PTH	Parathyroid hormone
PU	Passed urine/Peptic ulcer
PUD	Peptic ulcer disease
PUO	Pyrexia of unknown origin
PV/pv	Plasma viscosity/Per vagina
PVD	Peripheral vascular disease
qds	Quarter die sumendus (four times daily)
RA	Rheumatoid arthritis
RAST	Radioallergosorbant test
RAT	Regional action team
RBBB	Right bundle branch block
RBC	Red blood cell
RDW	Red cell distribution width
RF	Rheumatic fever
RH	Rhesus
RhF	Rheumatoid factor
RIF	Right iliac fossa
ROM	Range of movement
ROS	Review of systems
RR	Respiratory rate
RS	Respiratory system
RSI	Rapid sequence induction
RTA	Road traffic accident
RUQ	Right upper quadrant
RVH	Right ventricular hypertrophy
Rx	Prescription
s/sec	Seconds
SAH	Sub-arachnoid haemorrhage
SALT	Speech and language therapy
Sats	O_2 saturation
SBE	Sub-acute bacterial endocarditis
SBP	Systolic blood pressure
SC	Subcutaneous
SCBU	Special care baby unit
SCC	Squamous cell carcinoma
SCD	Sickle-cell disease
SD	Standard deviation
SE	Side-effects
SH	Social history
SHBG	Sex hormone-binding globulin
SHDU	Surgical high dependency unit
SHO	Senior house officer
SIADH	Syndrome of inappropriate antidiuretic hormone secretion
SL/Sl	Sublingual

SLE	Systemic lupus erythematosus
SOA	Swelling of ankles
SOB	Short of breath
SOBAR	Short of breath at rest
SOBOE	Short of breath on exertion
SOL	Space occupying lesion
SpO_2	Oxygen saturation in peripheral blood
SpR	Specialist registrar
SR	Slow release/Senior registrar
SSP	Statutory sick pay
SSRI	Selective serotonin reuptake inhibitor
Stat	Statim (immediately)
STD	Sexually transmitted disease
STEMI	ST-elevation myocardial infarction
STI	Sexually transmitted infection
STOP	Surgical termination of pregnancy
SVC	Superior vena cava
SVR	Systemic vascular resistance
SVT	Supraventricular tachycardia
Sx	Symptoms
SXR	Skull X-ray
Temp	Temperature
T_3	Tri-iodothyronine
T_4	Thyroxine
TACS	Total anterior circulation stroke
TB	Tuberculosis
TBG	Thyroxine-binding globulin
TCA	Tricyclic antidepressant
tds	Ter die sumendus (three times daily)
Teds	Thromboembolism deterrent stockings
Temp	Temperature
TENS	Transcutaneous electrical nerve stimulation
TFT	Thyroid function test
THR	Total hip replacement
TIA	Transient ischaemic attack
TIBC	Total iron binding capacity
TIPS	Transjugular intrahepatic porto-systemic shunting
TKR	Total knee replacement
TLC	Tender loving care/Total lung capacity
TOE	Transoesophageal echocardiogram
TPN	Total parenteral nutrition
TPR	Total peripheral resistance
TSH	Thyroid stimulating hormone
TTA	To take away
TTO	To take out

TURP	Transurethral resection of prostate
TWOC	Trial without catheter
Tx	Treatment
u/U	Units
U+E	Urea and electrolytes
UC	Ulcerative colitis
UMN	Upper motor neurone
UO	Urine output
URTI	Upper respiratory tract infection
US(S)	Ultrasound scan
USMLE	United States Medical Licensing Exam
UTI	Urinary tract infection
UV	Ultraviolet
V/Q	Ventilation/perfusion scan
VA	Visual acuity
VC	Vital capacity
VDRL	Veneral disease research laboratory (test)
VE	Vaginal examination/Ventricular ectopic
VF	Ventricular fibrillation
VMA	Vanillylmandelic acid
VP shunt	Ventriculoperitoneal shunt
VSD	Ventriculoseptal defect
VT	Ventricular tachycardia
VZV	Varicella-zoster virus
WB	Weight bear
WBC	White blood cell
WCC	White cell count
WHO	World Health Organisation
wk	Weeks
WPW	Wolff-Parkinson-White syndrome
wt	Weight
X-match	Crossmatch
yr	Years
ZN	Ziehl-Neelson

Introduction

Thank you for buying, or at least contemplating buying, the *Oxford Handbook for the Foundation Programme* – the first ever Foundation Programme handbook. This book is set out differently from others and taking 5min to read this page should help you to use it effectively.

Doing the job These six chapters cover the non-clinical side of being a junior doctor; each chapter starts with a contents list:

- ***The job*** (p1) essential kit, TTOs, ward rounds, being on-call
- ***Your career*** (p37) CVs, audits, exams, getting a job, moving on
- ***Communication*** (p71) breaking bad news, translators, languages
- ***Ethics*** (p85) death, confidentiality, consent
- ***When things go wrong*** (p95) errors, incident forms, hating your job
- ***Boring but important stuff*** (p103) NHS structure, money, benefits

Clinical presentations These cover common presentations and ward cover problems. They are arranged by symptom because you are called to see a breathless patient, not someone having a PE:

- ***Emergencies*** The inside back cover shows a list of emergencies according to symptom (arrest, chest pain, fitting) with page references. These pages give step-by-step instructions to help you resuscitate and stabilise an acutely ill patient.
- ***Symptoms*** The inside front cover shows a list of symptoms with page references. On the pages shown you will find causes, what to ask and look for, relevant investigations and a table showing the distinguishing features of each disease. The relevant diseases are described in the pages following each symptom.
- ***Diseases*** Once you know the disease you can also look it up on the list of diseases, p112. Each of these refers to a section showing the symptoms, signs and investigation results along with the management.

Specialities The specialities covered are shown on p301. They cover the key differences with history taking and examination along with common diseases unique to that speciality.

Procedures The procedures covered are shown on p455. Each one gives instructions on how to perform the procedure, the equipment needed and contraindications.

Interpreting results The results covered are shown on p497. Each one gives a guide to the important features to note and suggestions as to the cause of any abnormality seen.

At the back There are a number of useful pages before the index including contact numbers, weight and height conversion charts, blank timetables and phone number lists. Common drug doses we have shown after the index.

10 tips on being a junior doctor

(1) Book your annual leave Time off is essential. Make sure you spend it doing something you really enjoy with people you really like. It can be very difficult to book time off and it is your responsibility to swap the on-calls. The sooner you ask for swaps the easier it is.
(2) Take a break If you are unable to make decisions or get a cannula in you probably need a rest. Most decisions can wait, only acutely ill patients cannot and they will need an alert doctor. Get a drink, sit down and think about something else for 20min.
(3) Smile You cannot cure most diseases, you cannot make procedures pleasant, you cannot help the fact that you, the ward staff and the patients are stuck in the hospital, but smiling and being friendly can make all the difference.
(4) Never shout at anyone Shouting or being insulting is unprofessional. If you have a problem it should be addressed in private. The job rapidly becomes unpleasant if you get a reputation for being rude.
(5) Phone for senior help If you do not know what to do, or are unsure, then you should contact a senior. If it can wait then write it down to mention it next time you see them.
(6) Check in the *BNF* If you are not familiar with a drug then always check in the *BNF* before you give it. Trust nobody, it will be your name next to the prescription.
(7) Look at the obs It is difficult (but possible) to be acutely ill with normal obs, hence the use of scoring systems, eg MEWS p118. Do not dismiss deranged obs, try to find the cause and review the patient often.
(8) Trust your instinct If you or a nurse feel a patient is seriously unwell then they probably are. Do not dismiss this feeling, try to work out what it is that makes you uneasy and investigate accordingly. At the very least review the patient frequently and monitor their obs. If you can't figure it out, ask a senior.
(9) Be reliable If you say you are going to do something then make sure you do it. If you are unable to do it then let someone know.
(10) Prepare for the future Medicine is competitive, you need to give yourself the best chance. Over the first two years you should:

- plan your career
- keep your CV up to date
- get good referees and mentors
- undertake an audit
- present interesting cases to your team

The Foundation Programme

The concept

The Foundation Programme (FP) is a training programme for all doctors graduating from medical school. It is split into two years:

- F1 (foundation year one), equivalent to the PRHO grade
- F2 (foundation year two), equivalent to the SHO1 grade

After successfully completing F1, doctors will gain full registration with the General Medical Council (GMC) and start F2. Once F2 is successfully completed doctors can apply for specialist training (see p56).

The Foundation Programme has been introduced so that all new doctors receive training and assessment in the basic skills of being a doctor (both clinical and non-clinical). Before the FP junior doctor jobs varied widely in terms of supervision and feedback – hopefully this will improve.

Useful 'foundation terms'

Clinical supervisor	Senior member of staff who supervises your day-to-day learning and training
Educational supervisor	Doctor who will review your progress on a regular basis, check that your assessments are up to date and help you plan your career
Local administrator	A person in each trust or foundation school who keeps a record of all the assessments you complete and organises multi-source feedback
Foundation training programme director (FTPD)	The director of each foundation school who signs you off after each year
Unit of application (UoA)	A foundation school or deanery that you are applying to
Foundation school	The organisation that runs the Foundation Programme locally; it includes medical schools, deaneries, local hospitals (trusts) and PCTs

Other information

You can find more information about the Foundation Programme and future changes at www.mmc.nhs.uk. There are several documents to download including the Operational framework (the FP 'rules') and the Curriculum (full list of educational objectives) and Rough Guide to the Foundation Programme that are included in the FP induction pack.

After the Foundation Programme

The details of your future training have not been finalised yet; some of the likely features are described on p56. The speciality placements you undertake during your foundation training will not have a direct bearing on your selection to speciality training. To help you decide which training path to take, each foundation school should have careers advisors; see also p49 for careers advice.

FP applications

The application process has 3 stages:

1) Choose a UoA These are 'Units of Application' which simply means a foundation school (eg North West Thames) or a deanery (eg Trent). The exact application details and closing dates vary; details can be found on each UoA's website by following the links on www.mmc.nhs.uk in October. You need to make a list of UoAs you would be willing to work at in order of preference.
2) Apply Instead of sending a CV, all students will fill in the same application form. The competed form should be sent to your first choice of UoA according to the instructions shown on that UoA's website. You should also include:
   - The names and postal and email addresses of 2 referees
   - A letter from your medical school supporting your application to your first choice UoA
   - Your list of desired UoAs in order of preference
3) Wait. The application forms will be scored by a panel at the UoA it is sent to; national criteria will be used, so all UoAs should give you the same score. Your referees will be contacted at a later to date–they will not affect your score. If your score is good enough you will be told you have a place in January. Otherwise your details may be passed onto other UoAs on your list or you will be entered into clearing in the Spring.

Choosing you placements

The F1 year usually consists of 3 placements of 4 months; 2 of these will be general medicine and surgery. How these placements are allocated will be decided by the individual UoA; details should be shown on their websites (see above). Some will allocate placements alongside the UoA application procedure, while others will allocate them at a later date.

What happens in F2?

Most F2 posts will consist of 3 placements of 4 months. By 2007 one of these will be a GP placement for 80% of trainees. You can also arrange week long study leave 'tasters' in another specialty to help plan your career – to arrange these talk to your educational supervisor and a consultant in the relevant speciality.

Applying for an F2 post

The placement for your F2 year may have not been decided and you will need to apply for them 6–8 months into your F1 year. Once you are on a 2 year Foundation Programme you are guaranteed an F2 post in the same foundation school, but often in a different hospital. The allocation process will vary between foundation schools (eg CV, interview, random selection).

FP assessment and portfolios

Throughout the Foundation Programme you will be assessed to prove that you are learning the basic skills of doctoring. You will be given the Foundation Learning Portfolio at the start of the programme which will include examples of the various assessment forms.

Once you complete each assessment you should photocopy the form so you can keep one for your portfolio and send the other to your local administrator.

Assessments in the foundation programme	
Direct Observation of Procedural Skills (DOPS)	≥4 in F1, ≥6 in F2
A colleague should watch you perform a procedure (there is a list in the portfolio). The assessor simply ticks boxes about how well you did the various components.	
Initiated by yourself; you choose the time, place and assessor	
Mini-Clinical Evaluation Exercise (Mini-CEX)	≥4 in F1, ≥6 in F2
A colleague should watch you clerk a patient and tick boxes accordingly; they should also give you verbal feedback.	
Initiated by yourself; you choose the time, place and assessor	
Case-based discussion (CbD)	≥6 in F1, ≥6 in F2
You should present a case you have clerked to a doctor (SpR or senior) and discuss your choice of investigations and management. Once again boxes need ticking.	
Initiated by yourself; you choose the time, place and assessor	
Multisource feedback (MSF)	≥1 in F1, ≥1 in F2
This may be 'Mini-Peer Assessment Tool' (Mini-PAT) or a Team Asssessment of Behaviour (TAB). Both essentially involve 10–12 colleagues (consultants, SpRs, nurses, physios, GPs, etc) filling in a form about how you are doing.	
Initiated by your local administrator; you choose the assessors	

The 'Foundation Learning Portfolio'

Along with the assessment forms these are several other components to the portfolio that you need to complete:

- Self-appraisal-form – complete at the start of each placement before meeting with your educational supervisor
- Personal development plan (PDP) and Educational agreement – complete at the start of each placement in the meeting with your educational supervisor
- Induction meeting – complete at the start of each placement in the meeting with your clinical supervisor
- Reflective practice form and self-appraisal of learning – you do not have to complete any of these, but some consultants are very keen on them
- Summary of evidence presented – fill this in as you pass assessments to guide what areas further assessments need to cover
- Statement of health and probity – this should be completed at every appraisal

There are also forms to complete at the end of your F1 and F2 year to prove you have passed. It is important to keep your portfolio up to date and safe; it is essential that you can show evidence that you are competent to move onto the next level of training.

NCEPOD(2005)

NCEPOD or The National Confidential Enquiry into Patient Outcome and Death is part of the National Patient Safety Agency (NPSA). It is made up of representatives and observers from numerous organisations including the Royal Colleges, the Coroners Society and lay people. Its purpose is to improve the quality and safety of patient care.

An Acute Problem? NCEPOD(2005)[1] is a report based on the results of a survey of admissions to UK Intensive Care Units during a month in 2003.

The report is available on the internet[2] or in hard copy from NCEPOD. There are 29 main recommendations made, at least 10 of which have direct implications for the newly qualified doctor (see below). Each of these 10 points has been cross-referenced to the appropriate section in this handbook.

- More attention should be paid to patients exhibiting physiological abnormalities. This is a marker of increased mortality risk (p118–119)
- The importance of respiratory rate monitoring should be highlighted. This parameter should be recorded at any point that other observations are being made (p118)
- Education and training should be provided for staff that use pulse oximeters to allow proper interpretation and understanding of the limitations of this monitor. It should be emphasised that pulse oximetry does not replace respiratory rate monitoring (p118)
- It is inappropriate for referral and acceptance to ICU to happen at junior doctor (SHO) level (p19)
- Training must be provided for junior doctors in the recognition of critical illness and immediate management of fluid and oxygen therapy in these patients (p118 and 148)
- Consultants must supervise junior doctors more closely and should actively support juniors in the management of patients rather than only reacting to requests for help (p10)
- Junior doctors must seek advice more readily. This may be from specialised teams, eg outreach services, or from the supervising consultant (p26)
- Each hospital should have a track and trigger system that allows rapid detection of the signs of early clinical deterioration and an early and appropriate response (p118)
- All entries in the notes should be dated and timed and should end with a legible name, status and contract number (bleep or telephone) (p12)
- Each entry should clearly identify the name and grade of the most senior doctor involved in the patient episode (p12)

Readers are advised to study the report in full as there are numerous learning points for doctors of all grades and specialities.

[1] An Acute Problem? NCEPOD. 11th May 2005.
[2] http://www.ncepod.org.uk/2005.htm

Chapter 1

The job

Before you start

Important organisations

The prices quoted change frequently; they are intended as a guide.

General Medical Council (GMC) To work as a doctor in the UK you need GMC registration; a bargain at £100 for the PRHO year or £290 each year as an SHO or above.

NHS indemnity insurance This covers the financial consequences of any mistake you make at work, but no more. It automatically covers all doctors in the NHS so you do not need to subscribe or pay anything.

Indemnity insurance This is essential; do not start work without it. These organisations will support and advise you in any complaints or legal matters that arise from your work. They also insure you against work outside the hospital (eg locums, helping at a car crash). There are three main organisations, all offer 24h helplines (p524):

- Medical Protection Society (MPS) – £10 as a PRHO, £40–60 as an SHO
- Medical Defence Union (MDU) – £14 as a PRHO, £42–60 as an SHO
- Medical Doctors and Dentist Defence Union of Scotland (MDDUS) – £10 as a PRHO, £40–55 as a SHO

British Medical Association (BMA) Political voice of doctors; campaigns for better conditions, hours, pay and comments on health issues. Membership includes a weekly subscription to the BMJ and support in disputes with your employers. Costs £90 as a PRHO then £180 as an SHO.

Income protection Pays half your basic salary until retirement age if you become too ill to work as a doctor. NHS sickness benefits are poor (lasting only 1mth as a PRHO and 4mth the next year):

- Medical Sickness £18/mth as PRHO, rises afterwards according to age, pay, illness and risks; there are many others available

For more details on financial matters see p108.

NHS pension scheme This is the best pension available, do not opt out; a percentage of your pay will be automatically diverted to the pension.

Important documents for your first day

P45/P60 tax form When you leave a job you will receive a P45; if you continue in the same job you will receive a P60 every April. It is not a problem if you do not have a P45 to hand in, though you might have to pay emergency (extra) tax that will be refunded the next month.

Bank details Account number, sort code and address.

Hepatitis B You need proof of hep B immunity or vaccinations. You should be issued with an Occupational Health Smartcard.

GMC registration certificate To prove that you are a registered doctor.

Criminal Record Bureau (CRB) certificate Required for paediatrics, obs and gynae and A+E; if you do not have one you will need to fill in a form.

Induction pack and contract Sent by the trust before you start; otherwise contact human resources to find out where and when to meet.

On your first day (or before)

Leave plenty of time to find the right hospital and room on your first day. Many hospitals organise a fair to speed up the signing-in process. The following are the essentials:

House If you are living on site this is probably your top priority. Phone the accommodation office before you start to check their opening hours. Make sure they give you a key that works and opens the right flat. Try to avoid leaving your car filled with all your earthly possessions.

Pay roll It often takes over a month to adjust pay so it is vital to give the finance dept your bank details on the first day if you want to be paid later that month. Hand in your P45/P60 at the same time.

Parking Check with other staff about the best places to park and 'parking deals'; you will probably need to get several people to sign a form.

ID badge This may also be used to access secure sections of the hospital. If so, insist on getting access to all areas since you will be on the crash team. If the card doesn't give access to all wards return it and get it fixed.

Computer access This allows you to get results, access the internet and your NHS email. Write down all the passwords, usernames etc and keep any documents handed out. Ask for a phone number in case of difficulty.

Work rota Ideally this will already have arrived before the job starts.

Colleagues' mobile numbers This will probably be the last time you are all gathered in one place. Getting numbers makes social activities and rota swaps much easier. Asking for rota swaps on the first day is also easier.

Important places in the hospital

Try to get hold of a map; many hospitals have evolved rather than been designed. This can make navigation difficult. There are often short cuts.

Ward(s) Write down any access codes and find out where you can put your bag. Ask to be shown where things are kept including the crash trolley and blood-taking equipment. You may be able to meet your team and pick up your bleep.

Canteen(s) Establish where the best food options are at various times of day. Note the opening hours – this will be invaluable for breaks on-call.

Cash and food dispensers Hospitals are required to provide hot food 24h a day. This may be from a machine.

Doctors' mess Clearly essential. Write down the access code and establish if there is a freezer. Microwave meals are infinitely preferable to the food from machines.

On-call rooms/doctors' offices These are becoming scarce though.

Radiology Try to work out which radiological requests go where and which consultants deal with different imaging. Radiology secretaries are often a good source of information.

How to be a house officer

Being a house officer involves teamwork, organisation and communication – qualities that are not easily assessed during finals. As well as settling into a new work environment, you have to integrate with your colleagues and the rest of the hospital team. You are not expected to know everything at the start of your post; you should always ask someone more senior if you are in doubt.

As a house officer, your role includes:

- clerking patients (A+E, pre-op clinic, on-call or on the ward)
- updating patient lists and knowing where patients are (p6)
- participating in team ward rounds to review patient management
- requesting investigations and chasing their results
- liaising with other specialities/health-care professionals (p11)
- practical procedures
- administrative tasks eg theatre lists (p423), TTOs (p22), rewriting drug charts (p20), death certificates (p88)
- speaking to the patient and their relatives regarding progress/results

How to be efficient

- Fill in the blood bottle form on p460
- Make a list of common bleeps/extensions, p531
- Establish a timetable of your firm's activities, p530
- Make a folder/clipboard (see p6)
- See organisational tips, p6
- Prioritise your workload rather than simply working through jobs in order. Try to group jobs into areas of the hospital (ideally via the mess). If you're unsure of the urgency of a job, ask your seniors
- If you are working with another house officer split the jobs at the end of the ward round so that you share the workload
- If you have time fill in your details on spare request forms so there is less to write when you need them
- Fill out blood forms at the start/end of each day (find out what time the phlebotomists come); if a patient will need bloods for the next 3 days then fill them all out together with clear dates
- Be aware of your limitations eg consent should be done by the surgeon doing the procedure
- Get a copy of your hospital guidelines/protocols eg pre-op investigations, anticoagulation, DKA, pneumonia etc
- Get a map of the hospital if you haven't got your bearings

Breaks

Missing breaks does not make you appear hard-working – it reduces your efficiency and alertness. Give yourself time to rest and eat (chocolates from the ward are not lunch); you are entitled to 30min for every 4h worked. Use the time to meet other doctors in the mess, referring is much easier if you know them.

Know your limits

If you are unsure of something, don't feel embarrassed to ask your seniors – particularly if a patient is deteriorating. If you are stuck on simple tasks (eg difficult cannulation) take a break (the patient will welcome this) and try again or ask a colleague to have a go.

Your bleep

This quickly becomes the bane of your existence. When the bleep goes off repeatedly write down the numbers calling, sit down and answer them in turn. Try to deal with queries over the phone; if not make a list of jobs and prioritise them, tell the nurses how long you will be and be realistic. Encourage ward staff to make a list of routine jobs for when you pass by the ward instead of bleeping you repeatedly. The bleep should only be for sick patients and urgent tasks. Learn the number of switchboard since this is likely to be an outside caller waiting on the line. Crash calls are usually announced to all bleepholders via switchboard. If your bleep is unusually quiet, check the batteries. Consider handing over your bleep to a colleague when breaking bad news or speaking to relatives.

- ***Dropping the bleep in the toilet*** This is not uncommon; attempt to recover the bleep using non-sterile gloves. Wash thoroughly in running water (the damage has already been done) and inform switchboard that you dropped it into your drink
- ***Other forms of bleep destruction*** You will usually not have to pay for a damaged bleep; consider asking for a clip-on safety strap

Responsibility

As a house officer you will make innumerable difficult decisions, some with potentially serious consequences. Always consider the worst case scenario and how to avoid it (eg investigations, discuss with senior). Make sure you can justify your actions; document events and discussion with relatives carefully (p73).

Expectations

Seniors will expect you to know Mrs Jones' current medication dose, the details of the operation they performed yesterday (while you were chasing results) and the blood results from 5d ago. Initially this seems impossible, but with time your memory for such details will improve as you understand their relevance (emotional reaction to information = memory) and more importantly you will get a feel for what questions you will be asked.

Learning

You need to be proactive to learn interpretation and management skills as a house officer. Formulate a management plan for each patient you see and compare this with your senior's version; ask about any significant differences.

Getting organised

Your organisational abilities may be valued above your clinical acumen. While this is not why you chose to become a doctor, being organised will make you more efficient and ensure you get home as early as possible.

Folders and clipboards These are an excellent way to hold patient lists, job lists and spare paperwork along with a portable writing surface. Imaginative improvements can be constructed with bulldog clips, plastic wallets and dividers.

- ***Contents:*** spare clerking paper, drug charts, TTOs, blood forms, radiology forms, a list of phone/bleep numbers, job lists, patient lists, theatre lists, spare pen

Patient lists Juniors are often entrusted with keeping a record of the team's patients (including those on different wards, called 'outliers') along with their background details, investigation results and management plans. With practice most people become good at recalling this information, but writing it down reduces errors.

One means of keeping track is updating a ward-based computer spreadsheet; this also allows every member of the team to carry a copy. It can be invaluable for discussing/referring a patient whilst away from the ward. See p17. **These must be kept confidential and disposed of securely.**

Job lists During the ward round make a note of all the jobs that need doing on a separate piece of paper. At the end of the round these jobs can be allocated amongst the team members.

Serial results Instead of simply writing blood results in the notes try writing them on serial results sheets (with a column for each day's results). This makes patterns easier to spot and saves time. Some teams store all patients' results sheets in a single folder, though they must be transferred into the individual hospital notes at discharge.

Timetables Along with ward rounds and clinical jobs there will be numerous extra meetings, teaching sessions and clinics to attend. There are three blank timetables at the end of this book.

Important numbers It can take over 5min to get through to switchboard so carrying a list of common numbers will save you hours. At the end of this book there are three blank phone number lists for different attachments. Stickers on the back of ID badges can hold up to 15 numbers.

Ward cover equipment Finding medical equipment on unfamiliar wards wastes time and is frustrating. You can speed up your cannula visits by keeping a supply of equipment in a box (lunch boxes are surprisingly suitable and come in a range of attractive designs). Try to fill them with equipment from storerooms instead of clinical areas. Some doctors use pouches attached to their belts.

What to carry

Essentials

Pens These are the most essential piece of equipment. Always carry a backup and bear in mind that you need a biro for writing on blood bottles; all writing must be in black (allows photocopying).

Stethoscope A Littmann® Classic II or equivalent is perfectly adequate, however better models offer clearer sound. Common upgrades include Littmann's Cardiology III (£130) and Master Cardiology (£160).

Tourniquet Consider talking to a friendly drug rep. otherwise £4–7 over the internet. A tied glove can be used if your tourniquet is missing.

Money Out of hours, loose change is very useful for food dispensers.

ID badge This should be supplied on your first day.

Bleep This will be on the ward, at switchboard or with a colleague.

Optional extras

Clipboard folder see p6

PDA see p8

Pen-torch Very useful for looking in mouths and eyes; very small LED torches are available in 'outdoors' shops or over the internet and can fit onto a keyring (£3–7).

Tendon hammer These are mythical objects, rarely found on wards. Collapsible pocket-sized versions can be bought for £12–15 – try www.medshop.co.uk or www.medisave.co.uk and search for 'hammer'.

Ward dress

Patients and staff have more respect for well-dressed doctors, however it is important to be yourself. Try to find means of self-expression that are acceptable in hospital and be guided by comments from patients or staff.

Hair Long hair should be tied back.

Piercings Facial metal can be easily removed while at work; while ears are OK, lips and eyebrows ± noses draw comments.

Shoes A pair of smart comfy shoes is essential – you will be on your feet for hours and may need to run.

Scrubs Ideal for on-calls, especially in surgery. Generally they should not be worn for everyday ward work.

Mobiles Many doctors (and patients) carry mobile phones in hospital though their use is often banned. If you do carry one keep it on a silent setting and be subtle. Be aware that:
- they may affect some hospital equipment
- you should always turn your mobile off before entering ITU or HDU
- in theory you could be disciplined for breaking trust policy

Personal digital assistants (PDAs)

These simple to use pocket-sized computers can hold entire textbooks, medical calculators, Word and Excel documents, lists of contact numbers and almost anything else on your PC including pictures, games and mp3s. They are becoming increasingly popular with all doctors from PRHOs to Profs. A reasonable PDA can be bought for £150–200 though you'll spend at least £50 more on software.

The Basics PDAs measure about 11cm by 7cm (smaller than two credit cards) and are about 1.5cm thick. A touch-sensitive screen takes up the majority of this size. There is no keyboard – instead you write on the screen and this produces computer text. All PDAs come with basic functions including address books, calendars and to-do lists.

You can easily add in more advanced programs; there are currently about 20,000 available on the internet and these are transferred via a PC. PDAs link to PCs at the press of a button and can transfer files in both directions; they also back up their files by this means.

Which PDA? There is a huge range of PDAs on the market. It is worth reading reviews on the internet to get one suited to your needs. The most important considerations are:

- *Palm or Pocket PC* – these are the two main operating systems:
  - Palm tends to be cheaper and has many more medical applications available at present. It is currently the most popular
  - Pocket PC has better handwriting recognition and can do more, at least in theory. It may win the popularity contest eventually
- *operating system* – these are updated frequently. Try to buy the most up-to-date so that the PDA can run new programs
- *battery life* – this varies widely from 3d to 2wk. Palm and Pocket PC now last similar times though Palm used to last longer
- *memory* – 16Mb is plenty for ward use. The majority have a memory slot which is a cheap way to increase the memory to 128Mb or more
- *software* – check what programs each PDA comes with. Pocket PCs always link to Word and Excel. Palm needs Documents To Go or an equivalent (about £20) that is often included

Where to buy The internet is the cheapest source for PDAs; it also provides information and reviews about specific models. It is worth having a look at the individual PDAs in shops since they vary considerably in size, weight, style and screen performance.

Accessories There are plenty of add-ons for PDAs to use up your loan/salary. These include:

- ***cases*** – a metal case prevents broken screens (£20–30)
- ***screen protectors*** – thin plastic sheets to prevent scratches (<£5)
- ***memory cards*** – vital for textbooks and mp3s (£20–30 for 256Mb)
- ***others*** – keyboards, cameras, bluetooth, GPS, modems etc

PDA software

Software is available over the internet from the sites shown in the table below (amongst others); there are literally thousands of programs covering almost every conceivable need. Most programs offer a free trial. It is not possible to copy versions you have paid for to share with friends. The following are good, free medical programs:

- Diagnosaurous (differential diagnosis) – www.diagnosaurus.com
- Medcalc (medical calculator) – www.med-ia.ch/medcalc
- Eponyms (eponymous diseases) – www.eponyms.net
- EPocrates Rx (American version of *BNF*) – www.ePocrates.com

PDA software	Medical PDA software
www.palmgear.com	www.skyscape.com
www.pilotzone.com	www.pdamd.com
www.pocketgear.com	www.medspda.com
www.pocketpcsoft.net	www.doctorsgadgets.com
www.freewarepalm.com	www.collectivemed.com

PDA medical textbooks

Oxford Handbook The PDA version is a full copy of the *OHCM* including diagrams and tables. It is not as easy to use as the printed version, however it will always be in your pocket.

- costs £21.95, 1.1Mb (6Mb with pictures), www.oup.com/uk/medicine/handbooks

5 Minute Clinical Consult (5MCC) Contains over 1000 conditions with background, diagnosis and management. Easy to use and an excellent resource, though it does have a US bias. The Skyscape® version is better than the Handheldmed® one.

- costs $65, 4.3Mb (7.5Mb with pictures), www.skyscape.com

Harrison's Manual of Medicine A textbook of medicine with lots of background to diseases, but less practical information.

- costs $60, 1.3Mb, www.unboundmedicine.com

BNF on PDA

The *BNF* is published as a 32Mb SD card for use with Palm OS. It costs £116 for one year (after which it will stop running) and is available from www.pharmpress.com. There are plans to release a pocket PC version in the future. See 'ePocrates Rx' program mentioned above.

Patient records

There are several programs available for recording your patient's location, diagnoses and investigations (eg Patient Tracker, PatientKeeper). Most hospitals ban their use (Data Protection Act and security concerns) and in practice it is not efficient since you have to duplicate the patient's details. Bear in mind that only the patient's hospital notes are a legal record of care so these must be kept up-to-date.

The medical team

The medical team or 'firm' usually consists of a consultant, SpR, SHO and PRHO. Most firms have more than one doctor at each level. You may well work in a firm alongside other PRHOs under two or more consultants. This can cause some confusion, but make the most of the company and spread the work out between yourselves.

The Consultant is usually seen on their ward rounds, in outpatient clinics and in the operating theatre. They are responsible for your post and oversee your work. Reports on your behaviour, attitude and progress usually filter back to them from other members of staff. If the rest of your team is away and you need a management decision, don't be afraid to contact your consultant – they would much rather be informed about patients who are acutely unwell early on. Your consultant will also help you with audit projects, presentations and careers advice.

Specialist Registrars are in training, on the path to becoming a consultant. They are often involved in outpatient clinics, teaching, seeing inpatient referrals, undertaking procedures and operations. They usually lead daily ward rounds. If you don't understand their instructions, make sure you clarify what they want, otherwise you risk wasting time doing the wrong thing or being criticised for not understanding why an investigation is needed. Equally, their experience means they can teach you a lot, help you to improve your CV and offer useful interview tips.

Senior House Officers are often your first port of call for help, so it is important to get on with them. They are available to supervise you for practical procedures and can act as a ready source of hints and tips for both procedures and ward work. As they are more familiar with how hospital wards are run they can often help you prioritise your work. They may well be studying for exams, which means that you can get an insight into what preparation the exams require, courses and costs etc. If you get on well with them, they can be great to go out with socially too.

The House Officer (*also known as house plant or PRHO*)
As a PRHO, you have the opportunity to see and do as much as you want. You can learn by helping each other and discuss any difficult situations which have arisen. When altering on-call dates, try to be helpful and flexible wherever possible; you may need to swap an on-call in the future too. Those who don't pull their weight quickly become unpopular.

Other doctors on the team

- *Trust grade* this is a non-training SHO position
- *Staff grade* this is a non-training middle grade at senior SHO or registrar level often very experienced and respected
- *Clinical fellow* this is a middle grade at senior SHO or junior registrar level who is undertaking research
- *Associate specialist* a doctor with consultant-level ability and experience but without the accountability or management commitments; common in the surgical specialities

The multidisciplinary team

Optimal patient management involves looking at the impact of illness upon the patient's life and addressing non-medical issues affecting their welfare. This is usually discussed at weekly multidisciplinary meetings.

Nurses have a practical 'hands-on' role in hospital care, ranging from administering medications to attending doctors' ward rounds. You need to get on well with nurses as they can help you in ways which are not always obvious. Bear in mind you are working in a place they may have been at for much longer than you have. Don't be afraid to ask their advice – their training and experience means they can often help locate equipment and suggest further management options.

Specialist nurses include stoma, respiratory (asthma and COPD), pain, cardiac, diabetes, tissue viability and Macmillan nurses (provide hospital and community support to cancer patients). They can be a very important first point of call for junior medical staff.

Physiotherapists use physical exercises and manipulation to treat injuries and relieve pain. They are involved in acute care and rehabilitation and may be called out of hours to provide chest physiotherapy post-operatively or for patients with severe pneumonia. They also assess patient mobility and make sure the patient is able to walk adequately upon discharge (eg able to manage stairs).

Occupational therapists work with patients to restore, develop or maintain practical skills such as personal care. They assess and identify patients' needs/difficulties and may work in conjunction with speech and language therapists. They can decide if any alterations need to be made to the patient's accommodation once they are ready for discharge.

Social workers support patients' needs in the community. They assess patients and help decide/organise discharge packages (invaluable for care of the elderly patients). They can also liaise with other agencies and offer information on further help and support for patients and their families.

Pharmacists dispense drugs and advise you on choice of medication. They check the accuracy of every prescription that is written. Most hospitals have a drugs information line available for advice on prescribing and drug interactions. You may also need to contact the on-call pharmacist for an urgent prescription which is not available on the ward.

Phlebotomists are professional vampires who appear on the wards with the specific aim of taking blood. Beware – they can appear at unpredictable times and, depending on which hospital you work at, they may not come at all at weekends. Some can take blood from central lines and perform blood cultures while others can't. It is worth being nice to them as you'll often have a late additional request for blood taking.

Physicians' assistants are relatively new positions which involve taking over routine tasks and administration usually done by a junior doctor. They may be able to take blood, perform ABG, cannulate, request simple investigations and assist with procedures and operations.

Clinical notes

Most new house officers are unsure about writing in medical notes since this is rarely practised as a medical student. The medical notes are a written record of the patient's condition, and each 'consultation' with a doctor should be documented. There are a few rules which everyone, irrespective of grade, should conform to:

Note paper The patient's name, DoB and hospital number or address should identify every sheet.

Documentation Each entry should have the date and ideally the time of the consultation. It is often useful to have a heading such as 'WR SHO (Smith)' or 'Discussion with patient and family'. Sign every entry and write your surname and bleep number clearly.

What to write Document the condition of the patient, relevant changes to the history, obs or examination findings, the results of any new investigations and end with a plan. Write a summary of history, examination findings, obs and investigations and their results for complex patients; these are really helpful to others reading the notes. The notes should contain enough information so that in your absence someone else can learn what has happened and what is planned for the patient.

What not to write Patients can apply to read their medical notes and the notes are always used in legal cases. Never write anything that you do not wish the patient to read or that would be frowned upon in court. Documenting facts is accepted (eg obese lady), but not subjective material (eg annoying time-waster). Never doodle in the notes.

How to write Write clearly in black; poorly legible notes result in errors and are indefensible in court. Use only standard abbreviations and don't worry about length as long as sufficient information is documented. Always write in the notes at the time of the consultation, even if it means asking the ward round to wait a few moments.

Making changes If you wish to cross something out simply put a single line through the error and initial the mistake. Never cross it out so it cannot be read as this looks suspicious. Previous entries should not be altered, instead make a new entry indicating the change or difference.

Notes and the law It is unlikely that your notes will be used in court. If they are, you want them to show you as a caring and clear-thinking individual; make that clear from how you write. As far as a court is concerned, if it's not documented then it didn't happen.

Hints and tips Bullet points are a useful and clear means of documentation. It is acceptable to write about a patient's mood and it is useful to document if you have cheered them up or discussed some bad news (p77). It is also acceptable to document 'no change' if this is the case.

Medical reports The commonest medical report you will be required to complete will be the 'critical incident form'. Keep the report simple and document only the available facts. See p98.

Example of entries in medical notes

16/09/05 WR SpR (Ackerman)

10.20 Pt comfortable. No further chest pain.

PTO reg. BP 132/81. RR 15 Sats 99% on room air.

~~CXR shows bilateral pleural effusions~~ (Wrong patient CJF)

Rpt ECG (N) no new changes.

Imp

- A typical chest pain, unlikely to be cardiac.

(P)

- Await cardiac markers - if (N), (H) c̄ no f/u
- Pt wants to discuss risk factor when family arrive.

Dr C.J.Flint PRHO
Bleep 3294

16/09/05 d/w with Pt and wife

11.12

Pt wanted to talk about cardiac risk factor.

Given British Heart Foundation leaflet on risk factors and talked about lifestyle changes. Cardiac nurse will see Pt before discharge.

Rpt CE (N). Pt much relieved.

(H) later

Dr. C.J.Flint PRHO
Bleep 3294

16/09/05 Review, PRHO (Flint)

15.34 No change TTO written (H)

Dr C.J.Flint PRHO
Bleep 3294

Commonly used symbols/abbreviations (see also pxi at front)

Ⓗ	Home
Ⓝ	Normal
Ⓟ	Plan
Ⓛ	Left
Ⓡ	Right
Ⓣ	Temperature/telephone
dd/DD/$\delta\delta$/$\Delta\Delta$	Differential diagnosis
x/Dx	Diagnosis
Imp	Impression
Rx	Prescription/drugs
Sx	Symptoms
Tx	Treatment
O/E	On examination
–ve	Negative
+ve	Positive
+/–	Equivocal
+	Presence noted
++	Present significantly
+++	Present in excess
=	Equal to
d/w	Discussed with/discussion with
WR	Ward round
r/v	Review
f/u	Follow up
ATSP	Asked to see patient
IP	Inpatient
OP	Outpatient(s)
obs	Observations (pulse, BP etc)
c/o	Complains of/complaining of
Pt	Patient
$\bar{c}$	With
E+D	Eating and drinking
N+V	Nausea and vomiting
D+V	Diarrhoea and vomiting
BO	Bowels open
PUing	Passing urine
blds	Bloods
rpt	Repeat
°	No/negative (as in °free air under diaphragm)
1°	Primary
2°	Secondary

Daily ward duties

First thing

- Handover from doctor on nights
- Fill out any missing or extra blood/CXR/ECG requests
- Review new patients, consider writing a brief summary in the notes
- Write TTOs for any patients who might be going home

Ward round

- See p16 for ward round duties, try to keep a jobs list
- Attempt to do simple jobs during ward round

After the ward round

- Spend a few minutes comparing and allocating jobs with the other members of the team; try to group jobs by location in the hospital
- Radiology requests (USS, CT, MRI)
- Referrals to other teams eg surgery/dermatology/psychiatry
- Fill out TTOs and other paperwork
- Take bloods from patients the phlebotomists have been unable to bleed or that have been requested during the ward round

Lunch

- Is there anything you need to do, eg phoning, buying, booking, posting?
- You may have teaching/grand round/journal clubs

After lunch

- Review any patients you are worried about or who have deteriorated
- Check and record blood results; serial results sheets help a lot
- Check other results; consider chasing outstanding requests or results from other departments, eg radiology/referrals/microbiology
- Spend time talking to patients ± relatives
- Fill out blood, X-ray and ECG requests for the next day
- Check the patients' drug cards – do any need rewriting?

Before you go home

- Review results and outstanding jobs with other team members; make a note of anything that needs doing the next day
- Check that all warfarin doses have been written up
- Prescribe sufficient IV fluids for patients on IV infusions overnight
- Handover patients who are sick or need urgent results chasing to the on-call doctor; give their ward, name, DoB and hospital number and say exactly what you want the doctor to do

Before weekends

- Only write blood requests for patients who really need them
- Try to prescribe three days of warfarin doses
- Ensure that no drug cards will run out over the next two days, rewrite them if they will
- Write a weekend plan for each patient (especially those who are sick); include presenting complaint, relevant investigations and plan for the weekend (eg trial of oral fluids, stop IVs if tolerated, home next week)

Ward rounds

A smooth ward round requires preparation of notes, investigations and results. Try to predict requests and start the ward round armed with the appropriate answers. Consultant ward rounds may highlight details missed during the junior doctors' daily round.

Before the ward round

- Make an up-to-date patient list with patient details, location, summary of clinical problems/medical history, investigations/results and jobs (see opposite)
- Check notes, drug cards, obs charts, X-rays and bld results are present
- Clearly document all relevant investigation results and reports in the notes with a brief summary on your patient list
- Check all notes have continuation sheets headed with the patient's name, DoB and hospital number/address
- If your patients have moved, contact the bed manager to find out where they have been transferred to and phone the receiving ward to ensure they have arrived; make sure their notes, drug card, obs chart and X-rays (if relevant) have also arrived
- Find the dates/times for outstanding investigations; if a patient is not on the ward they may be having an investigation
- Learn your consultant's pet questions from your predecessor (eg pets, exposure to dyes)
- Consider multidisciplinary issues which may alter further management or delay discharge for the patient

During the ward round

- Ask a nurse to join you on the ward round
- If there are two junior doctors then one can prepare the notes, obs, drug cards and X-rays for the next patient while the other presents
- If you have a spare moment start filling in forms or doing the jobs generated on the ward round
- If you have any queries about the next step of management or investigation results, make sure you ask during the ward round
- Referrals made in the presence of your consultant are often more readily accepted and any queries can be discussed directly
- If you have not done something or are unsure, be honest; never make up results

After the ward round

- Sit down with the rest of the team and go through the jobs generated from the ward round over a cup of tea
- Prioritise the jobs
- Allocate the jobs between your team as appropriate
- If you are unsure of how to approach any of the jobs, ask your seniors
- Clarify any gaps in your understanding of the patients' management

Mr Johnston/Miss Jain's patient list 16-09-05

Patients Details	Problem list	Investigation/Detail	Jobs
Angel Ward			
Eleanor Rigby W876470 26/06/1922	Chest pain COPD Hiatus hernia	LBBB on ECG	Cardiac Marker TTO
Seabright Ward			
Annie Popple T589124 08/09/1935	Dysphagia Haematemesis Anaemia	3u Bld (15/09/2005) OGD - Ca stomach	Macmillan referral Gastro r/v

Sample patient list

16/09/05 WR: Mr Sutcliff (SpR)

0800 Day 1 post appendicectomy
Patient painfree; slept well overnight
No nausea/vomiting noted
Good urine output;
Obs (T) 36.5°C, BP 120/78, pulse 66
O/E

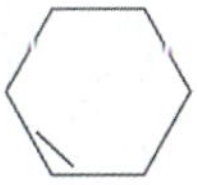

Soft
Non-tender
Bowel sounds present
Wound: clean, healing well;
no discharge/bleeding

PLAN: 1) FBC/U+Es check today
2) Sips, then light diet as able to tolerate
3) Aim for (H) later today/mane (OP in 6/52)

J. Smith
J. Smith
PRHO 6296

Sample ward round entry

Referrals

Doctors in other specialities will often be involved in the care of your patients. If you are asked to contact a specialist determine why the referral is necessary and what is desired (eg advice over the phone, full review or take the patient over). Phone the specialist middle grade directly.

Before referring make sure you have the following in front of you:

- hospital notes with patient's name, DoB, hospital number and ward
- latest set of obs and the patient's drug card
- most recent or serial results sheet

Start your referral with 'Please would you come and review this patient …' or by stating the specific question you want answered. Try to give just the details relevant to that specialist instead of a full history. Before you put the phone down determine exactly what action the specialist will do and when this will take place. Write the referral and outcome in the notes along with the specialist's name and bleep number.

Radiology This is the most common referral that junior doctors make and usually directly to the consultant. Make the referral as early in the day as possible (emergency lists get booked up early), take old X-rays and be aware of previous imaging and results. Make sure you are clear in your mind about why the investigation is required, how urgent it is and what action will be taken. Different modalities have specific questions:

- ***X-ray*** – exclude pregnancy first (<28d since LMP or –ve β-HCG)
- ***Ultrasound*** – may need a full bladder (especially transabdominal ultrasound); scan is unlikely to be of benefit if there is lots of bowel gas (obstruction) or severe tenderness
- ***CT*** – the patient needs to be able to lie still (confusion, children); exclude pregnancy (LMP or ideally β-HCG); can be claustrophobic
- ***Urgent CT head*** – be able to describe GCS, focal neurology, BP, pulse
- ***MRI*** – The patient needs to be able to lie still (confusion, children); exclude exposure to flying metal (grinding, hammering) or metal in their eyes – get an orbital X-ray if unsure; ask about metal implants (hips, pacemakers, metal stents); very claustrophobic
- ***Invasive radiology*** – exclude clotting problems (warfarin, heparin, NSAIDs, aspirin), jaundice suggests poor clotting
- ***Contrast imaging*** – contraindicated in renal failure
- ***Barium studies*** – will need soluble contrast if risk of perforation

Equivalent doses of radiological investigations

CXR = 2d background radiation

Investigation	Equivalent no. of CXRs
Limb X-ray	0.5
AXR	75
CT	100–400
Barium study	100–300

Dermatology previous rashes, onset, location, extent and character of the rash (see p321), treatments tried, new medications

ITU/HDU reversibility of disease, usual state (exercise tolerance, assistance, home help), severity of disease, current lines, O_2 requirements

Medicine Common questions include:

- ***Cardiology*** previous MIs, ischaemia, ECG results, cardiac risk factors (p127), chest pain (duration, character, speed of onset, present now?), aspirin, previous echo/angiogram/exercise tolerance test results
- ***Respiratory*** usual inhalers, nebulisers, home oxygen, ever been admitted/on ITU/ventilated, PEFR and usual PEFR, exercise tolerance, blood gas and saturations, O_2 requirements, CXR
- ***Gastro*** stool frequency (and normal frequency) and colour, alcohol intake (and intent to stop), NSAIDs, endoscopy results, vomiting (±blood)
- ***Endocrine*** type of diabetes, BM, ketones, ulcers, temp, dental hygiene

Microbiology pyrexia, swab/urine/stool/blood culture results, current antibiotics, allergies, renal/liver impairment, lines (central/peripheral), wounds

Neurology headaches, BP, pulse, focal neurology, LP or CT results

Obs and Gynae pregnancy excluded (always check β-HCG), urine dipstick results, previous pregnancies, births (NVD, assisted, LSCS) and miscarriages, previous gynae problems and operations, sexual history (past and present), contraception, usual periods, LMP. If abdo pain:

- is it worse on one side?
- is the pain worse with periods/opening bowels/eating?
- consider and exclude surgical problems (eg appendicitis)

Ophthalmology visual acuity (with or without glasses?), photophobia, pupil reflexes, eye movements, fundoscopy, previous/family glaucoma

Orthopaedics range of movement, swelling, tenderness, weight bearing, X-rays and results, suitability for surgery, neurology in legs, bowel and bladder function, perianal sensation

Paediatrics age (if ≥16yr and post GCSEs then no longer a paediatric patient), birth history, immunisations, family history, ears/throat exam

Psychiatry suicidal ideation/intent (previous attempts, plans), previous admissions/sections, previous diagnoses, medications, tests to exclude organic cause, hallucinations, illusions, sedation

Surgery recent food and drink, recent clear fluids (water, squash, black coffee/tea), previous operations (where, who and what), will they survive the anaesthetic, are they peritonitic (tenderness, guarding, rebound) or shocked (postural BP, pulse), G+S and clotting, PR findings

- ***GI*** bowel/vomit frequency and normal frequency
- ***Hepatobiliary*** jaundiced, INR, alcohol intake
- ***Vascular*** pulses and cap refill of limbs, warfarin and heparin, diabetes, previous MIs, exercise tolerance

Urology urine dipstick result, urine microscopy result, catheterised, if male: PR findings, PSA result

Prescribing

Knowing how drugs work and their common side-effects is very useful, but you must also be able to safely prescribe them to the patient. There are a few basic rules about prescribing; and if you are even slightly unsure ask the ward or hospital pharmacist. Always use the *BNF* if unsure.

The basics There are usually at least four drug sections on the drug card; once-only, regular and prn medications and infusions (fluids) (p263). Other sections might include oxygen, anticoagulants, insulin, medications prior to admission and nurse prescriptions.

Labelling the drug card As with the patient's notes, the drug card should have at least three identifying features: name, DoB, hospital number or address. There are usually spaces to document the ward, consultant, date of admission and number of drug cards in use (1 of 2, 2 of 2 etc).

The allergy box Ask the patient about allergies and check old drug cards if available. Document any allergies in this box and the reaction which was precipitated. If there are no known drug allergies, then record this too. Nurses are unable to give any drugs unless this box is complete.

Writing a prescription Use black pen and write clearly, ideally in capitals. Use the generic drug name (diclofenac, not Voltarol®) and clearly indicate the dose, route, frequency of administration, date started and circle the times the drug should be given. Record any specific instructions (such as 'with food') and sign the entry, writing your name and bleep number clearly on the first prescription.

Common abbreviations:

- IV – intravenous
- PO – by mouth
- IM – intramuscular
- SC – subcutaneous
- PR – by rectum
- INH – inhaled
- NEB – nebulised
- stat – immediately
- g – gram
- μg – microgram (avoid mcg)
- Ṫ, ṪṪ – one tablet, two tablets
- od – once a day/24h
- om – every morning
- on – every night
- bd – twice a day/12h
- tds – three times a day/8h
- qds – four times a day/6h
- iu – international units
- prn – as required
- mg – milligram
- ml – millilitre

Controlled drugs These are mainly strong opiate drugs (morphine, pethidine etc). Prescribe them as normal on in-patient drug cards, but the total amount must be written in words and numbers for TTOs (p22).

Changes to prescriptions If a prescription is to change do not amend the original; cross it out clearly and write a new prescription (see opposite). Initial and date any cancelled prescriptions and record a reason if appropriate (eg beta-blocker stopped in wheezy asthmatic patient).

Rewriting drug cards When rewriting drug cards ensure the correct drugs, doses and original start dates are carried over and that the old drug card(s) are crossed through and filed in the notes.

Drug PARACETAMOL			Date/Time	--/--/--	--/--/--
			0600		
Route PO/PR	Dose 1 g	Start 18.09.05	0800		
			1000		CJF
Additional instructions			1200		
			1400		
Signature Dr C.J.Flint	Pharmacy		1800		
			2200		
			0000		

Example of cancelled drug prescription for a regular medication

Drug IBUPROFEN			Date	18.09.05	
Route PO	Dose 400 mg	Start 16.09.05	Time	12:35	
Max frequency 8 hourly	Max dose/24hr 1.6 g		Dose	400 mg	
Indications for use Analgesia/fever			Route	PO	
Signature Dr C.J.Flint	Pharmacy		Given by	S.N.Jones	

Example of drug prescription for a PRN medication

Date	Drug	Dose	Route	Time	Prescribed	Given by	Time
16.09.05	ASPIRIN	300 mg	PO	STAT	C.J.Flint	S.N.Jones	15:35

Example of a once-only (stat) medication

Verbal prescriptions

You may prescribe common drugs over the telephone, but you must say the prescription to two nurses and sign for it as soon as possible. Try to avoid verbal prescribing, but it is occasionally necessary. Check your hospital policy first.

Self-prescribing

PRHOs can only prescribe on in-patient drug cards and TTOs. Post registration you can self-prescribe, but it is not recommended. Check with pharmacy first.

Discharge summaries (TTOs/TTAs)

'TTOs' or 'TTAs' (to take out or away) are a summary sheet usually written by doctors on the day of discharge for patients and their GPs, summarising what brought them to hospital and the course of the hospital admission. It comes with two or more carbon copies – as well as the patient's notes, one copy is for pharmacy and one is sent to the GP. The discharge letter (which provides a fuller and more formal account of the patient's hospital stay) is usually done by the SHO at a later date.

What information do TTOs contain?

- Patient's details
- Consultant and hospital ward
- Presenting complaint, relevant clinical findings and diagnosis
- Investigations/procedures/operations
- Treatment given
- Any complications
- Treatment on discharge and instructions to the GP
- Follow-up arrangements
- Your name, position and bleep number

When to write TTOs

TTOs should be written as soon as you know the patient will be discharged. This means the drugs can be dispensed from pharmacy without delay and the ward staff will not have to bleep you and call you back to do them.

- Carry TTO forms on ward rounds so that you can write them up during a gap in the ward round; you also have your team there if you have any queries
- Check the duration of the medication the patient is to be discharged with (eg antibiotics) and take the opportunity to reassess which drugs the patient no longer needs once discharged (eg prophylactic clexane)
- Check drug doses and frequencies to avoid being called by pharmacy. If you're unsure about any medications check the *BNF* or speak to your seniors, pharmacy or drug information
- If follow-up involves a clinic appointment check who will arrange this – the ward clerk usually organises the appointment date and time
- Contact the GP by telephone if the patient needs an early check-up, has a poor social situation or self-discharges
- If the patient is admitted for a day-case elective operation you could write the TTO whilst in theatre
- Hand the TTO, together with the patient's drug chart, to the nurse in charge or inform them that you have done the TTO to avoid being called later to do it
- If there is a query about whether the TTO has been done look at the original in-patient drug chart. Pharmacy usually tick a box on the drug chart to indicate TTOs have been dispensed
- Discuss the discharge plan with your patient; if they understand the management plan they are more likely to comply with it

Discharging with controlled drugs

Controlled drugs are those which are subject to the prescription requirements of the Misuse of Drugs Regulation 2001, eg morphine, diamorphine, pethidine and fentanyl. An out-patient prescription or TTO for these must be in the prescriber's own handwriting and include the name and address of the patient, the form and strength of the preparation, the total quantity of the preparation in words and figures and the dose. A maximum of 14d supply can be issued. Repeat prescriptions for controlled drugs cannot be issued using the previous form and prescriptions are valid for 13wk from the date written. Make sure you complete all the information requested, otherwise the pharmacist will not be able to dispense the medication.

Discharge form McBurney City Hospital

Name: *Eleanor Rigby*
DOB: 26/06/1922
Hospital number: W876470
Ward: E4
NHS/~~Private~~

Consultant: *Dr. Singh*
Date of admission: 15/09/2005
Date of discharge: 16/09/2005
Inpatient/~~Outpatient/Daycase~~

Presenting complaint: *Chest pain*
Diagnosis: *Musculoskeletal chest pain*
Investigations: *ECG shows LBBB, cardiac markers (N)*

Discharge Plan/Additional notes to GP: *Has had some toothache recently, advised her to see a dentist*

Discharge Medications:

Drug	Dose	Frequency	Duration	GP to continue?
Augmentin	*625mg*	*tds*	*5d*	NO
Paracetamol	*1g*	*prn*	*7d*	NO
Oramorph (10mg/5ml)	*10mg* Total=100mg (one hundred mg)	*bd*	*5d*	NO

Follow up? *No*
Print name *Flint*
HO/~~SHO/SpR~~

Date: 16-09-2005
Signature: *C.J. Flint*
Bleep number 3294

Sample TTO

Difficult patients

Alcoholism Many patients will drink over the daily and weekly recommendations (4 units/d for ♂ and 3 units/d for ♀), though not all of these will be 'alcoholics'. Defining alcoholism is a problem, but if drinking or the effects of drinking repeatedly leads to harm in work or social life, then this is clearly a problem. Answering 'yes' to three out of four of the *CAGE* questions suggests alcoholism: Ever felt you ought to **C**ut down on your drinking? Have people **A**nnoyed you by criticising your drinking? Ever felt bad or **G**uilty about your drinking? Ever had an **E**ye-opener to steady nerves in the morning?

Alcoholism management Have a low threshold for commencing benzodiazepine therapy to minimise risk of alcohol withdrawal (see suggested regimen below). In addition, start vitamin B_1 supplementation with either intravenous preparations (Pabrinex® 2 pairs/8h IV for 2d) or oral thiamine 200mg/24h PO and multi-vitamins (1–2 tablets/24h PO).

Suggested chlordiazepoxide doses to prevent alcohol withdrawal

Day 1	20mg/6h PO	Day 5	5mg/6h PO
Day 2	20mg/8h PO	Day 6	5mg/8h PO
Day 3	10mg/6h PO	Day 7	5mg/12h PO
Day 4	10mg/8h PO		

Elderly patients are often taking many medications, so interactions and side-effects are common. As renal function declines, drug excretion falls and lower doses can often be used for renally excreted drugs; equally, elderly patients handle fluid boluses less well and can easily go into heart failure from excessive IV fluids. Other issues to consider: more susceptible to infections, higher threshold to pain (can mask fractures or other acute pathology), atypical presentations of disease, poor thermoregulation (become hypothermic easily), consider malnourishment, history taking can be difficult if hard of hearing. Elderly patients can suffer with depression and other psychiatric illness (p400) and, like children, social circumstances must always be considered prior to discharge – liaise with OT, physio and social services.

Immunocompromised patients (p256) need to be protected from infection. They are reverse barrier nursed in isolation, so that equipment is sterilised before entering the room. Limit contact to essential staff. Before entering, wash hands and wear gloves, apron and mask; remove and dispose of these on leaving the room.

Infectious diseases Contagious infections require isolation and barrier nursing – equipment is sterilised or disposed of on leaving the room. Common reasons include gastroenteritis (especially *C. difficile*), chicken pox, shingles, TB (see below), MRSA (p255), meningitis. You should wear gloves, apron and mask before entering the room and wash hands on leaving.

Intravenous drug users (IVDU) are commonly admitted with infections (abscesses, cellulitis, endocarditis), DVTs or with pathology unrelated to IV drug abuse. Intravenous cannulation is often difficult and these patients often require temporary central access for prolonged antibiotic therapy. In some circumstances the patient will prefer to take blood samples themselves with a needle and syringe rather than have a junior doctor delving blindly into any potential vein. Treat all bodily fluids as high risk (see below) unless hepatitis and HIV status has been recently established as negative. IVDU patients should not be allowed off the ward unaccompanied with IV access *in situ*.

Paediatrics Drug doses vary with weight, look up the doses and use a calculator. Use anaesthetic cream and distraction to take blood samples, see the paediatrics section for details (p390).

Patient with tuberculosis If you suspect TB the patient must be nursed in isolation, ideally a ventilated side room. If TB is suspected or acid fast bacilli (AFBs) have been seen in their sputum then they and/or their visitor should wear a mask during all contact until three consecutive sputum samples are negative. Children, pregnant women or immunocompromised patients should avoid visiting. Treat sputum samples as high risk (see below). If the patient has to leave the ward for investigations and procedures they should wear a mask.

High-risk patient (hepatitis/HIV) (p193/260) Wearing gloves and meticulous handling of sharps (p33) should prevent transmission to yourself and others. Some doctors choose to wear two pairs of gloves (double gloving) when taking blood or using other sharps. All samples of bodily fluids sent for investigation should be labelled with high-risk stickers, as should the forms; they should be transported by porters, not by airtubes. The patient can be nursed on the open ward.

Psychiatric patients will often need admission to a medical ward; nurse in a bay in clear view of the nurses' station – see p400.

MRSA patient See infectious diseases opposite

Pregnant patient (p368) Avoid prescribing medications whenever possible; if a medication is necessary then check appendix 4 of the *BNF*. X-ray radiation should also be avoided, though the pelvis and lower abdomen can be shielded. Pregnant women have different normal values for some blood results – discuss with the laboratory or O+G.

Patients on regular steroids (>10d) are more prone to infections due to relative immunocompromise (p256), but also have suppression of their adrenocortical axis. Sudden withdrawal of (cortico)steroids in such patients can trigger an Addisonian-like crisis. Steroid therapy must be maintained or withdrawn slowly. During periods of illness, steroid treatment often has to be increased. If patients are nil by mouth, intravenous steroid preparations are available and equivalent doses can be calculated (p419).

Being on-call

Being 'on-call' will occupy at least a third of your time and may involve care of a different group of patients and a greater range of specialities than during the daytime work. Requirements, expectations and priorities are different.

What it's like

The standard on-call for newly qualified doctors involved an endless series of ward visits and trying to juggle the demands of countless bleeps whilst seeing patients with problems you'd never seen before and conditions you'd never heard of. 'I'd never felt so lonely' to quote one PRHO.

On-calls are still difficult but things have improved and with modest effort and following some simple rules they can be rewarding.

What's important

- Identify the sick
- Get help early enough
- Prioritise effectively
- Stay organised
- Eat
- Never be rude

How to handle the bleep when tired

It won't stop going off. Always try to answer it promptly, when you don't it will be the boss or someone really unwell.

Never get stroppy down the phone. Bad reputations take a moment to make, spread round a hospital in seconds and take years to improve.

Keep a record of all the bleeps that require action or thought. When busy you'll find you cannot remember who called you even 3min later.

Learn or note down the most common origins of your bleeps so you can spot the call from the switchboard, mess or your consultant's office.

Being organised on-call

This is the most responsibility you will have in your first year:

- document all your tasks, otherwise you **will** forget something
- have a means of identifying when you've done it and when it can be utterly forgotten (these may be very different)
- do not use scraps of paper, they will get lost; use a clipboard or PDA, see p6
- learn the times of important events – night drug round, post-take round, closing time of the canteen and local pizza delivery
- arrange to visit all the areas you cover in a logical order and tell the wards this is what you'll be doing; ask them to compile a list of tasks so you can do them all at once without multiple bleeps
- when you order a test on-call make a note to check the result, it's easy to forget

Prioritising

You will need to prioritise your tasks. The clinical pages include worrying features that should make you see the patient more urgently.

- sick patients need seeing first; if you have more than one really sick patient then tell your senior
- if the patient's condition is clearly life-threatening then ask the ward to bleep your senior while you're on your way there
- check if a task has a deadline (eg before pharmacy closes)
- does delaying the task risk making things worse?
- don't delay ordering investigations since everything else, including treatment, may depend on the results
- if you see an abnormal blood result check the patient/notes/previous blood results, see p497
- try to group tasks geographically, especially when covering a large area
- ask if a task can wait until you're next in that area; tell the staff when this will be and try to stick to it – they may even have a cup of tea waiting (to nurses reading this: ward cover is hell, seeing that someone is on your side can bring tears to the eyes of even hardened doctors)
- explain if and why you are going to be delayed

Taking breaks

You are entitled to a 30min paid break after every 4h of work. Whilst you must not ignore a sick patient there will be a constant supply of work that will not change for a short break. If you've been flat out and your remaining tasks can wait (most can) then take a break – you will be quicker and more efficient for doing so. Remain polite if you are disturbed, but explain/make an excuse and ask if it can wait.

Breaks are not just about food, they are essential to keep you going and prevent peptic ulcers. It is in your patients' interests that you allow yourself to recharge. Drink plenty (not alcohol!) – it is not just your patients who need maintenance fluids.

Where possible arrange to take breaks with the rest of the team – it allows you to catch up and stops you feeling isolated.

Nursing staff are not paid for their breaks and are reluctant to be disturbed during them.

The night shift

Few doctors look forward to their night shifts, especially if they are doing a whole week. That said, on nights you will be doing real medicine and will gain a lot of experience.

Things to take with you

- Food, both a main meal and several quick snacks – fruit is good
- Clinical kit, eg pentorch – there are fewer people to borrow from on nights (see list p7)
- Toothbrush/toothpaste
- Change for drinks machines etc
- Stuff for gaps in workload, depending on hospital policy these could include books for private study or a pillow

Things to check (on the first night)

- What areas of the hospital and specialities are you responsible for?
- What is the bleep policy? Can the wards bleep you directly?
- Who are your seniors and what are their bleep numbers?
- When and where is handover?
- What is the policy on short naps?

What is expected of you

- Turn up on time. Your colleague will have to stay late if you don't
- Work with the night-sister/nurse coordinator and your seniors; let them know what you are up to
- Prioritise your work according to urgency and explain this to those who will have to wait for you
- When bleeped to a sick patient ask for obs ±ECG to be done while you get there
- Tour the wards you are covering regularly; once nursing staff know you do this they will bleep you less for non-urgent tasks
- Only leave a ward once all the jobs are done or if there's a sick patient requiring urgent attention elsewhere
- Delegate simple tasks to support workers, find out which nurses can cannulate/take bloods
- Document all interventions in the notes to alert the regular teams of actions undertaken on their patients during the night
- Take regular breaks

Learning at night

The overnight period can be a very good learning opportunity. You can get direct supervision and you may get a chance to perform new procedures. Do not work beyond your competence without supervision. Ensure the other doctors on at night know if you have particular skills you wish to learn at that time (eg arterial blood gases or chest drains). They can then call you to observe or be supervised.

Working as a team will help you to learn and prevents the 'loneliness of nights'.

Pitfalls

Many more mistakes are made during night shifts than by day. If you are unsure, check. The following are some of the common problem areas:

- poor handover, ensure you understand which patients the day team are concerned about and what tasks need doing
- failing to appreciate how sick a patient really is and not calling for senior help; if unsure, check and if the nurses are unhappy with what you've done, discuss it with a senior colleague
- ignoring or dismissing abnormal obs or investigations, especially tachypnoea and tachycardia
- ignoring your gut instinct
- fluid prescriptions (eg failing to note wider history including renal/heart failure, diabetes, electrolyte imbalance)
- warfarin prescriptions with INRs coming back out of hours

How to cope

- It is easy to get very sleep deprived during nights; this will lead to increased errors
- Make sure you get adequate sleep during the day
- Try and go to bed for at least 7h each day, even if you don't sleep easily you'll rest
- You'll be most tired straight after the shift ends – try to sleep early. It's easy to waste 1–2h of life by faffing about because you're tired
- Make your bedroom dark – tape the curtains if need be
- Let others know you are on nights so they keep the noise down; foam ear plugs help in hospital accommodation
- Ensure the phone/mobile will not disturb you
- Eat enough; have a meal when you get up, before going in – the shift is always at its busiest early
- Travel safely; the Selby rail crash showed that it is the individual's responsibility to ensure they are fit to drive – if you feel too tired take a 20–30min nap first
- Avoid alcohol, it will make all the above worse
- Plan to see friends or arrange treats for the days off after the nights have finished – this will also help you recover
- Do not forget the rest of your life – open the post, pay the bills, ring the family
- If you are having problems adapting your sleep pattern during nights consider melatonin (pineal gland hormone); available over the counter in the USA (but not the UK)

Surviving

Many find the transition from medical school to junior doctor difficult. The learning curve appears vertical and the responsibility seems heavy. Medicine has always been a demanding profession and this takes time to get used to.

Attitudes

- Never, ever, even for one second consider shouting at a nurse
- Don't lose your cool when you're busy; remember – they didn't know you were doing something else or that you have other tasks to do as well. There will be times when you want to scream – avoid taking it out on the next person who irritates you
- Avoid arrogance. You may be a doctor now, but virtually everyone you come across has more experience than you. The very best doctors treat everyone as equals, from professors to porters
- Try to do things face to face at first. People like to put a face to a name. If you can remember peoples' names you'll make friends much faster
- Imagine yourself in your patients' shoes whenever possible. A little empathy goes a long way
- If you have time, just chat. One of the greatest privileges of medicine is it allows us insight into peoples lives
- Cynicism is often worn by slightly older colleagues as a badge of rank. It needn't be. All the authors enjoy medicine just as much as when they first started at medical school

Sleep

- Get enough
- Sleep deprivation is notoriously hard to appreciate in oneself. Signs include:
  - lack of energy
  - getting grouchy for little reason
  - difficulty concentrating and poor memory
  - loss of libido and even anhedonia
- Early nights give better rest than lie-ins
- Ensure your sleep is restful – this may mean eyepads and earplugs in shared accommodation
- You aren't superhuman, better to sleep through a precious weekend than risk your own health or that of your patients

Social aspects

- Keep in touch with friends and family
- Plan ahead; book trips to see things/people
- Do go out with colleagues for the ward nights out; people can be very different out of work and you'll find the job much easier when you know people better
- Groups of doctors who socialise together always get on far better at work

Stress and health

As well as sleep you need to make an effort to stay healthy and sane. Watch for signs of depression or stress, both in yourself and your colleagues. Doctors can have remarkably poor insight into their own problems. Look out for each other. A chat with understanding friends over a beer can be worth so much more than any prescription.

Whilst appreciating that the average medical student needs little advice on alcohol, clinical work is far less forgiving of hangovers. Be wary of allowing drinking too much for fun to drift into drinking too much out of need. Alcohol tends to make depression worse and can exacerbate stress. The GMC takes an exceedingly strong line on doctors who've been caught for drink driving.

A surprising number of doctors take up smoking either at medical school or in the first two years on the wards. Virtually all regret it.

Exercise is an excellent antidote to the stress of the wards, anything from a brisk walk at weekends to regularly attending a gym will make a difference. Consider getting into the countryside where the hospital problems seem more in perspective.

Do not ignore your own physical health. Register with a GP so you have a route to independent medical advice outside the hospital.

Coping strategies and support

Eat and sleep regularly, socialise with colleagues and friends often.

Talk to someone early if you are finding it difficult to cope. Avoid the jaded, super-cynical, slightly more experienced colleague. The senior nurses can often be very good sources of support – they've seen many generations of new doctors going through the same thing.

Start simple, talking to colleagues/seniors may help and need not go 'on record'. If your quality of work is being affected and you're having difficulty then get formal help early before things go too wrong. You are an essential part of the NHS; You might be surprised how far most deaneries will go to keep you working and healthy.

Formal support is available from several sources:

- ***your local deanery*** will offer support for those having difficulty and can be very helpful, especially if you feel overwhelmed about work
- ***your GP*** can sign you off work if you really do need to stop to recover
- ***occupational health*** can provide support and will need to be informed if you are off due to stress
- ***BMA counselling service*** anonymous and confidential 08459 200 169
- ***doctors for doctors*** provides support for doctors in distress and difficulty by helping them make informed decisions about their health. Contactable via the BMA website (www.bma.org.uk)
- ***other options*** p524

The laboratories

In your first year as a doctor you will probably spend more time sending samples to laboratories and acting on their results (p497) than you spend with patients. To be efficient (and go home on time) you must send correctly completed forms with labelled samples to the right places.

The forms Every form needs at least two (at least three for blood bank eg G+S) patient identification details (ie full name, DoB, hospital number, home address) along with the ward, date, who ordered the investigation (+ bleep no) and investigation requested.

- ***Clinical details*** It is important to distinguish between significant investigations that require a detailed history for interpretation (see box) and simple investigations that merit just a couple of words (eg 'PR bleed' for FBC, 'on diuretics' for U+E, 'pre-op' for G+S). Radiographers will refuse to take X-rays unless a suitable indication is written on the form

Forms that require in-depth clinical details

histology, pathology, genetics, CSF, CT, MRI, USS, blood cultures, endoscopy, blood film, antibodies, hormones (except thyroid), drug levels (doses and timing of doses)

Haematology The usual destination for FBC, haematinics (B_{12}, folate, ferritin), blood films, clotting screens and ESR. Samples must not be 'coagulated' (clotted); try gently mixing the blood tubes after filling.

Biochemistry Biochemistry receives the majority of blood tests not listed under the other headings including U+E, LFT, amylase, Ca^{2+}, PO_4^{3-}, HCO_3^-, cardiac markers, CRP, hormone levels and drug levels (except antibiotics). They also analyse other bodily fluids (including CSF, urine, stool and surgical drain fluid). Blood samples may be reported as haemolysed (burst cells); try taking the blood gently through a large needle.

Microbiology Receives urine, stool, swabs, pus, CSF and blood cultures, antibody levels and viral titres. There is a microbiologist (medical doctor) on-call 24h a day.

Blood bank Receives only the group and save/crossmatch sample, but sends out blood, fresh frozen plasma, platelets, clotting factors and salt-poor albumin amongst others (p276). G+S samples typically last about 10–14d. If you need a blood product urgently (<24h) then phone the lab.

Radiology Urgent USS, CT and MRI need to be discussed with a radiologist (p18). Give brief clinical details on all X-ray forms and include LMP (β-HCG if >28d) for females. NB Portable AXRs are rarely feasible.

Unlabelled/wrongly labelled samples You will forget to write a patient's details on a sample, usually from a patient who was uniquely difficult to bleed. Speak to the lab, they may agree to send the sample back (though you will be liable if it is the wrong sample). **Blood bank will never allow you to do this since transfusion errors can be fatal.**

Occupational health

Most hospitals have an occupational health department that is responsible for ensuring that the hospital is a safe environment for you and your patients. This includes making sure that doctors work in a safe manner. You can find your local unit at www.nhsplus.nhs.uk.

Common calls

During the Foundation Programme your contact with occupational health is likely to be one of the following:

- ***Hepatitis B booster*** You should have a booster every 5yr to maintain your immunity – this is often your first year as a doctor
- ***Needle-stick/sharps injury*** see next page
- ***Illness*** that affects your ability to work may require a consultation

Smartcards

NHS workers' occupational health records are being computerised and stored onto smartcards that are held by the staff member. These contain the details of all consultations including vaccination records.

Infection control

Hospitals are not clean environments. Patients are commonly infected by pathogens from the hospital and ward staff. The infections are more likely to be resistant to antibiotics and can be fatal. It is important to reduce the risk you pose to your patients:

- if you are ill stay at home, especially if you have gastroenteritis
- keep your clothes clean including white coats and ties
- clean your stethoscope with an alcohol swab regularly
- wash your hands or use alcohol gel after every patient contact, even when wearing gloves
- be rigorous in your use of aseptic technique
- stop unnecessary antibiotics after a full course

Sharps and bodily fluids

As a doctor you will come into contact with bodily fluids daily. It is important to develop good habits so that you are safe on the wards:

- Wear gloves for all procedures that could involve bodily fluids or sharps. Gloves reduce the risk of disease transmission when penetrated with a needle – consider wearing two pairs for high-risk patients
- Dispose of all sharps immediately. Take the sharps bin to where you are using the sharps to avoid walking around with contaminated needles; **always dispose of your own sharps**
- vacutainers are safer than a needle and syringe
- consider wearing goggles if bodily fluids might spray
- cover cuts in your skin
- avoid wearing sandals
- make sure your hep B boosters are up-to-date

Needle-sticks and blood-borne viruses

Most doctors have received needle-stick injuries without serious consequences. If you have just been exposed get, and take, advice asap.

Immediately

Stop what you are doing. If it is urgent phone your senior/colleague to do it. Your future health is your top priority.

- ***Percutaneous exposure*** (needle or sharp) Squeeze around the wound so that blood comes out and wash with soap and water; avoid scrubbing or pressing the wound directly
- ***Mucocutaneous exposure*** (eyes, nose, mouth, non-intact skin) Rinse with water (or 1l of 0.9% saline through a giving set for your eye/nose)

Within an hour a colleague should:

- ***talk*** to the patient and explain what has happened. Speak to them alone (without spouses, relatives and friends) and ask about:
  - injecting drugs
  - blood transfusions
  - tattoos or piercings in foreign countries
  - unprotected sex (particularly in last 3mth, in a developing country or, if male, with a man)
  - testing for hepatitis B+C or HIV and the results
- ***ask*** to take a blood sample for testing for hep B+C and HIV (p261)

You should:

- ***phone*** occupational health, microbiologist on-call or A+E and follow their advice exactly. This may include storing a sample of your own blood and taking post-exposure prophylaxis (see below)
- ***document*** the exposure in the patient's notes and on an incident form

Post-exposure prophylaxis

You may be prescribed anti-retrovirals (triple therapy, within 1h), 500u of hepatitis B immunoglobulin (within 24h) or hepatitis B booster (within 24h) according to the significance of the exposure. There is currently no post-exposure prophylaxis for hepatitis C.

	Hepatitis B	Hepatitis C	HIV
UK prevalence	<0.5%	<0.5%	<0.1%
Transmission risk	1 in 3 (without vaccine)	1 in 50	1 in 300
Vaccination	Vaccines at 1, 2 + 12mth	None	None
Post-exposure	Immunoglobulin or booster	None	Triple therapy

Over the next few weeks

The patient's blood tests should take <2d for HIV and hep B+C results. Following high-risk exposure you may be advised to have a blood test in the future (2–6mth); during this time you should practice safe sex (condoms) and not donate blood. **You cannot be forced to have an HIV test.** Discuss with occupational health about involvement in surgery.

Driving regulations

The DVLA issues strict regulations about which medical conditions affect your ability to drive. A summary of this information is shown below, the full guidelines are available on the DVLA website (www.dvla.gov.uk). This list is not exhaustive and a patient should stop driving if they, or their doctor, believe they are incapacitated.

Neurology	
Stroke (mild deficit)	Cease for 1mth
Disability	**Variable***
Chronic neurology	**Variable***
Meningitis	Drive if well
Seizure (or suspected)	**Cease for 1yr***
Severe head injury/intra-cranial bleed	**Cease for 6–12mth***
Brain tumours and mets	**Variable***
Neurosurgery	**Variable***
Visual field defects and dip-lopia	Cease driving (may be allowed if stable)
Visual acuity	Better than 6/12 corrected with both eyes
Fainting	Drive if well
Unexplained syncope	**Cease for 4wk***
Recurrent severe vertigo	**Once attacks controlled***
Diabetes	
Diabetes on insulin or tablets	**Must be able to recognise hypo***
Diabetes on diet only	Drive if well
Recurrent hypoglycaemia	Cease until controlled

Cardiology	
Stable angina	Drive if well
Unstable angina	Cease until stabilised
MI/ACS	Cease for 4wk
Angioplasty	Cease for 1wk
Pacemaker	**Cease for 1wk***
CABG	**Cease for 4wk***
Incapacitating arrhythmia	**Cease for 4wk after controlled***
Stable arrhythmia	Drive if well
Psychiatry and substance abuse	
Severe psychiatric illness	**Cease until stable for 3mth***
Alcohol abuse	**Cease until 6–12mth control***
Opioid, benzo + cocaine use	**Cease for 1yr after previous use***
Other recreational drugs	**Cease for 6mth after previous use***
Other	
COPD	Drive if well
Sleep apnoea + narcolepsy	**Cease until symptoms controlled***
Chronic renal failure	**Notify DVLA***
HIV	Drive if well

*** Patient must notify the DVLA**

If a patient refuses to notify the DVLA about a medical condition you have a duty to break confidentiality and inform the DVLA on their behalf.

Chapter 2

Your career

Continuing your education

Educational requirements During your PRHO (F1) year you will be allocated a clinical supervisor who will meet with you to talk about your progress. They should be able to answer any questions you may have about your training or career. Teaching sessions are mandatory and you should attend unless you are on nights, leave or bound by on-call commitments; failure to attend can result in failing the F1 year. Read the document on PRHO training provided by the university or postgraduate centre. Equally, teaching sessions are compulsory for SHOs and poor attendance can affect your study leave budget.

Study leave There is currently no formal provision for study leave for the F1 year and entitlement starts in F2. The number of days that can be taken vary, but commonly a maximum of 15d are allocated per six months. Study leave is for recognised courses and examinations, but you may be allowed to take private study leave which is most often used for revision prior to examinations. Check with your postgraduate centre.

Study expenses If your post is recognised by the postgraduate dean as a training post you are entitled to funding for courses including travel and subsistence. The amount you are entitled to varies, though most people receive between £300 and £400 for each 6mth period. Often you will have to pay for a course yourself and claim the money back after the course has taken place; check with your postgraduate centre. The cost of sitting examinations is not allowed to come out of your study budget; you will have to pay for these yourself (see p66).

Postgraduate courses There are literally hundreds of courses you could attend. The cost of courses vary – some are free, some cost over £500 per day, most are about £100–150 per day. Your study budget is limited, so plan ahead and spend your money on courses which are going to be valuable to you. Advanced Life Support (ALS) is a good course for everyone to attend and some hospitals provide this for free. Other courses specific to your speciality may be suggested by your seniors, but try to talk to others who have attended them before applying. Revision courses for examinations are popular, but again speak to people who have attended these. Check with the postgraduate centre for details of how to apply for courses and for funding. The BMA website lists many postgraduate courses (www.bma.org).

Exam planning Once you have decided on a career plan (p52), you will need to contact the appropriate Royal College (p525) and request a copy of the examination regulations (p66). There are prerequisites which one must fulfil before sitting the various components of the Colleges' examinations. Most of the Colleges' examinations consist of two parts; the first usually consists of basic science applicable to the speciality with some clinical content; the second part of the examination is usually much more clinically based. There is often an interval of a year between part one and part two. Preparation/revision for each part of the examination usually takes six months; it is a good idea to speak to others who have already passed to obtain hints and tips and maybe some books or notes.

Audits

Definition: '[The] examination or review that establishes the extent to which a condition, process or performance conforms to predetermined standards or criteria.'[1] NICE have produced an extensive document on clinical audit.[2] In essence, audit allows current practice to be compared to a standard (best practice or guidelines). Any deviation away from the standard is highlighted, causes identified and recommendations made. The audit is then repeated to check that improvements have occurred; this final step closes the 'audit cycle'. You will be expected to perform an audit as part of your F2 year.

An example of audit Guidelines state that all patients who present to A+E with chest pain should have an ECG taken within 20min. The audit looks at 100 patients presenting to A+E with chest pain and whether they have ECGs within 20min. The findings show that most do but a few take longer because they present to A+E at busy times. The solution is to ensure sufficient nursing staff are on at these busy times. Reaudit to measure success thereby completes the audit cycle.

Audit projects The best audits are simple ones which have important implications. If something has a guideline or standard then it can be audited. Here are some examples, though ask your supervisor before undertaking a project.

- Are Venflons replaced every 72h?
- Are drugs prescribed in accordance with local guidelines?
- Is there soap and alcohol gel in all dispensers?
- Do patients admitted with chest pain have their cholesterol measured?

Getting published

Having publications on your CV will certainly give you an advantage when applying for jobs. There are many ways to get your name in print and you don't have to write a book (which is not great for the social life).

Book reviews Get in touch with a journal and express interest in reviewing books for them; you don't have to be a professor to give an opinion on whether a book reads well or is useful.

Case reports If you have seen something interesting, rare or just very classical then try writing it up. Include images if possible; get a senior co-author and ensure you obtain patient consent.

Fillers Some journals have short stories or funny/moving one-liners submitted by their readers. Write up anything you see which others might be interested in; ensure you obtain patient consent.

Letters If an article is incorrect, fails to mention a key point or has relevance in another field then write to the journal and mention this; it might be worthwhile asking a senior colleague to co-author it with you.

Research papers If you have participated in some research then make sure you get your name on any publications that come out of it.

1 Stedmans Concise Medical Dictionary, 1997.
2 www.nelh.nhs.uk/nice_bpca.asp

Presentations and teaching

The thought of having to give an oral presentation provokes anxiety in most of us. Being able to relay information to an audience is a valuable skill and one which gets easier with time and experience, though it is helped by a logical approach.

Types of presentation In medicine there are four main types of presentation: audit, research, case presentation and a teaching session.

When is the presentation? If you have months to prepare then you can really go to town, whilst if you have only a few hours you need to concentrate on the essentials.

How long should it last? A 5min presentation will still need to be thorough, but less detailed than that lasting an hour. The length of the presentation will also aid you in choosing the topic.

What is the topic? Clarify as early as possible the topic you are to present and any specific aspect of the topic you should be discussing. If you can choose the topic, select something you either know about or are interested in researching.

Audience Are you presenting to your peers, your seniors or juniors? Is the audience ignorant of the topic or world experts in the field? This information will determine the level of depth you will need to go into.

Venue and means of delivery Are you expected to present with acetates on an overhead projector (OHP) or via a computer and projector? If you are going to use an OHP then you should still make your slides on computer and print them out.

Sources of information Do you already have any notes or books on the subject? Read about the topic on the internet by undertaking a search with an engine such as www.google.co.uk. Search *Medline* using keywords; review articles are often a good place to start.

If there is no information If you cannot find enough information to prepare your talk then it is likely you are not searching correctly; ask librarian staff for help. If there really is a lack of information then consider changing the topic, or choose an easier approach to it.

How many slides? On average allow one minute per slide.

Slide format OHP slides should be simple; avoid borders and complex graphics. PowerPoint has numerous pre-set designs, though remember it is the content of your talk the audience needs to be focused upon.

Presentation layout The presentation is in essence an essay which the speaker delivers orally. It should comprise a title page with the topic and speaker's name and an introduction which sets the scene and puts the rest of the presentation in context. The bulk of the presentation should then follow and be closed with either a summary or conclusion. Consider ending with a slide acknowledging thanks and a final slide with simply 'questions?' written on it to invite discussion.

Titles Give each slide a title to make the story easy to follow.

Font The font needs to be at least size 24. Ensure the colour of the text contrasts with the background colour as this will be easiest to read (eg yellow/white text on dark blue background). Avoid using lots of font effects; stick to one or two colours, **bold**, *italics* or underline features.

Graphics Use graphics to support the presentation; do not simply have graphics adorning the slide to make it look pretty.

How much information Avoid overcrowding each slide; it is better to use three shorter slides than one hectic one. Each slide should deliver one message and this should be presented in six points or less.

Bullet points Use these to highlight a few key words, not full sentences.

PowerPoint effects Keep the slides simple. Avoid text flying in from all directions and sound effects as these will distract the audience.

Rehearsing Go through the presentation a few times on your own so you know the sequence and what you are going to say. Then practice presenting it in front of a friend to check timing and flow.

Specific types of presentation

Audit Ensure you give a good reason why the audit was chosen and what existing research/audit has already been undertaken. State clearly your objectives, how you conducted your audit and its limitations. Use graphs to show numerical data and clearly summarise the findings of your audit. Identify how practice can be improved and conclude with plans of how to close the audit cycle and check improvements are effective. Invite questions/discussion. See audit section, p39.

Research This is simply an oral version of your write-up. Give a good introduction, explaining the background and why this research is important. Explain the methods used and their validity and then describe your research and findings. Discuss limitations and how your research may have been improved. Draw your conclusions and indicate where further research may be directed. Pay thanks to the appropriate parties. Invite questions/discussion. See research chapter, p43.

Case presentation The presentation should tell a story about a patient and let the audience try and work out the diagnosis as though they are clerking the patient for the first time. Name the talk something cryptic, eg 'headache in the traveller'. Present the history and physical examination. Invite audience suggestions for the diagnosis and management. Give the results of investigations and again invite the audience to comment. Give the diagnosis and discuss subsequent management. Summarise with an outline of the topic; end with a question/discussion session.

Teaching session It is often easiest to base a topic around a patient if this is appropriate. Aim to keep the session very interactive; have numerous question slides where the audience can discuss answers. Keep your teaching points very clear and slides very simple. Summarise with learning points; it is often helpful to provide a printed copy of your slides as a hand-out for people to take away.

Giving the presentation

Equipment Ensure that the projector and/or computer you will need are going to be available well in advance. Ideally check it works and leave enough time to find new equipment if there is a problem.

Timing Arrive early and check your presentation projects correctly. Leave the title page projected so the right audience sit before you.

Speaking You will need to talk loudly enough to be heard at the back of the room. This is often daunting, but a good presentation given inaudibly is more disappointing than a poor presentation delivered audibly.

Body language Stand at the front of the audience and avoid walking into the projected image. If there is a lectern then use that as your 'base'. Direct your talk at the audience, not the screen. This makes you appear more confident and also allows you to gauge if people are confused or bored.

Beginning Introduce yourself and your position, outline the topic you are going to talk about and explain why you chose the topic. This is a good time to interact with the audience; ask if people at the back can hear you.

To use notes or not You should not need notes to prompt you, but have them available; the key points on the slides should be sufficient.

Style Keep it professional, but show the audience you are human; it is acceptable to mention light-hearted aspects to make the audience laugh.

Pacing You probably speak quicker than you think; do not be afraid to take your time, pause and allow the audience to read all of your points.

Questions Decide in advance if you would like questions to be asked during your presentation or at the end. Anticipate what questions may be asked and prepare for these. Do not be afraid to say you do not know the answer, though offer to find out.

Feedback

Whenever possible ask for constructive criticism from someone who saw your presentation and try to learn from their comments.

Summary of points for a good presentation

- Plan well in advance
- Keep slides simple and clear
- Avoid unnecessary graphics
- Rehearse your talk
- Look at the audience, not the screen

Research and academia

Many consultants conduct research, but academics are employed specifically to lead a research group and teach alongside their clinical duties. While academia is not everyone's cup of tea it offers a diverse and challenging job in any speciality. The route to academic medicine begins long before becoming a consultant.

Foundation years Most departments are engaged in research of some form; if you express an interest and talk to your consultants there may be an opportunity to get involved. Look for case reports, carry out audits (see p39) and endeavour to get these published. You may be able to take a diploma or part-time masters (see below). Try to learn research design, basic statistics and presentation skills (p40). Some foundation programmes have academic attachments, though their content varies.

Post-foundation doctors interested in academia or entering competitive specialities often undertake a period of full or part-time research before or during their registrar jobs. Common taught courses include:

- *MA/MSc* (Master of Arts/Science) – a 1yr course usually with taught and research-based sections. Assessed by exams and a dissertation
- *Diplomas* – the length varies; similar to the taught section of a masters degree and assessed by exams

Research courses take longer, but have higher status:

- *MPhil* (Master of Philosophy) – lasts between 1 and 3yr and is assessed by a thesis of ~50,000 words
- *MD* (Medical Doctorate) – similar status, time frame and assessment to an MPhil, usually taken whilst continuing clinical work
- *PhD* (Philosophy Doctorate) – requires a period of research lasting at least 3yr and the production of an ~80,000 word thesis

Finding a project You need to actively seek out research projects. If you already have an idea for a project then try to identify a suitable supervisor through a literature search around the project (papers include contact details). Otherwise decide three things: (1) area of medicine (cardiology, surgery etc), (2) lab or patient based, (3) where you want to study. Contact consultants and universities around the area and ask about suitable projects – alternatively check the 'University, research and fellowships' section of *BMJ Careers*.

Funding One of the downsides of academic medicine is that you often need to raise funding to pay for yourself and your research. The process takes a long time (at least 6mth) and involves filling in vast numbers of forms (form filling is a transferable skill…). Common sources of funding include the Medical Research Council and Wellcome Trust (p524) and charities/societies with an interest in your chosen subject. There is a substantial list at www.omni.ac.uk/subject-listing/W20.5.

Medical statistics

Observational studies

Cross-sectional Looks at a sample of the population at one moment in time; used to highlight potential risk factors and determine prevalence.

Case–control (retrospective) Patients with a disease (cases) are asked about their previous exposure to potential risk factors. People without the disease (controls) are asked the same questions and the two groups are compared. Case–control studies are quick, relatively cheap and suitable for rare diseases.

Cohort study (prospective) A defined sample of the population is observed over time to see who develops diseases or complications and what risks they were exposed to. Cohort studies take a long time (years), are expensive and ineffective for rare disease.

Intervention studies/clinical trials

These are trials that compare new treatments against a placebo or the old treatment (as a control). Ideally the trials should be:

- ***randomised*** – allocating patients to a particular treatment by a random process
- ***blind*** – the patient is unaware which treatment they were given
- ***double-blind*** – both the patient and the researcher were unaware which treatment the patient was given

Meta-analysis

This is a powerful technique for answering clinical questions by mathematically combining the results from numerous similar trials into a single paper. The results are dependent on the quality of the trials included.

Level of evidence

Different study designs are ranked according to their 'level of evidence' (below), though a good cohort study may be much better evidence than a bad randomised controlled trial.

The level of evidence

High level	Meta-analysis
↑	Randomised controlled trial
	Clinical trial
	Cohort study
	Case–control
Low level	Cross-sectional

Population tests (Does one group differ from another?)
These are used to compare the averages of different groups, eg average life expectancy on treatment vs placebo. Choosing the correct test is difficult and is determined by the type of data and the number of groups.

This table acts as a guide; see definitions below and next page:

Type of data	Average	Distribution	Statistical test
Nominal	Mode	Variance	Binomial, Chi-squared, Fisher's
Ordinal non-numeric	Median	Variance	Mann–Whitney, Wilcoxon, Sign test
Ordinal numeric	Median	Range	Mann–Whitney, Wilcoxon, Sign test
Metric non-parametric	Median	Range	Mann–Whitney, Wilcoxon, Sign test
Metric parametric	Mean	Standard deviation	T test, ANOVA

Nominal (categorical) data consists of groups that cannot be arranged in order, eg blood types, eye colour.

Ordinal data consists of labels (non-numeric) or subjective numbers (numeric) that can be arranged in order, eg A-level grades, rate your pain out of 10.

Metric (interval) data consists of objective numbers. These should either have units, eg weight, or count observations, eg number of patients in clinic. The key consideration is that the numbers can be used mathematically: 2 × 35kg = 70kg (metric), but 2 × 2/10 for pain ≠ 4/10 for pain (ordinal).

Association tests (Does one variable change with another?)

These are used to investigate whether variables are related, eg survival time vs size of the tumour. The data should be plotted on a scatter graph to assess the shape. The association could be:

- ***positive*** – the two variables increase together, eg BP and age
- ***negative*** – one variable increases as the other decreases, eg life expectancy and smoking

Correlation is the measure of an association between two variables. It is shown as a coefficient called 'r' that is between –1.0 (negative association) and +1.0 (positive association). If there is no association the coefficient is 0. The data must be in a roughly straight line on the scatter graph. The significance of the correlation can be calculated from the coefficient using statistical tables. This table shows the correct test for calculating the correlation coefficient:

Type of data	Statistical test
One or both variables ordinal	Spearman's
Both variables metric	Pearson's

Regression This is the best-fit line on the scatter graph. Make sure the dependent variable is on the X-axis. The equation of the line can be calculated to predict other values.

Statistical definitions

Average A mid-point of the data, may be a mean, median or mode.

Continuous (cf discrete) Data with a full range of fractions, eg weight.

Dependent (cf independent) A measured variable that is affected by other variables.

Discrete (cf continuous) Data without fractions, eg number of patients.

Distribution How widely the data are spread about the average; may be a standard deviation, range or variance depending on the type of data.

Incidence (cf prevalence) Number of people developing a disease within a set time. Expressed as a number or a proportion of the population.

Independent (cf dependent) A variable that is altered by the researcher or one that causes another measured variable to change.

Level The number of categories in discrete data, eg gender = 2 levels.

Likelihood ratio The increased chance of having a disease based on a test result; calculated from sensitivity and specificity.

Matched When a control is chosen because their age/sex/height etc matches those of a case.

Non-parametric (cf parametric) Metric data that does not follow the 'normal distribution'. If in doubt assume non-parametric.

Number needed to harm (NNH) The number of patients receiving a treatment without detectable harm per patient receiving harm.

Number needed to treat (NNT) The number of patients who must receive a treatment for one of them to be identified as receiving benefit.

Odds ratio/relative risk The increased chance of contracting a disease following a specific exposure, eg 10:1 for lung cancer from smoking.

Paired When two or more observations are made on the same person.

Parametric (cf non-parametric) Metric data that follows the 'normal distribution'. A graph of frequencies in each group should be bell shaped.

Power calculations are used to design trials by calculating how many patients are required for a significant result based on previous findings.

Prevalence (cf incidence) The total number of people with a disease. May be expressed as a number or a proportion of the population.

Sensitivity Proportion of true positives correctly identified as positive, irrespective of false positives; ie a highly sensitive test will always rule-in those with the condition. D-dimers have a high sensitivity for DVT/PE.

Specificity Proportion of true negatives which are correctly identified as negative; ie a highly specific test can be used to safely rule-out those without the condition. D-dimers have a low specificity for DVT/PE.

95% confidence interval The range of values around the mean that represent where the true mean would lie with 95% confidence.

Keeping track

For the General Medical Council

GMC revalidation Since 01/04/05 doctors are required to prove they are up to date and fit to practise to the GMC on a regular basis. They must do this using evidence derived from their medical practice. This process (revalidation) is a condition of registration with the GMC. All doctors, including those in Foundation Programmes, need a licence to practise from the GMC. Doctors should compile folders of evidence derived from their practice which will be checked at a local level.

For your Royal College

Logbooks These are simply a record of what you have done, especially of practical procedures. They are almost impossible to compile retrospectively. Most Royal Colleges have logbook requirements for doctors training to become specialists. These are becoming electronic but many are still paper-based. During the Foundation Programme only a minority will know which College is likely to oversee their postgraduate training.

- If you are clear on future career plans, either:
  - register with the College and begin completing their logbook
  - or obtain copies of the relevant pages of the logbook from a senior colleague and complete them so that you have the data for your own logbook once registered
- If you are not clear on which speciality you wish to end up in:
  - keep a record of practical procedures
  - keep records of all appraisals etc (see below)

Data Protection Act

All data collected will be covered by the Data Protection Act. This means that you must not keep patient-identifiable data away from the hospital. The use of hospital numbers rather than names is considered acceptable.

Your 'portfolio'

Evidence for GMC revalidation includes the following:

- ***Appraisal*** This should be a comprehensive review of your training so far, your expectations and needs for the future and a chance to discuss areas of concern. It should take place at the start and end of each placement. It should be structured and agreed between the appraiser (educational supervisor) and trainee
- ***Objectives*** These should be a clear, realistic and personal list of what you hope to get out of a post. Agree them with your educational supervisor. These often form part of the appraisal process
- ***Competency*** As part of the Foundation Programme there will be an ongoing assessment of competency. Deaneries organise on this and will provide the assessment tool locally. It will remain your responsibility to highlight areas in which you need additional training. Do so and get trained

The portfolio itself

Roughly speaking, keep everything. You should end up with a box file containing the following:

- Up-to-date CV
- Proofs of qualifications
- Past appraisals
- If not in a logbook; procedures – when done and whether observing, performing or teaching
- Copies of presentations given
- Details of teaching you've done (with feedback if possible)
- Copies of audits you've been involved in
- Details of courses you've attended
- Copies of your publications
- Details of any complaints made against you and their resolution
- 'Triumphs' – difficult patients you've diagnosed/treated
- Praise – all thank you letters/cards

Important advice

- Start early (when you qualify)
- Keep it up-to-date
- Organise it by headings at least every 6mth
- Discuss it yearly with a suitable mentor

Choosing a job

Priorities Before looking for a job, write a list of your minimum requirements. Important considerations include:

- ***Partner/spouse*** Can they get a job nearby?
- ***Location*** Could you move or how far would you commute each day?
- ***Family/friends*** How far away are you willing to go?
- ***Career*** Is the job in the right speciality/specialities?
- ***Training*** Will a non-training post do?
- ***Rota/pay*** What banding and rota do you want or need?
- ***Type of hospital*** Large teaching hospital vs district general

If you have no firm career intentions then choose by location and rota since these will affect your life most over the next few months. With this in mind, try the website www.jobscore.co.uk where you can rate previous jobs (confidentially) and see what others thought of yours. Look for suitable jobs in *BMJ Careers* – the clinical alerts on the website are useful, if not 100% reliable. If you cannot find jobs then lower your expectations.

Staggering of jobs Not all the jobs come out together; some hospitals advertise over 6mth before the job, others less than 2. Once you accept a job you cannot change your mind (see below); this creates a tricky balance between waiting for the perfect job vs applying for acceptable ones. Hopefully the Foundation Programme will result in reform of this process, until then err on the side of applying to acceptable jobs.

Competition Medical jobs are competitive, often with hundreds of applicants for every post. The application process is something of a lottery – developing thick skin and applying for several jobs will help. See p58 to develop the perfect CV and application.

Researching a job Adverts rarely give a true reflection of a job. Phone up the hospital and ask to speak to the person doing the job at the moment. Quiz them on the hours, support, conditions and what their interview was like. Would they accept the job again? Try to visit the hospital and get a first-hand impression – this also looks good at interview.

Contacts With human resource departments and structured interviews, the days of jobs being just a consultant phone call away have gone. There is no doubt that some networking still occurs with mixed results. Senior contacts are useful for tailored career guidance, CV advice and giving realistic views of where your CV can get you.

Accepting a job Once you have accepted a job it is very bad manners to turn them down at a later date unless you have a valid reason (not another job). Doing so will often invoke angry letters from the interviewing consultants, possibly copied to your referees; it may make it difficult to get employment from that trust.

Specialities in medicine

Listed as currently accepted CCSTs:

- Main CCST
  - Sub-speciality CCST requiring additional training; where these can be accessed by more than one route, all have been listed

PMETB will change these to CCTs and may limit the list but this illustrates the breadth of posts available.

- Accident and emergency medicine
  - Paediatric accident and emergency medicine
- Allergy
- Anaesthetics
- Audiological medicine
- Cardiology (also known as cardio-vascular disease)
  - Stroke medicine
- Cardio-thoracic surgery (also known as thoracic surgery)
- Chemical pathology
  - Metabolic medicine
- Child and adolescent psychiatry
- Clinical cytogenetics and molecular genetics
- Clinical genetics
- Clinical neurophysiology
- Clinical oncology (also known as radiotherapy)
- Clinical pharmacology and therapeutics
  - Stroke medicine
- Clinical radiology (also known as diagnostic radiology)
- Dermatology
- Endocrinology and diabetes mellitus
- Forensic psychiatry
- Gastroenterology
  - Hepatology
- General adult psychiatry (also known as general psychiatry or psychiatry)
  - Liaison psychiatry
  - Rehabilitation psychiatry
  - Substance misuse psychiatry
- General internal medicine (also known as general medicine)
  - Acute medicine
  - Metabolic medicine
  - Stroke medicine
- General surgery
- Genito-urinary medicine (also known as venereology)
- Geriatric medicine (also known as geriatrics)
  - Stroke medicine
- Haematology
- Histopathology (also known as morbid anatomy and histopathology)
  - Cytopathology
  - Forensic pathology
  - Neuropathology
  - Paediatric pathology
- Immunology (also known as immunopathology)
- Infectious diseases (also known as communicable disease)
- Intensive care medicine
- Medical microbiology
  - Microbiology
  - Virology
- Medical oncology
- Medical ophthalmology
- Neurology
  - Stroke medicine
- Neurosurgery (also known as neurological surgery)
- Nuclear medicine

- Obstetrics and gynaecology
  - Community gynaecology
  - Gynaecological oncology
  - Maternal and fetal medicine
  - Sexual and reproductive health (previously reproductive medicine)
  - Urogynaecology
- Occupational medicine
- Old age psychiatry
- Ophthalmology
- Oral and maxillofacial surgery (basic medical and dental training)
- Otolaryngology (also known as ENT surgery)
- Paediatric cardiology
- Paediatric surgery
- Paediatrics
  - Community child health
  - Neonatal medicine
  - Paediatric clinical pharmacology
  - Paediatric endocrinology
  - Paediatric gastroenterology
  - Paediatric infectious diseases and immunology
  - Paediatric intensive care medicine
  - Paediatric nephrology
  - Paediatric neurodisability
  - Paediatric neurology
  - Paediatric oncology
  - Paediatric respiratory medicine
  - Paediatric rheumatology
- Palliative medicine
- Plastic surgery
- Psychiatry of learning disability
- Psychotherapy
- Public health medicine (also known as community medicine)
- Rehabilitation medicine
  - Stroke medicine
- Renal medicine (also known as renal disease and formerly known as nephrology)
- Respiratory medicine (also known as thoracic medicine)
- Rheumatology
- Trauma and orthopaedic surgery (also known as orthopaedic surgery)
- Tropical medicine
- Urology

Career structure – old

PRHO posts are followed by SHO rotations or stand-alone posts. By registration two-thirds of doctors have an idea what career they wish to pursue and can apply accordingly. Virtually all hospital specialities require College examinations (p66) and most SHO training is directed towards passing these. SHO training rotations are advertised in the *BMJ* and state their speciality usefulness (eg paediatrics or basic surgery).

Alternatively there are GP vocational training schemes, effectively a 3yr training rotation for general practice with 2yr in hospital and 1yr as a GP registrar. There rotations are also suitable for careers in public health as well as specialities which cross the community/hospital divide, eg psychiatry or family planning.

This system is difficult for the other one-third of trainees who don't know what they wish to do. These doctors tend to choose a more general rotation or a free-standing post such as A+E, hoping to make up their minds later.

The rotations tend to be very competitive, especially those in teaching hospitals and surgery. Many trainees take up non-training posts that do not count towards postgraduate exams and do not enjoy the same protection as SHO training jobs but improve their experience and CV. Whilst some are virtually identical to the SHO posts sharing the rota, some are little more than posts of abuse.

The SHO grade has no time limit; for those who wish to stay in training it ends when they obtain a national training number (NTN) and a speciality registrar post. The endless rounds of interviews and applications come to an end until at the CCT. Gaining access to an NTN is by (very) competitive application and interview. In many surgical fields a period of recognised and relevant research is essential; this prolongs the SHO time even more. Six years is not unusual for the more competitive specialities.
Therefore:

- try to decide on a career choice early (p52)
- take the relevant examination early (p66) and concentrate on passing first time
- give your CV an edge with extras (eg audits, publications, p39)
- do your homework and apply to good rotations (not necessarily in teaching hospitals)
- get a respected mentor to guide you

However, the system is changing in August 2007, see the next page.

The proposed MMC training ladder

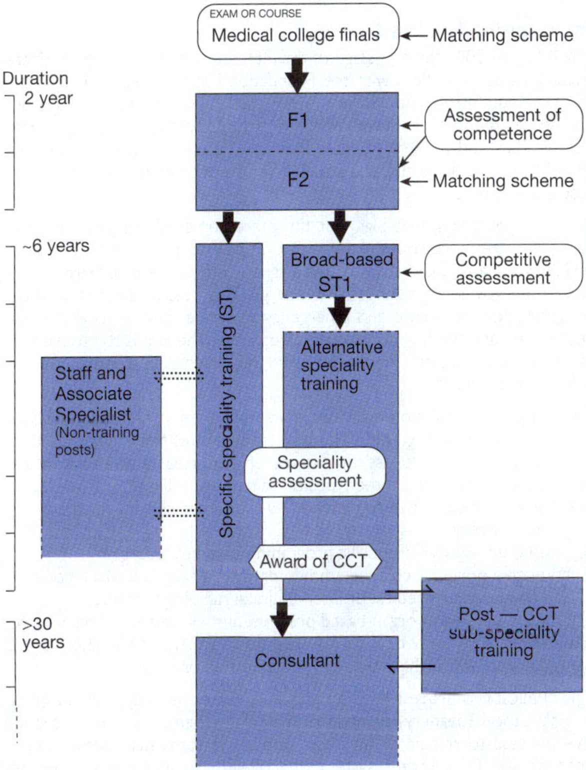

Career structure – new

Modernising Medical Careers

On 1 August 2005 the first stage of the MMC reforms of UK postgraduate training came into effect with the Foundation Programmes (FP) replacing the previous PRHO and 1st year SHO posts. The structure is far from finalised as the GMC is due to propose changes to the first postgraduate year in 2007 and the Postgraduate Medical Education and Training Board (PMETB) has yet to finalise the structure of the second year, especially the assessment process.

In short, you are guinea-pigs, but there are some advantages. The first two years are more coordinated than ever before and have a curriculum which you are expected to get signed off as you progress (via www.mmc.gov.uk or your local deanery). This curriculum has a heavy weighting towards acute and emergency medicine with an emphasis on recognising and treating acutely unwell patients. The aim is to ensure that all doctors, no matter which speciality they eventually choose, will be safe in an emergency.

Following the Foundation Programme you will enter continuous speciality training ('run-through grade'). The final shape of this training and particularly the application process for this are far from clear at the time of this book going to print, but three types of training seem likely:

- broad-based speciality programmes, eg acute medicine, paediatrics, general surgery
- focused end-speciality specific programmes, eg neurosurgery
- innovative organ-based programmes, eg vascular disease which could lead to a surgical, medical or interventional radiology career.

The broad-based and organ-based programmes will require choices to be made after one or two years to specialise further. These choices are likely to require a further competitive application process.

The applications process to enter a training programme is probably going to use a local (deanery) or national matching scheme. A more competitive process to remain in the most popular streams may occur after a year or so. The current system of College examinations is likely to change under the guidance of PMETB since these are career specific. Modular assessment with College-sponsored elements is one option.

We realise this is vague, but as you have found out by now, many of these changes are far from sorted.

Do not let the uncertainty stop you from seeking the best quality training you can get so that you can practice in your chosen field. No matter what changes take place you will need clinical experience.

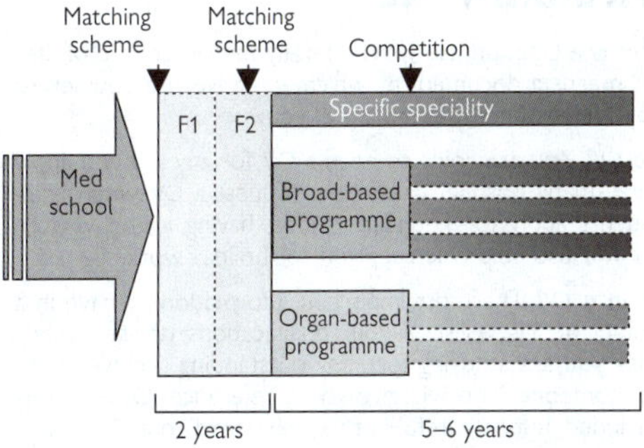

The training ladder from house officer to consultant

Your Curriculum Vitae

What is a CV? This is a Latin phrase which literally means 'course of life'. In modern days it means a document by which you advertise yourself to a potential employer; in essence, a summary of you.

When will I use a CV? You are going to need a CV for any job you apply for after graduating. Many hospital trusts now request a CV when final-year medical students apply for Foundation jobs; having a well-written and presented CV will also help when applying for holiday work.

What is included in a CV? The most important information to have in a CV are your contact details, a list of your qualifications (those already acquired and those you are studying for), any outstanding achievements, and the details of someone who will give you a reference. Other information is often included, but be careful not to overcrowd your CV.

CV philosophy Your CV should not be a static piece of work, it should evolve with you and reflect your changing skills and attitudes. It is important to keep your CV up-to-date, and from time to time reformat it to freshen it up. Use your CV to demonstrate how you have learnt from your experiences rather than just listing them; a potential employer will be much more impressed if you indicate you learnt about the importance of clear communication whilst working at a holiday resort, than by the actual job itself. Make it read in a positive light.

Getting help Career centres usually have advice on writing a CV, and often you can find people's CVs or templates on the internet by searching for 'CV'. Try to keep your CV individualised, so do not simply copy someone else's template.

Before writing your CV It is important to ascertain what a potential employer is looking for when sending in your CV. You need to alter the emphasis in your CV to match the position you are applying for eg, highlighting your communication skills or leadership experience.

Layout Your CV should look impressive; for many jobs over 200 CVs are received and yours must stand out above the rest. It must be word-processed. It needs to be clearly laid out and easy to follow. The key information and your most important attributes should stand out prominently. Think about the layout before you start writing.

Length Two sides of A4 paper is ideal for a basic CV (and an optional front page); add more as you progress up the ladder of seniority.

Front page You could have the first page of your CV with just your name and basic qualifications on; this looks smart, but means your CV will be one page longer.

Remember For most jobs, the candidates applying will have very similar qualifications and so the only way you will stand out to be short-listed for interview is via your CV. Make it as interesting as possible, without it looking ludicrous.

Personal details Name, address which you use for correspondence, contact telephone numbers (home, work, mobile), email address and date of birth are essential. You must state your type of General Medical Council membership (full/provisional) and number. Stating gender, marital status and other information is optional.

Personal statement This is very much an optional section. Some feel it gives you an opportunity to outline a little about yourself and where you see yourself in 10 years; others feel it is an irritating waste of space.

Education List your qualifications in date order, starting with the most recent or current and progressing backwards in time. Indicate where each was undertaken, the dates you were there and grade. Highlight specific courses or modules of interest. GCSE and A-level results are less important once you have graduated.

Employment and work experience List the positions you have held, work experience and volunteer work you have undertaken, starting with the most recent. Once you have qualified and done several jobs you should list the positions you held, the dates, the address of the employer and your supervising consultant. For those who have not yet qualified it might be easier to write a short paragraph, using bold text to highlight key words.

Interests An optional section which gives you a chance to outline what you like to do outside of medicine. A well-written paragraph here can show potential employers that you are interesting as well as intelligent.

Publications If you have not yet got your name in print try to get a letter in a medical journal (p39). If you have got publications put the most recent first; ensure they are referenced in a conventional style.

Referees Your referees should know your academic record as well as your ability to interact with others. State their relationship to you (such as personal tutor) and give contact address, telephone and fax numbers and email address. Ensure they are happy to provide a reference, give them a copy of your CV and tell them when you are applying for jobs.

Headers and footers Having the month and year in either a header or footer shows the reader you keep it up-to-date.

Photographs Some people include a small passport-sized photograph of themselves near the start of their CV; this is optional.

The finished CV Use the spell-checker and get a tutor and/or friend to read over it to identify mistakes and make constructive criticism; be prepared to make numerous alterations to get it just right.

Technical points Use just one clear font throughout. To highlight text of importance use the underline, **bold** or *italic* features. When printing your CV use good quality white paper and a laser printer if possible.

The covering letter Whenever you apply for a job, you must send a covering letter with your CV and application form. This should be short and to the point. Indicate the position you are applying for and briefly say why the job appeals to you.

Pre-Foundation Programme CV

Name	Charles J Flint
Address:	14 Abbeyvale Crescent McBurney's Point McBurney McB1 7RH
Home:	0111 442 985
Mobile:	0968 270 250
Email:	charles.flint@mcburney.ac.uk
Date of Birth:	12 June 1982 (age 23)

PERSONAL STATEMENT

I am an outgoing 23-year-old with an enthusiastic yet mature outlook. I have strong communication skills and experience of working independently, both as a team member and leader. I am conscientious, trustworthy, quick to learn and to employ new skills. My long-term aim is to practise an acute speciality within the hospital environment.

EDUCATION

2001–date

University of McBurney, McBurney's Point, McB1 8PQ

MBChB:	In my fifth and final year
BMedSci (Hons):	Upper Second Class, 2003
SSM:	*The effect of caffeine on the human platelet* Supervised by Professor McArdle
Dissertation:	*The epidemiology of multiple sclerosis* Supervised by Dr Lee
Elective:	*Drug resistant malaria in East Africa* Supervised by Dr Hope

Additional Information:

- President of Medical Society, 2002, 2003, 2004
- Awarded Lampter-Evans Prize for Anatomy, 2002

1999–2001

St Mary's College, Ainlee Road, Newamchester, NA68 1WD

3 A Levels:	Biology (B), Chemistry (A), Mathematics (A)
9 GCSEs:	Biology (B), Chemistry (A), Electronics (B), English Language (B), English Literature (B), French (C), Geography (A), Mathematics (B), Physics (A)

Additional Information:

- Awarded with the Wyn Gracetree Biology A Level Prize
- Raised £1000 for local children's charity by organising a 24-hr event

Employment History

During my undergraduate training I spent half a day every two weeks as a **voluntary worker** in a centre for children with **learning difficulties**, where I learnt much about child care and special needs.

For the last two years I have worked in the **University Union Bar** on Friday evenings, which I feel has helped improve my communication skills.

Prior to starting my undergraduate course, I shadowed a **junior doctor** at my local hospital and arranged a week helping out at my local **doctor's surgery**, both of which gave me better insight into the career I am entering.

Interests

I am a keen and active member of the university **rock climbing** society. I have attended several trips away to Scotland and one to Wales. I am interested in **medical journalism** and have spent a week in the editorial office of the International Journal of Thrombophlebitis.

I am an enthusiastic amateur cook and love entertaining with friends. I also enjoy black and white films, in particular the early horror movies of Vincent Price and Christopher Lee.

Publications

- **Flint CJ**. Letter: Student debt. *Medical Students Journal* 2004; **35**(2): 101
- **Flint CJ** & West DJ. Multiple sclerosis in social class three. *Journal of Social Medicine* 2003; **12**(9): 118
- Lee S, **Flint CJ** & West DJ. Caffeine as an activator of platelet aggregation. *International Journal of Thrombophlebitis* 2002; **54**(3): 99

References

- Dr William Bannister, Personal Tutor, Department of Respiratory Medicine, McBurney's Medical Centre, McBurney's Point, McBurney, McB1 7TS. Telephone 0111 709 979. Fax 0111 709 304. Email william.bannister@mcburney.ac.uk
- Professor Sarah Lee, Project Supervisor, Department of Neurology, McBurney's Medical Centre, McBurney's Point, McBurney, McB1 7TS. Telephone 0111 709 352. Fax 0111 709 245. Email sarah.lee@mcburney.ac.uk

Post-Foundation Programme CV

Name	Charles J Flint
Address:	14 Abbeyvale Crescent McBurney's Point McBurney McB1 7RH
Home:	0111 442 985
Mobile:	0968 270 250
Work:	0111 924 9924 bleep 1066
Email:	charles.flint@mcburney.ac.uk
Date of Birth:	12 June 1981 (age 24)
GMC:	0121231 (full)

PERSONAL STATEMENT

I am an outgoing 24-year-old with an enthusiastic yet mature outlook. I have strong communication skills and experience of working independently, both as a team member and leader. I am conscientious, trustworthy, quick to learn and to employ new skills. My long-term aim is to practise an acute speciality within the hospital environment.

EDUCATION

1998–2003

University of McBurney, McBurney's Point, McB1 8PQ

MBChB: 2003
BMedSci (Hons): Upper Second Class, 2001

EMPLOYMENT HISTORY

3 Apr 05–date	SHO to Mr Broom, Emergency Medicine Glenhaddock County Hospital
5 Dec 04–2 Apr 05	SHO to Dr Fungi, Microbiology St Steriles Hospital
31 Jul 04–4 Dec 04	SHO to Dr Golfer, General Practice Feelgood Health Centre, Speakertown
3 Apr 04–30 Jul 04	PRHO to Mr Grimshaw, General Surgery McBurney Royal Infirmary
5 Dec 03–2 Apr 04	PRHO to Miss Cracken, Gynaecology Buttery Community Hospital
31 Jul 03–4 Dec 03	PRHO to Dr Singleton, General/Renal Medicine McBurney City Hospital

Postgraduate Clinical Experience

During my first year of the Foundation Programme I developed my clinical and practical skills and became confident with the day-to-day organisation of emergency and elective admissions in both medicine and surgery.

Since commencing FP2 I have built upon these skills and now appreciate the wider role of the doctor in the smooth running of acute admissions and liaison with the community teams prior to, and after, hospital discharge.

Formal skills I have include:

- ALS provider (2005)
- Competent with chest drain insertion
- Have undertaken a two-day course on 'radiology in the emergency department'
- Basic surgical skills, including suturing and fracture management

Research and Audit

- I am currently involved in a research project comparing capillary blood gas analysis with arterial blood gasses in acute asthmatics
- I undertook an audit on MRSA screening on the surgical admission unit
- During my SSM I was involved in research investigating the role of caffeine upon platelet aggregation

Interests

I am a keen and **rock** and **ice climber** and have continued to improve my grade since leaving university. I have organised several climbing trips to Scotland and one to the Alps. I am interested in **medical journalism** and have spent a week in the editorial office of the International Journal of Thrombophlebitis.

Publications

- **Flint CJ.** Letter: ABGs: time for a change? BFS 2005; **82**(212): 63
- **Flint CJ.** Letter: Student debt. Medical Students Journal 2004; **35**(2): 101
- **Flint CJ** & West DJ. Multiple Sclerosis in social class three. Journal of Social Medicine 2003; **12**(9): 118
- Lee S, **Flint CJ** & West DJ. Caffeine as an activator of platelet aggregation. International Journal of Thrombophlebitis 2002; **54**(3): 99

References

- Dr William Bannister, Personal Tutor, Department of Respiratory Medicine, McBurney's Medical Centre, McBurney's Point, McBurney, McB1 7TS.
  Telephone 0111 709 979. Fax 0111 709 304.
  Email william.bannister@mcburney.ac.uk

- Miss Eve Cracken, PRHO Supervisor, Department of Gynaecology, Buttery Community Hospital, Buttery, BU20 2ER.
  Telephone 0110 132 677. Fax 0110 132 678.
  Email eve.cracken@buttery.net

Applying for jobs

- During the final year at medical school, most people enter the 'matching scheme' which allows individuals to apply for specific Foundation Programmes. As these Programmes draw to a close, you need to apply for the next training rotation
- Most people apply for 'rotations' where your contract is for between 2–6yr, and every 4–6mth you rotate/change speciality and potentially change hospital. Stand-alone 6mth jobs are likely to remain common, especially in emergency medicine
- Once you have passed the appropriate assessment (including postgraduate exams) and you have enough clinical experience you can apply to continue in speciality training. The majority of speciality training jobs are 'substantive', and you will rotate within one deanery (for example the London Deanery) until you are ready to apply for a consultant post

Job advertisements Most jobs are advertised in the *BMJ Careers* magazine, which accompanies the weekly *BMJ*; many people are members of the BMA and will receive this weekly, though most clinical libraries stock it, and it is available online (www.bmjcareers.com). The advertisements are divided into speciality and then subdivided into grade.

What to apply for? Competition for certain jobs and certain specialities is very high and some applicants are so keen to work within a particular field that they will apply for jobs all over the country. Others are keen to stay in a particular area and are less concerned about the speciality. It is useful to have a career plan, but not essential at an early stage (p52).

Applying for jobs Most adverts describe what the job entails, the duration of the post and often a little about the hospital and area, as well as the closing date for applications. A contact telephone number for further information or the application form is usually given; it is worthwhile clarifying any points about which you are unclear before applying. It is often useful to telephone and ask a few questions about the position, making sure you give your name, as you may be talking to someone who sifts through the applications and decides who should be interviewed.

Submitting your application Always follow the instructions on the advert exactly; if four copies of a two-sided CV are requested, then do just that – late applications are rarely accepted (consider recorded delivery). Tailor your CV to highlight the skills, qualifications and experience you have which are most appropriate for that position (p58). Always submit the completed application form and CV with a covering letter, explaining why you are interested in the job and why you would be a good person for it. You can apply for more than one job at a time, but if you accept a position you should withdraw all other applications.

Once submitted Wait two weeks; if there has been no news, telephone the medical personnel department and ask if you have been short-listed for interview. If you are unsuccessful then keep applying for other positions. If successful start preparing for your interview.

Interviews

Interview preparation Employers must allow you time off to attend the interview itself. Do some research about the hospital, the department and the type of patients and activities which go on there. This can easily be done on the internet. It's often worth speaking to someone who is currently in the position by phone or in person. Consider visiting the hospital before the interview to look around; you should arrange this with someone from the department you have applied to.

Interview day Arrive at the interview with plenty of time, allow for all sorts of delays on the roads or train, even if this means you have to read the newspaper for an hour. Relax and be yourself with the other candidates before you are called in; most of them will have similar qualifications and experience as yourself and will be just as nervous. Dress smartly in a simple suit and tie for men and suit for women (trouser or skirt).

The interview Relax. The very worst thing that can happen is that you are not offered the job, which is not the end of the world. There is no standard format to interviews; the panel may be as few as two or as many as 10 and can include management or medical personnel staff; they can last from five minutes to half an hour. Take a few moments to think about the questions and to formulate an answer. Ask for a question to be rephrased if you don't understand it or say that you do not know the precise answer, but then propose a potential answer/solution to demonstrate you can at least think on your feet.

Common questions It is impossible to predict the questions you will be asked, but they are likely to include questions about your CV, about the position you are applying for and about current medical affairs. Many questions will not have a correct answer and the panel just wants to see that you can communicate, are sensible and able to think for yourself.

- Tell us about yourself
- What are you most proud of on your CV?
- What is missing from your CV?
- What qualities can you offer our department?
- Why have you chosen this job? This hospital?
- What do you understand by 'clinical governance'?
- Have you been involved with audit and is this important?
- If you were the Secretary for Health, where would your priorities lie?
- How would you manage… (specific clinical scenario)?
- Where do you see yourself in 5, 10 years time?
- If you were the SHO/registrar in the hospital alone at night and you were struggling with a clinical problem, what would you do?
- Tell us about your teaching experiences. What makes a good teacher?

Results and feedback If you are offered the job and accept it, then you are morally obliged to take up that position and decline all further job offers, even if you think they might be better. If you are unsuccessful, try to obtain some verbal or written feedback about how you could improve your CV or your interview skills; just remember there are many more jobs than there are doctors, so you will find something.

Membership exams

To progress beyond the SHO level you need to complete the membership exams for your chosen speciality and gain experience in recognised training posts (check the BMJ careers advert, often written in bold, if in doubt check with the Royal College). Most membership exams take place 2–3 times a year. You need to apply about 2–4mth before each exam. For the contact details of the various Royal Colleges see p525.

Medicine Regional centres in London, Edinburgh, Glasgow and Dublin, however all centres use the same exams. The MRCP has three sections:

- Part 1 Written – basic science, £290, ≥18mth after finals
- Part 2 Written – clinical, £290, <7yr since part 1
- PACES – clinical skills, £470, <2yr and <3 attempts since part 2.

To become a SpR you need 2½ yr experience after graduation including ≥12mth in an acute medical job.

Surgery Regional centres in London, Edinburgh, Glasgow and Dublin, however all centres use the same exams. The MRCS has four parts, once you attempt part 2 you only have 3½ yr to complete the remaining parts:

- Part 1 Written – basic science, £190, eligible after graduation
- Part 2 Written – clinical, £190, eligible with part 1
- Viva – anatomy, physiology, pathology, £320, eligible with part 2
- OSCE – clinical and communication, £330, 1mth after successful viva

To become a SpR you need 2yr basic surgical training as a SHO. As a SpR you must pass an exit exam in your chosen speciality, eg ENT.

General practice You need to register with a vocational training scheme to take the MRCGP. There are four parts and no time limits:

- Two written modules (MCQ and short answer) – current evidence, appraisal of research, GP management and clinical, £275 each
- Consulting skills – assessment of videoed consultations, £275
- Viva – clinical, work place, political, ethical and legal issues, £275

To become a GP you need 2yr SHO experience and 1yr as GP registrar.

Other membership exams

Accident and Emergency (MFAEM) Two-part exam taken as a SHO, but MRCS, MRCP or FRCA also accepted; FFAEM exit exam after SpR.

Anaesthetics (FRCA) Primary exam is taken as a SHO with 1yr experience in anaesthetics; the final exam is completed as a SpR.

Obstetrics and Gynaecology (MRCOG) Part 1 (written) can be taken after graduation. Completed as a SpR after 4yr O+G experience.

Ophthalmology (MRCOphth) A three-part exam; part 1 can be taken after graduation; all must be completed before progressing to SpR level.

Paediatrics (MRCPCH) Similar structure to MRCP; part 1 can be taken after graduation; all must be completed before progressing to SpR level.

Pathology and Radiology Membership exams are taken as an SpR; it is possible to become a SpR with <12mth SHO clinical experience.

Psychiatry (MRCPsych) 12mth SHO psychiatry experience required before taking part 1 (written and clinical). Completed as a SpR.

Moving and finding a house

Finding a new place to live and moving can be very difficult when there is no gap between your old and new job. It is important to set aside time (often annual leave) to find somewhere suitable as this has a major impact on your future lifestyle.

Hospital accommodation

Most hospitals provide relatively cheap local accommodation. The prices and standards vary widely – view the room before you sign up. Prices usually include utility bills. It should conform to the minimum standards shown on the BMA website (p524). Apply early since rooms may be limited; they usually have information on other properties too.

Finding a house

Look through local papers which often have weekly property supplements, alternatively visit or phone estate agents and ask them to contact you if a suitable house is available. If you are not living near your new job then the internet is invaluable – make sure you always see the house before signing contracts. The following addresses may help:

www.propertyfinder.com	Renting and buying
www.ukpropertyshop.co.uk	Renting and buying
www.rightmove.co.uk	Renting and buying
www.naea.co.uk	Buying
www.lettingweb.com	Renting

Rental accommodation

Most rental contracts are for at least 6mth. You will usually need to pay electricity, water and gas bills and council tax on top of the rent.

Buying a house

On top of the house price you should expect extra costs of at least £3000, including: *Solicitor/conveyancing fees* (at least £400); *stamp duty* (≥1% of the value of the house); *surveying* – there are three types: valuation (best for houses <5yr old, £150), homebuyer's report (most popular, about £350), structural survey (for houses >40yr old, about £600); *land registry and searches* (£250).

NHS removal expenses

If you are taking up a job for 2yr or more, trusts may cover some of the cost of moving. This supplement of up to £8000 can include stamp duty, solicitor's fees, removal services and the cost of furnishing a new house. Search for 'removal expenses' at www.nice.org.uk for the NICE guidance.

Storage units You can store furniture and other possessions securely for about £50–100/mth. Use the internet to find a local company.

Van rental You can rent a decent sized van for about £50–100 a day. You need to have held a driving licence for ≥2yr and be ≥21yr.

Working in the UK (from abroad)

Europe Doctors who are European Economic Area (EEA) or Swiss nationals and trained within the EEA or Switzerland can apply for registration with the GMC without taking further exams.

Outside Europe There are three short cuts to obtaining limited registration with the GMC:

- ***sponsorship*** by a Royal College or University (requires at least 3yr clinical experience), see contacts on GMC website[1]
- completion of ***basic specialist training*** (2yr relevant clinical experience and completion of the Royal College membership exams)
- appointment to a UK ***specialist registrar*** post

Otherwise doctors must pass three exams:

- ***IELTS*** (International English Language Testing System) – a 3h test of academic English including speaking, reading, writing and listening. It costs about £85 and can be taken around the world. Doctors need to get 7/9 overall with at least 7/9 in speaking and at least 6/9 in all the other sections. See www.ielts.org for more details
- ***PLAB part 1*** (Professional and Linguistic Assessment Board) – a clinical MCQ that can be taken in test centres around the world for £145
- ***PLAB part 2*** – a 14-station test of clinical skills which must be taken in London and costs £430

The PLAB exams are organised by the GMC and application forms are on their website.[1] After passing these exams the doctor is entitled to limited registration with the GMC once they have evidence of being accepted for a job.

Limited registration costs £390 for 1yr. It entitles the holder to work in a supervised post in the NHS, but not as a consultant. If they wish to work outside the NHS they must contact the GMC.

Visa application See www.ukvisas.gov.uk for details by country.

Getting a job is the hardest part of obtaining limited registration. Foundation Programme, SHO and registrar jobs are competitive in the UK and many jobs require applicants to have at least 12mth NHS experience – it may be necessary to undertake unpaid clinical attachments. It is essential to have a well-presented CV (p58), good references and to apply for appropriate jobs. See p64 for more details. Consider applying through locum agencies (p525). This takes 14mth on average.

Job discrimination, including the job application process, is illegal in the UK. Trusts should have an equal opportunities policy that actively prevents such discrimination occurring. If you think that you have been or are being discriminated against then contact the BMA (p524).

Further information Search for the 'NACPME fact sheets' on www.britcoun.org, the 'Guide for doctors new to the UK' by the BMA at www.bma.org.uk and www.nlsandumrweb.co.uk.

1 www.gmc-uk.org

Working abroad (from the UK)

When to go The gap between the F2 year and basic specialist training provides an ideal opportunity for jobs abroad and travelling. It also gives more time to consider which career path to follow. There are no set rules and working abroad can be arranged at any stage. The longer you work the more you will be tied down by a rotation, finances or family.

Career impact Working abroad is viewed favourably by most employers, but will only count towards your training if the relevant Royal College agrees. This takes time so you must arrange the post well in advance. Ideally secure a job in the UK to return to by applying for deferred entry.

Australia and New Zealand These countries are the most popular choice; they are sunny, laid back and provide a reasonable salary for a 38h working week. The health service is similar to the NHS and no special exams are required. Posts may include a stint of working in a rural setting – be sure you know exactly where you will be expected to work.

Europe A British medical degree entitles you to work throughout Europe without extra exams, though obviously language may be a barrier.

USA You must pass the USMLEs which consist of two MCQs, basic sciences and clinical (£400 each in UK), and a language and clinical skills exam (£650 in USA only); apply at www.ecfmg.org. With these exams you can apply for a 3yr residency (SHO) or 4yr fellowship (SpR) post via the competitive internet matching scheme (ERAS, www.aamc.org). You will need to attend interviews in the USA. You must do both your residency and fellowship in the USA if you want to work there long term.

Canada The 'evaluating exam' (£450 in UK) and two 'qualifying exams' (£300 and £600 in Canada only) are required for registration.

Finding jobs Talk to your colleagues, many doctors have spent time abroad and may have contacts and ideas. *BMJ Careers* has a short international section. Alternatively the internet is an excellent place to search. Medics Travel (www.medicstravel.co.uk) is a good starting point. There are numerous companies willing to arrange work for doctors.

Developing world

Medecins Sans Frontieres (www.msf.org) offers placements of 6mth or more in challenging environments. You need at least 2yr post-registration experience, ideally post-membership.

Voluntary Services Overseas (www.vso.org.uk) Placements are of at least 2yr duration; you need at least 2yr post-registration experience. VSO will provide flights, a living allowance and accommodation.

NGOs and mission organisations These can provide diverse jobs all over the world. The Medics Travel website has a selection.

Other If there is a job you want then look for it, it will not look for you.

Chapter 3

Communication

Communication and conduct

Good communication with patients, your team and other health-care professionals is an essential part of the job.

Verbal communication

Your team Make sure you can provide a short summary/progress report for each patient on ward rounds:

- if you are worried about a patient or they deteriorate, bleep your SHO or registrar to let them know and ask for advice on what to do
- when asking a senior for help, state clearly what you want (ie advice, help), what you're worried about and why
- for details on referring patients to senior colleagues see p18
- never argue with colleagues in front of your patients
- if you don't know something never make the answer up; say you'll find out then do so

Your peers If you're working with another house officer make sure you know who is doing which jobs and what needs doing. Ideally, you should both know what's going on with all your patients:

- working with another house officer means you have a ready-made second opinion when you need it; help each other and 'share' any difficult tasks/patients
- it takes time to adapt to working with another house officer. If you are really having difficulties splitting the workload, then, as a last resort, you can divide the wards/bays so that you cover different patients

Your patient See p76; take time to establish a rapport and find out their problems and concerns;

- try to see things from their perspective and the effect on their quality of life
- listen and address their concerns; if you are busy arrange a time to come back for a proper chat
- use visual aids and simple language
- always be honest
- involve the patient in management decisions and update them with results of investigations
- if there is a language barrier then arrange an interpreter (p79)
- breaking bad news see p77

GPs may refer your team patients for admission:

- note down the patient's name, age, problem and likely time of arrival
- if you don't think the referral is appropriate then clarify the reason for the referral, be polite and don't forget that the GP has equivalent experience to a consultant

You may also be contacted by the GP regarding the information given on TTOs once the patient has been discharged. If you can't answer the query immediately then take down the patient's and the GP's details and contact them later once you have checked the patient's notes or discussed the patient with your team.

Other health-care professionals (HCP) Multidisciplinary meetings or ward rounds are a good opportunity to meet other HCPs and ask for their opinions on your patients. You can also clear up any queries you have. Get to know which aspects of patient care they focus on (see p11) and use them appropriately. Keep them informed of any changes, both for the patient's benefit and out of courtesy.

Referral letters You may be asked to write referral letters to residential homes or other speciality teams. The letter should be printed on hospital notepaper and include:

- patient and GP details
- relevant clinical history, investigation results and management
- the reason for referral
- your consultant, your name and your bleep number
- the date the referral is being made

Self-discharge If your patient decides to discharge themselves, try to explain why they need hospital management and what might happen if they leave (be blunt but honest). If you think the patient lacks the capacity (p93) to make this decision or requires sectioning (p415) then consult your seniors. If they still want to self-discharge and are capable to do so then ask them to sign a self-discharge form (saves a lot of paperwork for the nurses). If these are unavailable you can always write your own. You, the patient and a second witness should sign it, recording the time and date and the patient's decision. Keep it in the notes and inform the GP if relevant.

Sick notes Provide a brief explanation for the patient's sick leave without mentioning intimate details and give an appropriate amount of leave to recover. Remember to write the patient's name, sign and date it. If the patient is claiming state benefits you will need to complete and sign a DSS form – ask the ward clerk if you are unable to find one.

TTOs See p22.

Patients' relatives

- Organise a time when you can discuss the patient's progress at leisure in the relatives' room (ideally get a colleague to hold your bleep). To avoid repeating yourself, speak to the family collectively or ask them to appoint a representative
- Check the patient is happy to have their confidential medical details discussed (p92)
- Address concerns and answer each question in turn
- Be honest and aware of your limitations; if necessary ask them to arrange a time to meet with a senior
- If you are busy and unable to discuss everything, arrange a further time
- Keep the meeting professional
- If things get heated, excuse yourself, do an unrelated task and come back after calming down. If this doesn't work, speak to your SHO/SpR
- Always document in the notes the date and time, what was discussed and who was present

Giving information over the telephone

- Establish who the caller is and what they want to know
- If in doubt, take their number and offer to call them back
- Make sure you have the patient's permission before disclosing information on their progress to relatives
- If the relative wants further details, suggest arranging a meeting at the hospital
- If you are discussing the patient with another HCP or senior, try to use a private office to avoid being overheard
- If you are sending a fax referral, check the line is secure

Professional conduct

- Introduce yourself and wear your ID badge in hospital
- Learn the names of the people you are working with
- Avoid slang
- Never be rude to ward staff, you will get a bad reputation
- Do not gossip about your work colleagues; address any issues you have with a colleague directly and in private
- If you think it is not appropriate for you to do a job then run it by the ward staff or your seniors
- If you are going to be late, let the expecting team/ward staff know in advance so they can carry on with other jobs
- For difficult referrals make the effort to speak face to face
- Ask for help if you feel overrun with tasks
- When you do something wrong, apologise and learn from your mistake; it's a natural part of the learning curve

The importance of listening

Listening to your patient helps you gain an insight and appreciation about their worries. Their concerns may be things you can address and reassure them about, eg post-op pain.

Listening to colleagues and peers at work helps you develop your own style and pick up tips. Positive and negative feedback on your performance is important to make you a better doctor, no one starts off perfect.

Aggression and violence

The majority of patients have the deepest respect for NHS staff however under certain circumstances anyone can become aggressive:

- pain p282
- confusion or dementia, eg hypoglycaemia p231
- inadequate communication/fear/frustration
- intoxication (medications, alcohol, recreational drugs)
- mental illness or personality disorder p412

The aggressive patient Ask a nurse to accompany you when assessing aggressive patients. Position yourselves between the exit and the patient and ensure that other staff know where you are. The majority of patients can be calmed simply by talking; try to elicit why they are angry and ask specifically about pain and worry. Be firm, calm and do not shout or make threats. If this does not help, offer an oral sedative or give emergency sedation (below).

The aggressive relative Relatives may be aggressive through fear, frustration and/or intoxication. They usually respond to talking, though make sure you obtain consent from the patient before discussing their medical details. Consider offering to arrange a meeting with a senior doctor to discuss any issues that arise. If the relative continues to be aggressive, remember that your duty of care to patients does not extend to their relatives; you do not have to tell them anything or listen to threats/abuse. In extreme cases you can ask security or the police to remove the relative from the hospital.

Emergency sedation Any hospital doctor can give emergency sedation under common law if a patient is a risk to themselves or others. This can be done without their consent and under restraint. Start with a small dose, as shown, and repeat after 45min if necessary; lorazepam is kinder than haloperidol:

- lorazepam 2mg (1mg elderly/renal failure) PO/IM/IV stat
- haloperidol 4mg (2mg elderly) PO/IM/IV stat

Ask the nurses to monitor the patient regularly (at least every 15min for the next hour) and assess for pain and confusion once the patient is calm.

Violence Assault (the attempt or threat of causing harm) and battery (physical contact without consent) by a patient or relative is a criminal offence. If you witness an assault or are assaulted yourself, inform your seniors and fill in an incident form including the name and contact details of any witnesses. If no action is taken on your behalf inform the police yourself.

Abuse Patients of any age can be abused in hospitals or outside. Do not be afraid of asking patients how they received injuries or asking directly if someone caused them. Inform a senior if you believe a patient has been abused physically, sexually or by neglect.

Patient communication

A patient's perception of your abilities as a doctor depends largely on your communication (and phlebotomy) skills. Remember that patients are in an alien environment and are often worried about their health.

Introductions Always introduce yourself to patients and clearly state who you are. You are more approachable if you use your first name rather than Dr X. Check it is the right patient from their full name and date of birth (this also gives a rough guide to their mental state) and ask what they like to be called. Patients meet many staff members each day so it is important to reintroduce yourself each time you see them:

'Hello, my name is Charles and I'm one of the doctors working on this ward. Are you Doris Green?' 'Yes dear, but I like to be called Vera.' 'OK Vera, what's your date of birth...'

General communication Try to avoid using medical jargon. It is easy to get worse at this as your career progresses and you become more familiar with medical language. Patients may be unaware of the implications behind conditions; the phrases 'needing help to breathe', 'not reacting to pain' and 'hole in their bowel' could all sound quite innocent.

Honest replies Patients have a right to know what is going on with their body. If a patient asks you a direct question try to give a direct answer; if you are unable to do so then explain why. If you do not know the answer, say so and offer to find out; do not try to guess the answer.

Procedures You should fully explain all procedures and obtain informed verbal or written consent before starting them (p94). Your explanation should include why the procedure is necessary, how much it will hurt (be honest, blood gases are painful) and what the patient can do to help (keep still, sit up etc).

Results Explain why the investigation was performed, what it shows and what this means. If an X-ray or scan shows a clear image of the problem then show it to the patient. Showing other tests (especially ECGs) can cause more confusion than benefit.

Diagnosis Try to give the everyday name rather than a medical one (heart attack instead of MI). Explain why this has happened and if it is not something the patient has done, then say so. A patient who understands their condition is more likely to comply with medication and seek appropriate help if their symptoms change. Encourage them to learn about the condition and recommend good websites (p525) or support groups.

Prognosis Along with the obvious questions about life expectancy (p86), patients are most interested in how their life will be affected. Pitch your explanation in terms of activities of daily living (ADLs), walking, driving (p35) and working. Bear in mind that patients may want to know about having sex, but are often embarrassed to ask.

Breaking bad news

Ideally, breaking bad news should always be done by a senior at a predetermined time when relatives and friends ±specialist nurses can be present. In reality you are likely to be involved in breaking bad news, often whilst on-call. It can be a positive experience if done well.

Preparation Read the patient's notes carefully and ensure that all results are up-to-date. Be clear in your mind about the sequence of events and the meaning of the results. Think about what further investigations and treatments are required and the likely prognosis – discuss with a senior. Ask a colleague to hold your bleep and set aside suitable time (at least 30min), use a room where you will not be disturbed and take a nurse who has been involved in the patient's care with you.

Consent and confidentiality (p92) A patient has a right to know what is going on or to choose not to know. Ask before the investigations are done and document their response. If a patient does not want their relatives to know about their diagnosis you must respect this. Always ask, do not assume – many families have complex dynamics.

Warning shot Give a suggestion that bad news is imminent so it is not completely out of the blue, eg 'I have the results from … would you like anyone else here when I tell you them/shall we go to a quiet room?'

How to do it There is no set formula for breaking bad news, you should adapt to the patient, situation and yourself.

- Introduce yourself to all present and find out who they are
- *What do they know?* Patients often have an idea that something bad is afoot. Ask directly, 'What do you think is going on/what are you worried about?' It is also essential to find out what they know so far, again ask directly. This allows appropriate further information to be given
- *Brief summary of events* 'You came to this ward 7d ago with difficulty breathing. We have done some investigations including an X-ray, a scan of your chest and had a look in your lungs with a telescope and taken a sample'
- *Bad news* 'A doctor has had a look at the sample and I'm sorry to say it shows a cancer in your lung.' Give the information time to sink in and all present to react (shock, anger, tears, denial)
- *Prognosis* Give a summary of what this means and the further management. Keep it simple and be honest if you cannot answer
- *How long have I got?* This is a hard question. Explain how difficult this is to answer and what extra information is required for a better answer. Do not give exact times, go for hours, days, months or years
- Be realistic, but try to offer hope even if it is just an improvement in their symptoms or the chance to go home
- Arrange a time for further questions, ideally with a senior and yourself present. Give a clear plan of what will happen over the next 48h
- Document what has been said (diagnosis, prognosis, expectations) in the notes with your name and contact details

Patient-centred care

The traditional medical model has made the patient a passive recipient of care. Health care was done *to* people rather than *with* them. Most patients were entirely happy with this, but the patient should be able to be in charge of their own health care should they so wish.

Our task as clinicians is to find out our patients' expectations of their relationship with their doctors and then try to fulfill these. From 'whatever you feel is best doc' to reams of printouts and self-diagnoses from the internet, neither extreme is wrong and our task is to help.

Patient expectations Find out whether your patient wants guidance to be advised what treatment may be best.

Respect their right to make a decision you believe may be wrong. If you feel that they are doing so because they do not fully understand the situation or because of flawed logic, then alert your team to this so that things can be explained again.

Find out their other influences, these can be very powerful. Examples include: religious beliefs, friends, the internet and death/illness of relatives with similar conditions.

Treatment expectations Patients may have clear expectations of their treatment (eg an operation or being given a prescription). These expectations are important sources of discontentment when not fulfilled. Find out what their expectations are and why. Useful questions may include: 'What do you think is wrong with you? What are you worried about? What were you expecting we'd do about this?'

Yourself in their shoes Make time to imagine yourself in your patient's place. Isolation or communication difficulties will heighten fear at an already frightening time. Long waits without explanation are routine. Aggression from friends or relatives is often simply a manifestation of anxiety that not enough is being done. Ask yourself 'How would I want my family treated under these circumstances?' then do this for every patient.

Ensuring dignity Hospitals can rob people of their dignity.

- Wherever and whenever possible help restore this:
  - keep your patient covered in resus
  - ensure the curtains are round on the ward
  - make sure they have their false teeth in to talk and glasses on whenever possible
- Help them self-care when possible

Over-examination Patients are often clerked over four times for a single admission. This is frustrating for them and often seen as indicative of a lack of coordination within the hospital. Patients may need to be clerked and examined more than once, but the context of this should be explained carefully – is this to gain more insight about their condition or to allow a training doctor to learn? People rarely mind when they understand the reasons.

Keep examinations which are invasive or cause discomfort to an absolute minimum.

Cross-cultural communication

For patients who can't understand or speak the same language as you, the consultation can leave them feeling isolated, frustrated and anxious. You may have to rely on a third party to translate for you.

Family members as interpreters

Friends and relatives are commonly used as informal interpreters. The main drawbacks are the lack of confidentiality and the bias the relative may have on the patient's decision making – particularly when underlying family issues are present (you may be unaware of these).

Children can interpret for their parents from an early age, but again their views can bias the consultation and its outcome.
Address the patient directly and look carefully at the patient's response to gauge their understanding. Record the fact that a family member was used for interpretation in the notes.

Conflict of interests If you think the relative is biasing the conversation or it is an important issue then explain that you are professionally obliged to request a trained interpreter.

Consent Relatives cannot consent on behalf of adults, see p94.

Professional interpreters

Professional interpreters can be arranged before the appointment – ask ward staff or phone switchboard:

- allow extra time for the consultation and check the interpreter is acceptable to the patient
- address both the patient and the interpreter and look at the patient's non-verbal response to gauge their level of understanding
- ask simple, direct questions in short sentences to avoid overloading or confusing the interpreter; avoid jargon
- use pictures or diagrams to explain things wherever possible. Provide written/audiovisual material in the patient's own language to take away
- if you cannot organise an interpreter, you may be able to contact a telephone interpreting service who translate for you and the patient directly over the phone
- document that a trained interpreter has been used with their name and contact details so that the same interpreter can accompany the patient for future appointments
- never assume you know what the patient wants without asking them

Who can interpret

- Family
- Friends
- Hospital staff (switchboard may have a list)
- Hospital interpreters
- Local interpreting agencies
- Telephone service with which the hospital has a contract with

Languages

Ask the patient to point to their language below, which reads: 'I speak (this language)'

Albanian	Flas shqip
Arabic	أتكلم عربى
Bengali	বাংলা বলি
Bosnian	Govorim bosanski
Bulgarian	Говоря български
Cantonese	我 講廣東話
Chinese/ Mandarin	我說中國話
Croatian	Govorim hrvatski
Czech	Mluví m česky
Dutch	Ik spreek Nederlands
Farsi/Persian	فارسی حرف میزنم
French	Je parle français
German	Ich spreche Deutsch
Greek	Μιλώ ελληνικά.
Gujarati	હું ગુજરાતી બોલું છું
Hebrew	אברית (ה)דבר אני
Hindi	मैं हिंदी बोलता (बोलती) हूं
Indonesian	Saya cakap bahasa Indonesia
Italian	Parlo italiano
Japanese	日本話を語します

Korean	항국말을해요
Latvian	Es runāju latviski
Malay	Saya cakap Melayu
Polish	Mówię po polsku
Portuguese	Falo português
Punjabi	ਮੈਂ ਪੰਜਾਬੀ ਬੋਲਦੀ ਹਾਂ
Romanian	Vorbesc româneşte
Russian	Я говорю по-русски
Serbian	Говорим српски
Slovak	Hovorím slovensky
Somali	Waxaan ku hadlaa luuqada af Soomaliga
Spanish	Hablo español
Swahili	Nisema Kiswahili
Turkish	Turkçe bilirim
Urdu	میں اردو بولتا (بولتی) ہوں

Difficulties with using an interpreter

- The interpreters may misunderstand technical terms or distort your questions
- Your questions and the patient's response may not be translated correctly
- The interpreter may influence the patient's response
- The patient/interpreter may avoid sensitive issues

Other means of communication

The NATO phonetic alphabet is often used to prevent mistakes when relaying a list of letters or when spelling a word over radio or telephone; numbers are pronounced differently as well over radio and walkie talkie.

Alpha	November	1 WUN
Bravo	Oscar	2 TOO
Charlie	Papa	3 THUREE
Delta	Quebec	4 FOWER
Echo	Romeo	5 FIYIV
Foxtrot	Sierra	6 SIX
Golf	Tango	7 SEVEN
Hotel	Uniform	8 ATE
India	Victor	9 NINER
Juliet	Whisky	
Kilo	X-ray	
Lima	Yankee	
Mike	Zulu	

British sign language (BSL) is used predominantly by the deaf as a means of communication. Below are the hand positions for the English alphabet.

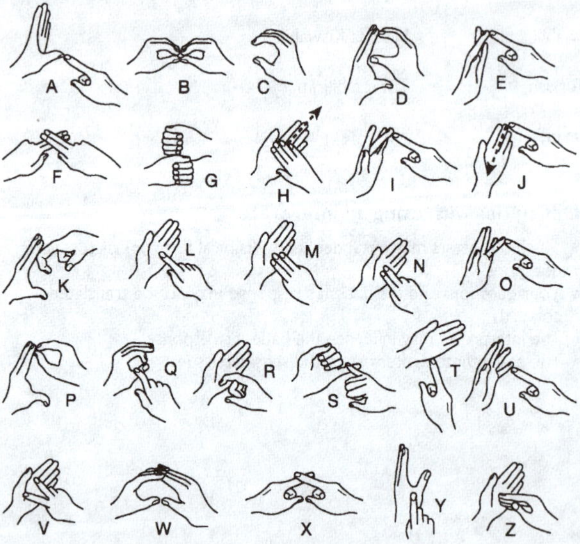

Outside agencies

Outside agencies who could enquire about your patients include: police, media, solicitors, fire brigade, ambulance services, general practitioner and the patient's employer. Patient confidentiality must be respected.

The rules:

- Do you really know who you are talking to?
- Check and arrange to call them back unless certain
- Do they have any right to the information they are seeking?
  - GPs and ambulance staff may well do, police have limited rights to information (see below), others do not
- Should you be the one discussing this or should a more senior member of the team?
- Do not talk to the media about a patient/your hospital unless:
  - you have the patient's permission
  - you have permission from your consultant/management (for trust issues)
  - you are accompanied by the trust public relations officer
- Do not 'chat' to a police/prison officer about a patient, no matter what the alleged circumstances; all patients have an equal right to privacy

Breaching a patient's confidentiality without good cause is treated as misconduct by the General Medical Council.

Confidentiality and the police

Immediate investigation of assaults The police may well ask the clinical condition of an assault victim. 'Is it life-threatening, doctor?' The purpose of this question is to know how thoroughly to investigate the crime scene. It is reasonable to give them an assessment of severity.

In the public interest In situations where someone may be at risk of serious injury, disclosure is permitted by the General Medical Council. This should be a consultant-level decision.

The Road Traffic Act Any person has a duty to provide the police with information which may lead to the identification of a driver who is alleged to have committed an offence under the Act. You are obliged to supply the name and address, not clinical details. Discuss with your registrar or consultant first.

Being a witness in court

Remember you are a professional witness to the court, you do not represent either side and your evidence should be an impartial statement of the facts. Do not get rattled by the barristers – stick to the facts, do not give opinions, explain the limits of your knowledge/experience. Address your remarks to the judge. Wear your best suit. Ensure you get an expenses form from the witness unit and get this stamped/signed.

Chapter 4

Ethics

Dealing with death

Fears

It is entirely natural for patients to have a fear of death and of dying. It is common to most of us. It should also be noted that many patients, especially the elderly, may be entirely at ease with the prospect of their own death. To quote one 90-year-old patient: 'Worried? No, each morning I wake up and think to myself "Good God, I'm still alive!" '

If your patient is afraid it can be important to establish exactly what they are afraid of, these may be different from your assumptions:

- loss of dignity
- loss of control
- symptoms, eg suffocating/pain
- their relatives seeing them suffering
- the unpleasant death of a relative years ago

Many of these can now be carefully managed or even entirely avoided. In the case of the last one, medicine, particularly in the field of palliation, has changed a great deal in recent years. Patients have often not explored what they are afraid of, talking it through with adequate time set aside can help.

When the death is not expected and the deterioration sudden (trauma for example) then your role in talking to the patient and allaying their fear cannot be overstated. This can be emotionally hard work.

Breaking bad news p77

Other sources of help

Even with sudden deteriorations there are many other sources of help. Use them or offer them to the patient:

- the palliative care team (see p398)
- the acute pain team (usually part of anaesthetics)
- Macmillan nurses
- the chaplaincy

Do not forget you're working with nursing staff who may know the patient and their wishes better than you, so discuss the patient's care with them.

Prognosis

You are strongly advised not to predict when someone is likely to die. You can give an idea of hours versus weeks or months but you'll be wrong as often as right. Some measure of prognosis allows patients to make any preparations they need, but don't let yourself be pressured into giving an exact prediction.

Patients may be concerned about their relatives and keen not to worry them. Setting aside the fact that everybody has usually guessed the likely outcome by this stage, the patient must remain in charge of who is told what. It can be helpful to explain that relatives will need time to prepare too.

Sorting arrangements

Obviously, marching in offering a priest and solicitor will be seen as insensitive. But be aware that the hospital will be able to provide legal support or an appropriate religious official if asked.

Many patients' strongest wish is to die in comfort, preferably in their own home. Get the Macmillan and/or palliative care team involved early and this can be arranged surprisingly often. Spending time in a hospice doesn't mean you have to die there but can offer an important respite for carers.

Do not resuscitate orders

This is a consultant-level decision. It should be clearly written in the notes/on a DNR form, signed, named and dated. This must be updated as the patient's condition changes. It should be discussed with the patients and/or their relatives. Tell the nursing staff.

Do not resuscitate is entirely different from do not treat. This difference is often understood well by the patients, especially the elderly, but misunderstood by relatives. It is worth explaining the difference between the highest quality care and futile heroism. Let them know that in the absence of other instructions you will try everything. Respect your patients' wishes – they may surprise you.

Requests for euthanasia

Deliberately quickening a patient's death is illegal. Relieving suffering to the extent that you allow someone to die naturally, with dignity, is not.

- Do not get drawn into discussions over euthanasia
- Explain you will always aim to minimise suffering
- Ensure you can justify your actions to the most hostile barrister
- Explain to relatives that relieving pain may hasten an inevitable death, before giving opiates
  - relieving pain removes the adrenergic stimulus which may appropriately lead to a natural death within a few minutes

An example of what to write in the notes when a patient dies

16.09.05 *Asked to verify death.*
03:35

No response to pain
Pupils fixed and dilated
No carotid pulse
No audible heart sounds } *for 60 seconds*
No audible breath sounds

Death declared at 03.40 on 16.09.2005.
No pacemaker palpable.

Dr CJ Flint
FLINT, PRHO
Bleep 3294

If your patient dies

The best medicine in the world can only delay death; it is inevitable for everyone. Patients often die in hospital and the following pages act as a guide for what you will be asked to do.

Declaring death

You will often be bleeped to declare a patient dead. This is not an urgent request, but the patient cannot be transferred to the morgue until it is done. There may be other members of staff who can do this. If you are uncomfortable ask a member of staff to accompany you. Check for:

- reaction to voice and pain (sternal rub or supraorbital nerve)
- pupil reflexes (eyes will be fixed and dilated with a dry appearance)
- central pulse for 1min (carotid or femoral)
- heart sounds for 1min
- respiratory movement and sounds for 1min (may hear gastro noises)

NB It is helpful to note if there is a pacemaker present (see p87)

In the notes Date and time, contacted to declare the patient dead at (time), summary of your examination, pacemaker present/absent. Remember to sign and print your name and bleep no.

What happens to the dead patient

When a patient dies the nurses prepare the body, including: lying them flat with one pillow and their eyes and jaw closed (may be propped closed), washing the body, packing orifices with cotton wool and removing attachments (eg fluids, pumps). Lines and tubes are not removed since these will be inspected if a post-mortem is required. The bed curtains are closed and the patient is covered with a sheet.

Once they have been declared dead they are taken to the morgue in a portable coffin. Screens are used to try and hide this from other patients.

Death certificates

Eligibility You should only fill in a death certificate if you have met the patient in the last 14d on their final admission, they are older than 18yr and you have a suitable understanding of what occurred. By signing a death certificate you are saying that you are confident enough about the cause of death to stand by it in court. Refer to a senior if you are unsure whether you meet these criteria.

Coroner Many hospital patients have to be referred to the coroner, see the box below. If you are in doubt, ring the coroner's office (hours vary but often only open during the daytime on weekdays) to discuss the case; they are usually friendly and helpful.

Inform the coroner if • death <24h since admission • suspicious, accidental or violent deaths (includes RTAs) • suicide • operation, anaesthetic or procedure in the last year (this includes endoscopy, chest drains, central lines etc) • death from acute effects of alcohol or drugs • death due to industrial disease (coal, asbestos, dust, dyes etc) • unknown cause of death

The coroner is often a lawyer, their job is to investigate suspicious deaths. For the majority of deaths you refer to the coroner's office you will be told to issue the death certificate. If you have referred the case to the coroner you need to circle the '4' on the front and the 'A' on the back. If you simply discussed the case then neither of these needs to be circled.

What to write Most of the entries are self-explanatory;

- **place of death** should be the ward, hospital and city
- write the same for your **residence** rather than your home address
- ring the **digit and letter** above causes of death, usually 3 or 4 + a or b
- tick the box below causes of death if industrial disease is suspected (there is a useful table on the back of the certificate)
- **qualifications**: this is your medical school degree, eg MBBS or MBChB
- remember to fill in the slips to the left and right and the back (you may need to circle 'A' or 'B')

Cause of death This is the hard bit. You must avoid using modes of death (how the patient died) in preference for causes of death (the disease that caused the mode of death). The table below offers common causes – there are many more. Once again the coroner's office can offer invaluable advice if you are unsure what to put.

You must fill in I(a), but the other three categories may be left blank if there is really nothing to put. Do not use abbreviations.

Causes of death	Modes of death
Myocardial infarction, arrhythmia	Cardiac arrest, syncope
Sepsis, hypovolaemia, haemorrhage, anaphylaxis	Hypotension, shock, off legs
Congestive cardiac failure, pulmonary oedema	Heart failure, cardiac failure, ventricular failure
Bronchopneumonia, pulmonary embolism, asthma, chronic obstructive pulmonary disease	Respiratory failure, respiratory arrest
Cerebrovascular accident	Collapse
Cirrhosis, glomerularnephritis, diabetic nephropathy	Liver failure, renal failure, uraemia
Carcinomatosis, carcinoma of the xxx	Cachexia, exhaustion

I (a) Direct cause of death, eg pulmonary embolism
  (b) Cause of I(a), eg fractured femur
  (c) Cause of I(b), eg steroid-induced osteoporosis

II Other disease or conditions that may have contributed, eg rheumatoid arthritis, congestive cardiac failure

Write in the patient's notes that you have completed the death certificate, whether they were referred to the coroner and the responses you gave for the categories I(a), (b), (c) and II so that the discharge letter can be written to the GP. You need to see the body to confirm identity.

On a separate piece of paper write down the patient's name, date and time of death, responses to categories I(a), (b), (c) and II, any operations and procedures in the last year (with date and doctor) and if it was referred to the coroner – this will be invaluable for the cremation form.

Post-mortem These used to be carried out regularly, however government legislation means they are now rare. They are usually only carried out if the disease was unusual (with relatives' consent) or if requested by the coroner.

Cremation form

If you are asked to fill in a cremation form you must see the body to check the patient's identity and whether they have a pacemaker. You will also have to sign that they do not have radioactive materials implanted – these are used for palliative treatment of some cancers (eg cervical, bone). The form is simple to complete if you have made a note of the information detailed above. You will be paid just over £55 for the certificate (see p109 re tax) – the money comes from the patient's relatives via the funeral director who keeps the money if you refuse the cheque.

Going to the mortuary

You need to check the identity (appearance and wristband) of all patients who you write death certificates for; use the opportunity to check for pacemakers. You are not checking if the patient is dead – this should now be beyond doubt. Use the patient's name rather than referring to 'the body', wear gloves and wash your hands afterwards.

Bereavement centres and funeral directors

Most hospitals have a bereavement centre that advises the relatives and deals with the paperwork following a death. They can usually arrange for relatives to see the body in the hospital chapel of rest. Further arrangements are made through a funeral director.

Coping with your patient's death

Death is a common, almost daily, occurrence on many wards. Usually the death is expected and peaceful, however this is not always the case. A patient's death can be totally unexpected, upsetting and shocking.

If a death has upset you the following may help:

- talk the case through with your colleagues and seniors
- talk to your relatives and friends – especially non-medical ones
- if you are unable to put it behind you then consider talking to your consultant, GP, the hospital bereavement office or chaplaincy

If you think you were responsible:

- you probably were not; you may have made mistakes, but they are unlikely to have had a significant impact
- read through the notes to get a better idea of what happened
- talk to a senior or colleague who you trust, tell them exactly why you think you were to blame
- if you are still seriously worried see p96 on making mistakes

Religion

Whatever your personal beliefs it is important to be aware of common religious beliefs as they will influence your patient's views.

Buddhism Started about 2500yr ago with the enlightenment and teachings of Siddharta Gautama. Buddists aim to leave the cycle of reincarnation through enlightenment by following the Dharma (teaching); belief in a god(s) varies. ***features*** no special dress, only monks wear saffron robes ***region*** Asia and Far East ***text*** numerous, eg Suttas ***building*** stupa/temple ***diet*** vegetarian ***festivals*** Wesak ***death*** no special arrangements

Christianity Began 2000yr ago with Jesus Christ whose life, teachings and resurrection guide followers and allows them to join God in heaven. Includes Catholics, Church of England, Protestants and many other denominations. ***features*** no special dress ***region*** predominantly Europe, Africa, Americas and Oceania ***text*** Bible ***building*** church ***diet*** no restraints ***festivals*** Christmas and Easter ***death*** no special arrangements

- ***Jehovahs' Witness*** A Christian denomination who believe that blood products are unacceptable. In adults this belief should be respected

Hindu Originated over 5000yr ago. Though exact beliefs vary widely, many believe in a supreme being (Brahma) who created many gods that perform different functions. Hindus aim to leave the cycle of reincarnation through good karma (consequences of actions) or enlightenment. ***features*** females may have a bhindi on their forehead ***region*** predominantly Asia ***text*** Baghavad Gita and Vedas ***building*** temple ***diet*** do not eat beef or pork, may be vegetarian ***festivals*** Diwali ***death*** cremation

Islam (Muslim) Founded 1400yr ago by the prophet Mohammed sent by Allah (God). Followers remain in the grave after death until the Day of Judgement when they may enter paradise. Muslim women may refuse male doctors. ***features*** most women cover their hair ***region*** predominantly Africa, Middle East and Asia ***text*** Quran ***building*** mosque ***diet*** halal meat, no pork ***festivals*** Ramadan (month of fasting) ***death*** burial

Judaism Jews follow the laws of God as written in the Torah about 3300yr ago. Some Jews await a saviour/Messiah. People become Jewish by birth (Jewish mother) or conversion; after death there is an afterlife. ***features*** males are circumcised and may wear a skullcap ***region*** predominantly Israel ***text*** Torah (first five books of the Bible) ***building*** synagogue ***diet*** kosher food, do not eat pork or shellfish ***festivals*** Hanukkah, Passover ***death*** do not leave the body alone and contact a family member

Sikhism Founded 500yr ago by Shri Guru Nanak due to Muslim and Hindu tensions. Sikhs believe in one god (Waheguru) and in reincarnation after death. ***features*** men wear a turban (uncut hair), ceremonial knife, underwear, comb and steel bracelet ***region*** mostly Punjab (India) ***text*** Shri Guru Granth Sahib ***building*** gurdwara ***diet*** may be vegetarian ***festivals*** Vaisakhi ***death*** do not move the body, cremation is preferred

Patient confidentiality

To breach patient confidentiality is unlawful and unprofessional. In essence, patient information held within your head or on a physical medium (paper or database) needs to be kept secret (Data Protection Act, p48). You should be careful when talking about patients in public places, including within the hospital environment, and only disclose patient information to recognised health-care staff as appropriate. Pieces of paper with patient information on must never leave the hospital and should be shredded if they are to be disposed of. **Do not leave patient lists lying around.** Personal electronic databases of patients should be disguised so individual patients cannot be identified.[1] You should never give any information (names or nature of injuries) to the police or press; ask your seniors to deal with these (see p83).

Publications Most medical journals now insist any article which involves a patient needs to be accompanied by consent from the patient for the publication of the material, irrespective of how difficult it would be to track down and identify the patient.

Presentations and images If you are talking about a patient to a group of health-care workers in your own hospital you do not need to obtain consent. If you are talking to an audience from outside your hospital it is advisable you seek the patient's consent. Equally, if you want to keep copies of radiographs or digital images, ensure these are made anonymous and if this isn't possible obtain the patient's consent.

Relatives Your priority lies with your patient and if a relative asks you a question about the patient, it is essential you obtain verbal consent from the patient to talk to the relative or offer to talk to the relative in the presence of the patient. The relatives do not have any rights to know medical information. If the patient lacks capacity then seek senior advice before talking to the relatives.

Children As above, if the child has capacity to give consent decisions (see 'Gillick competence', p93), you must seek verbal consent from the patient to tell the relatives (parents) about their health. If the patient refuses, then offer to talk to the patient about their condition in the presence of their relatives. If you sense the situation will be difficult, seek senior advice/support.

Telephone calls The ward will receive many telephone calls asking how patients are and if they have had tests or operations yet. The potential to break patient confidentiality here is great. In many hospitals now each bed has a telephone, so encourage relatives to speak to the patient directly. Otherwise, inform the patient who is on the telephone and simply relay a message from the patient to the caller. Apologise to the caller for not being able to offer any further information over the telephone, and suggest that you could talk things over with both themselves and the patient when they visit. See outside agencies, p83.

1 Electronic devices on which patient information is stored outside of the hospital should be registered under the Data Protection Act.

Capacity (OHAM2 p546)

Someone who has capacity can 'comprehend and retain information material to the decision, especially as to the consequences of not having the intervention in question, and must be able to use and weight this information in the decision-making process. They may have capacity to consent to some interventions and not others.'[1]

For a patient to have capacity they must:

- be able to take in and retain the information relevant to making the decision and consequences of refusal
- believe the information
- weigh up the information and arrive at a decision

Remember that:

- patients may have the capacity to make some decisions and not others
- capacity in the same patient may fluctuate over time

Capacity is most often impaired by chronic neurological pathology such as dementia, learning difficulties and psychiatric illness, but is also impaired by more acute states such as delirium, alcohol and drug intoxication (both recreational and iatrogenic).

Children and capacity Children under 16yr of age were once regarded as lacking capacity to give consent, but now if the child meets the criteria above then they are regarded as having 'Gillick' competence, and may give consent. It is always advisable, however, to involve the parent or guardian in discussions about the patient's care.

No capacity When the patient does not have capacity and is over 18, family and friends are not able to make a decision on the patient's behalf; their views should, however, be listened to. In this situation, the patient is treated under the 'doctrine of necessity', that is, doing what is in their best interests until they attain capacity to make the decisions themselves.

Gillick competence

Although 16 is the usual age at which young people are allowed to give their own consent, younger people can consent to most treatments or operations if they are capable. This follows a famous case in 1986 when Victoria Gillick went to the courts to get authority to be informed if her daughters sought contraceptive treatments. The law disagreed and decided that if the child was competent they could consent to treatment without their parents' knowledge – this is often referred to as being 'Gillick' competence when it matches the criteria in that case.

1 Department of Health reference guide to consent for examination or treatment.

Consent

Understanding consent and obtaining it satisfactorily can be difficult. If you are ever unsure seek senior help or refer to the many specialised texts on the subject.[1]

Obtaining consent The individual who obtains consent from the patient should be skilled in the procedure to be undertaken, be aware of the risks and benefits and be able to communicate the procedure in a language that the patient will understand. **If you do not regularly perform the procedure yourself then you must not obtain consent for it.**

Informed consent Consent should reflect the fact that the patient is aware of what is going to happen and why. They should be aware of the consequences of not undergoing the procedure, the potential benefits and any alternatives. The common risks and side-effects should be discussed, as should the potentially rare but serious consequences of the procedure. The patient should be provided with information well in advance of the procedure to allow them to think it over and prepare any questions they may wish to ask.

Types of consent There are four main types of consent:

- *implied;* the patient offers you their arm as you approach them with a needle and syringe to take blood
- *expressed – verbal;* you explain that you are going to site a chest drain to relieve a pneumothorax, by describing the procedure and potential complications and the patient agrees to have it done
- *expressed – written;* the patient is given an extensive explanation of the procedure and complications and informed of the alternatives. A record of the consultation is made which both patient and doctor sign. This document should be completed within 6mth prior to the planned treatment or procedure
- *consultant;* if the patient lacks capacity to give consent then two senior doctors can consider the case. If, having considered the opinions of the next of kin, they decide the procedure is in the best interests of the patient, they can jointly give consent for it. Eg amputation of a gangrenous toe which has rendered an elderly patient delirious

Difficult situations There are many situations where problems arise with consent issues. If in doubt seek senior advice or consult one of the medical defence unions (p524) which have 24h telephone support.

If a patient has capacity to give or withhold consent, and chooses not to receive treatment even in the face of death, then treating that patient against their will is potentially a criminal offence. This includes patients with psychiatric illness (OHAM2 p546).

HIV and consent Verbal consent needs to be obtained from patients to test for their HIV status unless they are unable to give consent (lack capacity or unconscious) and knowing their HIV status would alter their management or that of others following a needle-stick or other inoculation injury. Seek advice from a HIV physician if unsure (OHAM2 p342).

1 *Consent in Clinical Practice*. Margaret Mayberry & John Mayberry. 2003. Radcliffe Medical Press, Oxford.

Chapter 5

When things go wrong

Medical errors

Every doctor makes mistakes varying from the trivial and correctable to the severe untoward incident.

What to do at once/within an hour

- Do not compound the error by trying to cover it up or ignore it
- Correct where possible, apologising to the patient as appropriate
- Don't underestimate the seriousness of the situation; have a low threshold for asking for help to ensure things do not get any worse
- If serious and you have time, start documenting events, including times
- If, some time after an error, you realise you wish to add further details to the notes then do so **but** make it clear when these additions have been written by timing and dating them. This is perfectly acceptable
- Retrospectively altering notes, so as to appear more had been written at the time than was the case, is serious misconduct. Often by the time you are made aware of the problem the notes have already been copied, therefore any additions will be easy to spot

Serious untoward incidents

- An apology is not an admission of guilt, so apologise and explain to the patient early. Apologise that the event has taken place, it is not necessary to 'give confession' at this stage
- Inform your registrar/consultant
- If you believe your error has caused the patient significant harm then you should speak to your defence organisation (MDU/MPS etc). This is not an immediate priority

Disciplinary procedures

If you have made a really serious error the hospital may choose to suspend you. That is, to send you home at once and ask you not to return until they have carried out preliminary enquiries. They have the right to do so. It is not a judgemental act but is designed to allow calm and quick investigation. You must be informed why you have been suspended. You may be asked not to talk to others involved. If this happens to you, ring your defence organisation at once. You should be given a named person to contact in the hospital. You cannot be suspended for more than 2wk without a review. Go and stay with friends or family, don't be on your own. Let the hospital and others know how to get hold of you.

Less serious errors should be treated as a training issue and dealt with by your consultant initially or the trust clinical tutor/postgraduate dean. A period of close supervision or retraining may be appropriate.

Sources of help

- ***Clinical events*** Your consultant, the clinical tutor, the postgraduate dean, your defence organisation
- ***Non-clinical events*** Your consultant, the postgraduate dean, the BMA

Don't forget friends and family and remember that these events resolve extremely slowly, taking years in the big cases, so don't expect large numbers of answers in the first week.

Complaints

Every doctor has complaints made about them. These can be clinical or attitudinal, justified or spurious but they are inevitable, therefore do not feel your world has fallen apart when you are told a complaint has been made about you.

How the system handles complaints

There are two types of complaints – formal and informal. If a patient complains to you informally it is in everyone's best interest, and will save many hours of clinical time, if you are able to resolve the situation to the patient's satisfaction there and then. If you are unable to do so, but feel the problem may be solvable by more senior input, then call for help. Don't agree to do something which you are unable to carry out.

How to respond to a complaint

- All formal complaints are collated centrally. In the rare event you are sent a complaint personally, **do not respond** but pass it to the complaints department
- If a complaint has been made about the care of a patient you saw, you may be asked for a statement. This is an internal document and should be written as a memo, but bear in mind if the case goes to court this document could be requested by the patient's lawyers
- Simply state the facts as you see them, do not try to apportion blame. You may be able to expand on your notes, particularly the details of conversations which will not have been documented
- **Do not take it personally**
- If you feel it is clear how any error could be avoided in future then state this as well. Patients are often satisfied by knowing that any mistake they suffered will not be repeated for others
- All the statements made by the staff involved are then collated and a letter is written on behalf of the Chief Executive (and usually signed by them) to the patient. This usually ends the matter
- There are further steps, both with the trust and then regionally, if this is not enough

Serious errors

- Preventable death of a patient
- Significant harm to a patient, in a predictable way
- Disciplinary offences including
  - Taking recreational drugs
  - Being drunk on duty
  - Sexual/racial harassment

Critical incident reporting

A 'critical incident' is defined as:
- anything which harms patients' care or disrupts critical treatment
- an event which could potentially lead to harm if allowed to progress ('near misses'). They range from minor incidents, eg incorrect results, to life-threatening, eg wrong blood group in a blood transfusion

Critical incidents are not:
- incidents which involve staff, relatives or visitors
- complaints against individual behaviour

The aim of critical incident reporting is to highlight any adverse incidents or 'near misses', assess them and to review clinical practice as a result. Ultimately, it is designed to reduce clinical risks and improve the overall quality of patient care.

When a critical incident/near miss occurs:
- make sure the patient is safe
- complete a trust critical incident reporting form
- forward the form to the clinical risk coordinator
- inform staff involved of the outcome

Examples of common critical incidents:
- blood samples from two different patients being confused
- failure to report or follow up abnormal results
- equipment failure
- penicillin prescribed to patients who are allergic to penicillin
- delay in treatment/management

Completing incident forms

- Fill in an incident form as soon as you can after the event so that you don't forget any relevant information
- Check you are filling in the correct form
- Include the time, date, staff involved as well as the issues being reported
- Check if you need to get the consultant involved to fill in/sign the form
- If you are reporting an incident involving your colleagues, inform them and explain the situation. Learn from their mistakes without judging them

The critical incident form is copied to clinical risk directors for evaluation at panel meetings, where changes to clinical practice are discussed.

Hints and tips

- If a critical incident form is filed involving yourself, don't assume you're a bad doctor; use it as a learning experience
- Find out the reason and circumstances and clarify the situation with the person filing the report
- Go over the incident and review your actions, asking if there is anything you would change; if it helps, discuss it with a colleague

McBurney City Hospital NHS Trust

Clinical Incident Reporting Form

Serious untoward incident? ~~Yes~~/No *Near miss*

Hospital: *McBurney City Hospital*
Patient's name: *Eleanor Rigby*
Hospital number: *W876470*
Consultant: *Singh*

Name/grade of submitting staff member: *James Smith*
Signature: *J.Smith* Bleep: *3296* Date: *16/09/05*

Name of staff involved	Grade and speciality	Agency/locum
C. J. Flint	*PRHO.Medicine*	*N/A*

Brief details of incident:

Patient was prescribed augmentin 625mg/8h PO, despite penicillin allergy (this was stated on drug chart). This was noted by the pharmacist and the patient did not take any augmentin. The team PRHO was contacted and an alternative antibiotic was prescribed.

Severity of outcome: *Nil – action taken beforehand*

Location: *E4 ward* | Date: *16/09/2005* | Time: *16.00*

Immediate action taken: *As above*

Near miss? Yes/~~No~~
Are the file notes attached? *To follow*
Equipment failure? ~~Yes~~/No
FAX/POST THIS FORM TO THE CLINICAL RISK COORDINATOR
FOR INVESTIGATION – FAX99999 INTERNALLY

Example of a critical incident reporting form

Hating your job

Experiencing problems at work is common and is usually transient. If you find that things do not improve try to identify the problem. However difficult things are at work, you should always remain polite, punctual and helpful. If you don't you may be the one perceived to be the problem.

Stress at the workplace

With the responsibility that comes with being a doctor and an intense workload, the demands of your job can leave you physically and mentally exhausted. On top of this there is the pressure of litigation and high expectations from your peers and patients. If you feel things are getting on top of you, take a step back and assess your workload. Speak to colleagues to find out if there are easier ways of doing things. Take some annual leave and upon your return approach your work schedule differently to help regain control over things. Make sure you have plenty of time to relax away from the hospital and keep up your outside interests. If things continue to be stressful, talk to a friend, contact the BMA (p524) for advice (if you are a member) or discuss the situation with a senior.

Bullying at work

Bullying can be from your seniors, peers, other health-care professionals, patients and their relatives. If you feel you are being bullied, discuss it with someone, either at work or independently (eg the BMA). Speak to your predecessors to find out if they had similar difficulties and, if so, how they handled the problem. Keep a diary of relevant events, together with witnesses, and approach your consultant. If it is your consultant who is the problem, approach another trusted consultant or speak to the BMA.

Sexual harassment

This may start very innocently and gradually escalate into intimidating behaviour which may affect your work, social life and confidence. In the first instance make it clear that their advances are not welcome and confide in someone you trust. Find out if other colleagues are also being harassed and report the harassment to your personal tutor.

Discrimination

All employers must abide by an equal opportunities policy which includes standards on treating all employees. Before deciding to take things further confide in a senior colleague whom you trust. Keep a record of any events that stand out as being discriminatory, documenting dates, times and witnesses. Contact the BMA for advice (p524). You may have to submit a formal letter outlining your concerns, so make sure you are prepared to pursue a formal complaint before committing yourself on paper.

Handing in your resignation

If you can find no other option, you can always leave your job. Find out how much notice you are required to give from human resources and who to direct your letter of resignation to. During your last weeks, stay an active member of the team rather than taking a short-timer's attitude. Complete any outstanding work and tidy up loose ends before leaving. Check what happens with any leave owing to you and make sure you have contact details for colleagues who you intend to keep in touch with.

Colleagues and problems

Most of us have worked with a colleague who worried us professionally – 'I wouldn't want to be treated by Dr X'. When does this become enough to do something? And what do you do?

Clinical incompetence

- The GMC is quite clear that we all have a clinical duty to report colleagues who we believe to be incompetent. This does not equate to pointing out every fault of every other doctor but it does mean that you cannot ignore serious concerns if you believe patients are being put at risk of harm
- Serious concerns about a trainee should be passed to the relevant consultant. Ask to see them in private. It may be easiest to open the conversation with a question, to ask them to put your mind at rest, for example:
  'I don't know if you are aware that Dr X does not use chaperones. I've always been told we should use them for intimate examinations. I'm here because two women told me that they had felt uncomfortable with Dr X.'
- If the problem is with a consultant then you should either talk to another consultant or, if it is very serious, the medical director
- If you are unsure whether a problem exists, or how serious it is, then talk to a friendly senior colleague informally (eg your mentor for the FP, or a clinical lecturer you got on with at medical school)

Recreational drugs/alcohol

- There is a massive difference between the doctor who drinks too much at weekends or who smokes the occasional joint and one who helps themselves to controlled drugs
- Likewise, regardless of substance, there is a difference between what someone does that only affects themselves and actions which affect quality of patient care. The badly hungover colleague is better sent to the mess to recover and made to pay the favour back some other time than get drug dosages wrong on the ward
- Both being drunk on duty and theft of controlled drugs are serious disciplinary offences and acts of professional misconduct. They are better tackled early whilst solvable than left until they ruin a career
- It is unlikely that a colleague will change their behaviour simply because you have tackled them over it. Therefore consider discussing the situation with a trusted senior colleague as you may be helping them (in the longer term at least)

Psychological problems

- Every year doctors develop serious psychological illnesses just like the rest of the population and doctors are just as bad at self-diagnosis
- The more common problems include frank depression and hypomania, the rare include psychosis and schizophrenia; the symptoms often come on gradually such that even close colleagues may not notice the transition from mildly eccentric to frankly pathological
- Depression may also mask itself whilst at work
- Talk to your colleague if concerned about their health

Colleagues and problems

Chapter 6

Boring but important stuff

Pay and contracts

The number of hours you are allowed to work in a shift and the total for a given week are determined by two sets of rules: the European Working Time Directive (EWTD), which is incorporated into UK law, and the 'New Deal' on junior doctors' hours, which is an agreement between the BMA and all the UK Departments of Health.

EWTD

- Maximum of 58h of work a week until August 2007
- Maximum of 56h of work a week until August 2009
- Maximum of 48h of work a week from August 2009
- 11h of continuous rest each day or compensatory rest must be given
- 24h continuous rest each week or 48h in a fortnight

New deal

- Maximum of 56h of actual work (on your feet) a week
- Maximum of 72h (in total) of duty (including on-calls) a week
- 30min break for every 4h of continuous work
- The New Deal also has detailed requirements about the length of different shifts types. These are explained in the BMA *Junior Doctors' Handbook* or at www.bma.org.uk/ap.nsf/Content/TimesUp

Salary

Doctors in training are paid according to a banded contract which comprises

- a basic salary, which rises incrementally each year to reflect the trainee's greater experience
- a banding multiplier (see opposite) depending on the overall number of hours worked, the intensity of those hours and their antisociability

Monitoring and rebanding

- Monitoring of the actual hours worked by junior doctors is the main method of determining if the actual hours of the job mirror the theoretical hours of the rota
- All training posts have to be monitored for at least 2wk by all participants every 6mth. This is a contractual requirement
- If your post turns out to be monitored as a different band to the one you're paid then your pay can go up but is protected against going down
- Your rota cannot be changed in such a way as to affect your salary without the agreement of the majority of the doctors on the rota
- The rules for 're-banding' and for pay protection are complex and are available on the Department of Health or BMA websites:
  - www.dh.gov.uk/PolicyAndGuidance/HumanResourcesAndTraining/ModernisingPay/JuniorDoctorContracts/fs/en
  - www.bma.org.uk/ap.nsf/Content/Hubjuniordoctors

The structure of the NHS

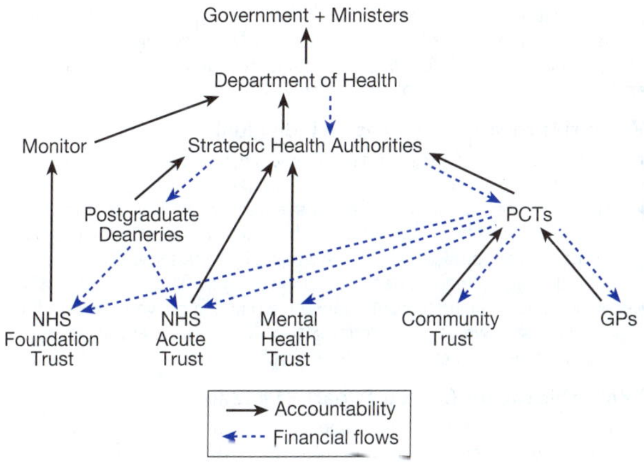

The Banding Contract

- Total hours of actual work over 56h/wk – Band 3
- Total hours of actual work <56h but >48h/wk – Band 2
- Total hours of actual work under 48h/wk – Band 1
- Bands 1 and 2 are further subdivided depending on the intensity and antisociability of the out-of-hours component (Bands 2A and 1A the most antisocial, then 2B and 1B, then 1C the least antisocial or intense)
- In 2004; Band 3 = 2.0xbasic, Band 2A = 1.8x, 2B = 1.5x, 1A = 1.5x, 1B = 1.4x, 1C = 1.2x. These rates are subject to annual review as part of the doctors' annual pay award

Clinical governance

DOH definition: 'Clinical governance is the system through which NHS organisations are accountable for continuously improving the quality of their services and safeguarding high standards of care, by creating an environment in which clinical excellence will flourish.'

What this means for you as an individual

- You are responsible for your clinical practice which you should be aiming to improve continuously
- You need a mechanism for assessing the standard of your practice. Whilst in training this is done for you by your consultant/trainer as part of your regular appraisal process. Additionally to this you may have audits and regular departmental meetings
- You should be aiming to continuously learn and improve your care for patients. Again, whilst still in training, this almost goes without saying. Revising for endless examinations and diplomas helps too

What this means for you as part of a team

- You should ensure you stick to departmental or hospital protocols and don't undertake procedures for which you have not been trained
- You will be asked to participate in regular departmental audits, usually of morbidity and mortality. These are used to ensure consistency of practice and to pick up problems early
- You should attend departmental and hospital-wide audit meetings and grand rounds to keep up to date with changes
- You should answer any responses to complaints promptly

Clinical governance mechanisms

The clinical governance structure in every hospital includes:

- audit of practice (eg reattendances within 1wk or wound infections)
- appraisal and revalidation structures
- regular departmental meetings (eg morbidity and mortality) to allow clinicians to compare their care and highlight common concerns
- clear routes of accountability for all staff. It can be obvious when these have broken down, leading to problems which everyone can identify but seemingly no one is responsible for fixing
- a risk management structure to identify practices which jeopardise high-quality patient care (critical incident reporting, p98)
- a complaints department to respond to complaints and ensure lessons are learned from them; may be part of the risk management dept
- a clinical governance committee/structure which oversees and ensures compliance with all of the above

Compliance with clinical governance mechanisms are measured both regionally and nationally.

NHS entitlements

As doctors working and training in the NHS you have certain entitlements, defined under your 'Terms and Conditions of Service'. Those relating to salary are discussed in Pay and contracts, p104. The others are listed here.

Accommodation

- In your first year after graduation you are entitled to free accommodation at your employing trust. This is defined in the Medical Act (1983), and is likely to be incorporated into the Terms and Conditions of Service during 2005
- In the following years hospital accommodation should still be available, though there may be a charge for it.
- The standards of accommodation have been agreed between the BMA and the DOH. They are explained on the BMA website (p524). Contact the BMA if you feel your accommodation is unacceptable and the hospital is unwilling to resolve this
- Substandard accommodation should be free

Medical staffing/human resources departments

- They are responsible for your employment. They sign you on the payroll and keep track of leave taken. They are the first port of call for employment problems

Leave entitlement

- Junior doctors are entitled to 5wk paid annual leave a year plus 2d for the old 'NHS stat days', a total of 27d/yr or 9d/4mth (13.5d/6mth). You are rarely allowed to carry leave over between academic years
- You will need to give 6wk notice for annual leave. Your form will need to be signed by your consultant
- Many posts have some or all leave fixed within the rota. Swaps may be possible, but difficult; ask your consultant or medical staffing
- You are allowed leave for bank holidays though not necessarily the days themselves. If you work any part of a bank holiday you are entitled to a day off in lieu

Maternity/paternity leave

- This is complex. In summary: all women are entitled to 26wk paid maternity leave and must be allowed to return to work after this. If you've been working over 6mth then you can apply for an additional 26wk unpaid leave. Fathers are entitled to up to 2wk paid paternity leave if they have worked for over 6mth. Some trusts try to claim you must have worked the 6mth with them (not just the NHS). This is ill-defined, talk to the BMA if you have a problem
- The detail is in the *Junior Doctors' Handbook* from the BMA

Less-than-full-time/flexible training

- Foundation Programme doctors are entitled to train less than full time if they have a valid reason
- A comprehensive list of valid reasons (eg having a baby or ill health) and advice on how to apply is available from your deanery

Money and debt

As the average medical graduate debt now exceeds £16,000, financial management priorities have changed. This section is not comprehensive but aims to give some important pointers and warnings.

Debt clearance

Most graduates have three different types of debt:

- Short-term high-interest debts (eg credit cards ± overdraft, if at full charge). Pay these back first and as fast as possible. Don't be tempted to extend them just because you have an income
- Medium-term commercial loans (eg a high street bank graduate studies loan). These should be paid back next, as spare funds allow
- Student loans at very low rates of interest – pay these back as slowly as you wish provided the APR (Annual Percentage Rate) remains ≤inflation

Pay close attention to the APR and charges attached to any loan arrangement. Interest-free loans or credit cards can help in the short term but ensure you don't get saddled with a high APR later. Loans are a very competitive market so shop around – especially for something like a car loan where the car dealer rarely offers the best rate.

Think 'total cost' not just 'monthly repayments'.

Financial advice

Since you now have a salary in the top 5% of earners, virtually guaranteed for life, finance companies will swarm round you like wasps round jam. Beware some very slick sharks – their aim is only to get you to buy their products. There is no altruism here.

- Truly independent financial advice is hard to obtain – ask how independent they really are
- Check what commission will be received for any product you choose, both to the individual who sold it to you as well as to their company
- Do not buy from the first or most persuasive salesperson, but take your time to consider what you really want and need

Some basic rules for financial planning

- Short term – clear debts with the highest interest as soon as possible. Try to accumulate about one month's salary as 'emergency' savings
- Medium term – think about trying to save for the deposit on a property (even if just £100/mth). If debt-free consider a medium-term saving scheme to reduce tax liability
- Long term – pension and mortgage

Documents to keep safe

P60 – sent every April to all employees
P45 – sent to you every time you change trust
Pay slips – issued every month
Record of additional income – eg locums
Annual interest statements from bank/savings/shares – issued annually

Financial and other products

Income support pays you some income (though less than your basic salary) if you are unable to work. Standard NHS benefits are poor especially for the first 2yr.

Critical illness gives a lump sum if you develop an incapacitating illness. Check if it still pays if you are capable of doing a less demanding job. Check if it pays for all conditions you may get at work.

Life insurance pays out a lump sum if you die, only really makes sense if you have dependents.

Pension Stay in the NHS pension scheme. Consider a top-up if you can afford one, eg Additional Voluntary Contributions (AVCs); these have performed badly over the last 10yr but should do better in the future. Starting early will cost you far less in the long term.

MDU/MPS Necessary additional protection for problems relating to clinical performance. NHS indemnity doesn't cover everything, eg good Samaritan acts.

BMA Advisable protection for non-clinical matters, eg wrong salary or poor accommodation. Trade Union for doctors.

Tax

Now that you are earning a salary you will be paying tax. Most will be collected by PAYE (Pay As You Earn). If you have no other sources of income then you can leave it at that. If you have any other income then you should ask for a tax return and complete it.

Tax codes The box on your first pay-slip will show you your tax code; it illustrates how many tens of pounds you are allowed tax-free (eg 474L = £4745, the basic allowance). You can add unavoidable expenses and subscriptions connected with your job to this, see below. The leaflet 'Understanding Your Tax Code' is available from the Inland Revenue.

Tax deductible Job-related expenses (eg stethoscope, keep receipts in case they check). Professional subscriptions – GMC, BMA, MDU/MPS, College if applicable. Claiming all these will save you money.

Tax returns A tax return is a long form asking for details of all the money you have received which may have tax owing on it. This includes your salary and other income whether earned (eg locum shifts or cremation fees) or unearned (eg lodger/flatmate, bank interest and dividend yields).

- If you get sent one, fill it in
- If you return it by the end of September then the IR will do the maths for you
- Do it after Jan and they'll fine you £100/6mth plus interest
- Claim your deductible allowances but also list your additional income

The IR has been known to ask an undertaker to list all payments to doctors and then cross-check. If your tax is simple then they're not hard to do, otherwise pay a company/accountant to do it for you.

Making more money

There are several ways to make money in addition to your basic income. It is crucial you keep records of all additional income and declare these when you complete your self-assessment to the Inland Revenue at the end of each tax year.[1]

Cremation certificates The cremation form has two parts (p90). The first is completed by a ward doctor (usually the PRHO) and the second by a senior doctor, often from another department. The first part takes about 10min to complete and the individual is rewarded about £55 for their trouble. The bereavement office usually handles the forms and issues the cheques. Make sure you see the body, checking identity and that there is no pacemaker; they do really explode!

Published articles Several journals and medical newspapers pay authors for articles which appear in print. The amount varies from between £25 to £250 depending on the length and importance. The journals' websites often outline payment and the types of articles they are after.

Research There are usually several research projects being undertaken in most hospitals which require volunteers to have experiments performed on them. These range from a 5min interview to a week-long study and in most circumstances the volunteers are rewarded financially (£5 book token to over £500).

Gifts The GMC are quite clear in their message that you should not encourage patients or their families to give, lend or bequeath gifts to yourself, others or to organisations.[2] If you are given a gift then it is acceptable to take it as long as it has negligible financial value. If you are given money then it is sensible to pass this onto the ward sister who can put it in the ward fund account.

Locums Most hospitals occasionally employ locum doctors to cover staff sickness or at very busy times. Locum doctors often already work for the hospital, but just work additional shifts outside of their normal hours for extra money; alternatively they may be from outside the hospital. It is important to remember that the hours you work as a locum should be added to your basic or regular hours and should not exceed the limits of the New Deal[3] or European Working Time Directive; some contracts may stipulate that you cannot work locum shifts in other hospitals or departments. There are many locum agencies that you can register with (p525), they are often advertised in *BMJ Careers*. Rates of pay vary, but a PRHO can expect pre-tax rates of £15–25 per hour, and SHOs £20–30. If your own hospital is employing you as a locum, you may be able to negotiate a better rate.

1 http://www.inlandrevenue.gov.uk/sa/
2 http://www.gmc-uk.org/standards/good.htm
3 *Junior Doctors' Handbook* 2003/04. British Medical Association.

Chapter 7

Clinical presentations

Contents by disease

These tables show where text on diseases is found; see the inside front cover for the clinical presentations list and inside back cover for the emergencies list.

History

A focused but thorough clerking is an essential skill as a junior doctor. See the individual speciality chapters (p301) for unique features in their clerking and p420 for pre-op clerking. The following two pages are a guide to taking and writing a standard clerking. It is helpful to use a similar format so that other doctors know where to find details.

Taking a history (OHCM6 p34)

- Make sure you are in a setting that offers privacy and has a bed.
- Establish the patient's name and age, check their date of birth.
- Introduce yourself and begin with open-ended questions.
- Find out how they were referred (eg GP, A+E, clinic).
- Never forget to ask about other medical problems, drugs and allergies.

Heading Your name, position, location, date, time, who was present

Dr C.J.Flint, medical PRHO, Ward D57
15/09/05, 22:15, Clerking from pt and son

Presenting complaint Why has the patient come to hospital? Write their main problem(s) in their own words along with duration and who referred them; if the referral letter has a different presenting complaint then document this too:

Eleanor Rigby, 83yr-old female with chest pain for 3 days, GP concerned about new onset of LBBB on ECG

Background Try to describe the patient's previous state in ≤3 lines; mention relevant medical history, drugs, social state and family history:

COPD – on inhalers, °home nebs, °LTOT
↑BP, ex-smoker (50 pk/yr), °previous IHD/MI
Lives alone, ET 100yd with stick, home help for cleaning

History of presenting complaint(s) Ask questions aimed at differentiating the causes of the presenting complaint and assessing its severity. Try to exclude potentially life-threatening causes first. Ask specifically about previous episodes and investigations/treatments. Use the SOCRATES questions for pain (site, onset, character, radiation, associations, timing, exacerbating/relieving factors, severity). Ask about the affect on their activities of daily living (ADLs). If there are multiple problems ask if they come on together or are related. Include any important negative or positive findings from the systems review.

Intermittent chest pain for 3/7, comes on suddenly at rest, gradual improvement over ~30min, heavy sensation, 5/10, worst 4hr ago, no change on exertion/breathing/movement, no radiation, mild SOB, no nausea/sweating, nil previous, no cough/leg pain, mild swelling of ankles

Coping at home, but unable to get to shops 2°SOBOE

Risk factors Document recognised risk factors for important differentials:

Previous IHD ×, ↑BP ✓, smoking ✓, FH ×, cholesterol ?, DM ×

Past medical history Ask about previous medical problems/operations and attempt to gauge the severity of each (eg hospital/ITU admissions, exercise tolerance (ET), treatment); use the drug history to prompt the patient's memory. Consider documenting specifically about asthma, diabetes, angina, ↑BP, MI, stroke, PE/DVT, epilepsy.

COPD – on inhaler, ° home nebs, ° LTOT, no recent change
↑BP on treatment °angina/MI/CVA/PE
Hiatus hernia and laparotomy 2° diverticular disease 1992

Drug history Document all drugs along with doses, times taken and any recent changes; always document drug allergies and the reaction.

Combivent inh ii/PRN
Becotide 100 inh ii/bd
Bendrofluazide 25mg/om
Lansoprazole 15mg/om
Lactulose 10ml/PRN
Allergic to penicillin, causes a rash

Family history Ask about relevant illness in the family (eg heart, cancer, epilepsy). Are other family members well at the moment?

Sister died of breast cancer aged 67, son alive and well

Social history This is essential ***home*** ask about who they live with, the kind of house (eg bungalow, residential home), any home help, own ADLs (cooking, dressing, washing) ***mobility*** walking aids (stick/frame), exercise tolerance ***lifestyle*** occupation, racial origins (if relevant), alcohol (units/wk), smoking (cigarettes/d and pack years), recreational drugs:

- *Alcohol* 1 unit = ½ pint of beer, glass of wine, measure of spirits bottle of wine = 9u, 1l of strong cider = 8.5u
- *Smoking* 1 pack year = 20 cigarettes/d for 1yr

Lives alone in a bungalow ET 100yd with stick, home help 2/wk for cleaning, ex-smoker for 30yr, 50 pack years

Systems review Relevant systems review will often be part of the HPC, a thorough systems review is only necessary if you are unsure what is relevant or are struggling to explain the symptoms. See OHCM6 p36.

CVS	Chest pain, palpitations, SOB, ankle swelling, orthopnoea
Resp	Cough (?bld), sputum, wheeze, SOB
Abdo	Abdo pain, nausea/vomiting, bowel habit (?bld), stool colour and consistency, distension, dysuria, frequency, urgency, haematuria
Neuro	Headache, photophobia, neck stiffness, weakness, change in sensation, balance, fits, falls, speech, changes in vision/ hearing
Systemic	Appetite loss, weight loss, fever/night sweats, malaise, stiff/swollen joints, fatigue, rashes/itch, sleep pattern

Summarising Ask if there are any other problems that have not been discussed and repeat back a summary of the history to the patient to check that they agree.

Examination

It is good practice to perform a brief CVS, RS, abdo and neuro exam on all patients but focus your examination according to their history. Check observations (temp, BP, pulse, RR, O_2 sats):

- ask a nurse to chaperone you if necessary
- ask permission before touching the patient and ask where it hurts
- assess whether the patient looks well or ill

Arm (OHCM6 p39)

- ***Look*** at the hands for signs of disease
- ***Pulse*** check the rate and rhythm

> **Nails** clubbing, pitting, koilonychia (concave, ↓iron), Beau's lines **hands** skin turgor, hyperpigmented folds, Dupuytren's disease, small muscle wasting, joint swelling, rheumatoid nodules (check elbows), ulnar deviation, Boutonniere's/swan neck deformity, trigger finger, sclerodactyly

Cardiovascular system (OHCM6 p40)

- ***Inspection*** JVP (very useful if visible), swollen ankles
- ***Palpation*** temp of hands, capillary-refill, carotid pulse (volume and character), apex beat, hepatomegaly
- ***Auscultation*** heart sounds, added sounds/murmurs (timing, volume, radiation), carotid bruits, basal crackles

> **General** clubbing, splinter haemorrhages, Janeway lesions, Osler's nodes, Quincke's sign (pulsing nail beds), Corrigan's sign (visibly pulsating carotids), de Musset's sign (bobbing of head), Roth's spots (retinal infarcts), xanthelasma, malar flush **chest** precordial scars, heaves, thrills (palpable murmur)

Murmur	Signs
Mitral stenosis	Mid-diastolic rumbling murmur, loud 1st HS, opening snap, malar flush, AF, tapping apex, left parasternal heave
Mitral regurgitation	Pansystolic murmur radiating to the axilla, soft 1st HS, 3rd HS present, thrusting apex, left parastenal heave
Aortic stenosis	Ejection systolic mumur radiating to the neck, 4th HS, reversed HS splitting, slow rising pulse, systolic thrill
Aortic regurgitation	Early diastolic murmur (best heard in expiration), collapsing pulse, wide BP, pistol-shot femoral pulse, Corrigan's sign, Quincke's sign, de Musset's sign

Respiratory system (OHCM6 p48)

- ***Inspection*** asterixis (flap), stridor, JVP, resp rate and effort (accessory muscles, recession), chest wall movement, peripheral oedema
- ***Palpation*** trachea, cervical lymphadenopathy, chest expansion
- ***Percuss*** right = left, hyperresonant, dull, stoney dull
- ***Auscultation*** reduced air entry, crackles, wheeze, bronchial BS, rub

> **General** clubbing, nicotine, asterixis (CO_2 flap), muscle wasting, peripheral or central cyanosis, purse-lip breathing, Horner's, (↓pupil, ptosis, ↓sweating), spine or chest wall deformity, cough **chest** scars, tactile vocal fremitus

Abdomen (OHCM6 p52)

- ***Inspection*** jaundice, scars, distension, hernias, peripheral oedema
- ***Palpation*** palpate each segment (start away from the pain) while watching the patient's face; feel for tenderness, peritonism (guarding, rebound, rigidity, percussion tenderness), masses, liver, spleen, kidneys and AAA (expansile mass), hernias, ±genitalia, PR (masses, stool, tenderness, blood/mucus/melaena)
- ***Percussion*** ascites (shifting dullness, fluid thrill), liver, spleen
- ***Auscultation*** bowel sounds (absent, reduced, increased, tinkling)

> **General** pallor, leuconychia (white nails, ↓albumin), palmar erythema, asterixis (liver flap), spider naevi, itching, bruising, tattoos, hepatic foetor (pear-drop breath), Virchow's node (left supraclavicular), gynaecomastia, hair distribution **abdo** visible pulsations/masses, caput medusa, striae, everted umbilicus, liver texture, tenderness, pulsatility, renal bruits, inguinal lymphadenopathy, radiofemoral delay

Peripheral nerves (OHCM6 p54)

See p224 for neuroanatomy.

- ***Inspection*** posture, movement of limbs
- ***Palpation*** tone, power (5 normal, 4 weak, 3 against gravity only, 2 not even against gravity, 1 twitch, 0 none), reflexes, plantars, sensation
- ***Coordination*** finger–nose, slide heel down opposite leg

> **Extras** involuntary movements, muscle wasting, fasciculations, clonus, light touch, pain, vibration, temperature, joint position, dysdiadochokinesis, Romberg's test

Cranial nerves (OHCM6 p56)

- ***Inspection*** GCS, alertness, mental state (p229), speech, posture
- ***Eyes*** (II, III, IV, VI) acuity, pupil reactivity, fields, movements, fundi
- ***Face*** (V, VII) sensation and power
- ***Mouth*** (IX, X, XII) tongue movements, palette deviation, cough
- ***Other*** (VIII) hearing, balance, gait (XI), shrug power, head movements

> **Extras** (I) familiar smells with each nostril (II, III, IV, VI) nystagmus, visual inattention, light and accommodation (V) corneal reflex, mouth muscles (VII) taste (VIII) Weber's, Rinne's, (IX, X) gag reflex, swallow

Differential diagnosis

Write a list of differentials in order of likelihood along with important diseases to exclude:

Imp 1 *Reflux pain 2° hiatus hernia*
2 *Musculoskeletal chest pain*
3 *Exclude MI*

Management plan

Write the important investigations and treatments the patient requires. Always include symptomatic relief (eg analgesia, antiemetics):

(P) *FBC, U+E, LFT, Cardiac markers, ECG, CXR*
O_2, GTN, Gaviscon, paracetamol
Admit overnight for repeat cardiac markers and ECG

Early warning scores

Early detection of the 'unwell' patient has repeatedly been shown to improve outcome.[1–3] Identification of such patients allows suitable changes in management, including early involvement of critical care staff or transfer to critical care areas (HDU/ITU) where necessary.

Identification of the 'at risk' patient relies on measurement of simple physiological parameters, which generally deteriorate as the patient becomes more unwell; these include respiratory rate, pulse, blood pressure, oxygen saturation, level of consciousness, urine output and temperature. Remember that the sick patient might not look that unwell from the bottom of the bed.

Scoring of these parameters can be carried out in many ways and is undertaken by nursing staff. One example, the Modified Early Warning Score (MEWS), is shown opposite. Normal observations are awarded a score of 0, whilst abnormal observations attract higher scores. The values for each physiological parameter are added together. If this total score reaches a 'threshold' value (eg 4 on the example opposite), the nursing staff should alert either a senior nurse or a doctor to review the patient, depending on local policy/guidelines.

Trends in physiological parameters are often more useful than one-off observations. Some patients may have abnormal scores even when they seem relatively 'well' because of compensatory mechanisms. These patients may be given higher thresholds, but are also likely to deteriorate much more quickly.

Patients who should be monitored by such scores include:

- emergency admissions
- unstable patients
- elderly patients
- patients with pre-existing disease (cardiovascular, respiratory, DM)
- patients who are failing to respond to treatment
- patients who have returned from ITU/HDU
- postoperative patients

Early warning scores are not used in all hospitals, though their principles can be used by anyone to help prioritise clinical need when faced with several referrals over the telephone or in an admissions unit.

ALERT™

Acute Life-threatening Events – Recognition and Treatment

This is an evolving course that aims to guide people in early recognition of the unwell patient and in their immediate resuscitation. This course complements the Immediate Life Support (ILS) and Advanced Life Support (ALS) courses (p122). Further information can be found at www.web.port.ac.uk/alert/

1 McGloin H 1999 *J R Coll Physicians* **33** 255.
2 McQuillan P 1998 *BMJ* **316** 1853.
3 Cooper N 2004 *student BMJ* **12** 12.

Adult Modified Early Warning System Observation Score (MEWS)

If score ≥4 notify junior doctor immediately. If any individual score = 3 notify junior doctor immediately.

Score	3	2	1	0	1	2	3
Respiratory rate		≤8	9–10	11–20	21–25	26–30	≥31
Pulse		≤40	41–50	51–100	101–110	111–130	≥131
Systolic BP (mmHg)	≤84	85–89	90–100	101–199		≥200	
SpO_2	≤87	88–91	92–94	95–100			
GCS or AVPU	≤8	9–13	14 New agitation or confusion	15 A	V	P	U
Temp °C		≤35.0	35.1–35.9	36.0–37.4	37.5–38.4	≥38.5	
Urine	≤10ml/h for 2h	≤30ml/h for 2h					

Peri-arrest

Airway	Check airway is patent; consider manoeuvres/adjuncts
Breathing	If no respiratory effort – **CALL ARREST TEAM**
Circulation	If no palpable pulse – **CALL ARREST TEAM**
Disability	If GCS ≤8 – **CALL ANAESTHETIST**

Airway – if irreversibly obstructed CALL ARREST TEAM
- **Look** inside the mouth, remove obvious objects/dentures
- Wide-bore **suction** under direct vision if secretions present
- **Listen** airway impaired if stridor, snoring, gurgling or no air entry
- **Jaw thrust**/head tilt/chin lift
- **Oropharyngeal** or **nasopharyngeal** airway as tolerated

If still impaired CALL ARREST TEAM

Breathing – if poor or absent respiratory effort CALL ARREST TEAM
- **Look** for chest expansion (does R = L?), fogging of mask
- **Listen** to chest for air entry (does R = L?)
- **Feel** for expansion and percussion (does R = L?)
- **Non-rebreath** (trauma) mask and 15l O_2 in all patients
- **Bag and mask** if poor or absent breathing effort
- **Monitor** O_2 sats and respiratory rate
- **Think** tension pneumothorax

Circulation – if no pulse CALL ARREST TEAM
- **Look** for pallor, cyanosis, distended neck veins
- **Feel** for a central pulse (carotid/femoral) – rate and rhythm
- **Monitor** defibrillator ECG leads and BP
- **Venous access**, send bloods
- **12-lead ECG**
- Call for **senior help** early if patient deteriorating

Disability – if GCS ≤8 or falling CALL ANAESTHETIST
- Assess **GCS** and check **BM**
- **Look** for pupil reflexes and unusual posture
- **Feel** for tone in all four limbs and plantar reflexes

Exposure
- **Remove** all clothing, check **temperature**
- **Look** all over body including perineum and back for rashes or injuries
- **Cover** patient with a blanket

Common causes

- Arrhythmia
- Myocardial infarction
- Hypovolaemia
- Sepsis (UTI/pneumonia)
- Hypoglycaemia
- Hypoxia
- Pulmonary oedema
- Pulmonary embolism
- Metabolic (↑↓K^+)
- (Tension) pneumothorax

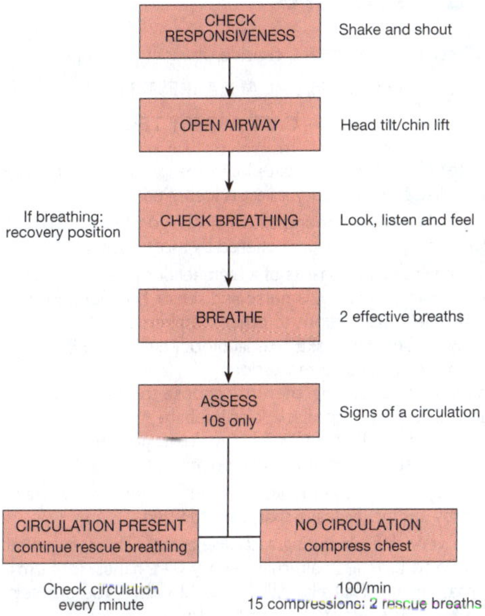

Adult Basic Life Support algorithm, 2000 guidelines

Reproduced by kind permission of The Resuscitation Council UK.

Advanced life support

Airway	Check airway is patent; consider manoeuvres/adjuncts
Breathing	If no respiratory effort – **CALL ARREST TEAM**
Circulation	If no palpable pulse – **CALL ARREST TEAM**

Basic life support (p121) should be initiated and the cardiac arrest team called as soon as cardiac or respiratory arrest is identified.

Advanced life support is centred around a 'universal algorithm' (opposite) which is taught on a standardised course offered by most hospitals.

The cardiac arrest team usually consists of a team leader (medical SHO or registrar), PRHO, anaesthetist, CCU nurse and senior hospital nurse:

- team leader – gives clear instructions to other members
- PRHO – provide BLS, cannulate, take arterial blood, defibrillate if trained, give drugs, perform chest compressions
- anaesthetist – airway and breathing, they may choose to bag-and-mask ventilate the patient, insert a laryngeal mask or intubate
- nurses – provide BLS, defibrillate if trained, give drugs, perform chest compressions, record observations, note time points and record ECGs.

Needle-stick injuries (p34) are commonest in times of emergency. Have the sharps box nearby and never leave sharps on the bed.

Cannulation can be very difficult during a cardiac arrest. The antecubital fossa is the best place to look first; alternatively try feet, hands, forearms, or consider external jugular if all else fails. Take bloods if you are successful, but don't allow this to delay the giving of drugs.

Blood tests are occasionally useful in cardiac arrests, especially K^+ which can often be measured by arterial blood gas machines. Use a blood gas syringe to obtain a sample (the femoral artery with a green needle is often easiest – NAVY, p464) and ask a nurse to take the sample to the machine. Other blood tests depend on the clinical scenario, if in doubt fill all the common blood bottles.

Defibrillation is taught on specific courses (eg ILS, ALS) and must not be undertaken unless trained. Automated External Defibrillators or AEDs (p474) are becoming more common and have been designed to be used by the lay person.

Cardiac arrest drugs are now prepared in pre-filled syringes: epinephrine (adrenaline) 1mg in 10ml (1:10,000), atropine 3mg in 10ml, amiodarone 300mg in 10ml. Always give a large flush (20ml saline) after each dose to encourage it into the central circulation. See inside back cover for further doses.

Cardiac arrest trolleys are found in most areas of the hospital. Know where they are for your wards. Ask the ward sister if you can open the trolley and have a good look at the equipment within it. They are often arranged so the top drawer contains **A**irway equipment, the second contains **B**reathing equipment, the third contains **C**irculation equipment and the lower drawer contains the drugs.

Advanced Life Support algorithm for the management of cardiac arrest in adults

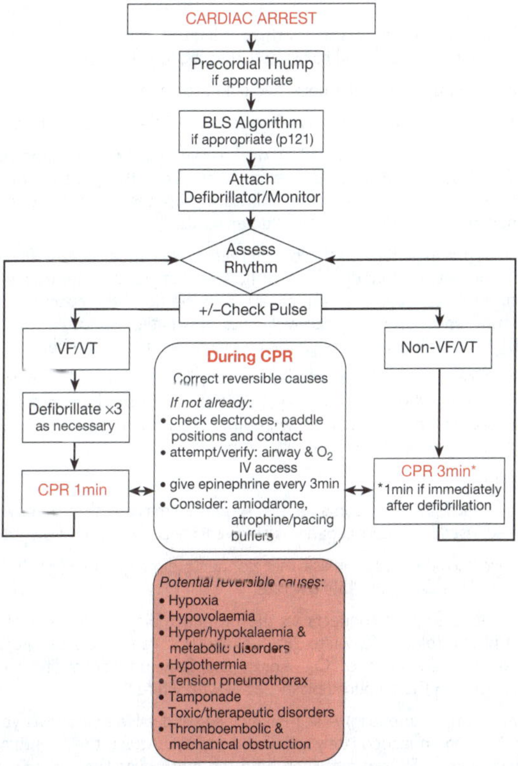

Adult Advanced Life Support algorithm, 2000 guidelines
Reproduced by kind permission of The Resuscitation Council UK.

Defibrillator energy levels for VF and VT

	Monophasic	Biphasic[1]
First two shocks	200J	150J
Third shock	360J	150J
Further shocks[2]	360J	150J

1 Different biphasic defibrillators use different energy levels, follow the maker's directions.
2 If a patient returns to sinus rhythm start again at the lower energy.

Arrest equipment and tests

Airways

Jaw thrust Pull the jaw forward with your index and middle fingers at the angle of each mandible. Pull hard enough to make your fingers ache.

Head tilt Gently extend the neck, avoid if C-spine injury risk.

Chin lift Pull the chin up with two fingers, avoid if C-spine injury risk.

Oropharyngeal airway (Guedel) A rigid, curved plastic tube; choose the size that reaches the angle of the mandible from the patient's mouth. Insert the smaller end with the hole facing up then rotate inside the patient's mouth until the hole faces downwards.

Nasopharyngeal airway A flexible, curved plastic tube, not to be used with significant head injury. Choose the size that reaches the tragus (triangular bit of ear separate from pinna) from the tip of the nose; insert by lubricating and pushing horizontally into the patient's nostril (not upwards). Use a safety pin through the end to prevent the tube being lost.

Suction Cover the hole on the side of a wide-bore suction catheter to clear secretions blocking an airway; this should only be done in the parts of the oropharynx that can be seen directly. A thinner catheter can be used to clear secretions in an intubated patient.

Breathing

Non-rebreath mask (trauma mask) A plastic mask with a floppy bag attached; used in acutely ill patients to give 85% O_2 with a 15l flow rate.

Standard mask A plastic mask that connects directly to oxygen tubing; delivers ~50% O_2 with a 15l flow rate.

Venturi A mask that connects to the oxygen tubing via a piece of coloured plastic (blue 24%, white 28%, yellow 35%, red 40%, green 60%) to give an accurate dose of O_2. Adjust the flow rate according to the instructions on the coloured plastic, eg 4l with white.

Bag and mask (Ambubag) A self-inflating bag and valve that allows you to force O_2 into an inadequately ventilated patient. Attach the O_2 tubing to the bag with a 15l flow rate then hold the mask over the patient's nose and mouth. Easiest with two people; one person stands at the head to get a firm seal with both hands whilst the other squeezes the bag. The mask can be removed to attach the bag to an intubated patient.

Pulse oximeter Plastic clip with a red light that measures blood oxygen saturations. Clip onto the patient's index finger. Do not rely on reading unless there is an even trace on the monitor and the patient has a pulse.

Nebuliser This is a 3cm-high cylinder that attaches beneath a mask. The cylinder is made of two halves that can be untwisted so that the nebulised fluid can be inserted. The nebuliser can be connected to a pump or directly to the O_2 supply or medical air.

Circulation

Defibrillator ECG leads Red to right shoulder, yellow to left shoulder and green to apex; turn the defibrillator onto 'monitor'.

Defibrillator paddles You can get a rhythm trace by holding the paddles in position (right paddle to right upper sternal edge, left paddle to apex) and turning the defibrillator onto 'monitor'.

Defibrillation (p474) Only defibrillate if you have been trained:

- check the gel pads are on the chest before you pick up the paddles
- never hold the two paddles in the same hand
- let someone else adjust the settings
- charge the paddles by pressing the charge button
- tell staff to stand clear and stand clear yourself
- check the O_2, staff and you are clear (O_2, top, middle, bottom, self)
- check the rhythm is still shockable then press the buttons on both paddles to deliver the charge.

Blood pressure Attach the cuff to the patient's left arm so it is out of the way and leave in place. If it does not work or is not believable (eg AF, arrhythmias) then ask for a manual reading.

Venous access Ideally a pair of brown/grey venflons in the antecubital fossae, however, get the best available (biggest and most central). Remember to take bloods (20ml syringe).

Disability

BMs Use a spot of blood from the venous sample or a skin prick to get a capillary sample.

Examination GCS, pupil size and reactivity to light, posture, tone of all four limbs, plantar reflexes.

Exposure

Get all the patient's clothes off, have a low threshold for cutting them off. Inspect the patient's entire body for clues as to the cause of the arrest, eg rashes, injuries. Remember to cover the patient with a blanket to prevent hypothermia and for decency.

Other investigations

Arterial blood gas Attach a green (23G) needle to a blood gas syringe, feel for the femoral pulse ($^1/_2$ to $^2/_3$ between superior iliac spine and pubic symphysis) and insert the needle vertically until you get blood. Check the blood is pulsing into the needle. Press hard on removal.

Femoral stab If no blood has been taken you can insert a green needle into the femoral vein which is medial to the artery (NAVY). Feel for the artery then aim about 1cm medially (p459). If you hit the artery take 20ml of blood anyway and send for arterial blood gas and normal blood tests, but press hard on removal.

ECG Attach the leads as shown on p471.

CXR Alert the radiographer early so that they can bring the X-ray machine for a portable CXR.

Chest pain emergency

Airway	Check airway is patent; consider manoeuvres/adjuncts
Breathing	If no respiratory effort – **CALL ARREST TEAM**
Circulation	If no palpable pulse – **CALL ARREST TEAM**

Call for **senior help** early if patient deteriorating

- **Sit patient up**
- **High-flow oxygen** in all patients
- **Monitor** pulse oximeter, BP, defibrillator ECG leads if unwell
- Obtain a full set of **observations** including BP in both arms and **ECG**
- Take brief **history** if possible/check **notes**/ask ward staff
- **Examine patient**: condensed CVS, RS, ±abdo exam
- Establish **likely causes** and rule out **serious causes**
- Consider **thrombolysis** (p133)
- Consider giving **aspirin** 300mg PO stat
- **Initiate further treatment**, see following pages
- **Venous access**, take bloods:
  - FBC, U+E, LFT, CRP, glucose, cardiac markers, D-dimer
- Request urgent **CXR**, portable if too unwell
- Call for **senior help** if no improvement or worsening
- **Reassess**, starting with A, B, C…

Life-threatening causes

- Myocardial infarction
- (Tension) pneumothorax
- Acute coronary syndrome
- Aortic dissection
- PE
- Sickle cell crisis

Chest pain

Worrying features ↑↓pulse, ↓BP, ↑RR, ↓GCS, sudden onset, sweating, nausea, vomiting, radiating to back or left arm, ECG changes

Think about ***most likely*** myocardial infarction, acute coronary syndromes, angina, pulmonary embolism, musculoskeletal, pneumonia ***other*** pneumothorax (tension or simple), aortic dissection, pericarditis, sickle cell crisis ***chronic*** reflux and peptic ulcer disease, anaemia

Ask about site (site of onset and radiation), quality (heavy, aching, sharp), intensity (scale of 1–10), timing (onset), associated symptoms (sweating, nausea, palpitations, breathlessness), exacerbating/relieving factors (breathing, position, exertion, eating), recent trauma/exertion ***PMH*** cardiac or respiratory problems, acid indigestion ***DH*** cardiac and respiratory medications, antacids ***SH*** smoking, exercise tolerance

Risk factors:
- *IHD* ↑BP, ↑cholesterol, FH, smoking, obesity, diabetes, previous IHD
- *PE/DVT* previous PE/DVT, immobility, ↑oestrogens, recent surgery, FH, pregnancy, hypercoagulable states, smoking, air travel
- *GI* acid indigestion, known peptic ulcer, alcohol binge

Obs pulse, BP (both arms), RR, sats, temp

Look for pulse rate/rhythm/volume, sweating, pallor, dyspnoea, cyanosis, ↑JVP, asymmetric chest expansion/percussion/breath sounds, chest wall tenderness, mediastinal shift, tracheal tug, swollen ankles, calf pain/swelling/erythema

Investigations ***ECG*** (p470/514 for procedure/interpretation) ***blds*** FBC, U+E, LFT, CRP, D-dimer (if PE suspected), cardiac markers ***ABGs*** taken on O_2 if patient acutely unwell (see p464/506 for procedure/interpretation) ***CXR*** if you suspect a tension pneumothorax, clinically, perform immediate needle decompression (p171), otherwise request a portable CXR if the patient is severely ill (poorer image quality) or standard CXR, see p508 for interpretation ***urgent echo***/CT if large proximal PE or aortic root dissection suspected (discuss with cardiologist on call)

Treatment High-flow (60–100%) O_2 in everyone initially. Consider intravenous opiates if pain is severe.

Diagnoses to exclude Even if you cannot confirm a diagnosis immediately, use the following criteria to rule out life-threatening causes:
- ***cardiac ischaemia*** – normal ECG, normal cardiac markers (p499)[1]
- ***PE*** – normal ECG, ABG, D-dimer, echo, low clinical risk for DVT/PE
- ***pneumothorax*** – clinically and radiologically no pneumothorax
- ***aortic dissection*** – no evidence of shock, left and right systolic BP differ by <15mmHg, no mediastinal widening on CXR, normal echo

Contact cardiology registrar on call for advice if necessary.

1 The various cardiac markers rise at different times, so check locally which you should assay for and at what time-point post onset of chest pain (p129).

	History	Examination	Investigations
STEMI	Sudden onset pain, radiating to left arm/jaw, >20min, breathlessness, sweating, nausea	Dyspnoea, ±arrhythmia, sweating, non-tender	ST elevation, ↑cardiac markers
NSTEMI	Sudden onset pain, radiating to left arm/jaw, >20min, breathlessness, sweating, nausea	Dyspnoea, ±arrhythmia, sweating, non-tender	ST depression or T wave inversion, ↑cardiac markers consistent with MI
Unstable angina	Anginal pain at rest or with ↑frequency, severity or duration	Dyspnoea, ±arrhythmia, sweating, non-tender	ST depression, T wave inversion, mild/modest ↑cardiac markers
Stable angina	Exertional pain, radiating to left arm/jaw, <20min, breathlessness, ↓by rest/GTN	Dyspnoea, tachycardia, non-tender, may be normal after pain resolves	Transient ECG changes, normal cardiac markers, +ve stress ECG + coronary angiography
Pericarditis	History of viral-like illness, pleuritic pain, ↑on lying, ↓sitting forwards	Pericardial rub, otherwise normal CVS and RS examinations	Saddle-shaped ST segments on most ECG leads, ↑CRP/ESR
Aortic dissection	Sudden onset severe interscapular pain, tearing in nature, breathlessness	Tachycardia, ↓BP, difference in brachial pulses and pressures, ↑RR	Mediastinum >8cm on CXR, aortic dilatation on echo/CT, aortic leak on angiogram
Pulmonary embolism	Breathlessness, PE risk factors, may have pleuritic chest pain and haemoptysis	Often normal, may have evidence of DVT (swollen red leg), tachycardia, dyspnoea, ↓BP	ABG: pO_2 ↔/↓, CO_2↓, clear CXR, ↑D-dimer, sinus tachycardia, $S_1Q_3T_3$ (rare), thrombus on echo
Pneumothorax	Sudden onset pleuritic pain, ±trauma, tall and thin, COPD	Mediastinal shift, unequal air entry and expansion, hyper-resonance	Pleura separated from ribs on CXR, other investigations often normal
Pneumonia	Cough, productive with coloured sputum, pleuritic pain, feels unwell	Febrile, asymmetrical air entry, coarse creps (often unilateral), dull to percussion	↑WCC/↑NØ/↑CRP, consolidation on CXR (p508)
Musculoskeletal chest pain	Lifting, impact injury, may be pleuritic, worse on palpation or movement	Tender, respiratory examination normal	ECG and CXR to exclude cardiac cause/pneumothorax in high-risk patients
GORD	Previous indigestion/reflux, known hiatus hernia, ↓by antacids	May have upper abdo tenderness, normal CVS and RS examinations	ECG to exclude cardiac cause, normal CXR, trial of antacids

Classification of spectrum of ischaemic heart disease

		Clinical	ECG	Markers
	Stable angina	Exertional pain	Transient ischaemia	↔
ACS	Unstable angina	Angina pain at rest	Ischaemic; ↓T waves	↔/↑
ACS	STEMI	Clinically MI	ST elevation; Q waves	↑↑
ACS	NSTEMI	Clinically MI	Ischaemic; ↓T waves	↑↑

Serum cardiac markers in suspected acute ischaemic heart disease

The term 'cardiac enzymes' is incorrect when referring to the troponins as these are structural/regulatory proteins and have no enzymic activity.

Creatine kinase (CK)	Enzyme found in all muscle and released in muscle cell lysis; not specific for cardiac muscle. Peaks within 24h post-MI and usually returns to normal within 48–72h.
CK-MB	Cardiac isomer of CK enzyme, so more specific than total CK. Rises and falls in similar fashion to total CK.
Troponins (I or T)	Identification of these in the blood is highly suggestive of myocardial injury, though they can be raised in PE, septicaemia and following tachyarrhythmias (but CK is seldom concurrently raised in these conditions). Detection is usually possible 6h after myocardial injury and levels remain elevated for up to 14d.
Aspartate aminotransferase (AST)	Intracellular enzyme found in many tissues, predominantly liver and muscles (skeletal and cardiac). Traditionally used to aid diagnosis of MI, but seldom used now with the advent of CK-MB and troponins. Rises 6–12h post-MI, peaks 24–36h post-MI and returns to normal 3–5d later.
Lactate dehydrogenase (LDH)	Intracellular enzyme found in most tissues. Traditionally used to aid diagnosis of MI, but seldom used now with the advent of CK-MB and troponins. Rises 8–12h post MI, peaks 3–5d post-MI and remains elevated for >10d.

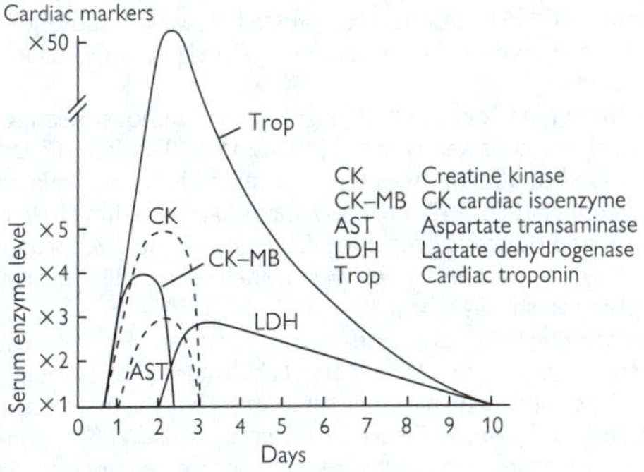

Changes in cardiac markers following an acute myocardial infection

STEMI (ST Elevation MI) (OHAM2 p12)

Symptoms central, crushing, heavy chest pain (>20min), ±radiating to left arm/jaw, shortness of breath, nausea, sweating, palpitations, anxiety
Risk factors smoking, obesity, DM, ↑BP, ↑cholesterol, FH, previous IHD
Signs tachycardia, cool and sweaty ('clammy'), ±LV failure or hypotension
Worrying signs features of LV failure (pulmonary oedema, hypotension)
Investigations *ECG* ST elevation, peaked T waves, new LBBB; subsequently Q waves (commonly), ±T wave inversion *CXR* cardiomegaly, signs of LV failure *cardiac markers* raised
Acute treatment O_2, aspirin (300mg), diamorphine (titrate 1mg boluses up to 5mg), antiemetic (p206), GTN (two puffs sublingually), thrombolysis (p133) – seek senior help to perform thrombolysis; alternatively consider for percutaneous transluminal coronary angioplasty (PTCA – see OHCM6 p118). Consider β-blocker and insulin sliding scale if elevated BM (DIGAMI regime, OHCM6 p783). Needs monitored bed.
Secondary prophylaxis assessment and reduction of modifiable risk factors (smoking, obesity, DM, ↑BP, ↑cholesterol), β-blockade, statin, aspirin, ACEi, symptom management (nitrates, Ca^{2+} channel antagonists)
Complications arrhythmias (heart block, bradycardia, VF/VT, non-VF/VT), LVF, valve prolapse, ventricular septal rupture, ventricular aneurysm formation, pericarditis (Dressler's syndrome, OHCM6 p722)

Sequential ECG changes following an acute STEMI

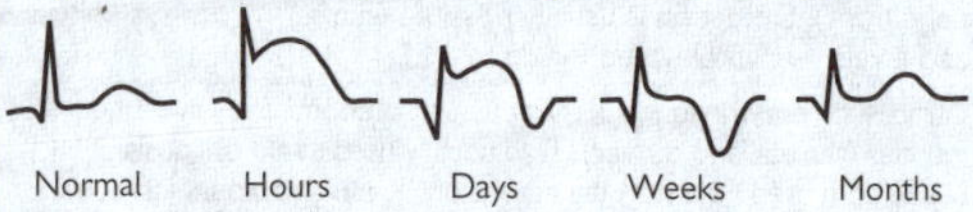

NSTEMI (Non-ST Elevation MI) (OHAM2 p46)

Symptoms central, crushing, heavy chest pain (>20min), ±radiating to left arm/jaw, shortness of breath, nausea, sweating, palpitations, anxiety
Risk factors smoking, obesity, DM, ↑BP, ↑cholesterol, FH, previous IHD
Signs tachycardia, cool and sweaty ('clammy'), ±LV failure or hypotension
Worrying signs features of LV failure (pulmonary oedema, hypotension)
Investigations *ECG* ST depression, inverted T waves; subsequently ±Q waves, ±T wave inversion *CXR* cardiomegaly, signs of LV failure *cardiac markers* raised
Acute treatment As for STEMI. If ongoing pain without meeting criteria for thrombolysis, consider IV nitrate infusion (0.05% Isoket® starting at 4ml/h increased to 10ml/h by increments of 2ml/h every 10min according to BP – keep systolic >90mmHg), anticoagulation with LMWH (p290), continue O_2 and opiates as required. Clopidogrel and glycoprotein IIb/IIIa inhibitors may be indicated under local guidelines (see *BNF*). Early referral for angioplasty to stratify risk.
Secondary prophylaxis assessment and reduction of modifiable risk factors (smoking, obesity, DM, ↑BP, ↑cholesterol), β-blockade, statin, aspirin, ACEi, symptom management (nitrates, Ca^{2+} channel antagonists)
Complications arrhythmias (heart block, bradycardia, VF/VT, non-VF/VT), LVF, valve prolapse, ventricular septal rupture, ventricular aneurysm formation, pericarditis (Dressler's syndrome, OHCM6 p722)

Unstable angina (OHAM2 p46)

Symptoms central, heavy chest pain radiating to left arm and jaw at rest or precipitated by minimal exertion and poorly relieved by rest or GTN, shortness of breath, nausea, sweating, palpitations; episodes lasting longer, more frequently and more severe than typical angina
Risk factors smoking, obesity, DM, ↑BP, ↑cholesterol, FH, previous IHD
Signs tachycardia, cool and sweaty ('clammy'), anxiety, pallor. Often no acute signs after episode has settled.
Investigations *ECG* ST depression, flat or inverted T waves, signs of previous MI *cardiac markers* troponin may be raised, but CK should be less than twice the upper limit of normal (otherwise NSTEMI). If resting ECG normal and no enzyme rise, consider exercise ECG (p472), thallium scan or coronary angiography.
Acute treatment As for STEMI until pain settles. If ongoing pain without meeting criteria for thrombolysis (p133), consider IV nitrate infusion (0.05% Isoket® starting at 4ml/h increased to 10ml/h by increments of 2ml/h every 10min according to BP (keep systolic >90mmHg)), anticoagulation with LMWH (p290), continue O_2 and opiates as required. Clopidogrel and glycoprotein IIb/IIIa inhibitors may be indicated under local guidelines (see *BNF*). Early referral for angioplasty to stratify risk.
Secondary prophylaxis assessment and reduction of modifiable risk factors (smoking, obesity, DM, ↑BP, ↑cholesterol), β-blockade, statin, aspirin, ACEi, symptom management (nitrates, Ca^{2+} channel antagonists)
Complications MI, arrhythmias (heart block, bradycardia, VF/VT, non-VF/VT)

Stable angina (OHCM6 p118)

Symptoms central, heavy chest pain (lasting <20min) radiating to left arm and jaw, precipitated by exertion and relieved by rest or rapidly by GTN (<5min), shortness of breath, nausea, sweating, palpitations
Risk factors smoking, obesity, DM, ↑BP, ↑cholesterol, FH, previous IHD
Signs tachycardia, cool and sweaty ('clammy'), anxiety, pallor. Often no acute signs after episode has settled
Investigations *ECG* transient ST depression, flat or inverted T waves, signs of previous MI *cardiac markers* normal at appropriate times, otherwise ACS (UA/STEMI/NSTEMI). If resting ECG normal and no enzyme rise, consider exercise ECG (p472), thallium scan or coronary angiography.
Acute treatment As for STEMI until pain settles. If ongoing pain without meeting criteria for thrombolysis (p133), treat as for NSTEMI/UA and consider IV nitrate infusion (0.05% Isoket® starting at 4ml/h increased to 10ml/h by increments of 2ml/h every 10min according to BP (keep systolic >90mmHg)), anticoagulation with LMWH (p290), continue O_2 and opiates as required. Glycoprotein IIb/IIIa inhibitors may be indicated under local guidelines (see *BNF*).
Primary prophylaxis assessment and reduction of modifiable risk factors (smoking, obesity, DM, BP, cholesterol), β-blockade, statin, aspirin, ACEi, symptom management (nitrates, Ca^{2+} channel antagonists)

Aortic dissection (OHCM6 p480 or OHAM2 p170)

Symptoms sudden onset severe chest pain, anterior or interscapular, tearing in nature, dizziness, breathlessness, sweating, neurological deficits
Risk factors smoking, obesity, DM, ↑BP, ↑cholesterol, FH, previous IHD
Signs unequal radial pulses, tachycardia, hypotension/hypertension, difference in brachial pressures of >15mmHg, aortic regurgitation, pleural effusion (L>R), neurological deficits from carotid artery dissection
Investigations *ECG* may be normal or show LV strain/ischaemia *CXR* classically widened mediastinum >8cm (rarely seen), enlargement of aortic knuckle and small left pleural effusion can develop from blood tracking down *echo* may show aortic root leak, aortic valve regurgitation or pericardial effusion. Also consider MRI/CT/conventional angiography.
Acute treatment If hypotensive, treat as shock (p148). O_2, two large-bore cannulas, crossmatch 10 units, analgesia (IV opiates), seek immediate cardiology/senior assessment
Chronic treatment surgery or medical management (OHAM2 p174)

Musculoskeletal chest pain (OHAEM2 p62)

Symptoms localised chest wall pain, worse on movement and/or breathing, recent trauma or exertion (eg lifting)
Signs focal tenderness, erythema, absence of other signs in CVS or RS
Investigations only investigate if you cannot satisfy yourself of the diagnosis on clinical grounds *ECG* normal (no ischaemia/MI) *CXR* normal (no pneumothorax) *D-dimer* normal
Acute treatment reassurance and simple analgesia (p282)
Chronic treatment should settle within 2wk, prevention from further injury (no more heavy lifting for a few weeks), adequate regular analgesia to allow activities of daily living to be carried out and to allow deep inspiration and coughing (to prevent chest infection), stop smoking

Pericarditis (OHCM6 p158)

Symptoms pleuritic chest pain, worse on lying flat and deep inspiration, relieved by sitting forwards, developed following a viral illnesses
Signs may be no abnormalities, ±pericardial rub
Investigations *ECG* saddle-shaped ST segments on most leads (concave upwards) *blds* ↑WCC and inflammatory markers, ±↑viral titres *echo* ±pericardial effusion
Acute treatment reassurance and analgesia (p282)

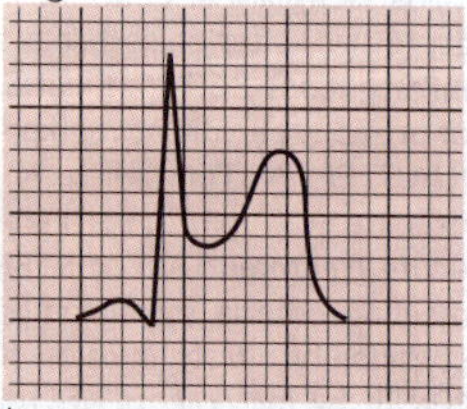

Chronic treatment should settle within 2–4wk; recurrence common

Bradyarrhythmia	p143	Reflux and gastric disease	p187
Tachyarrhythmia	p135	Pneumonia, PE, pneumothorax	p168

Symptoms still worsening or not resolving?

Obtain senior help. Reassess A, B, C; consider rechecking observations and investigations. Are you satisfied with the working diagnosis? Could this be something else or is there room for further analgesia/treatment?

Thrombolysis

If given within 12h of onset of chest pain, thrombolysis reduces immediate and subsequent morbidity and mortality; ideally given within 60min (OHCM6 p782).

Indications One of:

- ST elevation >2mm in two or more adjacent chest leads (V1–V6)
- ST elevation >1mm in two or more adjacent limb leads
- posterior infarct (p521)
- new onset left bundle branch block (LBBB – p516)

Contraindications Each patient must be assessed individually as there are no hard and fast rules about absolute and relative contraindications.

- Internal bleeding
- Prolonged/traumatic CPR
- Heavy vaginal bleeding
- Acute pancreatitis
- Active lung disease with cavitation
- Recent trauma or surgery (<2wk)
- Cerebral neoplasm
- Severe hypertension (>200/120)
- Suspected aortic dissection
- Previous allergic reaction
- Pregnancy or <8wk postnatal
- Severe liver disease
- Oesophageal varices/bleeding ulcer
- Recent head injury
- Haemorrhagic stroke
- Other CVA within 6/12

Streptokinase (SK) is a bacterial enzyme so can precipitate anaphylaxis. Give 1.5 million units in 100ml 0.9% saline over 1h IV. SE: nausea, vomiting, ↓BP, haemorrhage, stroke (1%), reperfusion dysrhythmias. Hypotension often resolves by slowing infusion. Do not give again after 4d due to risk of anaphylaxis/ineffective due to antibody response.

Recombinant tissue-type plasminogen activator (rt-PA) may be used if the patient has previously received SK and is the first-line agent in some institutions (eg alteplase, reteplase and tenecteplase). Dose depends on agent and is given as a bolus followed by heparin for anticoagulation.

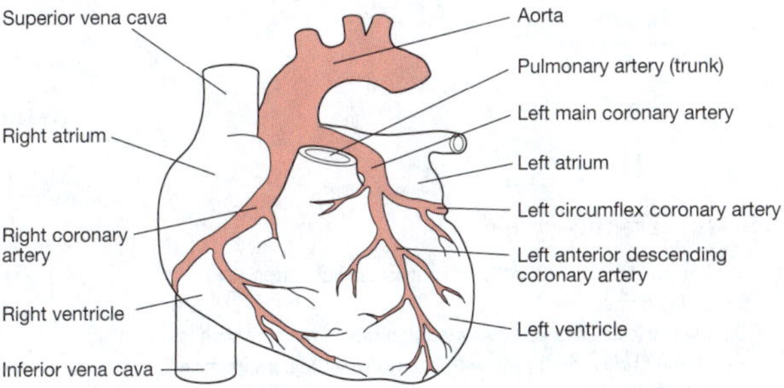

Structure of the heart and its coronary blood supply

Tachyarrhythmia emergency

Airway	Check airway is patent; consider manoeuvres/adjuncts
Breathing	If no respiratory effort – **CALL ARREST TEAM**
Circulation	If no palpable pulse – **CALL ARREST TEAM**

Call for **senior help** early if patient deteriorating
Pulse >100:

- **Sit patient up** unless hypotensive, then lay flat with legs elevated
- **High-flow oxygen** in all patients
- **Monitor** pulse oximeter, BP, defibrillator ECG leads if unwell
- Request full set of **observations** and **ECG**
- Take brief **history** if possible/check **notes**/ask ward staff
- **Examine patient**: condensed CVS, RS, ±abdo exam
- Establish **likely causes** and rule out **serious causes**
- **Initiate further treatment**, see following pages
- **Venous access**, take bloods:
  - FBC, U+E, LFT, CRP, D-dimer, cardiac markers, TFT
- Consider requesting urgent **CXR**, portable if too unwell
- Call for **senior help**
- **Reassess**, starting with A, B, C…

Life-threatening causes

- Ventricular tachycardia (VT) or ventricular fibrillation (VF)
- Torsades de pointes
- Supraventricular tachycardia with haemodynamic compromise
- Fast atrial fibrillation/flutter with haemodynamic compromise
- Sinus tachycardia
  - Secondary to shock, including PE
  - Iatrogenic (drugs)

Tachyarrhythmias

> **Worrying features** ↓GCS, ↓BP, ↑RR, chest pain, sweating, dizziness

Think about ***common*** sinus tachycardia, fast ventricular rate in AF, supraventricular tachycardia (SVT), atrial flutter ***other*** ventricular tachycardia (VT), re-entrant tachycardia (eg Wolff-Parkinson-White)

Ask about onset, associated symptoms (chest pain, shortness of breath, dizziness, palpitations, facial flushing, headache), previous episodes ***PMH*** cardiac problems (IHD, valvular lesions, hypertension), thyroid disease, DM ***DH*** cardiac drugs, thyroxine, salbutamol, anticholinergics, caffeine, nicotine, allergies ***SH*** smoking, alcohol, recreational drug use
AF risk factors ↑BP, coronary artery and valvular heart disease, pulmonary embolism, pneumonia, thyrotoxicosis, alcohol
Sinus tachycardia risk factors shock (hypovolaemic, cardiogenic, septic, anaphylactic, spinal), pain/anxiety, fever, drugs

Obs pulse (rate/rhythm/volume), BP, cap refill, RR, O_2 sats, GCS (or AVPU), temp

Look for sweating, tremor, pallor, dyspnoea, cyanosis, JVP, any precipitant of AF or sinus tachycardia (causes of shock, p150)

Investigations ***ECG*** P waves before each QRS imply sinus rhythm, irregular QRS without clear P waves implies AF, saw-tooth baseline implies atrial flutter, rate of ≥140 (narrow complexes) suggests SVT (including flutter with block), broad regular complexes suggests VT (always check for pulse) ***blds*** FBC, U+E, TFT, CRP, D-dimer (if PE suspected), cardiac markers, others as indicated by suspicion (eg crossmatch if haemorrhage) ***ABGs*** only when initial treatment has been initiated or results likely to alter management ***CXR*** only once initial treatment has been initiated or results are likely to alter management ***urgent echo*** only if large PE, acute valvular lesion or pericardial effusion is suspected

Treatment

In all patients

- Airway, breathing (with O_2), circulation (pulse, BP and capillary refill)
- IV access (two large bore cannula in both antecubital fossa)
- Obtain ECG or view trace on defibrillator to decide on rhythm
- If hypotensive or dizzy lay flat with legs up – call senior help
- If semi-conscious lay in recovery position – call senior/ARREST TEAM

Specific arrhythmias

- ***Sinus tachycardia*** Establish cause of sinus tachycardia, ?shock (p149)
- **AF** Is the patient normally in AF or is this new onset? (p137)
- ***SVT*** Usually time to call for help and get drugs ready (p139)
- ***VT no pulse*** Call ARREST TEAM and start BLS/ALS (p122)
- ***VT with pulse*** Call senior help and anaesthetist; cardioversion (p474). May respond to amiodarone (p138)

ECG features of tachyarrhythmias

	Rate	Regular	P waves	Broad/narrow
Sinus tachycardia	>100	✓	✓	Narrow (unless BBB)
Fast AF	>100	×	×	Narrow (unless BBB)
SVT	≥140	✓	✓	Narrow (unless BBB)
VT with pulse	≥150	✓	×	Broad
VT pulseless	As for 'VT with pulse'; always perform a pulse-check (carotid)			
VF	Chaotic irregular electrical activity. Never has a pulse			

Typical appearance of various tachyarrhythmias

	ECG, lead II view (rhythm strip)
Sinus tachycardia	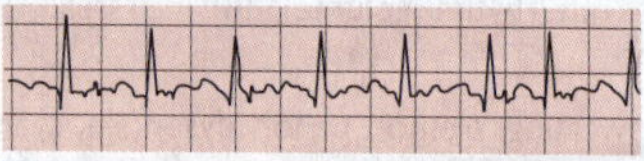
Fast AF	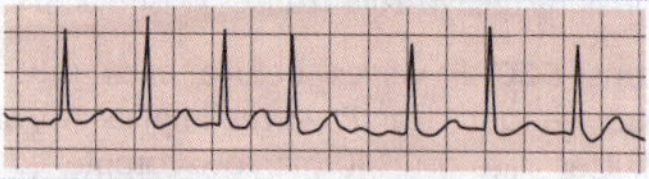
SVT	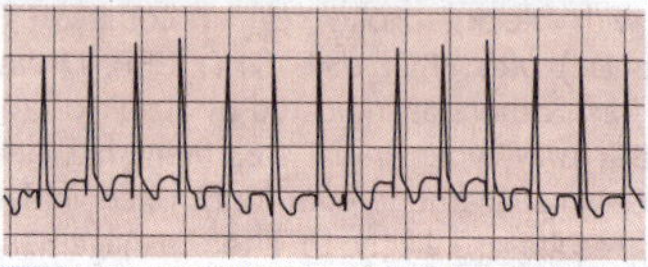
VT with or without a pulse	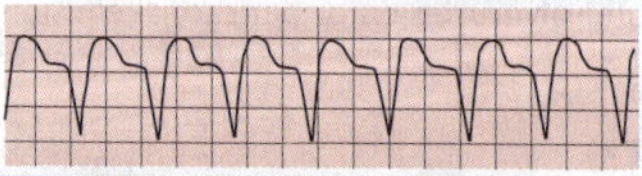
VF	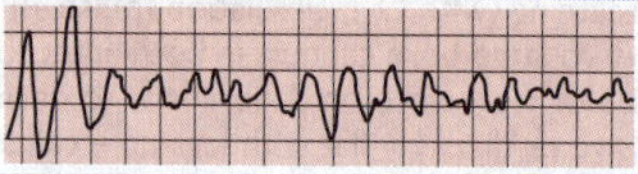

Fast atrial fibrillation (AF)/flutter (OHAM2 p84)

Symptoms palpitations, shortness of breath, dizziness, ±chest pains
Risk factors previous AF, ↑BP, IHD, valvular heart disease, PE, pneumonia, thyrotoxicosis, alcohol (acute excess, chronic use or withdrawal), dilated cardiomyopathy, ↑age, acute illness
Signs irregularly irregular pulse, hypotension if cardiovascular compromise, signs of concurrent/precipitant disease (pneumonia, thyrotoxicosis)
Worrying signs features of heart failure, hypotension or ↓GCS
Investigations *ECG* absent P waves, irregularly irregular QRS complexes in AF; saw-tooth appearance of baseline in atrial flutter *blds* FBC (↑WCC), U+E, TFT, alcohol, ±D-dimer (PE) *CXR* heart size, pulmonary oedema, pneumonia *echo* LV dilatation/impairment, valvular lesion
Acute treatment

- ***Haemodynamic compromise*** treat as shock (p149); O_2, IV access, needs rapid rate-control or restoration of sinus rhythm (DC cardioversion, see below). Seek immediate senior help
- ***Haemodynamically stable*** and AF present for >2d, load with digoxin (p138) and anti-coagulate with LMWH (p290). Seek senior advice
- ***Haemodynamically stable*** and AF present for <2d, aim to chemically cardiovert with flecainide, disopyramide or amiodarone and anti-coagulate with LMWH (p290). Seek senior advice for dosing regimen

Chronic management identify precipitant of AF (echo, stress ECG, TFT, CXR), anticoagulate, maintain sinus rhythm chemically or, if unsuccessful, consider elective DC cardioversion
Complications thrombo-embolic disease (eg ischaemic stroke commonly). Drug side effects (amiodarone, warfarin, β-blockers, digoxin etc).

DC cardioversion for arrhythmia with haemodynamic compromise

Call senior help. Check pulse. If no pulse commence BLS/ALS (p123)

Contraindications	Digoxin toxicity (start with lower energies) Electrolyte imbalance Inadequate anticoagulation in chronic AF (relative CI)
Sedation	Anaesthetist – short general anaesthetic with propofol
Paddles	Use hand-free paddles if available – safer
Starting energy[1] (monophasic)[2]	VT – 100J synchronised (100, 200, 360) AF – 100J synchronised (100, 200, 360) SVT – 100J synchronised (100, 200, 360) If initial shock unsuccessful increase energy as indicated in ( )
Unsuccessful	Change paddle position. Check contact with gel-pads
Complications	Asystole/bradyarrhythmia/ventricular fibrillation Thromboembolism Skin burns Aspiration

1 Advanced Life Support Guidelines 2004.
2 If using a biphasic defibrillator see local guidelines.

Starting digoxin therapy (OHAM2 p82)

Control of the ventricular rate in fast AF can be achieved with several drugs, as well as with DC cardioversion. The maintenance dose of digoxin depends upon ventricular rate (needs higher dose if rate poorly controlled) and patient factors (such as renal function).

Digoxin does not restore sinus rhythm, it merely slows conduction at the atrio-ventricular node, limiting the number of impulses passing from the atria through to the ventricles thus controlling ventricular rate.

Urgent loading as follows (also see *BNF*)

- Loading dose 500µg/over 30min IVI (in saline or glucose)
  - Use 250µg if patient very elderly, small or frail
- Repeat loading dose of 500µg/over 30min IVI 8h later
  - Use 250µg if patient very elderly, small or frail
- Commence maintenance dose (62.5 to 500µg/24h PO) 8h later

Non-urgent loading can be undertaken by commencing a likely maintenance dose (eg 125µg/24h PO).

Therapeutic monitoring can be undertaken if toxicity is considered or if compliance is questioned. Sample should be taken 6–12h post-oral dose (p569).

Digoxin toxicity (p146) is increased in ↓K^+, ↓Mg^{2+} or ↑Ca^{2+} and in renal impairment, therefore use a reduced dose.

Other anti-arrhythmics used in the treatment of tachyarrhythmias

Patient must be in a monitored bed during administration of these agents

Amiodarone (should be given via a central vein, but can be given peripherally in an emergency)	**Loading dose** 300mg/over 60min IVI via central line followed by 900mg/over 23h IVI via central line OR 200mg/8h PO for 1wk then 200mg/12h PO for 1wk **Maintenance dose** 200–400mg/24h PO
Disopyramide (rarely used)	2mg/kg/over 10min IV repeated every 5min to maximum 150mg OR 100–200mg/6h PO
Flecainide (caution if pt has IHD)	2mg/kg/over 10min IV (maximum 150mg) OR 100–200mg/12h PO
Procainamide (rarely used)	100mg/over 2min IV repeated every 5min to maximum 1g OR 250mg/6h PO
Verapamil (avoid if pt on β-blockers)	5mg/over 2min IV repeated every 5min to maximum 20mg OR 40–120mg/8h PO

Supraventricular tachycardia (SVT) (OHAM2 p78)

Symptoms palpitations, shortness of breath, dizziness, ±chest pains
Risk factors previous SVT, trauma, structural cardiac anomaly, alcohol
Signs tachycardia, anxiety, hypotension if haemodynamic compromise
Worrying signs one or more of: heart failure, hypotension or ↓GCS
Investigations ECG narrow complex tachycardia (unless concurrent BBB) with P waves (which may merge into QRS), regular QRS complexes, rate usually ≥140 *further investigations* only required if diagnosis in question, otherwise initiate treatment as below
Acute treatment O_2, large-bore IV access (antecubital fossa). Monitor rhythm on defibrillator.

- ***Vagal maneouvres*** get patient to strain down as though passing stool or attempt to blow the plunger out of a clean 10ml syringe from the narrow end. If this fails, gently massage each carotid artery in turn, about 1cm below and anterior to the angle for the jaw for 10s; never both at the same time
- ***Chemical*** adenosine 6mg fast bolus followed by rapid 5–10ml saline flush. If unsuccessful administer higher doses of 12mg, 12mg, 12mg at 1–2min intervals (relatively contraindicated in asthma); warn patient about transient flushing, chest tightness. Record rhythm changes on defibrillators printer, underlying AF may be revealed and transient asystole is common. If unsuccessful consider other agents (OHAM2 p82) under expert guidance (eg verapamil, β-blockers)

Chronic treatment if recurrent, seek cardiology advice as may require electrophysiological testing of cardiac conduction pathways
Complications hypotension, heart failure in individuals with existing cardiac disease, deterioration into more sinister arrhythmia

Accessory pathway tachycardias (re-entrant tachycardias)

Avoid digoxin and verapamil; may accelerate conduction down accessory pathway

Kent bundle (Wolff-Parkinson-White syndrome)

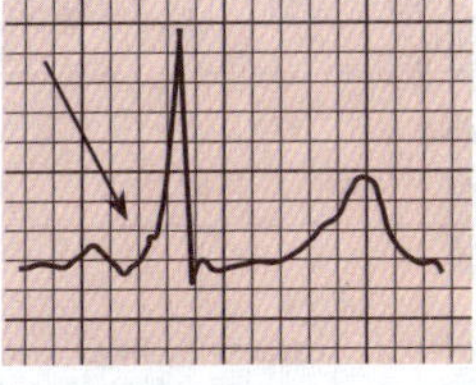

Short PR interval and delta (δ) wave (shown by arrow)

Three types:

A positive δ wave in V1–V6, not in lead I
B biphasic/negative δ wave in V1–V3, positive in lead I
Concealed no δ wave visible, conducts retrogradely

(δ wave represents aberrant conduction pathway between atria and ventricles)

Mahaim pathway
Pathway connects AV node to right bundle resulting in tachycardia with LBBB morphology

James pathway (Lown-Ganong-Levine syndrome)
Short PR interval but no δ wave
Pathway connects atria to AV node, His or fascicles

Ventricular tachycardia (VT) (OHAM2 p68)

Symptoms palpitations, dizziness, shortness of breath, ±chest pain, arrest
Risk factors IHD, trauma, hypoxia, acidosis, long QT
Signs tachycardia, anxiety, pallor, hypotension, ↓GCS, shock
Worrying signs one or more of: heart failure, hypotension or ↓GCS
Investigations *ECG* broad complex tachycardia, absence of P waves, rate usually >150 *blds* check urgent U+E (especially K^+) and Mg^{2+} *other investigations* should be directed by clinical situation though cardioversion is main priority at this stage
Acute treatment

- ***Pulseless VT*** Call ARREST TEAM, commence BLS/ALS (p122) after precordial thump
- ***VT with a pulse*** O_2, two large-bore IV cannula in antecubital fossa, call senior help. Restoration of sinus rhythm with either drugs (eg sotalol, amiodarone, magnesium) or DC cardioversion. Seek senior advice
- ***?SVT with BBB or VT*** Treat as VT

Chronic treatment may need drug therapy to maintain sinus rhythm, electrophysiological studies/ablation or implantable cardioverter/defibrillator (OHAM2 p70).
Complications may deteriorate into VF or other dysrhythmia.

Causes of prolonged QT interval

Normal QTc = QT/√(RR interval) = 0.38 – 0.46s (9 – 11 small sq.)	
Congenital	Jervell, Lange-Neilsen syndrome Romano-Ward syndrome
Drugs	Anti-arrhythmics (amiodarone, sotalol, quinidine) Antipsychotics (thioridazine, pimozide) Antihistamines (terfenadine, astemizole) Antimalarials (halofantrine) Organophosphate poisoning
Electrolyte disturbance	↓/↑K^+, ↓Mg^{2+}, ↓Ca^{2+}
Severe bradycardia	Complete heart block, sinus bradycardia
IHD	Ischaemia, myocarditis
Intracranial bleed	Sub-arachnoid haemorrhage

Shock/hypotension	p149	Hyperthyroidism	p239

Symptoms still worsening?

Obtain senior help or specialist cardiology input. Reassess A, B, C; consider rechecking observations and investigations. Are you satisfied with the working diagnosis?

Bradyarrhythmia emergency

Airway	Check airway is patent; consider manoeuvres/adjuncts
Breathing	If no respiratory effort – **CALL ARREST TEAM**
Circulation	If no palpable pulse – **CALL ARREST TEAM**

Call for **senior help** early if patient deteriorating
Pulse <50:

- **Sit patient up** unless hypotensive/dizzy, then lay flat with legs elevated
- **High-flow oxygen** in all patients
- **Monitor** pulse oximeter, BP, defibrillator's ECG leads if very unwell
- Request full set of **observations** and **ECG** with **rhythm strip**
- Take brief **history** if possible/check **notes**/ask ward staff
- **Examine patient**: condensed CVS, RS, ±abdo exam
- Establish **likely causes** and rule out **serious causes**
- Consider IV **atropine**, 0.3mg stat, repeat at 2–3min intervals (max 3mg)
- **Initiate further treatment**, see following pages
- **Venous access**, take bloods
  - FBC, U+E, LFT, CRP, cardiac markers, TFT
- Consider requesting urgent **CXR**, portable if too unwell
- Call for **senior help**
- **Reassess**, starting with A, B, C…

Life-threatening causes

- Complete (3rd degree) heart block (±following MI)
- Mobitz type II
- Pauses >3sec on ECG
- Hypoxia in children

Bradyarrhythmias

Worrying features systolic BP <90, pulse <40, heart failure, ↓GCS, chest pain, dizzy

Think about ***sinus bradycardia*** MI, drugs (including digoxin toxicity), vasovagal, hypothyroidism, hypothermia, Cushing's reflex (bradycardia and hypertension 2° to ↑ICP), sleep, physical fitness ***complete or 3rd degree atrioventricular (AV) heart block***

Ask about dizziness, postural dizziness, fits/faints, weight change, visual disturbance, nausea, vomiting ***PMH*** cardiac disease (IHD/AF), thyroid disease/surgery, DM, head injury or intracranial pathology, glaucoma ***DH*** cardiac medications (β-blockers, Ca^{2+} antagonists, amiodarone, digoxin), eye drops (β-blockers), allergies ***SH*** exercise tolerance

IHD risk factors ↑BP, ↑cholesterol, FH, smoking, obesity, diabetes, previous angina/MI

Obs pulse, BP, postural BP, RR, sats, temp, GCS

Look for pulse rate/rhythm/volume, pallor, shortness of breath, ↓GCS, drowsy, ↑JVP (cannon waves in 3rd degree AV block), signs of cardiac failure (↑JVP, pulmonary oedema, swollen ankles), features of hypothyroidism (myxoedema, hair loss, dry skin, slow reflexes – p239), signs of ↑ICP (papilloedema, focal neurology – p212)

Investigations ***ECG*** sinus bradycardia or complete heart block (see p144); evidence of ischaemia or infarction (p514) or of digoxin toxicity (p146) ***blds*** FBC, U+E, glucose, Ca^{2+}, Mg^{2+}, TFT, cardiac markers, digoxin level, coagulation (if considering pacing-wire) ***CXR*** unlikely to be helpful in the immediate setting, but may reveal heart size and evidence of pulmonary oedema ***head CT*** useful if you suspect raised intracranial pressure, though patient will be *in extremis* (about to cone, see p226) if ↑ICP causing bradycardia (speak to neuroradiologist and neurosurgeon on call)

Treatment

- Airway, breathing (with O_2) and monitor circulation
- If either ↓GCS or ↓BP (<90mmHg systolic), call for senior help or ARREST TEAM
- IV cannula and take bloods
- Consider giving IV atropine if systolic BP <90mmHg (0.3mg at 2–3 min intervals to a maximum of 3mg). Atropine is available in the cardiac arrest trolley and usually comes as 3mg in 10ml (0.3mg/ml); give 1ml increments for symptomatic bradyarrhythmias
- Check ECG to exclude myocardial infarction and to identify heart block or extreme sinus bradycardia or very slow atrial fibrillation

ECG features of bradyarrhythmias and types of heart block

Sinus bradycardia	P waves precede each QRS, rate <60
1st degree AV block	P–R interval >5 small squares (>0.2s)
Mobitz I (Wenkebach)	P–R interval lengthens until failure of AV conduction
Mobitz II	Intermittent P waves fail to conduct to ventricles, but P–R interval does not lengthen, unlike Mobitz type I
2:1, 3:1 AV block	Only 2nd or 3rd P wave conducts to the ventricle
3rd degree AV block	Complete dissociation between P waves and QRS
Digoxin effect/toxicity	Down-sloping ST segment (reversed tick), inverted T waves
Rate controlled AF	No P waves; irregular, irregular rhythm

Typical appearance of various bradyarrhythmias and types of heart block

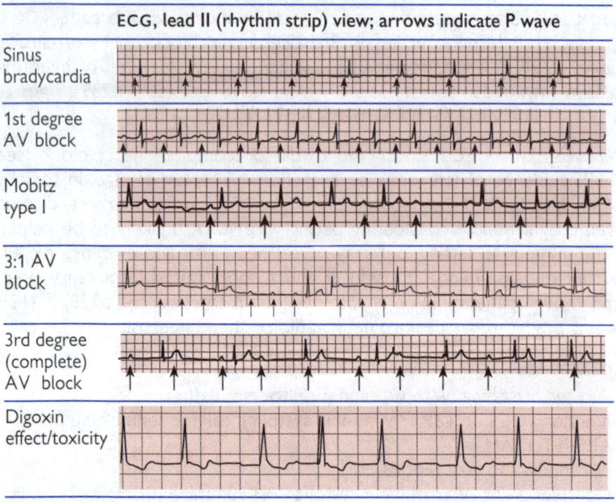

Sinus bradycardia (OHAM2 p102)

Symptoms asymptomatic, dizziness (±on standing), palpitations, shortness of breath, symptoms of either ↑ICP, hypothermia or hypothyroidism
Signs orthostatic ↓BP, hypothermia, evidence of ↑ICP (p212) or hypothyroidism (p239)
Worrying signs features of heart failure, hypotension, ↓GCS
Investigations *ECG* QRS complex will be preceded by a P wave, rate <60, QRS will be narrow unless BBB; exclude ischaemia/infarction *blds* FBC, U+E, Ca^{2+}, Mg^{2+}, TFT, cardiac markers, coagulation (if considering pacing-wire) *CXR* unlikely to be helpful in immediate resuscitation phase
Acute treatment if symptomatic (dizzy or GCS <15) or systolic <90mmHg, monitor heart rate on defibrillator, lay flat with legs elevated (as long as ↑ICP not suspected). O_2, secure IV access and take bloods. Call senior help/ARREST TEAM. Titrate 0.3mg atropine IV every 2–3min (to a maximum of 3mg) followed by a large flush, until HR improves. Identify and correct precipitant. Consider external pacing/pacing-wire via central line (p476) though seek senior advice first.
Chronic treatment may need permanent pacemaker (OHCM6 p134)
Complications bradycardia and high vagal tone can deteriorate into asystole so prompt treatment is required. Remember to regularly check for a pulse since PEA is common and the ECG trace will not change.

Vasovagal attacks

Sudden reflex bradycardia from unopposed parasympathetic inhibition upon heart rate is common and several factors are known to precipitate this.

Fear and pain (including needles)
Prolonged standing
Post-micturition (especially in men)
Nausea and vomiting
Dilatation of anal sphincter and cervix (during surgery)
Pulling of extra-ocular muscles and pressure on eye (during ophthalmic surgery)
↑intra-abdominal pressure (during laparoscopic surgery)

Drugs which can precipitate bradycardia

β-blockers	Reports of bradycardia from β-blocking eye drops
Digoxin	Rhythm likely to be AF, but may be sinus if reverted
Ca^{2+} antagonists	Verapamil and diltiazem slow heart rate
Amiodarone	Can cause conduction defects and bradycardia
α-agonists	Phenylephrine is mainly used by anaesthetists and can cause reflex bradycardia by increasing peripheral vascular resistance

Sick sinus syndrome

Dysfunction of the sinoatrial node, often precipitated by ischaemia/fibrosis. Results in bradycardia (±arrest), sinoatrial block or SVT with alternating bradycardia/asystole (tachy-brady syndrome). Needs pacing if symptomatic.

Complete (3rd degree) heart block (OHAM2 p106)

Symptoms asymptomatic, dizziness (±on standing), palpitations, shortness of breath, ±chest pain
Causes congenital, fibrosis, ischaemic, post-cardiac surgery, drug-induced (amiodarone, β-blockers, Ca^{2+}channel blockers), infective, neuromuscular
Signs ↓BP (and potentially ↓GCS), cannon waves in ↑JVP (due to asynchronous contraction of the right atria against a closed tricuspid valve), signs of heart failure, features of underlying disease
Worrying signs features of heart failure, hypotension, ↓GCS
Investigations *ECG* complete dissociation of P waves from QRS complexes; narrow QRS implies proximal lesion (may respond to atropine), broad QRS implies distal lesion (unlikely to respond to atropine); look for evidence of myocardial infarction *blds* FBC, U+E, cardiac markers, coagulation (if considering pacing-wire) *CXR* unlikely to be helpful in immediate resuscitation phase
Acute treatment if symptomatic (dizzy or GCS <15) or systolic <90mmHg, monitor heart rate on defibrillator, lay flat with legs elevated. O_2 supplementation, secure IV access and take bloods. Call senior help/ ARREST TEAM. Titrate 0.3mg atropine IV every 2–3min (to a maximum of 3mg), followed by a large flush, until HR improves. Identify and correct precipitant. Consider external pacing/pacing-wire via central line (p476) though obtain senior advice.
Chronic treatment likely to need permanent pacemaker (OHCM6 p134) and/or correction of precipitant
Complications severe bradycardia and high vagal tone can deteriorate into asystole so prompt treatment is required. Regularly check for a pulse since PEA is common and the ECG trace will not change.

Digoxin toxicity (OHAM2 p808)

Symptoms	Nausea, vomiting, confusion, diarrhoea, yellow and blurred vision
Bloods	Toxicity precipitated by renal failure, ↓K^+, ↓Mg^{2+} and ↓T_4 Check digoxin level (p569); toxic if >2.6nmol/l (>2µg/l)
ECG (p144)	Tachy- and bradyarrhythmias. ST depression/T wave inversion
Complications	↑K^+, cardiac dysrhythmias (tachy- and bradyarrhythmias)
Management	Airway, breathing, and circulation Continuous ECG monitoring Treat tachy- and bradyarrhythmias as described Consider *digoxin-binding antibody fragments* if cardiovascular compromise, resistant ventricular tachyarrhythmias or ↑K^+

Symptoms still worsening?

Obtain senior help. Reassess A, B, C; consider rechecking observations and investigations. Have you tried atropine (see above)? Consider external pacing[1] (OHAM2 p101).

1 Not all defibrillators can pace, so use the time waiting for senior help to get hold of a pacing-defibrillator (try CCU, A+E or theatres) and appropriate external pacing-pads.

Hypotension emergency

Airway	Check airway is patent; consider manoeuvres/adjuncts
Breathing	If no respiratory effort – **CALL ARREST TEAM**
Circulation	If no palpable pulse – **CALL ARREST TEAM**

Call for **senior help** early if patient deteriorating
Systolic <100:

- Lay patient flat and **elevate the legs** if dizzy
- **High-flow oxygen** in all patients
- **Monitor** pulse oximeter, BP, defibrillator ECG leads if unwell
- Request full set of **observations** and **ECG**
- Take brief **history** if possible/check **notes**/ask ward staff
- **Examine patient:** condensed RS, CVS, abdo and neuro exam
- Establish **likely causes** and rule out **serious causes**
- Large-bore **venous access**, take bloods:
    - FBC, U+E, LFT, CRP, D-dimer, cardiac markers, blood cultures
- Intravenous infusion of **1l 0.9% saline**, stat
- **Initiate further treatment**, see following pages
- **Arterial blood gas**, but don't leave the patient alone
- Consider requesting urgent CXR, portable if too unwell
- Call for **senior help**
- **Reassess**, starting with A, B, C…

Life-threatening causes

- Hypovolaemic/haemorrhagic shock
- Septic shock
- Cardiogenic shock (tamponade/tension pneumothorax/heart failure)
- Anaphylactic shock
- Neurogenic shock (spinal shock)

Hypotension (systolic<100)

Worrying features ↓GCS, ↑↓pulse, stridor, ↓O_2 sats, bleeding, chest pain, dizziness, low urine output, renal failure, severe back pain, non-blanching rash

Think about ***life-threatening*** shock (hypovolaemic/haemorrhagic, septic, cardiogenic, anaphylactic, neurogenic), dysrhythmia (brady- or tachyarrhythmia) ***other*** postural hypotension, vasovagal episode, Addison's disease/adrenal insufficiency, iatrogenic (β-blockers, ACE inhibitors, Ca^{2+}channel blockers, diuretics, nitrates)

Ask about palpitations, chest pain, shortness of breath, feeling faint/dizzy on standing, blood loss (haematemesis, melaena, PV bleeding), trauma, abdominal/back/loin pain, diarrhoea, vomiting, indigestion, polyuria, fever, sweats, cough, urinary symptoms, itch/urticaria, chest tightness, spinal trauma or anaesthetic, weight loss, skin darkening ***PMH*** AAA, gastroduodenal ulcers, pregnancy, diabetes insipidus and mellitus, infections (urinary, chest, cardiac, blood), immunocompromise, angina, MI, previous DVT/PE, Addison's disease, postural hypotension ***DH*** blood transfusions, antibiotics, cardiac medications (β-blockers, ACE inhibitors, Ca^{2+} channel blockers, diuretics, nitrates) heparin/warfarin, recent anaesthetics, steroids (?withdrawal) ***FH*** PE/DVT, Addison's/autoimmune disease ***SH*** smoking, alcohol, recreational drug abuse, IV drug use

Obs pulse, BP, postural BP, RR, sats, temp, GCS, fluid balance

Look for volume status (p262), pulse rate/rhythm/volume, evidence of diarrhoea or vomiting, source of bleeding (limbs, chest, abdomen, back, mouth, anus, vagina and head), palpable abdominal aortic aneurysm, abdominal guarding or tenderness, warm peripheries or fever, flushed appearance, sweating, urticaria, dyspnoea, focal signs in the chest (consolidation, pneumothorax (tension) or pulmonary oedema), calf swelling or tenderness, wasting of small muscles of the hands, ↑skin pigmentation

Investigations ***serial BP*** repeat BP manually to confirm diagnosis and check bilateral BP ***ECG*** arrhythmia, evidence of LVH/strain/MI ***blds*** FBC, U+E, LFT, glucose, G+S (crossmatch if haemorrhage), CRP, D-dimer, cardiac markers, clotting, blood cultures ***CXR*** do not request if you suspect tension pneumothorax – perform immediate needle decompression (p171); consolidation, mediastinal width ***urine*** catheterise, dipstix ±M,C+S, mast cell tryptase if anaphylaxis suspected ***urgent echo*** LV function, aortic root dilation/dissection, pericardial fluid (tamponade effect), massive PE, aortic/mitral valve prolapse ***other*** pelvic X-ray in trauma, CT chest may be necessary if aortic dissection suspected, central venous pressure monitoring may be needed via a central line, continuous arterial pressure can be monitored via an arterial line

Treatment

- Airway, breathing (with 100% O_2) and monitor BP; elevate legs
- IV access, 14G (orange/brown) cannulae in both antecubital fossa
- If bleeding give, IV colloids and consider blood
- Otherwise give 1l 0.9% saline stat
- Establish and treat likely cause
- Call for senior help early

Clinical markers in shock – how to differentiate between the types of shock

	Hypovolaemia/ haemorrhage	Sepsis	Cardiogenic	Anaphylaxis	Spinal
Pulse	↑	↑	↑	↑	↓
BP	↔/↓	↓	↓	↔/↓	↓
JVP	↓	↓	↑	↓	↓
Peripheries	Cool	Warm	Cool	Cool/warm	Warm

Main causes of shock – inadequate organ perfusion and tissue oxygenation

Haemorrhagic/ hypovolaemic	● External blood loss (eg scalp laceration) ● Internal blood loss (eg ruptured AAA/pelvic fracture) ● Severe dehydration • Inadequate fluid intake (eg starvation) • Excessive fluid loss (eg diarrhoea, sweating) • 3rd space loss (eg pancreatitis)
Septic	● Septicaemia • Blood-borne infection, ?source
Cardiogenic	● Pump failure/ineffective pump • Severe LV dysfunction • Outflow tract obstruction (eg aortic dissection) • Dysrhythmia (tachy- or bradyarrhythmia) ● Inadequate pump filling • Pulmonary embolism • Cardiac tamponade • Tension pneumothorax (or large simple)
Anaphylactic	● Systemic inflammatory response/dilatation • Anaphylactic or anaphylactoid reactions[1]
Spinal	● Loss of sympathetic (vascular) tone and ↓HR • Dilatation of arterioles/venous pooling • Loss of sympathetic drive of the heart (T1–T4)

Estimated blood loss – classification of haemorrhagic shock

Based on a 70kg adult man

	Class I	Class II	Class III	Class IV
Blood loss (ml)	<750	750–1500	1500–2000	>2000
Blood loss (% blood volume)	<15%	15–30%	30–40%	>40%
Pulse	↔/↑	↑	↑↑	↑↑
BP	↔	↔	↓	↓↓

1 Anaphylactic reactions are mediated by a specific IgE response, whereas anaphylactoid reactions are IgE-independent; clinically they are indistinguishable.

Hypovolaemic/haemorrhagic shock (OHAM2 p263)

Common causes

Haemorrhage	Trauma (external/internal bleeding), ruptured AAA, GI bleed
Salt + water loss	Diarrhoea, vomiting, burns, polyuria (DI and DM)
'3rd space' loss	Acute pancreatitis, ascites

Symptoms dizziness on standing (±lying), SOB, ±chest pain
Symptoms of underlying disease painful trauma to limb/chest/abdomen/pelvis, back/loin pain, melaena/haematemesis, diarrhoea, urinary frequency, epigastric pain radiating to back, abdominal swelling/bloating.
Signs BP <100mmHg systolic, tachycardia, weak/thready pulse, postural hypotension, cool peripheries/↓cap refill, ↓JVP, ↓GCS/restlessness, oliguria, mottled skin in severe hypotension
Signs of underlying disease obvious source of external (wound/GI bleed) or internal (haemothorax, ascites/tense abdomen, pelvic instability, swollen thighs) bleeding, burns, palpable AAA, tender epigastrium, Grey-Turners sign/Cullens sign, melaena on PR examination
Worrying signs BP<90mmHg, ↓GCS/restlessness, oliguria, mottled skin, unresponsive to fluid challenge, ongoing bleeding – call senior help
Investigations *blds* FBC (↓Hb, though may be normal in acute blood loss), U+E (↑urea in GI bleed, ↓K^+ in diarrhoea/vomiting), LFT, amylase, clotting, osmolality, crossmatch (in severe bleeding: 4 units O-negative + 4 units type-specific + 4 units full match) *ABG* acidosis in haemorrhage, DKA and pancreatitis, alkalosis in vomiting *ECG* ischaemia *CXR* haemothorax *pelvic X-ray* pelvic fracture *abdo USS* AAA (though if ruptured AAA likely to need theatre before USS) *Urine* Na^+ and osmolality in diabetes insipidus *stool* M,C+S (ova, cysts and parasites, *C. diff* toxin)
When to treat All hypotensive patients, especially if pulse >100. A BP of 100mmHg systolic may be critically low if the patient is normally hypertensive (eg elderly), use pulse and other clinical markers as a guide.
Acute treatment of severe haemorrhage O_2, 500ml colloid (eg Gelofusine®) stat, call senior help, lay flat and elevate legs if patient dizzy, attempt to stop bleeding by compression if appropriate, further 500ml colloid stat if no improvement in BP or slowing of pulse, identify likely cause of haemorrhage and commence appropriate management (see opposite). Early involvement of ITU, as may need inotropic support.
Acute treatment of non-haemorrhage hypovolaemia O_2, 1l 0.9% saline stat, call senior help, lay flat and elevate legs if patient dizzy, 500ml colloid stat if no improvement in BP or slowing of pulse, identify likely cause of hypovolaemia and commence appropriate definitive treatment (pancreatitis (see opposite), severe diarrhoea (p200), vomiting (p206), burns (OHAE2 p376), fever and sweating (p248), ascites (p193)). Early involvement of ITU.
Chronic treatment Once appropriate management initiated, recheck observations, including BM, and repeat U+E and FBC (±ABG); catheterise and monitor urine output; continually reassess starting with A, B, C.
Complications Hypotension results in underperfusion of vital organs and subsequent disruption in their physiology (brain – ↓GCS/coma, kidneys – renal failure, heart – myocardial ischaemia).

Severe GI bleeding (p174)

Haematemesis	Melaena/Fresh PR bleeding
A, B, C – call ARREST TEAM if compromised **Call for senior help** Give 100% O_2; lay flat with legs elevated if BP <100mmHg systolic Secure 14G cannulae in both antecubital fossa, take blood for 6 unit crossmatch 500ml colloid (Gelofusine®) stat, followed by 500ml colloid stat if no improvement	
Needs urgent upper GI endoscopy ?Sengstaken-Blakemore tube if varices Check U+E/LFT/clotting	Needs urgent upper GI endoscopy ±lower GI endoscopy Check U+E/LFT/clotting

Probable ruptured AAA (p188)

A, B, C – call ARREST TEAM if compromised
Call for senior help, vascular surgeon and anaesthetist
Give 100% O_2; lay flat with legs elevated if BP <100mmHg systolic
Secure 14G cannulae in both antecubital fossae, take blood for 8 unit crossmatch
500ml colloid (Gelofusine®) stat, aim to keep BP 90–100mmHg systolic
NEEDS THEATRE STAT

Severe external bleeding (p312)

A, B, C – call ARREST TEAM if compromised
Call for senior help
Give 100% O_2; lay flat with legs elevated if BP <100mmHg systolic
Apply pressure to bleeding source
Elevate bleeding source
Secure 14G cannulae in both antecubital fossa, take blood for 4 unit crossmatch
500ml colloid (Gelofusine®) stat, followed by 500ml colloid stat if no improvement
NEEDS THEATRE STAT

Pancreatitis (p198)

A, B, C – call ARREST TEAM if compromised
Call for senior help
Give 100% O_2
Secure intravenous access, take bloods, BM and ABG
1l 0.9% saline stat, followed by 1l 0.9% saline over 30min
Analgese with IV morphine as required
Catheterise; hourly urine measurement
Needs surgical input/surgical HDU bed

Septic shock (OHAM2 p270)

Common sources of infection resulting in septicaemia

Chest – pneumonia	**Intra-abdominal** – perforation/biliary tract
Skin/soft tissues – cellulitis/gangrene	**Urinary tract** – UTI/pyelonephritis
Heart – endocarditis	**Post-op** – wound infection, bowel leak

Symptoms dizziness on standing (±lying), SOB, ±chest pain.

Symptoms of underlying disease hot and cold, sweats, shivers, nausea and vomiting, breathlessness, cough, dysuria, urinary frequency, abdominal pain, wound/skin pain, headache, confusion

Signs fever, BP <100mmHg systolic, tachycardia, ±bounding pulse, warm peripheries, ↓JVP, ±↓GCS/restlessness, oliguria, mottled skin in severe hypotension, non-blanching petechial rash in meningococcal septicaemia. Signs of underlying disease such as cellulitis, consolidation in pneumonia or abdominal/loin/suprapubic tenderness in intra-abdominal infections.

Investigations *blds* FBC (↑WCC, ±↓Hb), U+E, LFT, ↑CRP/ESR, BM, clotting/fibrinogen *bld cultures* take 2–3 sets from different sites *ABG* acidosis, BE, lactate *ECG* ischaemia *urine dipstix* blood, protein, nitrites, leucocytes, M,C+S *Erect CXR* consolidation, free air under diaphragm sputum M,C+S *skin/wound swabs* M,C+S *echo* valvular lesion/vegetation (transoesophageal more sensitive than transthoracic) *other imaging* as appropriate

Worrying signs BP <90mmHg, ↓GCS, oliguria (renal failure), DIC, mottled skin, petechial rash, unresponsive to fluid challenge; call senior help

When to treat All hypotensive patients, especially if pulse >100. A BP of 100mmHg systolic may be critically low if the patient is normally hypertensive (eg elderly), use pulse and other clinical markers as a guide.

Acute treatment O_2, 500ml colloid (Gelofusine®) or 1l 0.9% saline stat, call senior help, lay flat and elevate legs If patient dizzy, give IV antibiotics appropriate to likely source of infection (see over and p254), repeat 500ml colloid bolus stat if no improvement in BP or slowing of pulse. Consider central line to monitor central venous pressure and arterial line for serial ABGs and invasive blood pressure monitoring. Early involvement of ITU, as may need inotropic/ventilatory support.

Chronic treatment Continue broad-spectrum antibiotic therapy until advised of alternative, more targeted therapy by microbiologist. Aggressive fluid therapy to ensure adequate tissue perfusion.

Complications Hypotension results in underperfusion of vital organs and subsequent disruption in their physiology (brain – ↓GCS/coma, kidneys – renal failure, heart – myocardial ischaemia) and in multi-organ failure. Sepsis can precipitate DIC which can result in necrosis and gangrene, as well as profound bleeding (p288).

Toxic shock is a specific form of septic shock, caused by the production of a toxin by Gram-positive bacteria. It is commonest amongst females and associated with menstruation and the use of tampons. Presents in similar fashion to other forms of septic shock, though sloughing of the skin off hands and feet is common 1–2wk after initial presentation. Treatment is the same: fluid resuscitation, broad-spectrum antibiotics initially, **remove source of infection/pus**, support impaired organ function.

Factors associated with a poor outcome in sepsis

Age >60yr
Disseminated intravascular coagulation (DIC)
Hospital-acquired infection
Hypothermia
Leucopenia
Liver failure
Multiple-organ failure (brain, heart, liver, kidneys)
Respiratory failure

Empirical antibiotic treatment in sepsis

For dosing regimens see p254	
Pneumonia	
Community-acquired	Co-amoxiclav or cefotaxime + clarithromycin
Hospital-acquired	Consult local guideline and discuss with microbiologist
Intra-abdominal	Cefuroxime + metronidazole
Biliary tract	Tazocin®[1] ±gentamicin (p569)
Meningitis	Ceftriaxone, discuss with microbiologist
Skin	Flucloxacillin 1g/6h IV, discuss with microbiologist
Urinary tract	
Community-acquired	Cefuroxime 1.5g/8h IV ±gentamicin (p569)
Hospital-acquired	Consult local guideline and discuss with microbiologist
Unsure of origin	Consult local guideline and discuss with microbiologist

Causes of lactic acidosis – metabolic acidosis with ↑lactate

Tissue hypoxaemia
- Inadequate perfusion
- Severe anaemia
- Severe hypoxia
- Catecholamine excess (↑SVR)
- Severe exercise

Non-hypoxaemic tissues
- Sepsis
- Renal and hepatic failure
- Uncontrolled DM
- Acute pancreatitis
- Paracetamol overdose

Drug-induced
- Metformin
- Methanol
- Ethanol
- Aspirin (salicylates)
- Cyanide

Rare hereditary causes
- Glucose-6-phosphatase deficiency
- Fructose-1,6-diphosphatase deficiency

1 Tazocin® 4.5g = piperacillin 4g and tazobactam 500mg.

Cardiogenic shock (OHCM6 p788)

Common causes

Pump failure	LV dysfunction (post-MI/ACS), aortic dissection, dysrhythmia
Inadequate filling	Pulmonary embolism, pneumothorax, cardiac tamponade

Symptoms dizziness on standing (±lying), SOB, ±chest pain
Symptoms of underlying disease chest pain, ±pleuritic, ±radiating to back/left arm/jaw, breathlessness, palpitations
Signs BP <100mmHg systolic (check both arms), tachycardia or bradycardia, weak/thready pulse, cool peripheries, ↑JVP, ±↓GCS, oliguria, mottled skin in severe hypotension
Signs of underlying disease stigmata of hyperlipidaemia, ↓O_2 sats, signs of pneumothorax (↓expansion, ↑percussion note, ↓breath sounds on affected side, tracheal deviation), pulmonary oedema, Beck's triad in cardiac tamponade (shock, ↑JVP, muffled heart sounds), pitting oedema
Worrying signs BP <90mmHg, ↓GCS/restlessness, oliguria (renal failure), mottled skin, chest pain, hypoxaemia; call senior help
Investigations If you suspect cardiogenic shock identify most likely cause and treat prior to undertaking investigations; seconds count. Most useful investigation will be immediate *echocardiogram* (bleep cardiologist on-call) for dissection, PE, cardiac tamponade, LVF *ECG* ischaemia, small complexes *CXR* pneumothorax, cardiomegaly *ABG* hypoxaemia *blds* FBC, U+E, BM, clotting, crossmatch *other imaging* as appropriate
When to treat All hypotensive patients, especially if pulse >100. A BP of 100mmHg systolic may be critically low for some normally hypertensive patients, so use pulse and other clinical markers as a guide.
Acute treatment 100% O_2. Further management depends on pathology.

Bradyarrhythmia	p142	Aortic dissection	p132
Tachyarrhythmia	p134	Pulmonary embolism	p169
Heart failure	p170	Pneumothorax	p170

Cardiac tamponade (OHCM6 p788)

Collection of fluid (usually blood) in pericardium resulting in external compression upon ventricles and inability for heart to fill/pump.
Causes trauma, pericarditis, post-MI, dissecting aortic aneurysm
Signs tachycardia, hypotension, Beck's triad (see above)
Investigations *echo* pericardial fluid, poor stroke volume *CXR* cardiomegaly, pulmonary oedema *ECG* small complexes, tachycardia, ischaemia
Acute treatment 100% O_2, IV access, needle pericardiocentesis

Emergency needle pericardiocentesis (OHCM6 p757) get senior help

- Monitor heart rhythm on ECG monitor, have drip running and defibrillator close
- Clean skin on chest/upper abdomen with antiseptic
- Long 18G cannula to 20ml syringe via a 3-way tap
- Advance needle to the left of xiphisternum, aiming for tip of left scapula
- Withdraw syringe as advancing, watching for ectopics on ECG
- Ectopics imply needle in myocardium, withdraw a little into the pericardial space
- Aspirating 20–40ml can improve BP, but fluid likely to reaccumulate
- Patient needs definitive cardiothoracic input urgently

Anaphylactic shock (OHCM6 p780)

Commoner precipitants

Drugs	Penicillins, anaesthetic drugs, contrast medium, blood products
Environmental	Latex, stings, eggs, fish, peanuts, strawberries

Symptoms chest tightness, wheeze, breathlessness, itching, swelling
Signs hypotension, tachycardia, tongue/periorbital swelling, wheeze, urticaria, erythema, cyanosis
Worrying signs BP <90mmHg systolic, ↓O_2 sats, chest tightness, stridor
Investigations If you suspect anaphylactic shock commence treatment; seconds count. Subsequently check for serum mast cell tryptase to confirm global mast cell degranulation consistent with diagnosis.
When to treat all patients with physical signs
Acute treatment call senior help; early involvement of ITU/anaesthetist.

- 100% O_2
- Secure airway if compromised (stridor p324)
- Remove precipitant (stop antibiotic IVI etc)
- Lay flat or with legs elevated if patient dizzy
- **Give 0.5mg epinephrine (adrenaline) IM (0.5ml of 1:1000)**
  - Every 5min until improvement in BP and respiratory symptoms
- Secure IV access, give 500ml colloid (Gelofusine®) stat
- Chlorpheniramine 10mg IV and hydrocortisone 200mg IV stat
- Salbutamol nebuliser 5mg
- Ensure senior help available

Chronic treatment follow-up by immunologist; may need EpiPen.

Epinephrine (adrenaline) preparations

1:1000	Preparation – 1ml ampoule. Give 0.5ml (0.5mg) IM 1mg in 1ml
1:10,000	Preparation – 10ml syringe in cardiac arrest drugs, or 10ml ampoule 1mg in 10ml

Spinal (neurogenic) shock

Common causes

Trauma	Traumatic transection of spinal cord at any level
Iatrogenic	Spinal anaesthesia

Symptoms usually has motor/sensory dysfunction below level of lesion, bowel and bladder dysfunction
Signs hypotension, warm peripheries, may not be able to mount tachycardia if lesion above T1/T2 (origin of sympathetic supply to the heart), focal neurology, up-going plantar relaxes, loss of anal tone
Investigations imaging of spinal cord as appropriate
When to treat BP <100mmHg systolic, symptomatic of ↓BP, organ failure
Acute treatment O_2, 500ml colloid (Gelofusine®) stat, call senior help, lay flat with legs elevated if patient dizzy. Catheterise. If trauma involve spinal/orthopaedic surgeons. If iatrogenic, (eg epidural) consult anaesthetist. Early involvement of ITU.

Postural (orthostatic) hypotension

Common causes

Volume depletion	Dehydration, anaemia, vasovagal
Iatrogenic	Antihypertensives, diuretics, nitrates, antidepressants
Autonomic neuropathy	DM, Guillain-Barré, syphilis, Parkinson's disease, ageing

Drop in the systolic BP of >20mmHg upon standing from sitting or lying position; can occur when sitting from a lying position in severe disease.
Symptoms dizziness, ±loss of consciousness (LOC) when standing
Signs fall in systolic BP of >20mmHg upon standing
Investigations lying/standing BP usually diagnostic. Other investigations as appropriate to investigate cause of syncope/collapse (p286).
When to treat all symptomatic patients
Acute treatment review medications and identify likely precipitants; can these be stopped or changed for a drug without this side-effect? Optimise control of diabetes. Identify and treat other precipitating disease (see above). Ensure patient is going to be safe in immediate period.
Chronic treatment advise simple lifestyle changes such as getting out of chairs slowly or holding onto something as one stands. Graduated stockings for lower legs may help if poor venous circulation. Steroids/mineralocorticoids may be useful in some situations, though benefit needs to outweigh risks.
Complications falls and subsequent bone and soft tissue injuries including intracranial bleeding and fractured neck of femur.

Addison's disease	p240	Hypothyroidism	p239
Anaemia	p272	Falls on the ward	p286

Hypertension emergency

Airway	Check airway is patent; consider manoeuvres/adjuncts
Breathing	If no respiratory effort – **CALL ARREST TEAM**
Circulation	If no palpable pulse – **CALL ARREST TEAM**

Call for **senior help** early if patient deteriorating
If **systolic >200** or **diastolic >120** (BP this high is often seen in clinic):

- **Sit patient up**
- **High-flow oxygen** in all patients
- **Monitor** pulse oximeter, BP, defibrillator ECG leads if unwell
- Request full set of **observations** and **ECG**
- Take brief **history** if possible/check notes/ask ward staff
- **Examine patient**: condensed RS, CVS, abdomen and eye examination
- Rule out **serious causes** and establish **likely causes**
- **Do not** give stat doses of antihypertensives without senior review
- **Initiate further treatment**, see following pages
- **Venous access**, take bloods:
  - FBC, U+E, LFT, cardiac markers, TFT, fasting glucose, cortisol
- Consider requesting urgent **CXR**, portable if too unwell
- Urinalysis and β-HCG
- Call for **senior help** for advice
- Re-assess, starting with A, B, C…

Life-threatening causes

- Pre-eclampsia/eclampsia
- Malignant hypertension >200/120
- Hypertensive encephalopathy
- Phaeochromocytoma
- Thyrotoxic storm

Hypertension (systolic >160 or diastolic >100)

Worrying features ↓pulse, ↓GCS, chest pain, retinal haemorrhages, systolic >200, diastolic >120, renal failure

Think about ***life-threatening*** malignant hypertension (BP>200/120), pre-eclampsia ***other*** anxiety, pain, primary (essential) or secondary hypertension (including thyroid storm and phaeochromocytoma)
Ask about visual symptoms, headache, chest/back pains, new motor weakness, facial flushing, diarrhoea, weight gain/loss, pregnancy (pre- or post-partum), change in hat size/change in facial features, haematuria; majority asymptomatic ***PMH*** previous hypertension, Cushing's syndrome, acromegaly, Conn's syndrome, phaeochromocytoma, coarctation, thyroid disease, DM, renal artery stenosis ***DH*** cardiac and antihypertensive medications, steroids, contraceptive pill, thyroxine/carbimazole, MAO inhibitors, antipsychotics, recreational drugs (cocaine, amphetamines) ***FH*** hypertension, endocrine disease, polycystic kidney disease ***SH*** exercise tolerance, smoking
Obs pulse, BP (both arms and postural), sats, temp, GCS, repeat BP after a period of relaxing (both arms and postural)
Look for ***signs of underlying disease*** radiofemoral delay, striae, buffalo hump, central obesity, large hands/feet/face, tremor, exophthalmos, thyroid mass/bruit, proximal myopathy, gravid uterus, renal bruits/polycystic kidneys ***signs of end-organ damage*** left ventricular hypertrophy (LVH – displaced apex beat), retinopathy (see table p161), Cushing's reflex (raised ICP) and proteinuria/haematuria
Investigations ***serial BP*** repeat BP manually to confirm diagnosis ***ECG*** features of LVH (see table p163) ***blds*** FBC, U+E, glucose, cholesterol, LFT ***urine*** blood, protein, β-HCG (<20wk) ***CXR*** unlikely to be helpful in the immediate setting, but may reveal heart size and aortic contours ***renal USS/arteriography*** small kidneys/stenotic renal arteries ***24h urine*** VMA (p505), cortisol (p239) ***24h ambulatory BP*** may reveal 'white-coat hypertension' which settles at home or during sleep

Treatment

- Airway, breathing (with O_2 if sats <95%) and monitor circulation
- If ↓GCS call for senior help, p226
- IV cannula and take bloods
- Check ECG to exclude myocardial infarction
- A sudden drop in BP can cause a stroke, aim to lower the BP gradually, see p161, unless benefits outweigh the risks (eg pregnancy, MI, aortic dissection or hypertensive encephalopathy)

Indications for admission

Diastolic persistently >120mmHg
Retinal haemorrhages
Newly diagnosed/recognised renal impairment

Malignant hypertension (OHAM2 p166)

Hypertensive emergency with acute retinopathy
Symptoms headache, visual loss, confusion and drowsiness
Signs BP usually >200/120, retinopathy (see p161), ↓GCS
Investigations as for hypertension in general (p159) to exclude a secondary cause and as a base-line investigation of renal function and size. Needs formal (ophthalmic) assessment for retinal disease.
Diagnosis relies on retinopathy being present, ±vasculitis, ±papilloedema, together with the symptoms and signs above. Additional features: renal failure, heart failure, microangiopathic haemolytic anaemia and DIC in severe cases.
Acute treatment needs admission to monitored area (HDU/ITU), with close monitoring of BP, ECG, neurological state and fluid balance (consider arterial line, central line, catheterisation). Aim to reduce diastolic BP to <100mmHg over first 24h (see opposite for treatment options). Patients with early features may be commenced on oral therapy, though late features need treating with IV agents. If no evidence of LVF use labetalol, though if LVF present commence furosemide (40–80mg IV) with either nitroprusside or hydralazine. Consider ACE inhibitor to counteract high circulating levels of renin.
Chronic treatment BP needs checking regularly once discharged from hospital. Ensure GP knows what investigations have been undertaken, their results and what the therapeutic plan/target BP is.

Hypertensive encephalopathy (OHAM2 p168)

Medical emergency. Cerebral oedema secondary to loss of autoregulation of cerebral blood flow. Rare in patients with chronic hypertension.
Symptoms headache, nausea, vomiting, confusion, visual changes/loss
Signs hypertension (BP rise only need be moderate), retinopathy (see opposite), confusion or ↓GCS, seizures, coma

Investigations as for hypertension in general (p159) to exclude a secondary cause and as a base-line investigation of renal function and size. Needs formal (ophthalmic) assessment for retinal disease and CT/MRI head to exclude other intracranial pathology.
Diagnosis of exclusion (stroke, encephalitis, tumour, bleeding, hypoglycaemia, vasculitis)
Acute treatment needs admission to monitored area (HDU/ITU), with close monitoring of BP, ECG, neurological state and fluid balance (consider arterial line, central line, catheterisation). Aim to reduce diastolic BP to <100mmHg over first 1–2h (see opposite for treatment options). Correct electrolyte abnormalities and give furosemide 40–80mg IV. Nitroprusside as first-line agent, labetalol and Ca^{2+} channel blockers as second-line agents. Avoid clonidine or methyldopa as these are sedating. Consider ACE inhibitor to counteract high circulating levels of renin.
Chronic treatment BP needs checking regularly once discharged from hospital. Ensure GP knows what investigations have been undertaken and their results and what the therapeutic plan/target BP is.

Emergency treatment of hypertension

Most cases of hypertension do not need emergency treatment and oral therapy is usually sufficient to control BP. Never use stat doses of sub-lingual nifedipine. If BP needs to be rapidly reduced use an intravenous agent in a high-dependency/critical care area.

Before commencing therapy confirm diagnosis by repeating BP and ensuring that the BP cuff is sited correctly and an appropriate size (width of the cuff should be at least 40% of the arm circumference and bladder of the cuff should be centred over brachial artery). Check baseline bloods and initiate investigations to exclude secondary causes.

IV antihypertensives for acute management of hypertension[1] (OHAM2 p164)

Patient must be in HDU/ITU, ideally with invasive BP monitoring. Intravenous therapy results in rapid falls in BP so drugs must be titrated slowly

Drug	Dose	Comment
GTN	1–10mg/h IVI	Venodilates. Useful in LVF and angina.
Hydralazine	5–10mg/20min IVI	Vasodilates, can cause compensatory rise in heart rate; use with a β-blocker.
Isoket® 0.05%[2] (500μg/ml)	2–10ml/h IVI (1–5mg/h)	Venodilates. Useful in LVF/angina. Easy for nurses to set up infusion. Drug of choice.
Labetalol	20–80mg/10min	Drug of choice in phaeochromocytoma or aortic dissection. Avoid in LVF.
Nitroprusside	0.25–8μg/kg/min	Rapid onset. Useful in LVF or hypertensive encephalopathy. Rarely used now.

Oral antihypertensives for acute management of hypertension[1] (OHAM2 p165)

Drug	Dose	Comment
Atenolol	50–100mg/24h PO	Many β-blockers available. Contraindicated in asthma, peripheral vascular disease, DM.
Hydralazine	25–50mg/8h PO	Vasodilator. Safe in pregnancy.
Nifedipine	10–20mg/8h PO	Avoid sub-lingual as rapidly drops BP. OK to use in conjunction with β-blocker (avoid verapamil or diltiazem with β-blockers).

Hypertensive retinopathy

Grade 1 Tortuous retinal arteries, silver wiring

Grade 2 Grade 1 + AV nipping

Grade 3 Grade 2 + flame-shaped haemorrhages and cotton wool spots

Grade 4 Grade 3 + papilloedema

1 Aim to reduce BP by 25% in 1–4h, then more slowly to a diastolic of <100mmHg.
2 Available as 50ml 0.05% solution (25mg in 50ml).

Essential (primary) hypertension (OHCM6 p140)

Accounts for 95% of cases of hypertension.

Symptoms most often asymptomatic, may present with end-organ damage (ischaemic heart disease, retinopathy, nephropathy, neuropathy).

Signs BP>160/90, ±retinopathy (see p161)

Investigations as for hypertension in general (p159) to exclude a secondary cause and as a base-line investigation of renal function and size. Needs formal (ophthalmic) assessment for retinal disease.

Worrying signs BP>200/120, signs of retinopathy or encephalopathy (p160)

When to treat BP>160/100 or BP>140/90 in diabetics

Acute treatment if BP<200/120 but >160/100 and no clear cause identified, commence oral antihypertensive therapy unless there are other indications to reduce BP more rapidly (eclampsia, MI, aortic dissection). If BP>200/120 consider commencing IV anti-hypertensive therapy (p161) in a monitored environment (HDU/ITU).

Chronic treatment BP needs checking regularly once discharged from hospital. Ensure GP knows what investigations have been undertaken, their results and what the therapeutic plan is. Inform patient about need to comply with medication regime and identify lifestyle changes and modifiable risk factors (opposite).

Antihypertensive drugs include: ACE inhibitors, β-blockers, Ca^{2+} channel blockers and diuretics

Complications end-organ damage, malignant hypertension

Secondary causes of hypertension

Renal (p269)	Intrinsic renal disease – glomerulonephritis, polycystic kidneys Renovascular disease – renal artery stenosis, AAA
Endocrine (p239)	Cushing's syndrome, Conn's syndrome, phaeochromocytoma, acromegaly, hyperparathyroidism, thyrotoxicosis
Drugs	Steroids, MAOi, oral contraceptive pill
Others	Coarctation, gestational, pre-eclampsia/eclampsia

Complications of hypertension

Blood vessels – atheroma

Eyes – retinopathy (see below)

Kidneys – nephropathy

CNS – stroke (haemorrhagic + ischaemic)

Heart – LVH, LVF, IHD, AF

Malignant hypertension (p160)

Hypertension accompanying acute stroke/intracranial bleed
(OHAM2 p166)

- Hypertension common during first 24–48h of stroke; usually settles
- Treat cautiously if diastolic >130mmHg (nitrate, labetalol, Ca^{2+} channel blockers)
- Avoid centrally acting agents as these will impair consciousness further
- In sub-arachnoid haemorrhage nimodipine may be useful to counteract vasospasm

ECG voltage criteria for left ventricular hypertrophy (LVH)

- Tallest R (V4–V6) + deepest S (V1–V3) >40mm
- Tallest R (V4–V6) >27mm
- Deepest S (V1–V3) >30mm
- R in aVL >13mm
- R in aVF >20mm
- Abnormal ST depression or T inversion in V4–V6

Lifestyle changes and modifiable risk factors

Lifestyle	Reduce stress and alcohol consumption Regular exercise
Modifiable risk factors (to limit risk of IHD/cVD)	Diagnose and aggressively treat DM Diagnose and treat dyslipidaemia Stop smoking

Starting an ACE inhibitor

Can be undertaken as in-patient, out-patient or by GP

Contraindications	Renal artery stenosis, aortic stenosis, hyperkalaemia, known allergy to ACEi, pregnancy/lactation
Side-effects	Dry cough, postural hypotension, renal impairment and hyperkalaemia, taste disturbance, urticaria and angioneurotic oedema
Before starting	Check U+E, document starting BP
First dose	Start with lowest dose and give at bedtime to limit any problems with first-dose hypotension
Day 4–7	Recheck U+E, ask about postural symptoms and check lying and standing BP
Day 10–14	Recheck U+E, ask about postural symptoms and check lying and standing BP
Week 3	Increase dose if tolerating and no new renal impairment
Week 4	Recheck U+E, ask about postural symptoms and check lying and standing BP
Week 5	Increase dose if tolerating and no new renal impairment. Continue weekly until target/maximal dose achieved

Phaeochromocytoma	p240	Cushing's syndrome/steroids	p239
Hyperthyroid	p239	Renal disease	p269

Breathlessness and low sats emergency

Airway	Check airway is patent; consider manoeuvres/ adjuncts
Breathing	If no respiratory effort – **CALL ARREST TEAM**
Circulation	If no palpable pulse – **CALL ARREST TEAM**

Call for **senior help** early if patient deteriorating

- **Sit patient up**
- **High-flow oxygen** in <u>all</u> patients
- **Monitor** pulse oximeter, BP, defibrillator's ECG leads if unwell
- Obtain a full set of **observations** including temp
- Take brief **history** if possible/check **notes**/ask ward staff
- **Examine patient**: condensed RS, CVS, ±abdo exam
- Establish likely causes and rule out serious causes
- Initiate **further treatment**, see following pages
- **Venous access**, take bloods:
  - FBC, U+E, LFT, CRP, bld cultures, D-dimer, cardiac markers
- **Arterial blood gas**, but don't leave the patient alone
- **ECG** to exclude arrhythmias and acute MI
- Request urgent **CXR**, portable if too unwell
- Call for **senior help**
- Reassess, starting with A, B, C...

Life-threatening causes

- Asthma/COPD
- Pulmonary oedema (LVF)
- (Tension) pneumothorax
- MI/arrhythmia
- Pneumonia
- Pulmonary embolism (PE)
- Pleural effusion
- Anaphylaxis/airway obstruction

Breathlessness and low sats

Worrying features RR >30, sats <92%, systolic <100mmHg, chest pain, confusion, inability to complete sentences, exhaustion, tachy/bradycardia

Think about ***life-threatening*** see box on previous page ***most likely*** COPD/asthma, pneumonia, pulmonary oedema (LVF), pulmonary embolism (PE), myocardial infarction (MI) ***other*** pneumothorax, pleural effusion, arrhythmia, acute respiratory distress syndrome (ARDS), sepsis, metabolic acidosis, anaemia, pain, panic, foreign body/aspiration ***chronic*** COPD, lung cancer, bronchiectasis, fibrosing alveolitis, TB, scoliosis

Ask about speed of onset, cough, sputum (quantity, colour and blood), chest pain (pleuritic (worse on deep inspiration or coughing), related to movement or tender), palpitations, dizziness, difficulty lying flat, recent travel, weight loss ***PMH*** cardiac or respiratory problems, malignancy, TB ***DH*** inhalers, home nebulisers, home oxygen, cardiac medication, allergies ***SH*** smoking, pets, exercise tolerance

- ***PE risk factors*** recent surgery/immobility/fracture/travel, oestrogen (pregnancy, HRT, the pill), malignancy, previous PE/DVT, recent stroke or MI, thrombophilia, varicose veins, obesity, central line

Obs temp, RR (11–20 is normal), BP, pulse, sats (should be >92%), O_2 requirements (improving or worsening?)

Look for confusion, cyanosis, CO_2 tremor, clubbing, rashes, itching, swollen lips/eyes, raised JVP, tracheal shift and tug, use of accessory muscles, abnormal percussion, unequal air entry, crackles, stridor, wheeze, bronchial breathing, swollen/red/hot/tender legs, swelling of ankles, cold peripheries

Investigations ***PEFR*** if asthma or COPD suspected (may be too ill) ***blds*** FBC, U+E, LFT, CRP, D-dimer (if PE suspected), cardiac markers, blood cultures ***sputum*** may need physio help, inspect and send for M,C+S; AFBs if TB risk ***ABGs*** see p506, keep on O_2 if acutely SOB ***ECG*** see p514 ***CXR*** see p508; portable if unwell, though image quality may be poor ***Spirometry*** this should be done once the patient has been stabilised to help confirm the diagnosis, see p512

Treatment

Sit all patients up and give high-flow (60–100%) oxygen – this saves lives. This can be reduced later and CO_2 retention in COPD takes a while to develop. Check sats and ECG in all patients:

- ***stridor*** – call an anaesthetist, p324
- ***wheeze*** – give nebulisers
- ***unilateral resonance with reduced air entry and shock*** – treat as tension pneumothorax (large cannula, 2nd intercostal, mid-clavicular)
- ***asymmetrical crackles and air entry*** – consider pneumonia
- ***symmetrical crackles and air entry with raised JVP*** – consider LVF
- ***normal examination*** – consider PE, cardiac and systemic causes

	History	Examination	Investigations
COPD	Known respiratory problems, smoker, cough worse than usual, pleuritic chest pain	±wheeze/crackles, ±cyanosed/purse-lip breathing, look for infection and pneumothorax	$\downarrow$PEFR; CXR hyperexpanded, exclude pneumonia and pneumothorax, flat diaphragms common in COPD
Asthma	Known asthma, recent cold or exposure to allergens	Wheeze ±crackles, look for signs of infection or pneumothorax	
Pneumonia	Productive cough, dark sputum, feels unwell, ±pleuritic chest pain	Febrile, asymmetrical air entry, crackles and percussion	$\uparrow$WCC/NØ/CRP, consolidation or blunted angles on CXR (p508)
Pulmonary embolism	PE risk factors, leg pain, ±pleuritic chest pain and haemoptysis	$\uparrow$JVP, $\uparrow$pulse, may have swollen red legs, can be severely shocked	Low pCO_2, ±hypoxia on ABGs, raised D-dimer, CXR often clear
Pulmonary oedema	Known cardiac problems, orthopnea, swollen legs	$\uparrow$JVP, symmetrical fine crackles, pink frothy sputum, oedema, cold peripheries	Big heart + signs of oedema on CXR (p508), ECG may show evidence of previous MIs
Pneumothorax	Sudden onset pleuritic chest pain, trauma, previous episodes, tall and thin	Unequal air entry and expansion, hyperresonant, displaced trachea (late)	Treat tension pneumothorax first, CXR shows pleura separated from ribs
Pleural effusion	Gradual onset breathlessness, ±pleuritic chest pain	Reduced expansion, stony dull base	Effusion on CXR
ARDS	Concurrent severe illness	Hypoxic	Bilateral infiltrates on CXR
Anaemia/MI/ arrhythmias	Chest pain, palpitations, dizziness, tiredness	Irregular or fast pulse, shocked, pale	Abnormal ECG (p514), $\downarrow$Hb, $\uparrow$cardiac markers
Anaphylaxis	Sudden onset, itching, swelling, urticarial rash, new drugs/food	Stridor, ±wheeze, shock, swollen lips and eyes, blanching rash	Treat with IM epinephrine (adrenaline) (p156)

Causes of lung disease

Restrictive

- Pulmonary fibrosis
- Chronic fibrosing alveolitis
- Sarcoidosis

Obstructive

- Asthma
- COPD

COPD/emphysema (OHAM2 p218)

Symptoms breathlessness, cough, ↑sputum, tight chest, confusion, reduced exercise tolerance, (ex-)smoker

Signs wheeze, cyanosis, barrel chested, poor expansion, tachypnoea

Investigations ↓*PEFR, ABGs* are often deranged in COPD, compare with previous samples and check the oxygen concentration. Repeat at 30min in seriously ill patients *CXR* hyperexpanded, flat diaphragm (look for evidence of infection, pneumothorax or bullae) *spirometry* low FEV_1, low FEV_1:FVC ratio

Acute exacerbation Sit the patient up and turn O_2 to 24–28%. Give salbutamol 5mg neb ±ipratropium (Atrovent®) 500μg neb and prednisolone 30–40mg PO (hydrocortisone 200mg IV if unable to take tablets). Get an ABG and CXR (portable if unwell). Use ABG results to guide management:

- ***Normal* ABG** (for them) continue O_2 and give regular nebs
- ***Worsening hypoxia*** 28–40% O_2, repeat ABGs <30min, watch for confusion or ↓RR which should prompt a repeat ABG sooner
- ***Worsening CO_2 retention*** continue or reduce O_2, ABG in 15min

Still worsening Call for senior help; give 5mg/kg IV aminophylline bolus over 20min unless the patient is on oral aminophylline or theophylline. If they are, use salbutamol 0.25mg IV over 10min instead and send blood for an urgent amino/theophylline level. Consider NIV, see below.

Antibiotics Consider prescribing antibiotics (amoxicillin 500mg/8h PO) if the patient has increased SOB, worsening cough or purulent sputum.

Chronic treatment See p339 or OHCM6 p188. Stop smoking, exercise, inhalers (p339 for colours and types), home nebulisers, long-term oxygen therapy (if pO_2 ≤8kPa), long-term oral steroids, antibiotics. Avoid giving O_2 >28% unless acutely SOB; this can reduce respiratory drive in some patients causing CO_2 retention and confusion.

Complications exacerbations, infection, cor pulmonale, pneumothorax, respiratory failure, lung cancer

Non-invasive ventilation (NIV)

These are machines that help ventilate patients through a tightly fitting mask instead of intubation. They are commonly used in COPD patients with a pH ≤7.25 and CO_2 ≥6.0kPa to get them through acute illness. BiPAP is the most common. CPAP is not a type of NIV since it does not give ventilation (see p170).

Asthma[1] (OHAM2 p210)

Severe	Incomplete sentences, PEFR <50% of best, pulse >100, RR >25
Life-threatening	As for severe plus any of: PEFR <33% of best, silent chest, pulse <60, systolic <100mmHg, confusion, sats <92%, PaO_2 <8kPa, poor respiratory effort, normal $PaCO_2$ (exhaustion), cyanosis
Near fatal	Any CO_2 retention – call an anaesthetist

Symptoms breathless, tight chest and wheezy episodes (exercise, allergens, cold), night and morning cough, excess sputum, previous wheeze, hayfever, eczema, relatives with asthma, previous admissions/ITU
Signs wheeze, prolonged expiration, tachypnoea, hyperinflation
Investigations *PEFR* reduced compared with their best *ABGs* normal to mild hypoxia with a low CO_2 due to hyperventilation *CXR* hyperexpanded, exclude pneumonia and pneumothorax *spirometry* low FEV_1, low FEV_1:FVC ratio
Acute exacerbation Sit up and 100% O_2. Give salbutamol 5mg nebs, ±ipratropium (Atrovent®) nebs 500μg and prednisolone 40mg PO (or hydrocortisone 200mg IV). Connect the nebuliser mask to the oxygen supply, do not use air. Repeat salbutamol 5mg nebs every 15–30min and monitor with 15–30min PEFRs and sats.

- ***No improvement*** discuss with a senior regarding magnesium infusion (1.2–2g IV over 20min), alternatively IV aminophylline or IV salbutamol. Recheck ABGs and consider calling an anaesthetist. Severe asthma may require intubation and ventilation.
- ***Improving*** gradually reduce the % of O_2 and frequency of salbutamol as tolerated – this can be done over several days.

Chronic treatment See p338 or OHCM6 p186. Avoid smoking and allergens, monitor PEFR, check inhaler technique, inhalers (see p339 for colours and types), oral steroids for exacerbations.
Complications exacerbations, infection, pneumothorax

Pneumonia (OHAM2 p194)

Symptoms cough, increased sputum (green), pleuritic chest pain, breathless, haemopytsis, fever, unwell, confusion
Signs ↑temp, ↑RR, ↑pulse, ↓sats, unequal air entry, bronchial breathing, dull percussion, reduced expansion
Investigations *blds* ↑WCC and NØ, ↑CRP *ABGs* hypoxic if severe with a low CO_2 due to hyperventilation *CXR* consolidation
Severity Pneumonia is treated as severe if ≥2 of the CURB-65 criteria are present: **C**onfusion, **U**rea >7mmol/l, **R**esp rate >30/min, **B**P <90/60mmHg, age ≥**65**yr. Sats of <92% or PaO_2 <8Kpa also suggest severe pneumonia.
Treatment Sit up and 100% O_2. Give antibiotics according to local policy or see p254 for empirical treatment. If admitting to hospital consider giving IV fluids if dehydrated to increase lung perfusion. If symptoms are not resolving within 3d consider repeating the CRP and CXR to exclude pleural effusion/empyema
Complications empyema (pleural effusion of pus), respiratory failure, sepsis, confusion

1 See BTS Asthma of guidelines.

Pulmonary embolism (OHAM2 p146)

Symptoms often none except breathlessness, may have pleuritic chest pain, haemoptysis, dizziness, leg pain, see risk factors below

Signs ↑JVP, ↑RR, ↑pulse, RV heave, hypotension, pleural rub, ±pyrexia

Investigations D-dimer these are raised by most inflammatory conditions, however a normal D-dimer makes a PE very unlikely *ECG* ↑pulse, RBBB, inverted T waves V1–V4 or $S_1Q_3T_3$ *ABGs* ↓CO_2, ±↓O_2 *V/Q scan*

Acute treatment Sit up and 100% O_2. If life-threatening get an urgent CT or echo followed by thrombolysis. Otherwise LMWH (p289), eg enoxaparin 1.5mg/kg/24h SC + pain relief; IV fluids if hypotensive.

Chronic treatment warfarin (INR 2–3) for 6mth or for life if second episode or thrombophilia. See p291.

Clinically assessing risk of pulmonary embolism[1]

Major risk factor	Minor risk factor
Recent major surgery	Indwelling central line
Late pregnancy	Oral oestrogens (OCP/HRT)
Fracture or varicose veins	Long distance travel
Malignancy	Obesity
Previous proven DVT/PE	Thrombotic disorder

(1) The patient must have:

- breathlessness and/or tachypnoea (±pleuritic chest pain, ±haemoptysis)

(2) If so, does the patient have:

- A) absence of another reasonable explanation for these symptoms?
- B) the presence of a major risk factor?

If the answer to A and B is 'yes' then there is HIGH probability of PE
If the answer to A or B is 'yes' then there is INTERMEDIATE probability of PE
If the answer to A and B is 'no' then there is LOW probability of PE

Management

HIGH probability; no D-dimer test required

- Start LMWH and request radiological imaging (CT-PA/VQ scan)

INTERMEDIATE or LOW probability; check D-dimer:

- If positive start LMWH and request radiological imaging (CT-PA/VQ scan)
- If negative no imaging required, identify alternative diagnosis

1 Adapted from British Thoracic Society guidelines for the management of suspected acute pulmonary embolism. *Thorax* 2003; **58**:470–84.

Pulmonary oedema (OHAM2 p112)

Symptoms breathless, frothy sputum, much worse lying down, usually sleeps with >2 pillows, swollen legs, previous heart problems

Signs raised JVP, tachypnoea, fine inspiratory basal crackles, wheeze, pitting oedema ankles and/or sacrum, cold hands and feet

Investigations *blds* FBC, U+E, LFT, CRP, cardiac markers, look specifically for anaemia, infection and MI *ABGs* may show hypoxia with ↑↓$PaCO_2$ *ECG* exclude arrhythmias and acute STEMI, may show old infarcts, LV hypertrophy or strain (p514) *CXR* cardiomegaly (not on portable), pulmonary oedema signs (p508) echo poor LV function

Acute treatment Sit up and 100% O_2. If the attack is life-threatening call an anaesthetist early since CPAP and ITU may be required. Otherwise monitor pulse, BP, RR and O_2 sats whilst giving diamorphine 1mg boluses IV (repeat up to 5mg, watch RR) and furosemide 40–120mg IV.

- ***Systolic >100*** Give 2 sprays of sublingual GTN followed by an IV infusion of GTN starting at 4mg/h and increasing by 2mg/h every 10min, aiming to keep systolic >100; usual range 4–10mg/h.
- ***Systolic <100*** The patient is in shock, probably cardiogenic. Get senior help as inotropes are often required. Do not give nitrates.
- ***Wheezing*** Treat as for COPD alongside above treatment.
- ***No improvement*** Give furosemide up to 120mg total (more if chronic renal failure) and consider CPAP (see below). Insert a urinary catheter to monitor urine output, ±CVP monitoring. Consider HDU/ITU.

Once stabilised they will need daily weights, ±fluid restriction, spironolactone can be prescribed in patients already on high dose of furosemide (monitor U+E). An echo should be performed to assess LV function and cardiac markers at >12h to exclude an MI. ACE inhibitors and β-blockers improve long-term life expectancy in heart failure

Continuous positive airway pressure (CPAP)

This is a machine that constantly blows air/oxygen via a facemask to prevent alveolar collapse at the end of expiration – similar to purse-lip breathing. It is used in the acute treatment of severe pulmonary oedema or the chronic treatment of sleep apnoea (may use nasal CPAP)

Pneumothorax (OHAM2 p236)

Symptoms breathless, ±chest pain

Risk factors *primary* tall, thin, male *secondary* COPD, asthma, infection, trauma, recent central line or pleural aspiration, mechanical ventilation

Signs hyperresonant on one side with reduced air entry on the same side, tachypnoea, may have tracheal deviation or fractured ribs

Investigations *CXR* lung markings not extending to the peripheries, line of pleura away from the periphery.

Treatment Sit up and 100% O_2. Chest drain/aspiration if breathing compromised (hypoxic, severe SOB) or large (>2cm from chest wall). See procedure and management, p480.

Tension pneumothorax (OHAM2 p242)

Symptoms breathless, ±chest pain

Signs hypotensive, tachycardia, tachypnoea, unilateral hyperresonance and reduced air entry, ↑JVP, may have tracheal deviation

Acute treatment Sit up and 100% O_2. This is an emergency, it will rapidly worsen if not treated; insert a large venflon (brown/grey) into the 2nd intercostal space, midclavicular line directly above the 3rd rib. Listen for a hiss and insert a chest drain on the same side. Treat immediately before CXR or further investigations. If there is no hiss remove the cannula, consider alternative diagnoses – a chest drain is usually still required.

Pleural effusion (OHAM2 p248)

Causes *transudates* (protein <30g/l) pulmonary oedema, cirrhosis, nephrotic syndrome *exudates* (protein >30g/l) malignancy, infection, vasculitidies, rheumatoid, haemothorax *empyema* (pH is <7.2) infection

Symptoms may be breathless with pleuritic chest pain

Signs stony dull to percussion with reduced air entry, tachypnoea

Investigations CXR loss of costophrenic angle with a meniscus, p508

Treatment Sit up and 100% O_2. Investigate the cause; if the effusion is large, pleural aspiration may relieve symptoms and aid diagnosis, see p478 (draining >1.5l/24h may cause pulmonary oedema).

Acute respiratory distress syndrome (ARDS) (OHAM2 p230)

Acute onset respiratory failure following a pulmonary insult (eg pneumonia, gastric aspiration) or systemic insult (shock, pancreatitis, sepsis).

Symptoms breathless, often multi-organ failure

Signs hypoxic, signs of respiratory distress and underlying condition

Investigations bilateral infiltrates on CXR

Treatment Sit up and 100% O_2. Transfer to HDU/ITU and treat underlying cause. Often requires ventilation, ±inotropes.

MI	p130	Bradyarrhythmia	p143
Anaemia	p272	Tachyarrhythmia	p135
Anaphylaxis	p156		

Cough

Causes of coughs

Acute	URTI, post-viral, post-nasal drip (allergy), pneumonia, LVF, PE
Chronic	post-nasal drip, oesophageal reflux, asthma, COPD, bronchitis, bronchiectasis, smoking, pneumonia, TB, parasites, interstitial lung disease, heart failure, ACE inhibitors, lung cancer, sarcoid, sinusitis, cystic fibrosis, habitual
Blood	***massive*** bronchiectasis, lung cancer, infection (including TB and aspergilloma), trauma, AV malformations ***other*** bronchitis, PE, pulmonary oedema, mitral stenosis, aortic aneurysm, vasculitidies, parasites

Haemoptysis Coughing up blood, ≥400ml is considered 'massive'.

Management FBC, U+E, clotting, G+S, sputum M,C+S and cytology, ABG, ECG, CXR. Sit up, 100% O_2. If massive: codeine 60mg PO (↓cough), good IV access (≥green), monitor pulse and BP, bronchoscopy.

Bronchiectasis (OHCM6 p178)

Causes cystic fibrosis, infection (pneumonia, TB, HIV), tumours, immunodeficiency, allergic bronchopulmonary aspergillosis, foreign bodies, rheumatoid arthritis

Symptoms chronic cough with purulent sputum, ±haemoptysis, halitosis

Signs clubbing, course inspiratory crepitations, ±wheeze

Investigations FBC, immunoglobulins, aspergillus serology *CF* blood or sweat test *sputum* M,C+S *CXR* thickened bronchial outline (tramline and ring shadows), ±fibrotic changes *CT thorax* bronchial dilatation *bronchoscopy* to exclude other diagnoses

Acute treatment O_2 ±BiPAP, as required, ±bronchodilators/corticosteroids. Infections likely to be *Pseudomonas* (consult local antibiotic guidelines). Chest physio to mobilise secretions.

Chronic treatment Postural drainage (chest physio), inhaled/nebulised bronchodilators/corticosteroids, surgery may be considered.

Complications recurrent pneumonia, Pseudomonal infection, massive haemoptysis, cor pulmonale

Lung cancer (OHCM6 p182)

Symptoms cough, haemoptysis, breathlessness, chest pain, recurrent pneumonia, anorexia, weight loss, bone pain

Risk factors smoking (active and passive), asbestos, radon gas

Signs clubbing, lymphadenopathy, pleural effusion, Horner's syndrome

Investigations *cytology* of sputum or pleural aspirate *CXR* ask for lateral views too *bronchoscopy* used to visualise and biopsy central lesions, bronchial washings may help diagnose lesions that are not visible *thoracoscopy* endoscopic visualisation of the pleura and peripheral lung via the chest wall *transthoracic biopsy* for peripheral lesions *CT/MRI* used to identify lung lesions and stage lung cancer

Bronchogenic lung cancer

Overall the prognosis is poor; 20% of patients survive 1yr from diagnosis.

Non-small cell

- ***adenocarcinoma*** usually peripheral; not smoking related
- ***squamous*** usually central
- ***large cell*** usually peripheral; rapid growth and early metastasis

Small cell usually central; very rapid growth and early metastasis, paraneoplastic complications are common.

Mesothelioma is a cancer of the pleural lining strongly associated with asbestos exposure. It presents in a similar manner to lung cancer though chest pain is more prominent. The prognosis is very poor.

Treatment

Surgery eg lobectomy and pneumonectomy offers a potential cure in non-small cell carcinoma. It is often not possible due to extensive local involvement (especially with central lesions) or distant metastasis.

Radiotherapy may be potentially curative or simply pallative.

Chemotherapy the main treatment for small cell tumours (though often used with radiotherapy), also used for some non-small cell tumours.

Complications

Metastases common sites include pleura, brain, bones, liver, adrenals

Recurrent effusion can be treated with pleurodesis, using talc

SVC or airway obstruction, see p378

SIADH small cell tumours, see p245

Cushing's syndrome small cell tumours may secrete ectopic ACTH

Hypercalcaemia bony metastases or ectopic PTH (squamous tumours)

Neuropathies including:

- ***Horner's syndrome*** unilateral sympathetic palsy to the head causing a closed eyelid (ptosis), constricted pupil and absence of facial sweating
- ***hoarse voice*** palsy of recurrent laryngeal nerve
- ***phrenic nerve palsy*** unilateral raised diaphragm on CXR
- ***peripheral neuropathy***

Lambert-Eaton small cell tumours, see p220

Myopathies proximal weakness or muscle pain

CNS brain metastases or non-metastatic confusion/seizures

GI bleeding emergency

Airway	Check airway is patent; consider manoeuvres/adjuncts
Breathing	If no respiratory effort – **CALL ARREST TEAM**
Circulation	If no palpable pulse – **CALL ARREST TEAM**

Call for **senior help** early if patient deteriorating

- Lay the patient **on their side** if vomiting
- **High-flow oxygen** in all patients
- **Monitor** pulse oximeter, BP, defibrillator's ECG leads if unwell
- Obtain a full set of **observations** including temp
- Take brief **history** if possible/check **notes**/ask ward staff
- **Examine patient**: condensed CVS, RS and abdo exam
- Two good (large) sites of **venous access**, take bloods:
  - FBC, U+E, LFT, clotting, urgent 4–8u crossmatch
- **0.9% saline** 1l IV, **colloid** 500ml IV stat or O –ve blood
- Correct clotting abnormalities if present (p288)
- **Arterial blood gas**, but don't leave the patient alone
- Initiate **further treatment**, see following pages
- Consider **serious causes** (below) and treat if present
- Give Glypressin® 2mg IV over 5min if **oesophageal varices** suspected

If bleeding is severe and the patient haemodynamically unstable:

- Request **urgent O –ve blood**
- Contact the on-call endoscopist and alert **surgeons**
- Call for **senior help**
- **Reassess**, starting with A, B, C…

Life-threatening causes

- Gastroduodenal ulcer
- Gastroduodenal erosions
- Vascular malformations
- Oesophageal varices
- Mallory-Weiss tears
- Upper GI malignancy

Upper GI bleeds (OHAM2 p608)

Worrying features ↓GCS, postural BP drop, ↑pulse, ↓BP, ↓urine output, continuous haematemesis, frank PR bleeding, chest pain, clotting abnormality, liver disease

Think about ***most likely*** gastroduodenal ulcer (NSAIDs, *H. pylori*), oesophagitis, gastroduodenal erosion, oesophageal varices, Mallory-Weiss tear, swallowed blood (eg epistaxis) ***other*** oesophageal or gastric cancer, coagulation abnormalities, vascular malformation

Ask about colour, quantity, mixed in or throughout vomit, frequency, onset, stool colour, pain on vomiting, chest pain, abdominal pain, pain on eating, palpitations, dizziness, fainting, sweating, shortness of breath, weight loss, difficulty swallowing ***PMH*** previous bleeding, clotting problems, liver problems (?varices), gastroduodenal ulcers, heartburn ***DH*** aspirin, NSAIDs, warfarin, iron, steroids ***SH*** alcohol consumption (duration if excess)

Obs pulse, BP, postural BP, GCS, RR, sats

Look for continued bleeding, colour of vomit, pale and cold extremities, sweating, pulse volume, bruises, other sources of bleeding (nose, mouth), abdominal tenderness, ±peritonitic, masses, signs of chronic liver disease (see p191) ***PR*** fresh blood/melaena

Investigations ***blds*** FBC, U+E, LFT, clotting, G+S or 4–8u crossmatch ***CXR***, ***ECG*** for ischaemia ***OGD*** within 4h if severe bleeding and shocked, diagnosis, biopsy, ±treatment

- ***Initial bloods*** may show a normal Hb, reticulocyte count and urea, despite a significant bleed. Check pulse, BP and postural BP

Rockall risk scoring system for GI bleeds

≤2 = low risk, ≥9 = high risk

Feature	0	1	2	3
Age	<60yr	60–79yr	≥80yr	
Systolic BP	>100mmHg	>100mmHg	<100mmHg	
Pulse	<100/min	>100/min	>100/min	
Co-morbidity	Nil major	Heart failure, IHD	Renal/liver failure	Metastatic disease
Diagnosis	Mallory-Weiss/none	Other	Upper GI malignancy	
Bleeding on OGD	Nil recent		Recent	

Management NBM for 24h, O_2, two good (≥green) sites of IV access, blood/colloids/fluids IV, regular obs (pulse, BP, postural BP, urine output), consider catheterisation, CVP line and HDU/ITU, admit for OGD

- ***Young patients*** with a postural drop and a pulse >90 may have lost a lot of blood

	History	Examination	Investigations
Gastroduodenal ulcers	Epigastric/chest pain, heartburn, melaena, previous ulcers, NSAIDs, alcohol	Epigastric tenderness, may be peritonitic if perforated	Ulcer on OGD, CLO test may be +ve
Oesophagitis/ gastritis	Heartburn, NSAIDs, alcohol, hiatus hernia	Epigastric tenderness	Inflammation/erosions on OGD, CLO test may be +ve
Oesophageal varices	Frank haematemesis, previous liver disease, alcohol	Epigastric tenderness, signs of chronic liver disease	↑INR, deranged LFT, varices on OGD
Mallory-Weiss tear	Normal coloured forceful vomit then bloodstained vomit	Epigastric tenderness	Tear seen on OGD if not resolving

Clotting abnormalities (p288)

Anticoagulated	FFP 2–4units (assess need eg heart valve)
↑ INR	Vitamin K 5mg IV
↓ Plts (↓30 x 10^9/l)	Platelets

Oesophageal varices (OHCM6 p226, OHAM2 p618)

Symptoms of chronic liver failure (p191), known liver disease, excess alcohol, varices are asymptomatic until they bleed

Signs of chronic liver failure (p191)

Investigations varices seen on OGD

Acute bleed resuscitate according to p174 then:

- ***Glypressin®*** 2mg/over 5min IV if not already given
- ***OGD*** (in <4h if shock) for sclerotherapy/banding
- ***Bleeding still uncontrolled*** consider a Sengstaken-Blakemore tube and transjugular intrahepatic porto-systemic shunting (TIPS)
- ***Antibiotics*** (eg ciprofloxacin 400mg/12h IV or cefuroxime 1.5g/8h IV) in all variceal bleeds

Once bleeding controlled Glypressin® 2mg/over 5min IV, 1–2mg/4h for up to 3d, propanolol, treat cause of liver failure, TIPS

Giving Glypressin®

Glypressin® is vasopressin (ADH); it must be given by a doctor though there is little scientific basis for this. The perceived risk is of arterial spasm leading to arrhythmia, angina, MI and acute limb ischaemia. Give slowly over 5min to reduce the risk.

Mallory-Weiss tear (OHAM2 p622)

Symptoms repeated forceful vomiting, initially bloodless, then bright red blood streaks or throughout vomit, often follows binge drinking

Acute bleed management as on p174, usually resolves spontaneously, may need an OGD, ±injection, a PPI may be used after OGD

Oesophagitis and gastritis

Symptoms as for GORD (p187) or gastroduodenal ulcer
Signs epigastric tenderness
Investigations OGD to identify inflammation and CLO test for *H. pylori*, 24h oesophageal pH study
Acute bleed management as on p174, PPI (PO or IV) after OGD
Treatment weight loss, stop smoking, reduce alcohol, *H. pylori* eradication if present (below)

Gastroduodenal ulcer (ulcer diathesis) or erosions

(OHCM6 p214)
Causes *H. pylori*, NSAIDs, alcohol, smoking, stress
Symptoms epigastric pain related to eating, heartburn, chest pain, improves with antacids, bloating, melaena
Signs epigastric tenderness
Investigations ↓Hb, ↑urea, urea breath test for *H. pylori* (does not need OGD), ulcer on OGD, normal biopsy, CLO test on OGD for *H. pylori*
Acute bleed management as on p174, PPI (PO or IV) after OGD
Treatment Treat *H. pylori* infection (below), PPI (eg lansoprazole, omeprazole), avoid NSAIDS and aspirin, stop smoking, weight loss, reduce alcohol intake, avoid spicy food
Follow-up continue PPI and repeat OGD in 6–8wk

H. pylori infection and eradication

- Diagnosed by urea breath test (no OGD) or CLO test (OGD)
- Treat with triple therapy for 1wk, eg lanzoprazole 30mg/12h PO, amoxicillin 1g/12h PO, clarithromycin 500mg/12h PO

Lower GI bleeds

Worrying features continuous bright red PR bleeding, postural drop, ↑pulse, ↓BP, dizziness, ↓GCS, abdominal pain, weight loss, abdominal swelling, vomiting

Think about ***most likely*** polyps, diverticular disease, angiodysplasia, haemorrhoids, anal fissure, inflammatory bowel disease, colon cancer, upper GI bleed (p175) ***other*** aorto-enteric fistulae, ischaemic colitis, Meckel's diverticulum

Ask about onset, quantity, colour (red, black, clots), type of blood (fresh bleeding, mixed with stool, streaks on stool or toilet paper), abdominal pain, pain on eating, vomiting (colour), pain on opening bowels, straining, constipation, diarrhoea, change in bowel habit, anorexia, weight loss, bloating, palpitations, chest pain, dizziness, fainting, sweating, shortness of breath, tiredness ***PMH*** gastroduodenal ulcer, heartburn, liver disease, previous bleeding, inflammatory bowel disease, aortic surgery ***DH*** aspirin, NSAIDs, warfarin, steroids, iron ***FH*** inflammatory bowel disease, bowel cancer ***SH*** alcohol consumption (duration if excess)

Obs pulse, BP, postural BP, GCS, RR, sats

Look for pale and cold extremities, sweating, pulse volume, bruises, other sources of bleeding (nose, mouth), abdominal tenderness, ±peritonitic, masses, signs of chronic liver disease (see p191), distension, absent/tinkling bowel sounds ***PR*** blood, melaena, palpable mass ***proctoscopy*** haemorrhoids

Investigations ***blds*** FBC, clotting, U+E, LFT, glucose, G+S or 4–8u crossmatch ***ABG*** if unwell ***OGD*** to exclude upper GI bleed, urgent if shocked ***ECG*** if age >50yr ***sigmoidoscopy/colonoscopy*** for investigation, biopsy and treatment, may require ***mesenteric angiography*** if bleeding source cannot be identified

Management Lower GI bleeding is usually treated by surgeons whilst upper GI bleeding is usually a medical condition. Some patients' bowels do not realise this and upper GI bleeding may present with PR bleeding.

- ***Diagnosis*** It is rarely possible to tell the cause of significant lower GI bleeds from history and examination alone, investigations are essential
- ***Fresh blood on toilet paper*** or streaking stool only and patient well, treat as haemorrhoids/anal fissure (exclude Ca)
- ***Mild bleeding*** (no evidence of shock) NBM for 24h, O_2, two good (≥green) sites of IV access, blood/colloids/fluids IV, regular obs (pulse, BP, urine output), reassess if worsens or further bleeding
- ***Moderate bleeding*** (postural drop, ↑pulse) transfuse blood/colloids until haemodynamically stable, catheterise, hourly fluid balance, discuss with senior, may need urgent OGD
- ***Severe bleeding*** (fresh bleeding/clots, ↓BP) treat as upper GI bleed, fast bleep senior, transfuse O –ve blood, call anaesthetist, on-call endoscopist and surgical SpR

	History	Examination	Investigations
Upper GI bleed	Fresh PR bleeding, clots or melaena, epigastric pain	Liver disease or epigastric tenderness, PR blood or melaena	↓Hb, ↑urea, lesion on OGD
GI cancer or polyps	Change in bowel habit, weight loss, abdominal pain	PR blood or melaena, mucus/palpable mass	↓Hb, lesion on sigmoidoscopy/ colonoscopy
Inflammatory bowel disease	Abdominal pain, diarrhoea, weight loss, mouth ulcers	↑temp, abdo tender ±peritonitic, PR blood, mucus, melaena	↓Hb, ↑WCC, ↑CRP, lesions on sigmoidoscopy/ colonoscopy
Diverticular disease	Abdominal pain, fever, change in bowel habit	Tenderness, ±peritonism, PR blood, mucus	↓Hb, diverticulae on colonoscopy
Bowel ischaemia	Abdo pain, previous arterial disease	Shock, generalised tenderness	↑WCC, acidotic, ±AF or previous MI on ECG
Angio-dysplasia	Often asymptomatic, old age, recurrent fresh blood or melaena	PR blood or melaena	↓Hb, lesion on colonoscopy, consider angiography
Haemor-rhoids	Painless, fresh red blood on toilet paper, perianal itching, constipation	Often not palpable on PR, perianal tags, may have rectal prolapse	Lesions seen on proctoscopy
Anal fissure	Pain on defaecating, fresh red blood on toilet paper, constipation	Posterior/anterior PR tear, perianal tags, tenderness	Proctoscopy to visualise lesions

Chronic gastrointestinal blood loss

Causes oesophagitis, gastric erosions, gastritis, drugs, gastroduodenal ulcer, gastric/bowel cancer, polyps, lymphoma, inflammatory bowel disease, angiodysplasia

Symptoms unexplained anaemia, melaena, anorexia, weight loss, tired, faint, change in bowel habit, vague intermittent abdo discomfort

Signs pale, cachexic, mild abdo tenderness ***PR*** blood, palpable mass

Investigations stool for faecal occult blood (FOB), ova, cysts and parasites, bloods for FBC (↓Hb, ↓MCV), iron, ferritin, B_{12}, folate, U+E, LFT, OGD, sigmoidoscopy, colonoscopy/Ba enema, may need a barium follow through if small bowel disease suspected

Treatment investigate and treat the cause, treat anaemia with ferrous sulphate 200mg/8h PO, consider admission for transfusion if Hb <8g/dl or if symptomatic with anaemia

Colorectal cancer and polyps (OHCM6 p506)

Causes sporadic, familial, genetic syndromes

Symptoms intermittent abdo pain, altered bowel habit, blood or melaena in stool, tenesmus, weight loss

Signs abdo tenderness ***PR*** palpable mass, blood, mucus

Investigations ↓Hb, lesion on sigmoidoscopy/colonoscopy/Ba enema

Treatment polypectomy (send for histology), multiple polyps may need colonic resection or regular colonoscopy follow-up

Haemorrhoids (OHCM6 p522)

Dilated and displaced perianal vascular tissue (anal cushions)

Symptoms and risk factors painless, recurrent fresh red blood on toilet paper or streaking stools, may bleed enough to fill the bowl, pruritus ani, constipation with straining, multiple vaginal deliveries

Signs not palapable unless prolapsed ***PR*** blood, otherwise normal

Investigations proctoscopy to visualise haemorrhoids, sigmoidoscopy to identify other pathology (eg malignancy)

Treatment high-fibre diet, topical Anusol®, injection of sclerosants, band ligation, coagulation, cryotherapy, may need haemorrhoidectomy

Strangulated haemorrhoids Painful, tender mass, unable to sit down, treat with ice packs, stool softeners, regular analgesia and bed rest. Once stable, inject piles and consider elective haemorrhoidectomy.

Anal fissure (OHCM6 p520)

Symptoms new onset pain on opening bowels, fresh red blood on toilet paper, history of constipation and straining, may be Crohn's or cancer

Signs anal tear visible posteriorly on the anal margin (10% anterior), perianal ulcers, fistulae ***PR*** blood, tender

Investigations sigmoidoscopy if suspicious of cancer

Treatment *conservative* high-fibre diet, 5% lidocaine ointment, 0.2–0.3% GTN ointment, botox injection, lateral internal sphincterotomy

Angiodysplasia (OHCM6 p482)

Submucosal arteriovenous malformations, often in the ascending colon

Symptoms elderly, recurrent blood in the stool, abdo pain is rare

Signs may be normal; pallor ***PR*** blood

Investigations faecal occult blood (FOB), Ba enema/colonoscopy, mesenteric angiography

Treatment embolisation (via angiography), electrocoagulation (via endoscopy), surgical resection, treat anaemia eg ferrous sulphate

Inflammatory bowel disease	p203	Upper GI bleed	p175
Bowel ischaemia	p187	Diverticular disease	p188

Gastrointestinal cancer

Oesophageal cancer

Risk factors smoking, excess alcohol, obesity, reflux oesophagitis, Barrett's oesophagus, achalasia, strictures, coeliac disease
Symptoms and signs weight loss, appetite loss, general malaise, dysphagia, hoarseness, cough, haematemesis, retrosternal chest pain, lymphadenopathy, hepatomegaly
Investigations OGD, Ba swallow, CT thorax and abdo
Treatment surgical resection, stenting, radiotherapy, chemotherapy

Stomach cancer

Risk factors *H. pylori* infection, gastroduodenal ulcer, pernicious anaemia, blood group A, atrophic gastritis, gastric resection, Japanese origin
Symptoms and signs weight loss, appetite loss, general malaise, dyspepsia, epigastric pain, epigastric mass, Virchow's node
Investigations FBC, OGD and biopsy, Ba meal, CT abdo
Treatment gastrectomy, ±lymphadenectomy; chemotherapy if metastases

Colon cancer

Risk factors low-fibre diet, polyps, inflammatory bowel disease, FH
Symptoms and signs may present with obstruction or perforation:

- ***Right side*** weight loss, abdo pain, melaena, anaemia
- ***Left side*** altered bowel habit, tenesmus, PR bleeding, ±mass

Investigations faecal occult blood (FOB), FBC, CEA, CA 19-9, Ba enema, sigmoidoscopy/colonoscopy and biopsy, CT thorax/abdo/pelvis
Treatment may need chemotherapy if severe (eg Dukes C), surgery:

- Ascending, transverse, descending colon, high sigmoid – hemicolectomy
- Low sigmoid, high rectum – anterior resection

Rectal cancer

Risk factors polyps, inflammatory bowel disease, FH
Symptoms and signs rectal bleeding, constipation, tenesmus, pain on defaecating, mucus discharge, weight loss, appetite loss, general malaise, PR shows mass, mucus and/or blood
Investigations CEA, CA 19-9, sigmoidoscopy, Ba enema, CT abdo/pelvis
Treatment may need radiotherapy as well as:

- Upper 2/3 – anterior resection
- Lower 1/3 – AP excision with colostomy

Anal cancer

Risk factors syphilis, anal warts, vulval cancer
Symptoms and signs PR bleeding, pain on defaecating, constipation, pruritus ani, anal stricture, anal fistulae
Investigations CEA, CA 19-9, anal biopsy, sigmoidoscopy
Treatment Anorectal excision and colostomy or radiotherapy and chemotherapy

Abdominal pain emergency

Airway	Check airway is patent; consider manoeuvres/adjuncts
Breathing	If no respiratory effort – **CALL ARREST TEAM**
Circulation	If no palpable pulse – **CALL ARREST TEAM**

Call for **senior help** early if patient deteriorating

- **High-flow oxygen** in all patients
- **Monitor** BP, pulse oximeter, defibrillator's ECG leads if unwell
- Obtain a full set of **observations**, are they haemodynamically stable?
- Take brief **history** if possible/check **notes**/ask ward staff
- **Examine patient**: condensed RS, CVS, abdo, ±wound exam
- Consider **serious causes** (below) and treat if present
- Initiate **further treatment**, see following pages
- **Venous access**, take bloods:
  - FBC, U+E, LFT, amylase, CRP, clotting, crossmatch 4u, bld culture
- Give IV **fluids** if hypovolaemic or shocked (p148)
- **Analgesia** as appropriate
- **Arterial blood gas**, but don't leave the patient alone
- **Erect** CXR (portable if unwell) and **plain** AXR (cannot be portable)
- **Urine dipstick** and **β-HCG** (all pre-menopausal women), ±catheter
- Keep patient **NBM** if likely to need theatre
- Call for **senior help**
- **Reassess**, starting with A, B, C...

Life-threatening causes and emergencies

- Perforation
- Bowel infarction/ischaemia
- Bowel obstruction
- Acute pancreatitis/cholangitis
- Appendicitis
- Leaking abdominal aortic aneurysm (AAA)
- Strangulated hernia
- Testicular torsion
- Ruptured ectopic pregnancy
- Referred pain (MI, aortic dissection)

Abdominal pain

Worrying features sudden onset, ↑pulse, ↓BP, ↓GCS, distension, peritonism, expansile mass, recurrent vomiting, haematemesis, frank PR bleeding

Think about ***life-threatening*** see box on previous page ***common*** gastroenteritis, gastroduodenal ulcer, gastro-oesophageal reflux disease (GORD), constipation, inflammatory bowel disease (IBD), irritable bowel syndrome (IBS), diverticular disease, adhesions, mesenteric adenitis, renal colic, UTI, urinary retention, biliary colic ***obs/gynae*** ectopic pregnancy, ovarian cyst, accident, pelvic inflammatory disease, endometriosis, labour ***other*** MI, heart failure, pneumonia, sickle-cell crises, DKA, renal disease, psoas abscess, trauma

Ask about nature of pain (constant, colicky, changes with eating/vomiting/bowels), duration, onset, frequency, severity, radiation to the back, dysphagia, dyspepsia, abdominal swelling, nausea and vomiting, stool colour, change in bowel habit, urinary symptoms, weight loss, breathlessness, rashes, lumps, chest pain, recent surgery, last period ***PMH*** DM, inflammatory bowel disease, ischaemic heart disease, jaundice, pancreatitis ***DH*** NSAIDs ***SH*** alcohol

Obs temp, pulse, BP, RR, sats, BM, urine output

Look for jaundice, sweating, pale, pulse volume, lung air entry, clubbing, leuconychia (white nails), lymphadenopathy (Virchow's node), abdominal scars, distension, ascites, visible peristalsis, abdominal tenderness, peritonitis (tenderness with guarding, rebound and/or rigidity), loin tenderness, hepatomegaly, splenomegaly, masses (assess if expansile/pulsatile), check hernial orifices, examine external genitalia (if male examine for testicular vs epididymal tenderness), femoral pulses, bowel sounds (absent, reduced, normal, increased) ***PR*** perianal skin tags, fissures, warts; feel for tenderness, masses, prostate hypertrophy, stool, check glove for blood, mucus, pus, melaena and stool colour

Investigations ***urine*** dipstick, β-HCG in all pre-menopausal women of reproductive age, MSU ***blds*** FBC, U+E, LFT, amylase, Ca^{2+}, glucose, ±cardiac markers, clotting, bld cultures ***ABGs*** if the patient is unwell ***ECG*** to exclude MI ***erect CXR*** to exclude perforation ***plain AXR*** to exclude bowel obstruction ***KUB or IVU*** for renal colic ***USS*** especially if hepatobilary cause suspected, portable USS may help diagnose leaking AAA or identify peritoneal fluid ***CT abdo*** discuss with senior

Treatment

Give all patients O_2, adequate analgesia and anti-emetics; insert a urinary catheter if unwell. Keep them NBM until urgent surgery is ruled out:

- ***Shocked*** resuscitate with IV fluids, urgent senior review
- ***Peritonitic*** resuscitate with IV fluids, IV ABx, urgent senior review
- ***>50yr with severe pain*** consider AAA, IV fluids, urgent senior review
- ***Abdo pain and vomiting*** consider obstruction, IV fluids, NG tube, AXR, p510, urgent senior review
- ***GI bleed*** resuscitate with IV fluids, see p174, urgent senior review

See diagram on next page

	History	Examination	Investigations
Perforation	Short onset, severe abdominal pain	Peritonitis, no bowel sounds	Gas under diaphragm, acidotic
Bowel obstruction	Pain, distension, nausea, vomiting, constipation	Distension, tenderness, absent/tinkling bowel sounds	Dilated loops of bowel on AXR
Bowel ischaemia/ infarction	Sudden onset, severe pain, previous arterial disease	Shock, generalised tenderness	↑WCC, acidotic, ± AF or previous MI on ECG
Appendicitis	RIF pain, anorexia, nausea, vomiting	Slight temp, RIF tenderness, ±peritonitic	↑WCC, ↑CRP
Strangulated hernia	Sudden onset pain, previous hernia	Shocked, tender hernial mass	Needs urgent surgery
GORD/ gastroduodenal ulcer	Dyspepsia, heartburn, anorexia, NSAIDs	Epigastric tenderness	Seen on OGD, +ve CLO test
Gastro-enteritis	Rapid onset, vomiting, diarrhoea	↑temp, epigastric tenderness, no peritonitis	↑WCC, ↑CRP
Inflammatory bowel disease	Weight loss, mouth ulcers, PR bleeding, vomiting, diarrhoea	Distended, tender, ±peritonitis	↑WCC, ↑CRP, dilated bowel on AXR, lesions seen on colonoscopy
Diverticular disease	Pain, diarrhoea, constipation, PR bleeding	Tenderness, ±peritonitis	↑WCC, ↑CRP, diverticulae on colonscopy
Acute pancreatitis	Constant epigastric pain radiating to back, vomiting, anorexia, ↑alcohol or gallstones	Shock, epigastric tenderness, ↓bowel sounds	↑↑↑amylase, ↑WCC, ↑CRP, ↑glucose, ↓Ca^{2+}
Abdominal aortic aneurysm (AAA)	Abdominal and back pain, collapse/faint, previous heart disease/↑BP, age >50yr	Expansile mass, unwell, often ↓BP, ↓leg pulses	Straight to theatre if leaking, may be seen on portable USS
Renal colic	Sudden severe colicky flank pain, radiates to groin, nausea/vomiting	Sweating, restless, loin tenderness	90% of stones visible on KUB, lesion on IVU
Hepatobiliary disease	Constant or colicky RUQ pain, gallstones	RUQ tenderness, ±jaundice	Deranged LFT
Obs/gynae disease	Lower abdo pain, PV bleeding, irregular/ absent periods	Lower abdo tenderness, PV exam abnormal	β-HCG +ve, lesions seen on USS
Testicular torsion	Sudden onset severe unilateral groin pain	Tender testicle, ±swelling	Urgent surgery

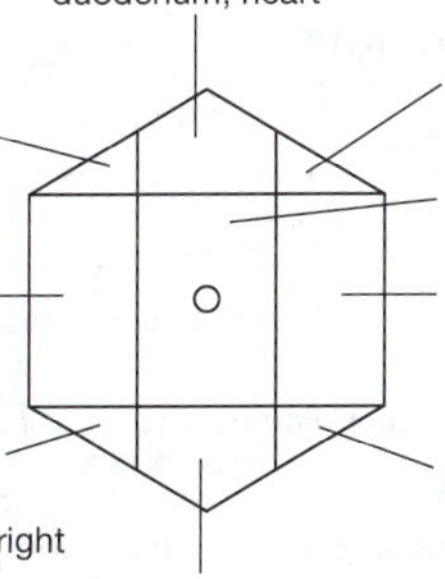

GI bleed	p175	Testicular torsion	p435
Inflammatory bowel disease	p203	Hernias	p434
Irritable bowel syndrome	p202	Renal disease	p269
Gastroduodenal ulcer	p177	Obs and gynae	p350
Hepatobiliary disease	p196	Gastroenteritis	p201

Perforation (OHCM6 p474)

Causes gastroduodenal ulcer, appendicitis, diverticulitis, inflammatory bowel disease, bowel obstruction, GI cancer, gall bladder
Symptoms acute abdominal pain worse on coughing or moving ***PMH*** gastroduodenal ulcer, cancer, inflammatory bowel disease ***DH*** NSAIDs ***SH*** alcohol
Signs ↑pulse, ±↓BP, ↑RR, peritonism (abdo tenderness, guarding, rebound, rigidity), reduced or absent bowel sounds
Investigations ↑WCC, ↓Hb, ↑amylase, erect CXR shows air under the diaphragm, ±obstruction on AXR, acidosis on ABGs
Management resuscitate with IV fluids, 100% O_2, good IV access (large × 2), analgesia (eg morphine 5–10mg IV with cyclizine 50mg/8h IV), NBM and urgent crossmatch 2–4u: IV antibiotics (cefuroxime 1.5mg/8h, metronidazole 500mg/8h) insert NG tube and catheterise, prepare for laparotomy (↑mortality with delay, may need ECG)

Bowel obstruction (OHCM6 p492)

Causes of intestinal obstruction

Outside the bowel	Adhesions, hernias, masses, volvulus
Within the bowel wall	Tumours, IBD, diverticular disease, infarction, congenital atresia, Hirschsprung's disease
Inside the bowel	Impacted faeces, foreign body, intussusception, strictures, polyps
Paralytic ileus (pseudo-obstruction) (ileus)	Post-op, electrolyte imbalance, ureamia, DM, anticholinergic drugs

Symptoms vomiting (may be faeculant), colicky abdo pain, pain improves with vomiting, constipation (±absolute – no flatus or stool), bloating, anorexia, recent surgery

Signs ↑pulse, ±↓BP, ↑RR, swollen abdomen, absent or tinkling bowel sounds, peritonitis, scars from previous surgery, hernias, PR masses

Investigations mild ↑WCC and ↑amylase, ±acidosis, look for dilated bowel (?small or large) or volvulus on supine AXR (p510), erect CXR to exclude perforation

Treatment may need fluid resuscitation and analgesia, treat according to the type and location of the obstruction:

- ***Strangulated*** Constant severe pain in an ill patient with peritonitis (acute abdomen); can be small or large bowel. This will require urgent surgery especially if caused by a hernia. See p435
- ***Small bowel*** Early vomiting with late constipation, usually caused by hernias, adhesions or Crohn's. Treated conservatively with NBM, an NG tube and IV fluids (0.9% saline 1l/4–6h) – often referred to as drip and suck – until the obstruction resolves. K^+ is often lost into the bowel and needs to be replaced in fluids (eg 20mmol/l)
- ***Large bowel*** Early absolute constipation with late vomiting, usually caused by volvulus (sigmoid or caecal), tumours, faeces or diverticulitis. IV fluids, NBM and refer to a senior surgeon. Urgent surgery may be required if the caecum is >8cm across on AXR otherwise a colonscopy or water-soluble contrast enema may be ordered to investigate the cause. Surgery is usually required except for:
  - Sigmoid volvulus – sigmoidoscopy and flatus tube insertion
  - Faecal obstruction – laxative enemas, see p204
- ***Paralytic ileus*** Loss of bowel motility can mimic the signs and symptoms of a mechanical blockage. It is a response of the bowel to inflammation locally (eg surgery) or adjacently (eg pancreatitis). The main distinguishing feature is the relative lack of abdo pain, however the pathology responsible for the ileus may cause abdo pain itself. An USS abdo, contrast enema or CT may be required to exclude mechanical obstruction. Treat conservatively with NBM, NG tube, IV fluids (0.9% saline 1l/4–6h) until the underlying pathology improves. K^+ is often lost into the bowel and needs to be replaced in fluids

Complications strangulation, bowel infarction, bowel perforation, hypokalaemia, hypovolaemia

Adhesions

Causes previous surgery, abdominal sepsis, inflammatory bowel disease, malignancy, endometriosis

Symptoms and signs chronic intermittent abdominal pain and tenderness, may develop bowel obstruction (distension, vomiting, constipation)

Treatment analgesia and stool softeners; may need division of adhesions, but this may lead to new adhesions forming

Bowel ischaemia/infarction (OHCM6 p488)

Symptoms unwell, sudden onset severe constant abdominal pain *PMH* MI, heart failure, polycythaemia, AF

Signs ↑pulse (?irregular), ±↓BP, ↑RR, ↑temp, cold extremities, generalised tenderness but few specific signs

Investigations ↑WCC, ↑amylase, acidotic (metabolic), ±AF on ECG

Treatment NBM, resuscitate with IV fluids; analgesia, IV antibiotics (cefuroxime 1.5g/8h, metronidazole 500mg/8h), anticoagulate with IV heparin (p290) and treat AF if present (digoxin, p138), consider ITU care, laparotomy is often necessary. Very poor prognosis.

Appendicitis (OHCM6 p476)

Differential UTI, diverticulitis, gastroenteritis, mesenteric adenitis, perforated ulcer, inflammatory bowel disease, diverticulitis *Gynae* ectopic pregnancy, ovarian cyst accident, salpingitis

Symptoms central, abdominal colicky pain worsening over 1–2d then developing into constant RIF pain, worse on moving, anorexia, nausea, vomiting, may have constipation, diarrhoea, dysuria, oliguria

Signs ↑temp, ↑pulse, ±↓BP, RIF tenderness ±guarding/rebound/rigidity, RIF pain on palpating LIF (Rovsing's sign), PR tender on right

Investigations ↑WCC, ↑ESR, ↑CRP, blood cultures (if pyrexial), G+S

Treatment NBM, IV fluids, analgesia, IV antibiotics (cefuroxime 750mg–1.5g/8h and metronidazole 500mg/8h). If peritonitic for immediate surgery, otherwise reassess frequently, continue ABx, fluids and analgesia whilst awaiting surgery.

Gastro-oesophageal reflux disease – GORD (OHCM6 p216)

Common risk factors smoking, alcohol, obesity, pregnancy, hiatus hernia

Symptoms burning retrosternal or epigastric pain, worse on bending and lying, waterbrash (excess saliva), acid reflux, nausea, vomiting, nocturnal cough, symptoms improved by antacids

Signs epigastric tenderness (no peritonitis)

Investigations endoscopy if symptoms persistent, difficulty swallowing or weight loss; 24h ambulatory pH monitoring

Treatment *conservative* weight loss, avoid foods/drugs which exacerbate symptoms *medical* Gaviscon®, ranitidine, regular PPI (eg lansoprazole), *surgery* fundoplication (rarely) if severe

Diverticular disease (OHCM6 p482)

- ***Diverticulosis*** diverticulae (outpouchings) present in the large bowel
- ***Diverticulitis*** inflammation of diverticulae; usually acutely symptomatic

Symptoms abdominal pain/cramps (usually left sided, improves with bowel opening), irregular bowel habit, flatus, bloating, PR bleeding

Signs ↑temp, ↑pulse, ±↓BP, LIF tenderness, ±peritonitis, distension

Investigations *blds* ↑WCC, ↑CRP, diverticulae may be seen on barium enema (may lead to perforation in diverticulitis) or colonoscopy

Treatment *diverticulosis* high-fibre diet, antispasmodics (eg mebeverine), laxatives (eg senna, p204) *diverticulitis* NBM, analgesia, fluids and antibiotics (cefuroxime 1.5g/8h IV, metronidazole 500mg/8h IV)

Complications obstruction, perforation, abscess, adhesions, strictures, fistula, PR bleeding (usually painless)

Abdominal aortic aneurysm – AAA (OHCM6 p480)

If you suspect a ruptured/leaking AAA:

- fast-bleep for senior help and vascular surgeon immediately
- order urgent O–ve blood and urgent crossmatch 8u.

Symptoms severe constant or colicky abdominal pain radiating to the back, collapse or feeling faint

Risk factors ↑age, male, ↑BP, smoking, heart disease, ↑cholesterol

Signs expansile abdominal mass (pushes hands apart, not just pulsing) – examination will not cause rupture, ↑pulse, ±↓BP, ↑RR, pale, sweating, cool extremities, distension, tenderness, ↓peripheral pulses

Investigations none if the patient is unstable; seniors may order an urgent USS/CT abdo if diagnosis is doubted

Management *emergency* give O_2, resuscitate, IV access for bloods and stat infusion of colloid/blood; once senior help arrives get the patient to theatre; *if the patient is stable/not leaking* keep NBM, prep for theatre, with observations every 15min

Renal colic (OHCM6 p264)

Exclude a AAA (if the patient is >50yr) and other causes of abdominal pain especially if no previous renal stone disease

Symptoms acute onset severe unilateral colicky loin pain, nausea and vomiting, sweating, haematuria, dysuria, strangury (frequency as the stones pass); iliac fossa or suprapubic pain suggests another pathology

Signs ↑pulse, sweating, patient restless and in severe pain, usually no tenderness on palpation unless superimposed infection

Investigations blood/haemoglobin on urine dipstick (~90% of cases), imaging (KUB, IVU, CT according to local policy), check FBC and U+E, pregnancy test in ♀

Treatment analgesia (NSAID first, then opiates), if <5mm should pass spontaneously. If evidence of infection give IV antibiotics (check local policy). If evidence of infection and hydronephrosis refer urgently to urologist for nephrostomy or stent depending upon local expertise.

Complications pyelonephrosis, renal dysfunction

Liver failure emergency

Airway	Check airway is patent; consider manoeuvres/adjuncts
Breathing	If no respiratory effort – **CALL ARREST TEAM**
Circulation	If no palpable pulse – **CALL ARREST TEAM**
Disability	If GCS ≤8 – **CALL ANAESTHETIST**

Call for **senior help** early if patient deteriorating

Altered mental state and **coagulopathy** in the presence of **jaundice**:

- Lay the patient **flat** with legs elevated
- **High-flow oxygen** in all patients
- **Monitor** pulse oximeter, BP, defibrillator's ECG leads if unwell
- Obtain a full set of **observations** including GCS, BM and temp
- Take brief **history** if possible/check **notes**/ask ward staff
- **Examine patient:** condensed CVS, RS, abdo, ±neuro exam
- Consider **serious causes** (below) and treat if present
- Initiate **further treatment**, see following pages
- **Venous access**, take bloods:
    - FBC, U+E, LFT, INR, CRP, glucose, amylase, Ca^{2+}, Mg^{2+}, PO_4^{3-}, bld cultures, paracetamol levels, viral serology
- Give 1l of **5% glucose** over 4–6h
- **ECG** to exclude arrhythmias and acute MI
- Request urgent **CXR**, portable if too unwell
- **Arterial blood gas**, but don't leave the patient alone
- Call for **senior help**
- **Reassess**, starting with A, B, C…

Causes of liver failure

Acute liver failure	Paracetamol overdose, drugs, toxins, viral hepatitis, autoimmune hepatitis, malignancy, ischaemic hepatitis (heart failure and shock), Budd-Chiari
Acute decompensated chronic liver disease	Infection, GI bleeds, alcohol excess, metabolic disturbances, sedatives, diuretics, acute illness, surgery

Liver failure

Worrying features ↑pulse, ↓BP, drowsiness, ↓GCS, bleeding, slurred speech, any neurology symptoms/signs, tremor/flap, renal failure

Think about ***emergencies*** acute liver failure, decompensated chronic liver disease, hepatic encephalopathy ***acute liver failure*** paracetamol overdose (p311), viral hepatitis (A, B, C, CMV, EBV), pregnancy, medications (see below), toxins (eg poisonous mushrooms), vascular disease (eg Budd-Chiari), sepsis, abscess, right heart failure ***chronic liver failure*** alcohol, idiopathic, autoimmune, hepatitis B+C, malignancy, Wilson's disease, haemochromatosis, α_1-antitrypsin deficiency

Drug-induced jaundice Antibiotics (augmentin, flucloxacillin, minocycline), NSAIDs, psych drugs (chlorpromazine, SSRIs), anti-epileptics (phenytoin, valproate), anti-TB drugs, statins, oestrogens

Ask about tiredness, jaundice (+onset), abdo pain, drowsiness, ±confusion, bruising, bleeding (skin, nose, bowel, urine), distension, ankle swelling, vomiting, rashes, recent infections (sore throat), weight loss, hair loss, darkening skin ***PMH*** previous jaundice, gallstones, breathing problems, transfusions ***DH*** paracetamol ***FH*** liver disease, recent jaundice ***SH*** alcohol, IVDU, tattoos, piercings, foreign travel, sexual activity (?abroad)

Obs temp, pulse, BP, RR, sats, GCS, BM, urine output

Look for volume status p262 ***acute liver failure*** drowsiness, confusion, slurred speech, jaundice, flapping tremor (asterixis), poor co-ordination, bruising, foetor hepaticus (pear drop smell), lymphadenopathy, abdominal tenderness, hepatomegaly, ascites ***chronic liver disease*** cachexia, palmar erythema, clubbing, xanthelasma, spider naevi, caput medusa, gynaecomastia, muscle wasting, splenomegaly, genital atrophy, track marks (IVDU), pneumonia/chronic lung disease, darkened skin

Investigations ***urine*** MSU ***blds*** FBC, clotting, iron, ferritin, U+E, LFT, hepatitis serology (A, B+C), EBV and CMV serology, caeruloplasmin (if <50yr), autoimmune screen (antimitochondrial, anti-nuclear and anti-smooth muscle antibodies, p194), bld cultures ***urgent USS abdo*** looking for metastases and dilated ducts ***ascitic tap*** (p486) if ascites present ***liver biopsy*** (percutaneous or transjugular) and ***CT abdo***

Grading of hepatic encephalopathy

Altered mood or behaviour	Grade I
Mild drowsiness, confusion, slurred speech	Grade II
Stupor, very confused and restlessness, incoherent	Grade III
Coma	Grade IV

	History	Examination	Investigations
Hepatic jaundice	New jaundice	Jaundiced, ±RUQ pain and hepatomegaly	↑mixed bilirubin, ↑ALT/AST
Acute liver failure	New jaundice, drowsy, unwell	Signs of acute liver failure, altered mental state	↑mixed bilirubin, deranged LFT, ↑INR
Chronic liver failure	Previous liver problems, excess alcohol	Signs of chronic liver disease	Deranged LFT

Acute liver failure (OHAM2 p658)

Hepatic encephalopathy and coagulopathy in the presence of jaundice:

Types of acute liver failure

Liver failure <7d of disease onset	Hyperacute fulminant hepatic failure
Liver failure 1–4wk of disease onset	Acute fulminant hepatic failure
Liver failure 4–12wk of disease onset	Subacute fulminant hepatic failure
Liver failure 12–26wk of disease onset	Late-onset hepatic failure

Symptoms jaundice, bruising/bleeding, drowsy, ±confusion, abdo pain

Signs ↑pulse, ↓BP, ↓sats, ↓BM, ↓urine output, signs of acute liver failure (p191)

Investigations ↑INR, deranged LFT, ↑bilirubin, ↑WCC, ↓glucose, ↓Mg^{2+}, ↓PO_4^{3-}, respiratory alkalosis, metabolic acidosis (bad sign), abnormal results specific to cause of liver failure

Treatment Discuss with a senior early, often needs ITU/HDU with invasive monitoring, may need transfer to a specialist liver centre. Regular obs and BMs; insert a catheter and monitor fluid balance.

- ***Raised INR*** give one-off dose of vitamin K 10mg IV:
  - Never give FFP without discussing with a senior because INR is used to monitor disease progress; it may be indicated if the patient is bleeding or needs invasive procedure
- Stop aspirin, NSAIDs and ***hepatotoxic drugs*** (see p191) and check other drugs in appendix 2 of the *BNF*
- ***Antibiotic*** prophylaxis in all patients (eg cefotaxime) ±antifungals
- Daily ***bloods*** (FBC, U+E, LFT, INR)
- ***Lactulose*** 30–50ml/8h in all patients
- ***Hypotensive*** IV fluids, avoid sodium if chronic liver disease/ascites – salt-poor albumin is often used, contact blood bank
- ***Hypoglycaemia*** IV glucose, see p230

Complications cerebral oedema, bleeding, sepsis, renal failure, respiratory failure, ↓glucose, ↑Na^+, ↓K^+

Vascular liver disease

Diagnosed by Doppler USS; these diseases can cause hepatic jaundice or acute liver failure, often treated by endovascular methods:

- ***Budd-Chiari*** hepatic vein obstruction
- ***Portal vein obstruction***
- ***Liver ischaemia*** due to hypotension and/or hepatic artery stenosis

Acute viral hepatitis (OHCM6 p576)

Causes hepatitis A, B, C and E, cytomegalovirus (CMV) and Epstein–Barr virus (EBV)
Symptoms flu-like symptoms: fever, malaise, anorexia, fatigue, nausea, vomiting, arthralgia, sore throat; jaundice, rash, diarrhoea, abdo pain
Signs may have no signs, ↑temp, urticarial rash, jaundice, hepatomegaly, splenomegaly, lymphadenopathy
Investigations ↑WCC, ↑bilirubin, ↑AST/ALT, ±↑INR, hepatitis serology
Management avoid alcohol, supportive treatment, monitor for progression to acute liver failure (opposite) which may need interferon-α
Complications acute liver failure, chronic disease

Chronic viral hepatitis (OHCM6 p576)

Lasts >6mth, *causes* hepatitis B (±D) and C
Symptoms and signs usually asymptomatic, signs of chronic liver disease
Investigations deranged LFT, ±↑INR, USS shows cirrhotic change, persistent raised viral serology
Treatment avoid alcohol, consider interferon-α therapy and ribavirin
Complications cirrhosis, hepatocellular carcinoma

Decompensated cirrhosis (chronic liver failure) (OHCM6 p232)

Symptoms jaundice, abdominal distension, itching, haematemesis, melaena; may be asymptomatic
Signs signs of chronic liver disease (p191), malnourished
Investigations LFT, FBC, clotting profile, immunoglobulins, autoantibodies, ferritin, transferrin saturation and α1 antitrypsin, ultrasound abdomen, ascitic tap, liver biopsy
Treatment avoid alcohol, NSAIDs, sedatives and opioids, refer to gastroenterologist and dietician may need liver transplant
Ascites low salt diet, daily weights, spironolactone 100mg/24h PO increasing dose every 48h to 400mg/24h, may need furosemide, ascitic tap for diagnosis (p486) and to exclude spontaneous bacterial peritonitis, may need therapeutic paracentesis
Complications portal hypertension, bleeding varices, encephalopathy, hepatocellular carcinoma

Spontaneous bacterial peritonitis

Symptoms abdominal pain in the presence of ascites, associated with confusion, unwell, fever
Signs fever, ↑pulse, ±↓BP, abdo tenderness, ± peritonitic
Investigations ↑WCC, ↑CRP, >250 white cells/mm^3 on ascitic tap
Treatment cefuroxime or ciprofloxacin

Autoimmune liver disease (OHCM6 p240)

Causes primary biliary cirrhosis, primary sclerosing cholangitis, autoimmune hepatitis (type I and II); primary biliary cirrhosis and type I autoimmune hepatitis may overlap
Symptoms often asymptomatic, may have fever, malaise, rash, joint pain or symptoms of chronic liver disease
Signs of chronic liver disease
Investigations deranged LFT, ±↑INR, USS and liver biopsy, autoantibodies (see table)
Treatment *autoimmune hepatitis* prednisolone 30mg/24h PO initially then azathioprine *other diseases* see p197
Complications acute liver failure, cirrhosis, hepatocellular carcinoma

Autoantibodies and HLA tests in autoimmune liver disease

Primary biliary cirrhosis	Anti-mitochondrial (AMA)
Primary sclerosing cholangitis	Anti-smooth muscle (SMA), anti-nuclear (ANA), p-ANCA
Autoimmune hepatitis type I	Anti-smooth muscle (SMA), anti-nuclear (ANA)
Autoimmune hepatitis type II (children only)	Anti-liver/kidney microsomal type 1 (LKM1)

Haemochromatosis (OHCM6 p234)

Autosomal recessive disease causing excess iron absorption
Symptoms fatigue, lethargy, arthralgia, hyperpigmentation, diabetes, family history of haemochromatosis
Signs arthralgia, hepatomegaly, signs of chronic liver disease, cardiac failure, osteoporosis
Investigations ↑AST/ALT, ↑glucose, ↑↑ferritin, ↑transferrin saturation, liver biopsy (iron loading and severity), ECG, echo if ?cardiomyopathy, genetic test
Treatment Venesection (1unit/wk) until ferritin normalises then every 3–6mth. Transferrin saturation can be used to screen relatives.

α_1-antitrypsin deficiency (OHCM6 p236)

Genetic disease with complex inheritance causing liver and lung damage
Symptoms breathlessness, liver failure, family history
Signs emphysema, signs of chronic liver disease
Investigations ↓α_1-antitrypsin levels, liver biopsy, genetic test
Treatment stop smoking, may need liver transplant, COPD treatment

Wilson's disease (OHCM6 p236)

Autosomal recessive disease; copper accumulates in the liver and CNS

Symptoms tremor, slurred speech, abnormal movements, clumsiness, depression, personality change, psychosis, liver failure, family history

Signs Kaiser-Fleischer rings in eyes, signs of liver failure

Investigations ↓caeruloplasmin, ↓serum free copper, ↑24h urinary copper excretion, copper on liver biopsy, positive genetic test

Treatment lifelong penicillamine, may need liver transplant, screen relatives

Jaundice

Worrying features ↑pulse, ↓BP, drowsiness, ↓GCS, bleeding, slurred speech, poor coordination, tremor/flap, renal failure, weight loss

Think about

- *Pre-hepatic* Gilbert's syndrome, haemolysis, malaria
- *Hepatic* paracetamol overdose, viral hepatitis, alcohol, chronic liver disease, pregnancy, medications (p191), toxins (eg poisonous mushrooms), vascular disease (eg ischaemia, Budd–Chiari), sepsis
- *Cholestatic* choledocholithiasis (gallstones in common bile duct), ascending cholangitis, pancreatitis, pancreatic cancer, cholangiocarcinoma, primary biliary cirrhosis, primary sclerosing cholangitis

Ask about tiredness, jaundice (+onset), abdo pain, itching, dark urine, pale stools, drowsiness, confusion, bruising, bleeding (skin, nose, bowel, urine), bloating, vomiting, rashes, recent infections (sore throat), weight loss, generalised aching, hair loss, darkening skin, joint pain ***PMH*** previous jaundice, gallstones, breathing problems, transfusions ***DH*** paracetamol and medications on p191 ***FH*** liver disease, recent jaundice ***SH*** alcohol, IVDU, tattoos, piercings, foreign travel, sexual activity (?abroad)

Obs temp, RR, pulse, BP, urine output, O_2 sats, BM, GCS

Look for volume status p262, bruising, evidence of bleeding, drowsiness, confusion:

- *Pre-hepatic* splenomegaly, pale conjunctiva, breathlessness
- *Hepatic* signs of acute or chronic liver failure p191
- *Cholestatic* abdominal tenderness, ±peritonsim, Charcot's triad (fever, jaundice and abdo pain = cholangitis), palpable gallbladder

Initial investigations ***urine*** MSU, bilirubin, urobilinogen ***blds*** FBC, reticulocytes, blood film, clotting, U+E, LFT, amylase, paracetamol levels, hepatitis serology (A, B+C), EBV and CMV serology, bld cultures ***urgent USS abdo*** looking for dilated ducts, cirrhosis and metastases

	Urine	Liver tests	Other tests
Pre-hepatic jaundice	Urobilinogen	↑unconjugated bilirubin	↓Hb, ↔MCV, ↓haptoglobulin, ↑reticulocytes
Hepatic jaundice	Urobilinogen	↑mixed bilirubin, ↑ALT/AST	May have positive hepatitis serology or ↑paracetamol levels
Obstructive jaundice	Bilirubin, dark urine	↑conjugated bilirubin, ↑ALP, ↑γGT	Dilated biliary ducts on USS
Cholangitis	Bilirubin, dark urine	↑conjugated bilirubin, ↑ALP, ↑γGT	↑WCC, ↑CRP, dilated biliary ducts

Haemolysis	p274	Hepatic jaundice	p191
Acute liver failure	p191		

Gilbert's syndrome

Common genetic disease causing a rise in unconjugated bilirubin with acute illness, no progression to liver failure

Biliary colic (OHCM6 p484)

Contraction of the gallbladder or cystic duct around gallstones
Symptoms recurrent colicky or constant RUQ/epigastric pain, especially on eating fatty foods, nausea, vomiting, bloating
Signs RUQ tenderness, non-peritonitic
Investigations bloods normal, USS shows gallstones
Treatment analgesia and elective cholecystectomy
Complications gallstone rarely passes into common bile duct where it may cause cholestatic jaundice, cholangitis or acute pancreatitis

Acute cholecystitis (OHCM6 p484)

Gallstone impacted in the neck of the gallbladder with inflammation
Symptoms continuous RUQ/epigastric pain, unwell, vomiting
Signs ↑temp, RUQ tenderness and peritonitis, Murphy's sign (pain on inspiration if two fingers placed on RUQ, not present on LUQ)
Investigations ↑WCC, ↑CRP, USS shows gallstones
Management NBM, analgesia, cefuroxime 1.5g/8h IV and metronidazole 500mg/8h IV; consider cholecystectomy

Cholangitis (OHCM6 p484)

Infection of the bile duct with Charcot's triad: fever, jaundice, abdo pain
Symptoms unwell, abdo pain, rigors, jaundice
Signs ↑temp, ↑pulse, ±↓BP, RUQ tenderness
Investigations ↑WCC, ↑CRP, ↑bilirubin, urgent USS
Management cefuroxime 1.5g/8h IV and metronidazole 500mg/8h IV, may need an urgent ERCP if gallstones are in the common bile duct

Primary biliary cirrhosis (OHCM6 p238)

Inflammation and damage of the interlobular bile ducts
Symptoms and signs fatigue, itching, cholestatic jaundice, cirrhosis
Investigations ↑ALP, ↑γGT, ±↑bilirubin, anti-mitochondrial antibodies (AMA), ↑IgM, USS, ERCP, liver biopsy shows granulomas
Treatment ursodeoxycholic acid, replace fat-soluble vitamins (A, D, E, K) colestyramine 4–8g/24h PO for itching, may need liver transplant

Primary sclerosing cholangitis (OHCM6 p238)

Inflammation and fibrosis of intra- and extrahepatic bile ducts
Symptoms and signs chronic biliary obstruction leading to cirrhosis
Investigations ↑ALP, ±↑bilirubin, ↑immunoglobulin levels, anti-smooth muscle antibodies (SMA), anti-nuclear antibodies (ANA), p-ANCA, HLA-A1, B8 + DR3, ERCP shows multiple strictures, fibrosis on liver biopsy
Treatment steroids, ursodeoxycholic acid may help symptoms, may need stenting or liver transplant

Acute pancreatitis (OHCM6 p478)

Varies from a mild self-limiting illness to severe and life-threatening

Causes 'GET SMASHED': gallstones, ethanol, trauma, steroids, mumps, autoimmune, scorpion bites, hyperlipidaemia/hypercalcaemia, ERCP, drugs (eg thiazide diuretics)

Symptoms constant severe epigastric pain radiating to the back, improved with sitting forward, nausea, vomiting, anorexia

Signs ↑pulse, ±↓BP, ↑temp, cold extremities, epigastric tenderness with peritonitis, abdominal distension, ↓bowel sounds, mild jaundice, Cullen's (bruised umbilicus) or Grey–Turner's (bruised flanks) sign

Investigations ↓Hb, ↑WCC, ↑↑↑amylase (usually >3x normal values), ↑glucose, ↓Ca^{2+}, deranged clotting (can have DIC, p288), deranged LFT *USS* gallstones *CT* pancreatic necrosis

Treatment resuscitate with IV fluids and O_2, analgesia, insert NG tube and urinary catheter, monitor fluid balance, NBM, if the patient is unwell and haemodynamically compromised call for senior review, may need ITU/HDU. Monitor obs and BMs regularly along with daily U+E, FBC, CRP. Prophylactic LMWH see p289.

Complications DIC, renal failure, respiratory failure, haemorrhage, thrombosis, sepsis, pseudocyst, abscess, thrombosis, chronic pancreatitis

Chronic pancreatitis (OHCM6 p252)

Causes usually alcohol, but can be due to gallstones (which may also cause recurrent pancreatitis), familial, cystic fibrosis, hyperparathyroidism

Symptoms general malaise, anorexia, weight loss, recurrent epigastric pain radiating to back, steatorrhoea, bloating, diabetes

Signs cachexia, epigastric tenderness

Investigations glucose (exclude diabetes, p236), USS, endoscopic USS, ERCP, CT abdo

Treatment analgesia, advise to stop drinking alcohol *diet* refer to dietician: low fat, high calorie, ↑protein with fat-soluble vitamin supplements *pancreatic enzymes* eg Creon® before eating *surgery* coeliac-plexus block, stenting of the pancreatic duct, pancreatectomy

Causes and management of itching (pruritus)

Dermatological urticaria, dry skin, contact dermatitis, allergic reaction, skin infestations (eg scabies), infection, dermatitis herpetiformis, lichen planus

Systemic causes cholestatic jaundice, chronic renal failure, diabetes, thyroid disease, hyperparathyroidism, leukaemia, polycythaemia rubra vera, malignancy (eg Hodgkin's lymphoma), drug allergy, psychological

Management avoid allergens, treat infections/infestations, symptomatic relief: cold compresses, moisturisers, chlorphenamine 4mg/6h PO, terfenadine 60mg/12h PO, calamine lotion 12h topically, colestyramine (for biliary obstruction only) 4–8g/24h PO

Hepatobiliary and pancreatic cancer

Metastatic liver cancer (OHCM6 p242)

The liver is a popular site for metastases and suggests widespread disease. Treatment and prognosis depends on the primary lesion. Solitary lesions may be resectable.

Hepatocellular carcinoma (OHCM6 p242)

Risk factors hepatitis B+C, cirrhosis, (alcoholic liver disease, non-alcoholic fatty liver disease, haemochromatosis), schistosomiasis, aflatoxin (fungi)

Symptoms and signs malaise, weight loss, anorexia, RUQ pain, jaundice, hepatomegaly, ascites

Investigations FBC, clotting, LFT, hepatitis serology, α-fetoprotein, USS, CT

Treatment surgery, radio frequency ablation, chemoembolisation, liver transplant

Cholangiocarcinoma (OHCM6 p242)

Tumour of the bile duct

Risk factors liver flukes, biliary surgery

Symptoms and signs fever, weight loss, anorexia, malaise, abdominal pain, jaundice

Investigations ↑ALP, ↑bilirubin, LFT, CA 19.9, USS, ERCP, ±biopsy

Treatment surgery, palliative stenting by ERCP

Pancreatic cancer (OHCM6 p248)

$^2/_3$ occur in the head of the pancreas and present with cholestatic jaundice; cancer in the body/tail presents later. May secrete hormones.

Symptoms general malaise, weight loss, epigastric pain radiating to back, vomiting, dyspepsia, jaundice

Signs cachexia, epigastric mass, hepatomegaly, jaundice, gallbladder

Courvoisier's law in the presence of jaundice an enlarged gallbladder is unlikely to be due to gall stones (exclude Ca).

Investigations FBC, U+E, LFT, glucose, amylase, Ca^{2+}, USS/CT abdo, ERCP, ±biopsy, ±stent

Management Often symptomatic/palliative since prognosis is poor; may be suitable for Whipple's procedure.

Diarrhoea

Worrying features ↑pulse, ↓BP, low urine output, PR blood, weight loss, abdo pain

Think about ***acute*** gastroenteritis, antibiotics, laxatives, drugs, pseudomembranous colitis, overflow diarrhoea (secondary to constipation), post-chemotherapy ***chronic*** inflammatory bowel disease, irritable bowel syndrome, colon cancer, diverticular disease, chronic pancreatitis, alcoholism, malabsorption disorders (eg coeliac), thyrotoxicosis, bowel resection, bowel ischaemia parasitic/fungal infections, autonomic neuropathy, carcinoid, ischaemic colitis, Addison's disease

Traveller's diarrhoea *E. coli, Salmonella, Shigella, Campylobacter*, giardiasis, amoebic dysentery, cholera, tropical sprue

Ask about normal bowel habit and frequency, onset/frequency of diarrhoea, recent constipation, stool character (floating, greasy, bloody, mucus), colour, abdominal pain, pain better/worse on opening bowels, nausea, vomiting, flatus, fluid intake, weight loss, mouth ulcers ***PMH*** diabetes, colon cancer, inflammatory bowel disease, diverticular disease, irritable bowel syndrome, surgery ***DH*** recent antibiotics, immunosuppression ***SH*** travel abroad, occupation (food, healthcare), alcohol

Medications causing diarrhoea antibiotics, laxatives, colchicine, digoxin, iron, NSAIDs, ranitidine, propanolol, PPIs

Obs temp, pulse, BP, postural BP, RR, sats, fluid balance

Look for volume status (p262), cachexia, mouth ulcers, clubbing, jaundice, rashes, pale conjunctiva, thyroid mass, abdomen tenderness, ±peritonitis, masses, distension, surgical scars ***PR*** faecal impaction, pain, masses, stool colour, consistency

200

Investigations ***stool*** M,C+S x3, *C. diff* toxin, ova, cysts and parasites (OCP) ***blds*** FBC, U+E (check K^+), glucose, LFT, Ca^{2+}, TFT, CRP, bld cultures ***AXR*** obstruction, ±faecal impaction ***sigmoidoscopy*** ±biopsy if not improving ***colonoscopy/Ba enema*** if cancer suspected

General treatment

- ***Conservative*** increase fluid intake, avoid dairy products, encourage mobilisation, review drugs: consider alternatives without GI side-effects
- ***Infective*** isolation and barrier nursing, antibiotics if systemically unwell
- ***Medical*** anti-diarrhoeal drugs should be avoided in infective diarrhoea, acute ulcerative colitis or pseudomembranous colitis

Anti-diarrhoeal drug	Dose
Loperamide	2mg/loose stool PO, max 16mg/d
Codeine	30mg/6h PO, max 240mg/d
Colestyramine (Crohn's/ileal resection)	4g/6h PO, max 36g/d

	History	Examination	Investigation
Gastro-enteritis	Sudden onset, ±vomiting, abdominal cramps	↑temp, sweating, abdo tenderness	↑WCC, ↑CRP, +ve microbiology on stool sample
Inflammatory bowel disease	Crampy abdo pain, weight loss, blood in stool, mouth ulcers	Abdo tenderness, ±peritonitis, PR blood/mucus, iritis/uveitis	↑WCC, ↑CRP, megacolon on AXR, lesions seen on sigmoidoscopy
Irritable bowel syndrome	Bloating, abdominal cramps, mucus in stool	Abdo tenderness, non-peritonitic, PR mucus	Diagnosis of exclusion; normal investigations
Malabsorp-tion disorders	Weight loss, pale greasy stools, tired, anaemia	Pale, abdo tenderness, oedema, bloating, PR pale stool	↓Hb, ↓albumin, ↓Ca^{2+} ± anti-endomysial antibodies
Bowel cancer	Abdo pain, weight loss, fresh blood or melaena	PR blood or melaena, mucus/palpable mass	↓Hb lesion on sigmoidoscopy/ colonoscopy
Diverticular disease	LIF pain, PR bleeding	LIF tenderness, ±peritonitis	↑WCC, ↑CRP, diver-ticulae on colonoscopy
Pseudomem-branous colitis	Recent antibiotics (days/weeks), crampy abdo pain, green watery stool	↑temp, abdo tenderness, PR green, foul smelling, ±blood	↑WCC, ↑CRP, *C. diff* toxin +ve
Overflow diarrhoea	Constipation, poor mobility, abdominal pain	Abdo distension and tenderness, PR palpable stool	AXR may show faecal loading
Drugs	Antibiotics, laxatives, colchicine, digoxin, iron, NSAIDs, ranitidine, propanolol, PPIs, thiazide diuretics		

Gastroenteritis (OHCM6 p556)

Symptoms rapid onset, recent vomiting and/or diarrhoea, patient may implicate a certain food, feels unwell, crampy abdominal pain, flu-like symptoms, pyrexia

Appearance of stool bloody (*Campylobacter, Shigella*); watery 'rice' stool (*cholera, E. coli*), green (typhoid)

Signs ↑temp, ↑pulse, dehydrated, flushing, sweating, abdominal tenderness, general malaise *PR* tenderness, peri-anal erythema

Investigations *stool culture* positive (takes ≥48h) *blds* ↑WCC, ↑CRP, may have ↑urea

Treatment isolation/barrier nursing, increase oral fluids, anti-emetics (p206), IV fluids if not tolerating oral fluids despite anti-emetics, antibiotics if symptoms severe, bloody diarrhoea or following stool culture (see table overleaf), advise rigorous hand-washing for nurses, doctors and visitors, some causes of infective diarrhoea are notifiable, see p253

Prolonged check stool for *C. diff toxin*, ova, cysts and parasites, *sigmoidoscopy*, consider alternative diagnosis

Common antibiotic choices in gastroenteritis – discuss with microbiology

Organism/source	Antibiotic therapy
C. difficile (see below)	Metronidazole PO or vancomycin PO
Campylobacter	Ciprofloxacin/erythromycin
Cholera	Tetracycline
Shigella	Ciprofloxacin/trimethoprim
Typhoid	Ciprofloxacin/cefotaxime/chloramphenicol

Organisms usually requiring supportive treatment only

Bacteria *Salmonella, C. perfringes* (type A), *bacillus cereus, E. coli*

Viral causative agent not usually identified

Pseudomembranous colitis

Overgrowth of *Clostridium difficile* following antibiotic use

Symptoms usually 3–9d after antibiotic therapy (can be 24h–6wk), rapid onset of high-quantity green, foul-smelling stool, crampy abdo pain

Investigations stool *C. difficile* toxin, M,C+S; ↓K^+

Treatment isolation and barrier nursing, rehydrate with oral/IV fluids and correct electrolyte abnormalities, metronidazole 400mg/8h PO and/or vancomycin 250mg/6h PO (oral route targets the GI tract)

Complications toxic megalcolon, perforation

Irritable bowel syndrome – IBS (OHCM6 p248)

Need to exclude bowel cancer and other causes of GI pathology

Worrying features acute onset, >40yr, weight loss, anorexia, PR blood

Symptoms central/lower abdo pain relieved by opening bowels, bloating, altered bowel habit, intermittent constipation and/or diarrhoea, exacerbated by stress, small amount of mucus in stool

Signs often normal or generalised abdo tenderness

Investigations FBC, ESR, LFT, TFT, anti-endomysial antibodies, urine M,C+S, consider sigmoidoscopy, colonoscopy/Ba enema, other tests according to associated symptoms (eg OGD, parasites)

Treatment reassure and explain, mebeverine 135mg/8h PO, loperamide or Fybogel® according to symptoms, consider low-dose antidepressants

Malabsorption disorders (OHCM6 p252)

Causes coeliac disease, chronic pancreatitis/pancreatic tumours, tropical sprue, cystic fibrosis, small bowel/gastric resection, alcohol liver disease

Symptoms diarrhoea, ±steatorrhoea, weight loss, tiredness, SOB, dizziness, bruising, swelling, vomiting, dairy/lactose/wheat/gluten intolerance, abdo pain

Signs cachexia, pale, dehydrated, mouth ulcers, sore tongue, abdo tenderness, oedema, bruises

Investigations ↓Hb, ↓MCV, ↓Ca^{2+}, ↓albumin, ↓iron, ↓folate, anti-endomysial antibodies +ve in coeliac disease, intestinal biopsy

Treatment nutrient supplements, refer to dietician and gastroenterologist, may need permanent gluten-free diet

Inflammatory bowel disease – IBD (OHCM6 p244)

Ulcerative colitis (OHCM6 p244), **Crohn's disease** (OHCM6 p246)

Symptoms recurrent episodes of diarrhoea, ±blood, ±mucus associated with abdo pain, malaise, tiredness, anorexia and weight loss
Admit if bowels open ≥6/24h, severe abdo pain, pyrexia, hypovolaemic
Signs ↑temp, ↑pulse, ±↓BP, pale, abdo tenderness, ±peritonitic, abdo swelling (toxic megacolon), malnourished, fistulae, fissures

Extra-intestinal signs clubbing, mouth ulcers, erythema nodusum, pyoderma gangrenosum, conjunctivitis, episcleritis, iritis, large joint arthritis, sacroiliitis, ankylosing spondylitis, fatty liver change, primary sclerosing cholangitis, cholangiocarcinoma

Investigations ↑WCC, ↑CRP, ±abnormal LFT, ↓Ca^{2+}, ↓iron, ↓folate, ↓B_{12} (terminal ileal disease), bld cultures *AXR* toxic megacolon >6cm *sigmoidoscopy* cobblestone appearance, ulcers, thickened bowel wall *Ba enema* (never during an attack episode) rose thorn ulcers, strictures, loss of haustra *biopsy* see table small bowel *enema* if Crohn's suspected

Differentiating factors between ulcerative colitis and Crohn's

Feature	Ulcerative colitis (UC)	Crohn's
Symptoms	Diarrhoea and PR blood/mucus prominent	Diarrhoea, abdo pain and weight loss prominent
GI involvement	Rectal involvement, may extend along the colon only	Anywhere along GI tract, most commonly terminal ileum or proximal colon
Sigmoidoscopy	Inflammed mucosa, continuous lesions from rectum proximally	Inflammed, thickened mucosa, normal mucosa in between (skip lesions)
Histology	Mucosal and submucosal inflammation, crypt abscesses, reduced goblet cells	Inflammation extends beyond the submucosa, granulomas present

Treatment resuscitate with IV fluids as needed (pulse, postural BP)

- ***Mild*** (<6 motions a day and systemically well) prednisolone 30mg/24h PO, oral fluids, consider prednisolone enema in UC
- ***Severe*** (≥6 motions a day, systemically unwell, marked PR bleeding, pulse >100), NBM, IV fluids, ±blood transfusion if severe anaemia, hydrocortisone 100mg/6h IV, if ↑temp give cefuroxime 1.5mg/6h IV and metronidazole 500mg/8h IV, avoid analgesia if possible, frequent (≥twice daily) abdo exam (tenderness, distension, bowel sounds), daily FBC, U+E, CRP, ±AXR (toxic megacolon >6cm), discuss with senior

Other therapies rectal steroids, elemental diet, sulfasalazine, mesalazine, azathioprine, methotrexate, ciclosporin, infliximab, bowel resection
Complications toxic megacolon, bowel obstruction, perforation, malabsorption, fistulae, fissures, strictures, malignancy

Overflow diarrhoea

Symptoms and signs elderly, immobility, poor diet, recent constipation, nausea, vomiting, bloating, abdo pain and tenderness, indentable stool filled bowel palpable ***PR*** hard, palpable stool, liquid stool in lower rectum
Treatment treat as constipation (p204)

Constipation

Worrying features abdominal pain, distension, nausea/vomiting, ↑pulse, ↓BP, absent/tinkling bowel sounds, weight loss, PR bleeding

Think about ***serious*** bowel obstruction, bowel cancer ***common*** opiates and other medications, poor diet, paralytic ileus, dehydration ***other*** anal fissure/stricture, pelvic mass, immobility, spinal/pelvic nerve injury, hypothyroid

Ask about abdominal pain, nausea, vomiting, date bowels last opened and frequency, normal bowel habit and frequency, stool consistency and colour, blood in stools, pain on opening bowels, straining, bloating, flatus, fluid intake, weight loss, tenesmus, recent surgery ***PMH*** inflammatory bowel disease, diverticulosis, hernias, previous surgery, colon cancer, hypothyroidism ***DH*** opiates, TCAs, iron ***SH*** mobility, diet

Obs temp, pulse, BP, fluid balance

Look for volume status (p262), tenderness, ±peritonism, abdominal distension, masses, absent/tinkling bowel sounds, hernias, scars ***PR*** anal fissures, rectal masses, faecal impaction, melaena/blood

Investigations ***blds*** FBC, U+E, TFT, Ca^{2+} ***AXR*** to exclude obstruction ***sigmoidoscopy*** ±biopsy if sub-acute onset ***colonoscopy/Ba enema*** if cancer suspected

Common laxative agents – drugs with different mechanisms can be prescribed together

Mechanism	Name	Dose
Bulking agents	Fybogel®	1 sachet/12h PO
	Normacel®	1 sachet/12h PO
Stimulants	Senna	2 tablets/24h (at night) PO
	Bisacodyl	5–10mg/24h (at night) PO
	Glycerol suppositories	Single suppository PR
Softener/stimulant	Sodium docusate	200mg/8h PO
Osmotic	Lactulose	15ml/12h PO
	Movicol®	1–3 sachet/24h PO
	Phosphate enema	Single enema PR

Common choices of laxatives according to degree of constipation

Mild	Senna or lactulose
Moderate	Senna and sodium docusate
Severe	Senna and sodium docusate and movicol/glycerol suppositories
Very severe	Phosphate enema, manual evacuation, Picolax® bowel prep

	History	Examination	Investigation
Bowel obstruction	Pain, distension, nausea, vomiting, constipation	Distension, tenderness, absent/tinkling bowel sounds	Dilated loops of bowel on AXR
Paralytic ileus	Absence of flatus, recent operation	Distended abdomen, absent bowel sounds	Distended bowel loops on AXR, ↑↓U+E
Bowel cancer	Abdo pain, weight loss, fresh blood or melaena	PR blood or melaena, mucus/ palpable mass	↓Hb, lesion on sigmoidoscopy/colonoscopy
Recto-anal pathology	Fresh red blood on toilet paper, ±pain	Perianal tags, may have a tear or tenderness	Proctoscopy or sigmoidoscopy
Poor diet	Anorexia (eg post-op), low-fibre diet	Cachexia	↓Hb, ↓MCV, ↓Ca^{2+}
Drugs	Opiates, diuretics, aluminium/Ca^{2+} based drugs, iron, calcium channel blockers, tricyclic antidepressants and anticholinergics		

Treatment

- ***Conservative*** good fluid intake, high-fibre diet, encourage mobilisation, review drugs – are there alternatives that do not affect bowel habit?
- ***Medical*** see laxatives opposite
- ***Manual evacuation*** literally scooping the hard faeces out of the rectum, should only be performed if requested by a senior

Poor diet

Aim for regular high-fibre meals, with good fluid intake

Symptoms nausea, vomiting, post-op, alcohol excess, malabsorption

Signs thin, dehydrated

Investigations FBC, U+E, TFT, Ca^{2+}

Treatment review diet, refer to dietician

Hints and tips

- Prescribe prophylactic laxatives for patients at risk of developing constipation (eg regular opiates, post-op).
- Exclude obstruction before prescribing a laxative.
- Reassess if constipation does not resolve.
- Consider malignancy in all patients >40yr presenting with altered bowel habit (see p181).

Anal fissures/haemorrhoids	p180	Bowel obstruction	p186
Inflammatory bowel disease	p203	Polyps	p180
Irritable bowel syndrome	p202	GI cancer	p181

Nausea and vomiting

Worrying features ↑pulse, ↓BP, ↓GCS, recurrent vomiting, severe pain (head, chest, abdomen), head injury, constipation, blood/coffee grounds, risk of inhalation

Think about ***severe*** raised intracranial pressure (ICP), meningitis, MI, bowel obstruction, acute abdomen, diabetic ketoacidosis ***most likely*** post-op pain, drug induced (opioids), gastroenteritis, other infection, alcohol ***other*** paralytic ileus, pregnancy, electrolyte imbalance (Ca^{2+}, Na^{+}), migraine, labyrinthitis, Ménière's, chemotherapy, Addison's, bulimia

Ask about frequency, timing, relation to food or medications, content, colour, blood, coffee grounds, melaena, dizziness, diarrhoea, constipation, flatus, abdo pain, chest pain, other pain, headaches, head trauma, visual problems, weight loss, altered bowel habit ***PMH*** previous surgery, migraines, diabetes ***DH*** opioids, chemotherapy, digoxin ***SH*** alcohol

Obs temp, fluid balance, pulse, BP, BM, GCS

Look for assess volume status (p262), respiratory creps, SOB, distended abdomen, tender abdomen, peritonitis, tinkling bowel sounds, hernias, scars from previous operations, mouth ulcers, neck stiffness, rash, photophobia

Investigations Vomiting without the worrying features usually does not require urgent investigation. If vomiting is recurrent check ***U+E*** for signs of dehydration or electrolyte imbalance and ***AXR*** if bowel obstruction suspected. Otherwise investigate according to related symptoms, consider: ***blds*** FBC, U+E, LFT, glucose, amylase, Ca^{2+}, blood cultures ***CXR*** aspiration ***ABGs*** if acutely unwell ***CT brain*** if head trauma, p309.

Common anti-emetic drugs

Drug[1]	Indications	Contraindications	Dose
Cyclizine (Antihistamine)	Most causes	Low GCS, severe heart failure	50mg/8h PO/IM/IV
Prochlorperazine (Phenothiazine – Stemetil®)	Post-op or drug induced	Low GCS, severe COPD	5–10mg/8h PO or 10–20mg PO one-off dose
Metoclopramide	Gastroenteritis, hepatobiliary disease, drug induced	<25yr, GI obstruction/perforation/haemorrhage, <4d post GI surgery	10mg/8h PO/IM/IV
Domperidone	Drug induced, less sedating	None. Not ideal post-op or for chronic use	10–20mg/6h PO, 30–60mg/6h PR
Ondansetron ($5HT_3$ antagonist)	Post-op, severe vomiting, chemotherapy	Tight budget	4mg/4–8h IM/IV

1 Different types of anti-emetics can be prescribed together except metoclopramide and phenothiazines which are very similar and can both cause dystonic reactions (eg spasms), especially at the extremes of age.

	History	Examination	Investigations
Raised ICP/ meningitis	Headache, blurred vision, dizzy, feels ill, drowsy	Febrile, neck stiffness, photophobia, rash, Cushing's reflex or shock, low GCS	↑WCC/NØ/CRP, abnormal CT brain or CSF results
Bowel obstruction	Colicky abdo pain, constipation, absence of flatus, brown vomit	Distended tender abdomen, tinkling bowel sounds, empty rectum	Distended bowel loops on AXR, see p510
Paralytic ileus	Constipation, absence of flatus	Distended abdomen, absent bowel sounds	Distended bowel loops on AXR, see p510
Acute abdomen	Severe abdo pain, feels ill	Tender, rigid, guarding, rebound, shock	Pneumoperitoneum on CXR
Upper GI bleed	Fresh blood or coffee-ground vomit	Tender abdomen, PR melaena	↓Hb, ↑urea
Gastro-enteritis	Vomiting after eating, diarrhoea, feels better after vomiting	Febrile, epigastric tenderness, not peritonitic	↑WBC, ↑LØ or NØ, positive stool culture
Labyrinthitis/ Ménière's	Dizziness is main feature, difficulty standing, tinnitus	Unable to stand	Acute investigations normal, see p208
Migraine	Visual aura, headache	Photophobia, visual field defects	Acute investigations normal
Drug induced	Many medications can induce vomiting, particularly opioids, chemotherapy and digoxin toxicity		

Treatment

Vomiting should be seen as a marker of disease severity and the diagnosis comes mostly from the associated symptoms; investigate and treat the underlying disease. Vomiting is very distressing for patients so try to relieve the symptoms with anti-emetics.

Headache	p210	Pregnancy	p356
Abdominal pain	p182	Electrolyte imbalance	p243
Upper GI bleed	p175	Dizziness	p208

Gastroenteritis (p201) Vomiting is often an early feature of bowel infections, especially those derived from food. Maintain good hydration with plenty of oral fluids ±rehydration solutions eg Dioralyte®, IV fluids may be required if vomiting is severe.

Dizziness

Worrying features ↑pulse, irregular pulse, hypoxia, ↓BP, ↓glucose, chest pain, sudden onset, unable to stand

Think about ***faint*** shock, arrhythmia, MI, postural hypotension, anxiety, hyperventilation, syncope, epilepsy, hypoglycaemia, reaction to pain, numerous medications ***vertigo*** labyrinthitis, benign positional vertigo, trauma, ototoxic drugs, Ménière's, CVA, multiple sclerosis, acoustic neuroma ***imbalance*** alcohol intoxication and toxicity, CVA, cerebellar space occupying lesion, intracranial infection

Ask about world moving or spinning, sudden or gradual, duration, position when attack came on, ringing in the ears, new hearing problems, blacking out, loss of consciousness, nausea/vomiting, falling, head injury ***PMH*** previous dizziness, hypertension, diabetes, MS, epilepsy ***DH*** anti-hypertensives, diuretics, aminoglycosides ***SH*** alcohol

Obs temp, pulse, lying and standing BP, BM, GCS

Look for ability to stand, standing with eyes shut (Romberg's, +ve if falls with eyes shut), ability to walk, change with position, cerebellar signs (DANISH – dysdiadochokinesis, ataxia, nystagmus, intention tremor and past pointing, slurred speech, hypotonia; nystagmus is found with many peripheral and central causes of vertigo), focal neurology, appearance of ear through an otoscope (effusion, perforation)

Investigations The type of dizziness (vertigo, imbalance, fainting) should be determined from history alone; beyond ***postural BPs*** acute investigation is rarely required. In the long term a ***tilt table test*** and ***audiometry*** may be considered and a ***CT scan*** if a CVA or tumour is suspected or there are cerebellar signs.

	History	Lesion
Fainting	Light-headed, no sensation of movement, anxious, palpitations, sweating, may have loss of consciousness	Shock, arrhythmia, MI, postural hypotension, anxiety, syncope, epilepsy, ↓glucose, reaction to pain; see p287 (falls)
Vertigo	Sensation of the world or patient moving, better when still, no loss of consciousness	Labyrinth, vestibular nerve, central connections of vestibular nerve, eg brainstem
Vertigo and hearing change	As above with either tinnitus (ringing/buzzing) or hearing loss	Labyrinth or vestibular nerve (VIII)
Imbalance	Inability to stand or walk straight, no sensation of movement, may have cerebellar signs (above)	Peripheral nerve, dorsal/posterior columns, cerebellum; lesion will be Romberg –ve

Fainting/syncope see p286

Vertigo (OHCM6 p346 and OHCS6 p546)

The sensation of vertigo can be treated with the same drugs used for nausea and vomiting (p206), especially since these are often effects of vertigo. Cyclizine 50mg/8h PO or betahistine 16mg/8h PO are good first-line agents though the underlying cause should be determined.

Benign positional vertigo Sudden onset vertigo following movement of the head and lasting seconds. Treated with the Epley Manoeuvre and referral to physiotherapy for vestibular exercises.

Labyrinthitis Sudden onset vertigo often following an URTI or febrile illness; vertigo may be severe and last days; there should be no focal neurology. Attacks gradually resolve over 2–3wk. Use the medications described above.

Ménière's Severe vertigo with tinnitus, nausea and vomiting lasting hours. Treat with the medications above and refer to ENT.

Motion sickness Rarely encountered in hospital, however cinnarizine 30mg PO or cyclizine 50mg PO 2h before journey are more effective than other anti-emetics.

CVA see p222

Imbalance/ataxia

Cerebellar disorders The cerebellum can be affected by the same diseases as the rest of the brain resulting in the DANISH signs (see opposite). Common causes include CVA, multiple sclerosis, infection, space occupying lesions and alcohol toxicity. Treat as a type of focal neurology and investigate the cause according to p218.

Spinal disease Romberg's positive; joint position sense is carried in the dorsal tracts which can be impaired by compression of the spinal cord secondary to infection, tumours and skeletal disease. Assess for other features of spinal disease (p223) and order an urgent MRI spine if new.

Peripheral neuropathy Romberg's positive; damage to the sensory nerves from the joints can result in imbalance, see p220.

Headache

Worrying features ↓GCS, rapid onset, severe headache, recurrent vomiting, photophobia, rash, neck stiffness, focal neurology, papilloedema

Think about ***emergencies*** intracranial haemorrhage (subarachnoid, subdural, extradural) meningitis, encephalitis, raised intracranial pressure (ICP), temporal arteritis, acute glaucoma ***common*** dehydration, tension, infection, migraine, trauma, post-LP, post-nitrates, extracranial (sinuses, eyes, ears, teeth) ***other*** cluster, hypertension, hypoglycaemic, hyponatraemic

Ask about severity, location, bilateral vs unilateral, speed of onset, character, change with coughing, nausea and vomiting, rashes, trauma, visual changes (before or currently), dizziness, seizures, joint pain, recent LP, sweating, malaise ***PMH*** previous headaches, migraines (and usual symptoms) ***DH*** nitrates, antihypertensives, insulin, oral hypoglycaemics ***SH*** recent stressors

Obs temp, GCS, BM, pulse, BP, fluid balance
- ***Cushing's reflex*** is a late sign of raised ICP: ↓pulse and ↑BP

Neuro obs GCS, limb movements, pupil size and reactivity, pulse, BP, RR, temp

Look for volume status (p262), neck stiffness, photophobia, Kernig's (fully flex hip and passively extend knee, +ve if painful in head or neck), visual and eye problems including tenderness (press on closed lid) and papilloedema, focal neurology, temporal artery tenderness and pulsatility, tender over sinuses, head trauma, dental hygiene, ear pathology, non-blanching rash (check whole body)

Investigations In the absence of worrying features it is appropriate to give pain relief without investigations; otherwise secure IV access and send ***blood*** for FBC, ESR, U+E, LFT, glucose, CRP, clotting and bld cultures ***ABG*** especially if GCS is reduced. Discuss with a senior whether a ***CT head***, ±***LP*** are required (LP procedure and contraindications p488). An ***EEG*** may help diagnose encephalitis.

Treatment

Exclude emergencies and treat other causes with simple analgesia (p282); ask to be contacted if symptoms fail to improve or worsen:
- ***new onset GCS <15:*** see p226
- ***new onset focal neurology:*** treat as meningitis, encephalitis or ↑ICP: O_2, consider antibiotics – call a senior urgently
- ***sudden (<2min), severe and constant:*** treat as subarachnoid: O_2, lie flat – call a senior urgently
- ***unwell, deranged obs:*** could be meningitis/sepsis, classic symptoms present in <30%: O_2, IV fluids, antibiotics – call a senior urgently
- ***red, painful eye with ↓acuity:*** glaucoma: refer urgently to ophthalmology
- ***temporal tenderness:*** temporal arteritis: O_2, high-dose prednisolone, ESR and urine dipstick – call a senior urgently

	History	Examination	Investigations
Sub-arachnoid or warning bleed	Rapid onset, severe pain, vomiting, low GCS if severe	May be normal, neck stiffness, photophobia, focal neurology	Bleed seen on CT or red cells and xanthochromia in CSF
Meningitis ±septicaemia	Unwell, irritable, drowsy, feels ill, ±rash, darkened room	Febrile, ±septic, neck stiffness, photophobia, ±non-blanching rash	↑WCC, ↑CRP, neutrophils in CSF
Raised ICP	Vomiting, progressive, blurred vision, dizzy, drowsy, seizures, worse on coughing/bending	Small or big pupils, focal neurology, papilloedema and Cushing's reflex are late signs	Abnormal CT, large ventricles, may have a focal lesion
Encephalitis	Drowsy, confused, vomiting, seizures, preceding flu-like illness, non-specific symptoms	Pyrexia, may have focal neurology, neck stiffness, photophobia and papilloedema	↑LØ and protein in CSF, ±RBCs, cerebral oedema on CT or MRI
Temporal arteritis	Age >55yr, visual disturbances, ill, weight loss, polymyalgia, jaw pain when eating	Tender, palpable, non-pulsatile temporal artery, tender scalp	↑CRP and ESR with anaemia, ↑plts and ↑ALP
Migraine	Similar to previous migraines, visual aura, usually unilateral, throbbing, nausea, ±vomiting	Photophobia, visual field defects, may have focal neurology	None
Tension	Bilateral, band-like pressure, worse when stressed	May have scalp tenderness, otherwise normal	None
Sinusitis	Frontal pain, blocked/runny nose	Tender above or below eyes	May have ↑LØ, NØ or EØ
Acute glaucoma	Age >50yr, blurred vision, pain in one eye, often occurs at night	Reduced visual acuity, dilated, ±oval pupil, red around cornea, tender	↑intraocular pressure
Drug induced	Many medications can induce headaches, particularly nitrates, Ca^{2+} channel antagonists and metronidazole with alcohol		

Sub-arachnoid haemorrhage (OHAM2 p466)

Suspect if over 40yr with recurrent vomiting and severe headaches.

Symptoms rapid onset (<2min), severe and continuous (>2h) headache, often occipital, vomiting, dizziness, may have seizures

Signs neck stiffness, drowsy, focal neurology, ↓GCS, photophobia

Investigations urgent CT head; if normal, LP to exclude small bleeds

Treatment 100% O_2, analgesia (codeine 60mg PO or 5–10mg morphine IV) and anti-emetic, eg metoclopramide 10mg IV/IM. Reassess often and request neuro obs. Lie the patient flat and advise not to get up or eat. If GCS is low or diagnosis confirmed involve an anaesthetist and neurosurgeon early and consider transfer to HDU/ITU. Use fluids to keep systolic >100mmHg, but try to avoid sudden increases in blood pressure. Focal neurology or reduced GCS carry a worse prognosis.

Complications cerebral ischaemia, rebleeding, hydrocephalus

Meningitis and septicaemia (OHAM2 p432, OHCM6 p368)

Symptoms headache, neck pain, photophobia, seizures, unwell

Signs ↑pulse, ±↓BP, ↑temp, ↓GCS or abnormal mood, neck stiffness, ±rash, focal neurology

Investigations ↑WCC, ↑CRP, CT scan then LP (p488), treat first

Treatment Resuscitate as needed (p158). 100% O_2, IV fluids and contact a senior. Start benzylpenicillin 2.4g/6h IV (or chloramphenicol 12–25mg/kg/6h IV if allergic to penicillin) and ceftriaxone 2g/24h IV immediately if you have a clinical suspicion of bacterial meningitis. Contact public health regarding contact tracing.

Complications ↑ICP, hydrocephalus, seizures, focal neurology

Encephalitis (OHAM2 p442)

An uncommon disease with non-specific symptoms that is hard to diagnose. It is caused by numerous viruses including herpes.

Symptoms not acting as normal, seizures, drowsy, headache, neck pain

Signs altered personality, ↓GCS, focal neurology, neck stiffness, ↑temp

Investigations CT followed by LP (p488), send CSF for viral PCR, EEG may show temporal lobe changes

Treatment aciclovir 10mg/kg/8h IV (10d) and ABx as for meningitis

Complications ↑ICP, seizures

Raised intracranial pressure – ICP (OHAM2 p452)

Causes CVA, tumours, trauma, infection (including abscess), cerebral oedema (eg post hypoxia), electrolyte imbalance, benign

Symptoms headache and vomiting (worse in morning and coughing/bending over), tiredness, visual problems, seizures

Signs altered GCS, papilloedema (late sign), focal neurology, Cushing's reflex (late sign ↑BP, ↓pulse)

Investigations urgent CT head to assess cause and severity

Treatment Elevate the head end of the bed to 40° and correct hypotension with 0.9% saline. Discuss with a senior before giving mannitol or dexamethsaone (tumours only) to reduce the ICP. Involve a neurosurgeon/neurologist early.

Complications herniation of the brain (coning)

Temporal arteritis (OHAM2 p760)
This is a medical emergency.
Symptoms headache, jaw pain on eating, visual problems, aching muscles
Signs temporal artery and scalp tenderness, pulseless or nodular temporal artery
Investigations ↑ESR (>50mm), ↑CRP, ↑plts, ↓Hb
Treatment Start 40–60mg/24h prednisolone PO and strong analgesia. Phone on-call surgeon to arrange a temporal artery biopsy within 5d (signs will resolve). Discuss with an ophthalmologist if visual symptoms are present. Dipstick urine.
Complications blindness, stroke, MI

Migraine (OHCM6 p342)
New migraines are uncommon, exclude underlying pathology (CT)
Symptoms visual aura (flashing lights, zigzag, loss of visual field) followed by throbbing one-sided headache (worse on exertion), nausea, vomiting, pain from light and sound
Signs visual field defects, focal neurology
Investigations normal
Treatment Treat with simple analgesia (see p282), ±anti-emetic and rest. If attack is severe consider triptan or ergotamine (see BNF or OHCM6 p342). Ask nurses to contact you if symptoms worsen and consider other diagnoses.

Sinusitis (OHCS6 p554)
Symptoms blocked nose, runny nose (clear/yellow/green), headache worse on bending
Signs tender over sinuses (above medial eyebrows, bridge of nose, below eyes), ↑temp
Treatment Try a mixture of saline nebs 5ml/2–4h, beclometasone nasal spray 2 sprays to each nostril bd and/or ephedrine nasal drops 1–2 drops in each nostril/6h (7d max). If severe (eg purulent mucus, systemically unwell) prescribe amoxycillin 500mg/8h PO.
Complications local spread of infection

Acute glaucoma See p385, this needs an urgent ophthalmology review.

Post LP (OHCM6 p753) Usually within 24h of LP, but up to 7d; advise the patient to lie flat, treat with analgesia and increase fluid intake.

Other headaches Prescribe simple analgesia, see p282. If the patient is dehydrated prescribe appropriate fluids (p263); if hypoglycaemic see p230; if profoundly hypertensive see p158.

Seizures and fits emergency (for adults)

Airway	Check airway is patent; consider manoeuvres/adjuncts
Breathing	If no respiratory effort – **CALL ARREST TEAM**
Circulation	If no palpable pulse – **CALL ARREST TEAM**

Call for **senior help** if >5min

0–5min, start timer

- Insert a **nasopharyngeal airway**
- **High-flow oxygen** by mask in all patients
- Keep patient safe and put into **recovery position** if possible
- **Monitor** pulse oximeter, BP, defibrillator's ECG leads, temp
- **Venous access** (after 3–4min). Take **bloods:**
    - FBC, U+E, LFT, Ca^{2+}, glucose, bld cultures, anticonvulsant levels
- **Check BM**: if <3.5mmol/l give 100ml of 20% glucose stat

5–20min

- Call for **senior help** and attach a cardiac monitor
- **Lorazepam** 4mg IV over 2min, repeat at 10min if no effect
- **OR diazepam** 10mg PR if no IV access, repeat up to 30mg
- Ask ward staff about **history**/check **notes**/ask word staff
- If alcoholism/malnourished give **Pabrinex**® 2 pairs IV over 10min

20–40min

- Call for **anaesthetist**
- **Phenytoin** 15mg/kg IV at 50mg/min, unless already taking phenytoin
- If taking phenytoin give **paraldehyde** 10ml IM
- **Monitor** ECG, BP and temperature

>40min

- **Phenobarbitone** 20mg/kg IV at 100mg/min on ITU/HDU
- **Transfer to ITU** for general anaesthetic and EEG monitoring

Life-threatening causes

- Hypoxia/cardiac disease
- Hypoglycaemia
- Metabolic (↓Ca^{2+}, ↓↑Na^{+})
- Trauma
- Meningitis, encephalitis, malaria
- Raised ICP and CVA
- Drug overdose
- Hypertension/eclampsia (pregnancy)

Seizures and fits

Worrying features preceding headache or head injury, recent depression (overdose), duration >5min, prolonged post-ictal phase, adult onset

Think about ***life-threatening*** see box on emergency page ***most likely*** idiopathic (>50%), epilepsy, alcohol withdrawal, hypoglycaemia, hypoxia, trauma ***other*** kidney or liver failure, pseudoseizures, overdose of tricyclics, phenothiazines, amphetamines ***non-seizure*** brief limb jerking during a faint, rigors, syncope, arrhythmias

Ask about get a detailed description of the fit from anyone who witnessed the episode (see below), headache, chest pain, palpitations, SOB ***PMH*** previous seizures, diabetes, alcoholism, cardiac, respiratory, renal or hepatic disease, pregnant ***DH*** anticonvulsants, hypoglycaemics ***SH*** alcohol intake, last drink, recreational drugs, recent travel ***FH*** epilepsy

Obs GCS, temp, BM (recheck), BP, sats

Look for sweating, tremor, head injury, tongue biting, neck stiffness, papilloedema, focal neurology, urinary or faecal incontinence, pregnancy, infection, limb trauma, posterior dislocation of shoulder

Investigations if a known epileptic or acute withdrawal from excess alcohol it is often appropriate to do none, see below for investigation of a first fit. Consider ***urine*** β-HCG if pre-menopausal female (–ve after 22wk gestation) ***blds*** FBC, U+E, LFT, glucose, Ca^{2+}, Mg^{2+}, blood cultures, anticonvulsant levels ***ABG*** if hypoxia or metabolic upset suspected ***ECG*** to exclude arrhythmia ***CT*** may show a focal lesion, raised ICP, haemorrhage or infarction ***MRI*** may be required to exclude small lesions ***LP*** if meningitis or encephalitis suspected ***EEG*** may help to exclude encephalitis or out-patient EEG to investigate epilepsy

Witnessing/describing a seizure

- ***Onset*** position, activity, any warning, starting in one limb or all over, presence of tonic phase (arched back, muscle spasm)
- ***During*** reaction to voice and pain, limb movements, eye movements, jaw and lip movements, breathing, peripheral or central cyanosis, sounds (may scream as air forced out of lungs), incontinence (urinary and faecal), duration, pulse and rhythm
- ***Afterwards*** tongue trauma, sleepy, limb weakness (Todd's paresis, p221), muscle pain, headache

First fit

History Detailed account from a first-hand witness
Investigations FBC, U+E, LFT, glucose, Ca^{2+}, Mg^{2+}, PO_4^{3-}, clotting, medication levels, urine and serum toxicology screen (including paracetamol and salicylate), CT, consider LP after CT, may need an MRI if a lesion is suspected
Management Admit for 24h unless GCS 15 and alert, decision regarding seizure status and driving (see p35, 1yr ban), follow up with neurology (first fit clinic)

	History	Examination	Investigations
Seizure	Sudden onset, muscle pain, post-ictal confusion	Often normal, may have tongue or limb trauma	Often normal, may have focal lesion or metabolic cause
Alcohol withdrawal	>50u/wk alcohol consumption, last drink >24h ago	Anxious, sweating, tachycardic, tremor, liver disease	↑MCV and γGT, may have a mild anaemia
Pseudo-seizures	Unusual features, short duration of active movements, memory of event	Responsive to pain, normal respiration, no injuries	Normal investigation
Meningitis or encephalitis	Drowsy, confused, irritable, vomiting, headache	Febrile, ±septic, neck stiffness, photophobia, non-blanching rash, focal	Abnormal CSF, see p503
Trauma, raised ICP and CVA	Prolonged drowsiness/confusion, headache, vomiting, blurred vision, dizzy, weakness	Falling/low GCS, focal neurology, papilloedema, neck stiffness, head injury	Abnormal CT
Transient arrhythmia/Stokes-Adams	Sudden LOC, any posture, palpitations, pale, ±limb jerking, rapid full recovery with flushing	Evidence of cardiac disease, injury following fall, weak/irregular/absent pulse during attack	May have arrhythmia or heart block on ECG, 24h ECG and BP monitoring
Rigors	Coarse shaking, felt cold/hot, no LOC, symptoms of infection	Febrile, source of infection eg UTI, pneumonia, viral illness, no injury	↑WBC, NØ or LØ and CRP, +ve urine dipstick
Syncope	Rare lying down, ±fine limb jerking, ±urinary incontinence, rapid recovery, no postictal phase	Bradycardia and hypotension during episode, GCS 15/15 within min, no focal neurology	Postural drop (systolic drop of 20mmHg or more)

Treatment

General Stop the seizure using the treatment outlined on p214. Correct any metabolic upset (glucose, Ca^{2+}, Na^{+}) and exclude life-threatening causes, try to establish the cause. Get an ***urgent CT*** if the patient has a persistent GCS <15 post-fit, focal neurology or if the seizure was <4d post-trauma. Secure airway if still fitting or GCS ≤8.

Partial seizures are more likely to have a focal source. Diagnosing limb jerking as a seizure could prevent the patient driving for one year. If in doubt write a detailed description and allow senior staff to decide.

Epilepsy (OHCM6 p378)

Symptoms Diagnosis is mainly from the history. There are many types:

- ***Partial*** Seizure that involves only one cerebral hemisphere, only one side of the body will be affected. Can be motor, sensory or both:
  - *Simple* Partial seizure without altered consciousness, eg jerking/spasm of left side or spreading of jerking (Jacksonian)
  - *Complex* Partial seizure with altered consciousness, eg temporal lobe epilepsy (altered mood, hallucinations, stereotyped movements)
- ***Generalised*** Seizure involving both cerebral hemispheres:
  - *Tonic-clonic* Initial muscle spasm of whole body (tonic) followed by jerking phase (clonic); LOC throughout
  - *Absences* Sudden stopping of activity with staring or eye rolling, lasts <45s, most common in children
- ***Secondary generalised*** Partial seizure that spreads to both hemispheres

Signs ↓GCS, tongue trauma, limb weakness, incontinence

Investigations often normal, may have an abnormal CT or EEG if there is a focal lesion

Treatment Follow the treatment plan on p214. There is no specific treatment required post seizure. Do not alter the patient's regular medication yourself, but make sure the patient is able to take their medication (consider NG medications) and is doing so. See OHCM6 p380 for ongoing management.

Alcohol withdrawal (OHAM2 p500)

Symptoms anxiety, shaking, sweating, vomiting, seizures *3–4d post-alcohol* confusion, delusions, hallucinations, amnesia, encephalopathy

Signs hypertension, tachycardia, pale, sweaty, tremor *3–4d post-alcohol* pyrexia, nystagmus, past pointing, ataxia, hypoglycaemia

Investigations may have ↓Mg^{2+} or ↓PO_4^{3-}

Treatment Any patient who consumes >50u a week needs a reducing dose of chlordiazepoxide (see p24) with thiamine 25mg/24h PO and multivitamins one tablet/24h PO.

If >100u a week replace the thiamine with Pabrinex® 2 pairs/8h IV infusion over 10min for 5d, this is a high-potency combination vitamin B and C that may rarely cause an anaphylactic reaction. Monitor blood pressure and BM.

Complications seizures, coma, encephalopathy, hypoglycaemia

Post-traumatic Needs an urgent CT scan. If haematoma seen, contact a neurosurgeon, otherwise hourly neuro obs and reassess if GCS falling.

Raised ICP	p212	Hypertension	p158
Hypoglycaemia	p230	Syncope	p286
Hypocalcaemia	p246	Tachy/bradyarhythmias	p135/143
Hyper/hyponatraemia	p243/244	Hypoxia	p165
Pre-eclampsia	p375	Meningitis/encephalitis	p212

Focal neurology

Worrying features ↓pulse, ↑BP, ↓GCS, hypotension, hypertension, severe headache, pyrexia, neck stiffness, photophobia, vomiting, papilloedema

Ask about weakness, clumsiness, tingling, pain, numbness, double vision, blurred vision, talking problems, swallowing problems, balance problems, speed of onset, weight loss, fever, cough, headache, nausea, vomiting (early morning), photophobia, neck stiffness, rashes, recent infections, behavioural change, tiredness ***PMH*** previous neurology, migraines, epilepsy, eye problems, blood pressure, irregular heart, diabetes ***DH*** antipsychotics, isoniazid ***SH*** alcohol and cocaine ***FH*** nerve or muscle problems

Obs BP, pulse, GCS (see p226 if low), BM

Neuro obs GCS, limb movements, pupil size and reactivity, pulse, BP, RR, temp

Look for perform a complete neuro exam including cerebellar signs (p221), CVS exam for AF and carotid bruit

Investigations These should be determined by the location of the lesion determined by clinical examination. Investigations include ***blood*** tests and autoimmune markers, ***nerve conduction studies, CT/MRI*** imaging and ***LP*** (procedure p488, interpretation p503)

Urgent CT brainstem or cerebral (lateralising) signs, persistent ↓GCS, sudden onset headache lasting >2h, head injury with loss of consciousness and recurrent vomiting or seizures

Lesion location

The aim is to determine which region of the nervous system is affected to allow further investigation and diagnosis. With motor symptoms there are three main areas:

- ***lower motor neurone (LMN)*** – peripheral nervous system; wasting, fasciculations, reduced reflexes and tone, forehead included if CN VII
- ***upper motor neurone (UMN)*** – central nervous system; increased tone and reflexes with upgoing plantars, forehead spared if CN VII
- ***mixed*** – consider cord compression of the conus, motor neurone disease, Friedreich's ataxia, syphilis (taboparesis), sub-acute combined degeneration of the cord

The following table offers a simplified guide to locating the lesion in patients with focal neurology. Due to the complexity of the nervous system diseases can present with atypical features that do not fit these patterns. Acute intracranial pathology may present with decreased tone and reflexes before the characteristic UMN signs develop.

	Motor	Sensory	Reflexes and tone	Features
Myopathy	Proximal > distal	Normal	Normal/↓	Bilateral
NMJ	Proximal > distal	Normal	Normal/↓	Bilateral, fatigability (or reinforcement)
Neuropathy	Distal > proximal	Tingling or numbness	Normal/↓	Unilateral or glove and stocking, atrophy and fasciculations
Radiculopathy	Distal > proximal	Painful with tingling or numbness	Normal/↓	Unilateral, painful, atrophy and fasciculations
Myelopathy	Distal > proximal	↓ below sharp level	↑	Bilateral, urinary retention
Brainstem	Whole leg/arm/face	Whole leg/arm/face	↑	Crossed, cranial nerve lesion (not II)
Cerebrum	Whole leg/arm/face	Whole leg/arm/face	↑	Unilateral, dysphasia/inattention
Cerebellum	Normal	Normal	Normal/↓	Cerebellar signs

Common causes

- ***Myopathy (muscle)*** alcohol, hypothyroid, inflammatory (eg polymyositis), medication (eg statins), muscular dystrophy, myotonic dystrophy
- ***Neuromuscular junction (NMJ)*** myasthenia gravis (fatigability) or Lambert-Eaton (reinforcement), botulism toxin
- ***Peripheral neuropathy (nerve)*** diabetes, trauma, vitamin B_{12}/folate deficiency, alcohol, renal failure, inflammatory (eg Guillain-Barré, SLE), hypothyroid, carcinoma, motor neurone disease, Bell's palsy, nerve entrapment syndromes (p298)
- ***Radiculopathy (nerve root)*** disc protrusion (usually L4, L5, S1), spondylosis, spinal stenosis, NB sciatica is a radiculopathy affecting the sciatic nerve (L4, L5, S1); cauda equina syndrome is a radiculopathy affecting all the cauda equina nerves and is an emergency
- ***Myelopathy (spinal cord)*** multiple sclerosis, infection, neoplasia, epidural haematoma, syringomyelia, spinal stenosis, spondylosis, central disc herniation, NB cord compression is an emergency
- ***Brainstem*** CVA, neoplasia, multiple sclerosis, abscess
- ***Cerebrum*** CVA, neoplasia, multiple sclerosis, migraine, abscess
- ***Cerebellum*** CVA, neoplasia, multiple sclerosis, alcohol, abscess
- ***Also consider*** hypoglycaemia, hyponatraemia, meningitis, encephalitis, raised intracranial pressure, focal seizure, autoimmune

Specific conditions

Inflammatory myopathy *see p417*

Muscular dystrophy genetic diseases causing progressive muscular weakness, eg Duchenne's (X-linked recessive)

Myotonic dystrophy slow relaxing muscles (myotonia), autosomal dominant congenital form is most common – slow hand shake release

Myasthenia gravis (OHCM6 p400, OHAM2 p506)
Symptoms weakness on exertion, diplopia, dysarthria, symptoms worse in evening than morning
Signs muscle fatiguability, especially on upward gaze, normal reflexes
Investigations antibodies to ACh receptor, improvement with edrophonium (perform in resuscitation area only), CT of thymus
Treatment anticholinesterase (eg pyridostigmine), immunosuppression, surgical removal of thymus gland, plasmapheresis (removes antibodies from the blood), immunoglobulins
Myasthenic crisis Myasthenia symptoms can worsen rapidly due to illness, surgery and some medications. The patient may develop respiratory failure requiring ventilation due to diaphragm fatigue; assess with spirometry (FVC). Treatment is with immunosuppression, anticholinesterase, immunoglobulins and urgent plasmapheresis.

Lambert–Eaton Autoimmune disease caused by small cell lung cancer showing improved strength with repetition (reinforcement) including reflexes. Trunk affected more than face and reflexes reduced.

Mononeuropathy (OHCM6 p390)
Bell's palsy (OHCM6 p388) Rapid onset mononeuropathy of the facial nerve (VII). Usually recovers spontaneously within weeks, prednisolone and/or aciclovir may be used (no evidence of benefit). Tape the affected eye closed at night and use regular artificial tears (p384) with sunglasses.
Carpal tunnel syndrome (OHCS6 p662) Mononeuropathy of the median nerve causing aching and tingling of the hand (especially thumb, index and middle fingers) that is worse at night. Nerve conduction studies may aid diagnosis; treated with steroid injections or surgery.

Peripheral neuropathy (Polyneuropathy) (OHCM6 p392)
Causes see p219
Symptoms clumsiness, weakness, tingling, numbness
Signs usually glove and stocking distribution
Investigations urine dipstick, FBC, B_{12}, folate, U+E, LFT, glucose, TFT, ESR, serum electrophoresis, ANCA, ANA, CXR, nerve conduction studies
Treatment treat or remove the cause if possible
Complications wounds, ulcers, joint abnormalities eg Charcot joint

Guillain–Barré (OHAM2 p512) post-infectious proximal neuropathy that can rapidly progress to respiratory failure; use spirometry (FVC) to assess severity and progression, consider early ventilation and immunoglobulins if developing respiratory failure or FVC falling.

Motor neurone disease (OHCM6 p394)
Symptoms stumbling, poor grip, muscles quivering, speech and swallowing problems, aspiration pneumonia
Signs mixture of LMN and UMN signs, normal sensation, fasciculations
Investigations electromyography (EMG)
Treatment mostly symptomatic, life expectancy is usually 3–5yr
Complications aspiration pneumonia, respiratory failure, spasticity

Syringomyelia (OHCM6 p404) central tubular spinal cord cavities seen on MRI; weakness and loss of pain/temp sensation in the arms

Cervical/thoracic spinal stenosis caused by degenerative changes or spondylosis resulting in a radiculopathy or myelopathy

Todd's paresis transient focal neurological symptoms following a seizure, typically limb weakness; lasts minutes to hours so mimics a TIA

Parkinson's (OHCM6 p382)
Symptoms shaking, difficulty getting up, slow walking, depression
Signs resting tremor (pill rolling), rigidity, bradykinesis (slow movement), monotonous voice, expressionless face, altered handwriting
Investigations clinical diagnosis, MRI and CT not usually required
Treatment levodopa (reduced effectiveness after 5yr, start if symptoms interfere with life), peripheral dopa-decarboxylase inhibitor eg carbidopa, dopamine agonists eg cabergoline, anticholinergics eg benzatropine
Complications depression, dementia

> ***Causes of dystonia*** (involuntary movement) Parkinson's, Wilson's, multiple sclerosis, CVA, trauma, antipsychotics, levodopa, metoclopramide, anticonvulsants, Huntington's chorea, Sydenham's chorea, ataxia telangiectasia, syphilis, AIDS, CJD

Multiple sclerosis (OHCM6 p384)
Symptoms recurrent weakness (in different nerves), numbness, tingling, vision loss, ataxia, urinary incontinence, (dysphasia and seizures are rare)
Signs any focal neurology, especially spastic limb paralysis and vision loss
Investigations areas of inflammation on MRI, slowed nerve conduction, CSF may show oligoclonal bands (p503)
Treatment *acute* steroids, baclofen, diazepam or botulinium toxin to relieve spasticity *disease modifying drugs* β-interferon, glatiramer
Complications incontinence, relapse, pain

Space occupying lesion (OHCM6 p386)
Causes tumour, aneurysm, abscess, chronic subdural haematoma
Symptoms focal neurology, seizures, behavioural change, early morning headache and vomiting
Signs focal neurology, papilloedema
Investigations CT, MRI (brainstem/cerebellum), do not perform an LP
Treatment for raised ICP see p212, surgical removal of tumour/lesion

Cerebellar dysfunction (causes p219)
Symptoms clumsiness, imbalance, speech problems
Signs DANISH: dysdiadochokinesis, ataxia (truncal and gait), nystagmus, intention tremor (past pointing), slurred speech (dysarthria), hypotonia

Stroke (OHCM6 p354, OHAM2 p478)

Causes haemorrhage (20%) or infarction (80%, eg AF, carotid stenosis)
Symptoms sudden onset focal neurology though onset can be stuttering
Signs Check for irregular heartbeat and carotid bruit. Determine region:

- *total anterior circulation* (TACS) – all three features shown in the table
- *lacunar* (LACS) – affects the internal capsule causing profound weakness and/or anaesthesia without other defects
- *partial anterior circulation* (PACS) – similar features to TACS or LACS, but not fulfilling the full criteria
- *posterior circulation* (POCS) – affects the brainstem or cerebellum.

	TACS	LACS	PACS	POCS
	All of following	**Any abnormality listed**		
Motor and/or sensory defect	Unilateral in ≥2 out of face, arm and leg	Face with arm and/or leg	Unilateral, <TACS or LACS criteria	Bilateral or associated with cranial nerve defect on opposite side
Eyes	Homonymous hemianopia[1]	Normal	Variable	Homonymous hemianopia or new diplopia
Ataxia	Absent	Ataxic hemiparesis[2]	Absent	Present, other cerebellar signs
Higher cerebral[3]	Present	Normal	Present	Normal or ↓ GCS

1 Visual field defect on same side in both eyes, eg right sided vision in right and left eyes for a the left side of brain stroke.

2 Unilateral weak and ataxic arm and leg without other cerebellar signs.

3 Higher cerebral dysfunction includes dysphasia (right side of brain) or visuospatial disorder, eg inattention (left side).

Prognosis LACS, PACS and POCS have a similar prognosis with 15% mortality by 1yr while 60% live independently; TACS are worse with a mortality of 60% at 1yr with only 5% living independently.
Investigations FBC, U+E, LFT, glucose, ESR, lipids, clotting, ECG, CXR, urgent CT head if GCS persistently low or evidence of raised ICP; otherwise within 48h, consider non-urgent echo and carotid doppler
Treatment Aspirin 300mg PO unless high suspicion of haemorrhage (severe headache, meningism, persistent ↓GCS). Nil by mouth with IV fluids if swallow affected (requires SALT assessment). Monitor BP, but do not try to lower-BP without discussing with a senior. Admit to stroke ward for rehabilitation with multidisciplinary team.
Prevention Aspirin (75mg/24h PO), control BP, statin, stop smoking, exercise, warfarin (AF) or carotid endarterectomy (stenosis)
Complications Aspiration pneumonia, dependent lifestyle, further CVA
Transient ischaemic attack (TIA) Sudden onset stroke symptoms and signs resolving completely in less than 24h. Take seriously. Give aspirin 300mg PO, investigate and start preventative measures as for stroke.

Back pain (OHCS6 p618–27)

Worrying features bilateral leg neurology or pain, bladder/bowel changes, progressive/night pain, weight loss, age <20yr or >55yr, steroids, thoracic or non-mechanical pain, previous Ca, altered perianal sensation

Causes ***serious*** cord compression, cauda equina syndrome, metastases, myeloma, infection, fracture, aortic aneurysm ***common*** mechanical back pain (see table), bruising, sprain

Types of mechanical back pain	
Disc prolapse	'Slipped disc', may compress the nerve root causing a unilateral radiculopathy (sciatica)
Spondylosis	Degenerative changes of the spine, eg osteoarthritis
Spondylolysis	Recurrent stress fracture leading to a defect in the vertebrae
Spondylolisthesis	Slippage between lumbar vertebrae as a result of spondylosis or spondylolysis
Lumbar spinal stenosis	Narrowing of the spinal canal due to osteoarthritis, causes leg aching and heaviness on walking (spinal claudication)

Examination ***Look*** scoliosis (sideways curvature), kyphosis (forwards curvature) ***Feel*** press each vertebral body to elicit tenderness, repeat next to spine ***Move*** flexion, extension, lateral flexion, rotation, compress iliac crests together (sacroiliac joints) ***Straight leg raise*** if shooting pain is brought on by raising straight leg <45° suggests a mechanical radiculopathy ***Neuro exam*** full examination of leg power, sensation and reflexes ***PR*** if suggestion of cauda equina syndrome

Investigations FBC, ESR, CRP, Ca^{2+}, ALP, PSA, spine X-ray if centrally tender post trauma or with risk of pathological fracture, urgent MRI spine if cord compression or cauda equina suspected, bone scan

Treatment

- ***Mechanical back pain*** early mobilisation, avoid lifting and maintain good posture, analgesia (p282), consider diazepam 2mg/8h PO for servere muscular spasm, refer if symptoms not improving at 6wk
- ***Non-mechanical back pain*** refer to orthopaedics

Emergencies (OHAM2 p508)

Cord compression weakness and anaesthesia of legs (arms and legs if cervical), reflexes increased below the level of the lesion, reduced at the lesion and normal above, bladder and bowel problems are late features

Cauda equina bilateral radiculopathy (sciatica), painless urinary retention, perianal anaesthesia and reduced anal tone

Causes degenerative changes, central disc prolapse, tumours, infection, haematoma, trauma

Investigations urgent MRI spine especially if rapidly progressing

Treatment refer immediately to orthopaedics, often requires surgery (<6h)

Complications paralysis, anaesthesia and sphincter dysfunction

Essential neuroanatomy

Root levels of main limb movements

Joint	Movement	Root	Joint	Movement	Root
Shoulder	Abduction	C5	Hip	Flexion	L1–2
	Adduction	C5–7		Adduction	L2–3
Elbow	Flexion	C5–6		Extension	L5–S1
	Extension	C7	Knee	Flexion	L5–S1
Wrist	Flexion	C7–8		Extension	L3–4
	Extension	C7	Ankle	Dorsiflexion	L4
Fingers	Flexion	C8		Plantarflexion	S1–2
	Extension	C7	Big toe	Extension	L5
	Abduction	T1			

Root levels of reflexes

Reflex	Root	Reflex	Root
Bicep	C5–6	Knee	L3–4
Supinator	C5–6	Ankle	S1–2
Tricep	C7–8		

Spinal tracts and anatomy

Tract	Modality	Crosses (decussates) at
Anterior and lateral corticospinal (pyramidal)	Motor	Medulla
Posterior columns (dorsal)	Light touch, vibration, position	Medulla
Spinothalamic	Pain, temperature	Level of entry to the cord

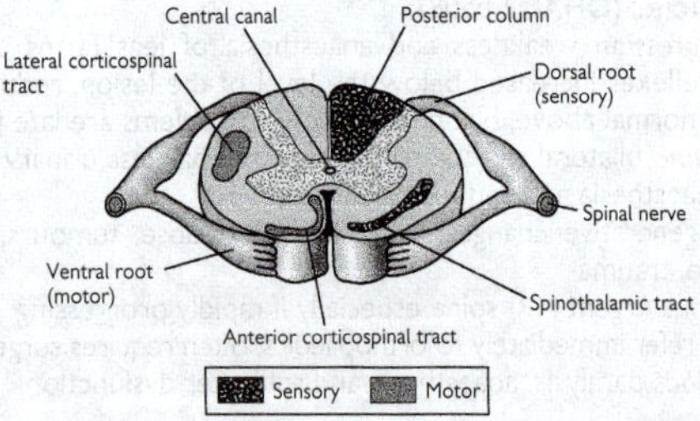

Dermatomes

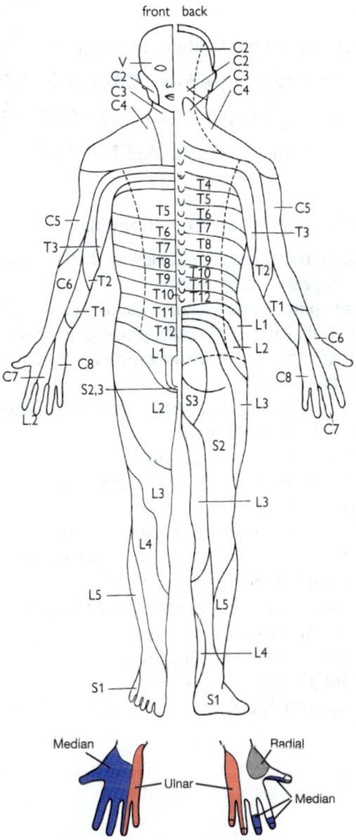

Innervation of hand movements

Movement	Nerve
Finger abduction and adduction	Ulnar
Thumb opposition and abduction	Median
Finger extension	Radial

Coma and reduced GCS emergency

Airway	Check airway is patent; consider manoeuvres/adjuncts
Breathing	If no respiratory effort – **CALL ARREST TEAM**
Circulation	If no palpable pulse – **CALL ARREST TEAM**
Disability	If GCS ≤8 – **CALL ANAESTHETIST**

Call for **senior help** early if patient deteriorating

- **Oropharyngeal** or **nasopharyngeal airway** if tolerated
- Give **high-flow oxygen** in all patients
- Stabilise **cervical spine** if there is any risk of injury (eg fall)
- **Monitor** BP, defibrillator's ECG leads, pulse oximeter
- Get nurses to take a full set of **observations** including **BM** and **temp**
- **Venous access**, take bloods:
  - FBC, U+E, LFT, glucose, Ca^{2+}, cardiac markers, clotting, bld cultures, paracetamol and salicylate levels
- Start **IV fluids** if blood pressure ≤140/80
- **ECG** and treat **arrhythmias**, tachy p134, brady p142
- **Control seizures**, p214
- Ask ward staff for a brief **history** or check **notes**
- **Examine patient** brief RS, CVS, abdo and neuro exam:
  - brainstem, lateralising or meningeal signs
- **Arterial blood gas**, but don't leave the patient alone
- Request urgent portable **CXR**
- **Stabilise** and **treat**, see following pages
- Call for **senior help**
- **Reassess**, starting with A, B, C…

Life-threatening causes

- Hypoxia
- Hypotension
- Metabolic
- Toxins
- Infections
- Structural lesions

Stabilisation

- Get **senior help**
- Treat **hypoxia** with O_2, airway aids, ±ventilation
- Treat **arrhythmias** and **hypotension** urgently
- Start broad-spectrum **antibiotics** if sepsis suspected (?meningitis)
- Treat simple **metabolic/intoxication** abnormalities:
  - **BM <4**, 20% glucose 100ml IV stat
  - **BM >20**, 0.9% saline 1l IV stat and consider DKA/HONK
  - **Opioids** (pinpoint pupils and ↓RR), naloxone 0.4mg IV/IM stat
  - History of excess **alcohol**, Pabrinex® 2 pairs IV over 10min
  - **Benzodiazepine** overdose **alone**, flumazenil 200μg IV over 15s

Hypoxia	p164	Hypoglycaemia	p230
Hypotension	p148	Hyperglycaemia	p232
Hypertension	p158	Liver failure	p190
Tachyarrythmia	p134	Metabolic	p242
Bradyarrhythmia	p142	Pyrexia	p248
Meningitis	p212	Overdose	Toxbase

Further management

- Check brainstem function (see table below):
  - ***normal*** – stabilise the patient and get an urgent CT head
  - ***gradual onset dysfunction*** – consider mannitol and urgent CT head
  - ***rapid onset dysfunction*** – give mannitol, hyperventilate on ventilator and contact a neurosurgeon urgently; the patient's brain is probably herniating due to raised intracranial pressure
- If **CT normal** proceed to lumbar puncture to test for meningitis or encephalitis
- If **CT and LP normal** the cause is probably metabolic or intoxication

Cause	Signs
Intoxication	May have shallow, slow breathing, pinpoint pupils suggests opioids, ↑↑RR suggests salicylates
Brainstem dysfunction	• **Eyes** dilated or slow reacting pupil (unilateral or bilateral), absent corneal reflex, eyes looking in different directions (III, IV, VI lesion), eyes fixed – 'doll's head' movements (not drifting back to forwards gaze when neck rotated) • **Swallow** water not swallowed spontaneously/no gag reflex • **Respiration** apnoeas, gasping, irregular or Cheyne-Stokes breathing (alternating rapid breathing and apneoas) • **Body** increased tone and upgoing plantars unilaterally/bilaterally/crossed
Lateralising (cerebral dysfunction)	Facial asymmetry, asymmetrical tone and plantar responses
Meningism	Neck stiffness, photophobia

Coma and reduced GCS

Think about

- ***No focal neurology*** hypoxia, hypotension, metabolic (glucose, Na^+, Ca^{2+}, K^+, acidosis, alkalosis, renal failure, liver failure), overdose (alcohol, opioids, benzodiazepines), epilepsy, hypothermia, pyrexia, hypothyroid, malignant hypertension
- ***Brainstem dysfunction or lateralising signs*** CVA, tumour, abscess, haematoma, hypoglycaemia or rarely other metabolic abnormalities
- ***Meningism*** meningitis, encephalitis, sub-arachnoid

Ask about (notes, relatives, nurses) speed of onset, headache, chest pain, palpitations, vomiting, seizures, weight loss ***PMH*** cardiac, respiratory, diabetes, kidney, liver, psychiatric ***DH*** elicit past medical history from medications, consider the possibility of overdose ***SH*** alcohol, recreational drugs

Obs GCS, temp, BP, pulse, sats, O_2 requirements, RR

Neuro obs GCS, limb movements, pupil size and reactivity, pulse, BP, RR, temp

Look for heart rate and rhythm, respiratory rate, depth and distress, breathing equal on both sides, soft abdomen, check for pulsatile mass, organomegaly, pupil reflexes, papilloedema (late sign), limb tone, plantar reflexes, check skin all over for rashes or trauma

Investigations ***blds*** FBC, U+E, LFT, Ca^{2+}, glucose, cardiac markers, CRP, clotting, bld cultures, toxicology screen (paracetamol and salicylate) ***ABGs*** $\downarrow O_2$ or $\uparrow CO_2$ ***ECG*** arrhythmias ***CXR*** aspiration ***CT*** if the patient has focal neurology or there is no clear diagnosis then an urgent CT head is required, the patient may need to be intubated first ***LP*** after a CT scan if CT normal

GCS scoring (3/15 minimum)

Eyes	Open spontaneously	4	**Motor**	Obeys commands	6
	Open to command	3		Localises pain	5
	Open to pain	2		Flexes/withdraws to pain	4
	No response	1		Abnormal flexion to pain	3
Voice	Talking and orientated	5		Extension to pain	2
	Confused/disorientated	4		No movement	1
	Inappropriate words	3			
	Incomprehensible sounds	2			
	No vocalisations	1			

Acute confusion

- ***Confusion*** acute deficit in thinking, short-term memory and orientation in time/place with reduced awareness
- ***Dementia*** chronic deficit in thinking, memory and/or personality
- ***Delirium*** acute onset confusion with hallucinations or illusions
- ***Psychosis*** hallucinations or illusions without confusion

Think about ***emergencies*** hypoxia, MI, sepsis, intracranial bleed, meningitis, encephalitis, raised ICP, CVA ***common*** infection, metabolic (glucose, Na^+, Ca^{2+}, kidney/liver failure), drug toxicity (opioids, benzodiazepines, post-GA), heart failure, head injury, alcohol withdrawal/intoxication, endocrine, malignancy, post-ictal, vitamin deficiency (thiamine, B_{12}) ***chronic*** dementia

Ask about use direct questions about how they are at the moment; further history from the ward staff, relatives or notes: speed of onset, chest pain, cough, sputum, dysuria, frequency, incontinence, head injury, headache, photophobia, vomiting, dizziness ***PMH*** diabetes, heart, lung, liver or kidney problems, epilepsy, dementia, psychiatric illness ***DH*** benzodiazepines, opioids, steroids, NSAIDs, β-blockers, psychiatric medication ***SH*** alcohol, recreational drugs, usual mobility and state

Obs GCS, temp, pulse, BP, RR, sats

Look for cyanosis, pulse (rate and rhythm), unequal air entry, bronchial breathing, creps, abdo pain, signs of head injury, neck stiffness, photophobia, focal neurology, pupil responses, papilloedema, tone and reflexes, record score on abbreviated mental test score

Investigations urine dipstick, M,C+S ***blds*** FBC, U+E, LFT, CRP, glucose, Ca^{2+}, cardiac markers, blood cultures, consider amylase, magnesium, TFT, B_{12}, folate ***ABGs*** $\downarrow O_2$ or $\uparrow CO_2$ ***ECG*** arrhythmias ***CXR*** infection or aspiration ***CT*** if focal neurology or non-resolving confusion ***LP*** if CT normal

Abbreviated mental test score (AMTS) ≥8 is normal for an elderly patient

Age	1	Recognise two people (eg Dr, nurse)	1
Date of birth	1	Year World War Two ended (1945)	1
Repeat: 42 West Street	0	Who is on the throne (Elizabeth II)	1
Year	1	Count backwards from 20 to 1	1
Time (nearest hour)	1	Recall: 42 West Street	1
Name of hospital	1	Total:	/10

Management

- Nurse in a well-lit, quiet environment
- Ensure patient is visible from nurse's desk to prevent falls/accidents
- Ask relatives/friends to stay with them
- See p75 if sedation is required for investigation and treatment
- Investigate and treat the cause, infection is the most common

Hypoglycaemia emergency

Airway	Check airway is patent; consider manoeuvres/adjuncts
Breathing	If no respiratory effort – **CALL ARREST TEAM**
Circulation	If no palpable pulse – **CALL ARREST TEAM**
Disability	If GCS ≤8 – **CALL ANAESTHETIST**

Call for **senior help** early if patient deteriorating

BM/glucose is normally >3.5mmol/l

Poorly controlled diabetics can be hypoglycaemic with a BM >3.5mmol/l

Coma or low GCS with low BM

- Protect airway
- **High-flow oxygen** by mask in all patients
- Establish **venous access** unless already present
- Give IV **glucose** stat (50ml of 50%, 100ml of 20% or 200ml of 10%)
- For large insulin overdoses give 1mg **glucagon** SC/IM/IV
- Begin to follow **emergency protocol** on **p226** (low GCS)
- If hypoglycaemia is responsible, GCS should return to 15 in <10min
- Start **1l 10% glucose/4–8h IV**, adjust rate to keep BM >5mmol/l
- **Monitor BMs** 30min–1h until patient stable
- Attempt to determine the **cause** of the hypoglycaemia
- Call for **senior help**
- **Reassess**, starting with A, B, C; if no improvement see p226

GCS 15/15 with low BM

- Give 120ml Lucozade or a single dose of **Hypostop® gel** orally
- **Monitor BMs** 1–2h until stable, aim for BM >5mmol/l
- For persistent hypoglycaemia give **1l 10% glucose/6–8h IV**
- Attempt to determine the **cause** of the hypoglycaemia

Life-threatening causes

- Insulin overdose
- Oral hypoglycaemia overdose
- Sepsis
- Alcohol excess
- Acute liver failure

Hypoglycaemia

Worrying symptoms unconscious, low GCS, recurrent, not diabetic

Think about ***most likely*** excess insulin or oral hypoglycaemics in a diabetic or accidental dose in non-diabetic, alcohol, missed meal ***other*** dumping syndrome (post gastric surgery), liver failure, adrenal failure (Addison's), pituitary insufficiency, sepsis, insulinomas, other neoplasia, malaria

Ask about sweating, hunger, exercise, recent food, previous hypos, usual BMs, seizures, weight loss, tiredness, anxiety, palpitations ***PMH*** diabetes, gastric surgery, liver or endocrine disease ***DH*** insulin dose, oral hypoglycaemic dose ***SH*** alcohol

Obs pulse, GCS, recent and current BMs

Look for pale, sweating, tremor, slurred speech, focal neurology (can be severe, eg hemiplegia), low GCS, abdo scars, pigmented scars, jaundice, spider naevi, hepatomegaly

Investigations *BM* A quick and easy test – if the result is unexpected (eg non-diabetic) ask for a repeat on a different machine and send a blood sample in a fluoride (p460) tube for an accurate glucose result. If the patient is ***not diabetic*** send a sample for FBC, U+E, LFT, glucose, insulin and C-peptide levels prior to correcting hypoglycaemia; consider thick and thin films for malaria

Further investigations Hypoglycaemia is very rare in a non-diabetic in the absence of alcohol. The investigation of choice is glucose, insulin and C-peptide levels after a 72h observed fast. Gut hormones may also be requested. See OHCM6 p300

Treatment

Follow the treatment plans on the opposite page.

Diabetes A single episode of mild hypoglycaemia should not prompt a change of medication. If the patient is having regular hypos then consider a dose reduction. Reduce insulin doses by 20%, consult *BNF* to reduce the doses of oral hypoglycaemics. Ensure the patient is aware of the sick day rules (p236).

Alcohol Hypoglycaemia following alcohol should not be recurrent unless alcohol consumption is recurrent. Once the patient's BMs are stable they can be discharged unless there are other problems.

Dumping syndrome Fast passage of food into the small intestine following gastric surgery can cause fluid shifts and rapid glucose absorption. Excessive insulin secretion results in rebound hypoglycaemia 1–3h after a meal. A diet low in glucose and high in fibre will improve the condition.

Neoplasia Refer to surgeons.

Addison's/pituitary failure	p240/241
Sepsis	p153
Acute liver failure	p192

Hyperglycaemia emergency

Airway	Check airway is patent; consider manoeuvres/adjuncts
Breathing	If no respiratory effort – **CALL ARREST TEAM**
Circulation	If no palpable pulse – **CALL ARREST TEAM**
Disability	If GCS ≤8 – **CALL ANAESTHETIST**

Call for **senior help** early if patient deteriorating

Diabetic ketoacidosis (DKA) – type 1 diabetes, pH <7.3, ketonuria

- **High-flow oxygen** by mask in all patients
- Establish **venous access**, take bloods:
  - FBC, U+E, glucose, osmolality, HCO_3^-, bld cultures
- Give **1l 0.9% saline IV** stat
- Check **BM** and dipstick **urine** for ketones
- Start a **sliding scale**, see p235
- **Arterial blood gas** if pH <7.0; get senior help
- **Monitor** U+E, glucose and HCO_3^- hourly, K^+ will fall unless replaced
- Further management, p234; attempt to **determine the cause**
- Call for **senior help**
- **Reassess**, starting with A, B, C…

HONK coma – type 2 diabetes, plasma osmolality >340 mosmol/kg, BM >35mmol/l

- **High-flow oxygen** by mask in all patients
- Establish **venous access**, take bloods:
  - FBC, U+E, glucose, osmolality, bld cultures
- Give **1l 0.9% saline IV** over 30min
- Check **BM**
- Start a **sliding scale** if BM still raised after 1h of fluids, see p235
- **Monitor** U+E and glucose
- Further management, p234; attempt to **determine the cause**
- Call for **senior help**
- **Reassess**, starting with A, B, C…

Life-threatening precipitants of DKA/HONK

- Sepsis
- MI
- Trauma/surgery
- Other acute illness

Hyperglycaemia

Worrying symptoms ↓GCS, ketones in urine, acidosis, vomiting

Think about ***emergencies*** diabetic ketoacidosis (DKA), hyperglycaemic hyperosmolar non-ketotic coma (HONK) ***common*** after sugary food, steroids, non-compliance with diabetic treatment, infection or acute illness in diabetics, severe illness

Ask about tiredness, thirst, polyuria, frequency, dysuria, urgency, weight loss, vomiting, breathlessness, rashes, lumps, teeth problems, cough, sputum, chest pain, abdo pain, recent surgery ***PMH*** diabetes ***DH*** insulin dose, oral hypoglycaemic dose, steroids ***SH*** alcohol

Obs temp, RR, GCS, recent and current BMs, fluid balance

Look for volume status (p262), signs of infection, check skin thoroughly (including perineum) for abscesses or rashes, look in mouth for dental infection, sweet smelling breath, chest for poor air entry or creps, abdominal tenderness

Investigations ***BM*** repeat if result unexpected ***urine*** ketones and evidence of infection, MSU if unwell ***blds*** send blood tests if the patient is unwell, has persistent hyperglycaemia (over 48h) or has ketones in the urine (type 1 DM), request FBC, U+E, LFT, osmolality, HCO_3^- blood cultures ***ABGs*** if the patient is unwell, look for pH <7.3 in type 1 diabetes ***ECG*** if treatment has been required ***CXR*** if treatment has been required

Treatment

A single episode of mild hyperglycaemia in an otherwise well patient is unlikely to suggest underlying pathology. DKA takes hours to days to develop whilst HONK takes days to weeks.

Type 1 diabetic Check BM and urine. BMs are usually high in DKA but may be transiently normal soon after a dose of insulin. Assess the patient's volume status (p262) and check if the urine contains ketones. If they are unwell proceed with the treatment plan for DKA opposite. Otherwise send a venous sample for pH/HCO_3^-, if normal this excludes DKA. Persistent hyperglycaemia should prompt a change to the insulin regime by increasing doses by 20% and monitoring BM.

Type 2 diabetic Check BM and urine. The BM must be raised for a diagnosis of HONK. If the patient is unwell follow the treatment plan for HONK initially. Otherwise monitor glucose levels every 6h for 48h, increase oral/IV fluid intake and reassess. DKA can occur in type 2 diabetics on insulin but it is very unusual (a small amount of insulin inhibits ketone production). For persistent hyperglycaemia increase the dose of hypoglycaemic medication or insulin with frequent BM checks.

Non-diabetic patients New diabetics often present with DKA/HONK; have a low threshold for starting the treatment plans opposite. Hyperglycaemia can also be precipitated by steroids and stress, eg severe illness or surgery. Investigate persistent hyperglycaemia as shown above.

DKA post-emergency (OHAM2 p556)

Stabilise the patient as shown on the treatment plan, p232:

- continue IV fluids, see regime below or ask a senior
- monitor U+E every 1–2h and add 20mmol/l KCl after the first litre of fluid even if the plasma K^+ is normal, the patient is likely to be K^+ depleted from their illness. Use 40mmol/l KCl if hypokalaemic
- monitor glucose, osmolality and HCO_3^- every 1–2h
- repeat ABG if not improving
- if severely ill: catheterise, consider admission to HDU or ITU and an arterial and/or central line
- NG tube if GCS <15 to prevent aspiration
- nil by mouth for at least 6h
- infection is common and may be asymptomatic, check blood cultures, MSU and CXR; have a low threshold for starting antibiotics (p254)
- check an ECG to exclude MI as a precipitant
- give prophylactic LMW heparin SC if immobile (p289)
- convert to SC insulin once eating and urinary dipstick ketones ≤1

Excess or excessively fast fluid replacement can lead to cerebral oedema

DKA fluids 1l stat, 1l over 1h, 1l over 2h, 1l over 4h and 1l over 6h; tailor to the patient according to volume status and weight. Initially use 0.9% saline and convert to glucose and saline or 5% glucose if BMs <15mmol/l. Add 20–40mmol/l KCl to second and following bags as determined by U+E, hypokalaemia will develop otherwise. Monitor fluid balance and assess volume status (p262) for signs of overload.

Precipitants of DKA/HONK infections (chest, UTI, abscesses, dental problems), MI, CVA, surgery, trauma, acute illness, poor compliance/incorrect insulin dose, alcohol

HONK post-emergency (OHAM2 p562)

Stabilise the patient as shown on the treatment plan, p232:

- continue IV fluid replacement at about half the rate used in DKA
- monitor U+E, glucose and osmolality every 2h
- may have spurious hyponatraemia due to excess glucose, call senior help if Na^+ is above normal at any stage
- if severely ill: catheterise, consider admission to HDU or ITU and an arterial and/or central line
- NG tube if GCS <15 to prevent aspiration
- nil by mouth for at least 6h
- septic screen and antibiotics as indicated
- ECG and look for an underlying cause (see box)
- give prophylactic LMW heparin SC if immobile (p289)
- convert to insulin/oral hypoglycaemics when BM <12mmol/l

Sliding scales

These give strict monitoring and control of a diabetic patient's glucose levels. They are used in the treatment of DKA, HONK and for surgery on diabetics (see below). They are also used when serious illness disrupts diabetic control, eg post MI.

You need to prescribe both the insulin infusion with appropriate IV fluids on the infusions section of the drug card. Use 5–10% glucose with 20mmol/l KCl, unless you are treating DKA or HONK in which case 0.9% saline is used until the BM is <15mmol/l. Further IV fluids can be prescribed alongside a sliding scale at a slower rate to allow for the extra IV fluid infusion (p263).

Date	Route	Fluid	Additives	Vol	Rate	Signature
18/09/05	IV	0.9% saline	50iu Actrapid	50ml	Sliding scale	Dr CJFlint
18/09/05	IV	5% glucose	20mmol KCl	1l	8h	Dr CJFlint

Example of sliding scale regime, check local policy

Insulin	Date	Start time	BM (mmol/l	Rate (ml/h)
Actrapid	18/09/05	13:45	<4	Stop-call doctor
Dose	Route	Check BM	4-7	1
1iu/ml	IV	1h	7.1-11	2
Signature			11.1-20	4
Dr CJFlint			>20	7-call doctor

If the sliding scale is not controlling blood glucose levels then check the infusion pump and cannula; if no problems found double the doses and check venous bicarbonate (type 1) or osmolality (type 2). If the BM is <4mmol/l check that there is 5–10% glucose running, increase the fluid rate and/or glucose concentration (up to 10%); recheck BM in 30min. If persistently <4mmol/l consider halving the doses. If BM<2 see p230.

Prescribing insulin

Most hospitals have separate drug cards for prescribing insulin. Check the patient's usual doses and write up accordingly, for example:

	Insulin	Dose	Route	Start
Breakfast	Mixard 30	18iu	SC	18/09/05
	Insulin	Dose	Route	Start
Night	Mixard 30	10iu	SC	18/09/05

Diabetes mellitus

- *Type 1* (insulin dependant – IDDM) an autoimmune disease that can occur at any age – always needs lifelong insulin
- *Type 2* (non-insulin dependent – NIDDM) caused by insulin resistance, ±hyposecretion – tends to occur in the elderly and overweight
- ***Impaired glucose tolerance (IGT)*** abnormal glucose tolerance test but below diabetic criteria – often develops into diabetes
- ***Impaired fasting glucose (IFG)*** raised glucose levels after an overnight fast, but below criteria for diabetes – may develop into diabetes
- ***Gestational*** transient insulin resistance during pregnancy (p375)

Acute type 1 DM (OHCM6 p292)

Symptoms tiredness, weight loss, thirst, polyuria, abdo pain, vomiting
Signs cachexia, sweet smelling breath, shock, acute abdomen
Investigations Random glucose >11.1mmol/l, fasting blood glucose ≥7mmol/l (eg after an overnight fast). Check plasma HCO_3^- or ABG and urine (glucose, ketones) to exclude DKA. Islet cell antibodies and HbA_{1C}.
Treatment Resuscitate and investigate for DKA initially; monitor BM ≥4 times a day after starting a suitable insulin regime (discuss with a senior). Refer to a diabetic nurse specialist and arrange out-patient follow-up.

Properties of common subcutaneous insulins

Name	Type of insulin	Onset	Peak	Duration
Short-acting				
Novorapid®	Aspart	15min	0.5–1.5h	5h
Humalog®	Lispro	15min	0.5–1.5h	5h
Actrapid®	Soluble	30min	2–4h	8h
Intermediate and long-acting				
Insulatard®	Isophane	2h	6–12h	24h
Ultratard®	Zinc suspension	4h	12–18h	28h
Lantus®	Glargine	1h	1–24h	24h
Levemir®	Detemir	1h	1–24h	24h
Mixtures				
Mixtard 30®	30% soluble 70% isophane	30min	2–12h	24h

Sick day rules

Educate diabetic patients what to do if they are feeling unwell:
- never stop taking your insulin or tablets (may need to increase dose)
- test your blood for glucose at least 4 times a day
- test your urine for glucose (and ketones if on insulin)
- drink plenty of fluids
- if not eating try milk, soup, cereals, fruit juice or fizzy drinks instead
- contact your GP or diabetes team if you cannot keep fluids down

Acute type 2 DM (OHCM6 p294)

Symptoms as for type 1, but can also present with complications, eg visual problems, neuropathy, MI, claudication, confusion, coma

Signs foot ulcers, infections, peripheral neuropathy, poor visual acuity and diabetic retinopathy, evidence of cardiovascular disease

Investigations Suspect if a random glucose/BM is >11.1mmol/l or glycosuria. Confirm with a fasting blood glucose ≥7mmol/l (eg after an overnight fast); an HbA_{1C} >7% makes diabetes very likely. If there is any doubt or the fasting glucose is ≥6.1mmol/l and <7mmol/l perform an oral glucose tolerance test.

Oral glucose tolerance test Check fasting blood glucose after an overnight fast then give the patient 75g glucose in 300ml water. Repeat the blood glucose 2h after the drink.

Interpretation of oral glucose tolerance test

Fasting glucose	Glucose after 2h	Diagnosis
Any	≥11.1mmol/l	Diabetes
≥7mmol/l	Any	Diabetes
<7mmol/l	7.8–11.0mmol/l	Impaired glucose tolerance (IGT)
6.1–6.9mmol/l	≤7.7mmol/l	Impaired fasting glucose (IFG)
<6.1mmol/l	≤7.7mmol/l	Normal

Treatment Type 2 diabetes may initially be controlled by a healthy diet with minimal rapid release carbohydrates (eg sugary drinks, cakes, sweets) and weight loss. Oral medications and insulin may be required.

Common oral hypoglycaemics for type 2 diabetes

Class	Examples	Comment
Biguanides	Metformin	Increase glucose uptake and reduce appetite; avoid if any renal failure
Sulphonylureas	Gliclazide	Stimulate remaining β cells but cause weight gain
Thiazolidinediones	Pioglitazone	Reduces insulin resistance

Treatment options in IGT and IFG and diabetes

Insulin				✓	✓
Oral hypoglycaemics			✓	✓	
Diet and exercise	✓	✓	✓	✓	✓
	IGT and IFG	**Step 1**	**Step 2**	**Step 3**	**Type 1**
		Type 2			

Diabetes long term (OHCM6 p296)

- Education including what to do if feeling ill (see 'sick day rules', p341)
- Promote exercise, weight loss, healthy diet, smoking cessation
- Strict glucose control, aim for HbA_{1C} of ≤7.4%, this will reduce complications; hard to achieve as type 2 diabetes progresses
- Aim to control blood pressure (<140/90), ACEi to reduce nephropathy
- Monitor cholesterol and prescribe a statin if raised
- Regular ophthalmology review for retinopathy (often photographed for comparison), may need photocoagulation
- Regular chiropody and treat ulcers early

Complications of type 1 + 2 diabetes

DKA/HONK, atheroma (MI, limb ischaemia, bowel ischaemia), CVA, neuropathy, nephropathy, retinopathy, glaucoma, cataracts, retinal bleeds, leg ulcers, infections, hypoglycaemia

Diabetes and surgery

Taking insulin

- Check U+E and ECG pre-op
- Put the patient first on the theatre list
- Admit the evening before surgery and omit usual long-acting insulin
- If on morning list do not give morning SC insulin or breakfast
- If afternoon list give usual SC short-acting insulin dose with breakfast, but no long-acting insulin
- Start a sliding scale at least 2h before surgery (see above)
- Monitor BM hourly until stable post-op then 2h, check U+E if >12h
- Stop sliding scale once tolerating food, restart usual insulin regime

Type 2 DM on oral hypoglycaemics

- If fasting BM >10mmol/l or having major surgery treat as type 1 DM
- Put the patient first on the theatre list
- Check U+E and ECG pre-op
- Omit morning hypoglycaemics
- Give hypoglycaemics post-op with a meal
- Check BMs

Type 2 DM diet controlled

- Check U+E and ECG pre-op
- No extra treatment pre-op
- Check BMs post-op
- Avoid 5% glucose IV unless hypo

More information on diabetes care or pre-op management see:

- www.nottinghamdiabetes.nhs.uk/gppages.html

Endocrine disease

Hyperthyroid (OHCM6 p304)

Excess of thyroxine.

Symptoms weight loss, agitation, anxiety, psychosis, sweating, heat intolerance, diarrhoea, tremor, oligomenorrhoea

Signs thin, ↑temp, tachycardia, irregular pulse, warm hands, tremor, goitre, ±nodules, lid lag

Investigations ↑T_4 or T_3, ↓TSH (if raised suspect pituitary tumour), thyroid autoantibodies, ECG, may need a thyroid scan

Treatment Propanolol 40mg/6h for symptoms (unless asthmatic or co-existent heart or vascular problems – see BNF), 4wk of oral carbimazole to suppress thyroid. May also be treated by surgery or radioiodine.

Complications AF, ophthalmopathy, osteoporosis

Thyrotoxic storm Caused by infection, severe illness, recent thyroid surgery or radioiodine. Presents with tachycardia, ±AF, agitation, confusion or coma with a raised T_4 or T_3. Resuscitate as required (p226) and get senior help. Propanolol, carbimazole and hydrocortisone are the main treatments. See OHCM6 p820 or OHAM2 p590.

Hypothyroid (OHCM6 p306)

Deficiency of thyroxine.

Symptoms tiredness, lethargy, weight gain, depression, dementia, cold intolerance, constipation, menorrhagia, infertile

Signs obese, bradycardia, ↓temp, cold/dry hands, non-pitting oedema, goitre, peripheral neuropathy, slow relaxing reflexes

Investigations ↓T_4, ↑TSH, thyroid autoantibodies

Treatment Thyroxine 100µg/24h PO OD if young, 25µg/24h PO OD if elderly or heart problems. Check TFT and increase dose 4–12wkly to relieve symptoms whilst maintaining TSH in normal range. TFT yearly once stable. Consider propanolol 40mg/6h PO if they have ischaemic heart disease.

Complications angina from treatment

Myxoedema coma Caused by infection, severe illness, stroke, previous thyroid surgery or radioiodine. Presents with bradycardia, hypothermia, confusion or coma with a low T_4. Resuscitate as required including warm blankets (p310) and get senior help. T_3 and hydrocortisone are the main treatments, beware of worsening ischaemic heart disease or heart failure following treatment.

Cushing's syndrome (OHCM6 p310)

Cushing's syndrome is an excess of glucocorticoids (cortisol); Cushing's disease is an excess of glucocorticoids from an ACTH-producing pituitary tumour. A patient on steroids may be 'Cushingoid'.

Symptoms weight gain, depression, psychosis, tiredness, weakness, oligo or amenorrhoea, hirsutism, impotence, infections, diabetes

Signs central obesity (buffalo hump), moon face, water retention, ↑BP, thin skin, striae, bruising, peripheral wasting, hyperpigmentation only in Cushing's disease or ectopic ACTH production

Investigations ↑glucose, 24h urinary cortisol >280nmol, plasma ACTH, see OHCM6 p310 for further tests

Treatment Remove source of cortisol or reduce steroid dose. If steroid dependent give bone protection with bisphosphonate and vitamin D, eg alendronic acid 70mg once a week (empty stomach, full glass of water, sit up for at least 30min) and Calcichew® D3. Monitor for ↑glucose.
Complications osteoporosis, diabetes, infection, poor healing, infertility. Stopping long-term (>2wk) steroids suddenly may cause an Addisonian crisis; taper the close gradually (p419), especially below 7.5mg/d.

Addison's disease (OHCM6 p312)
Deficiency of cortisol and aldosterone.
Symptoms tiredness, lethargy, weight loss, weakness, dizziness, depression, abdo pain, diarrhoea or constipation, vomiting, aches and pains
Signs vitiligo, postural hypotension, hyperpigmentation of creases, scars and mouth (buccal)
Investigations ↓Na^+, ↑K^+, ↑urea, may have abnormal FBC and LFT. If suspected perform short Synacthen® test: order 250µg Synacthen® from pharmacy, once this arrives send a blood sample for cortisol and ACTH levels, give the Synacthen® IM (p468) and repeat cortisol levels in 30min. Addison's is excluded if initial cortisol >140nmol/l or second cortisol >500nmol/l.
Treatment Hydrocortisone 20mg PO om and 10mg PO on, may need fludrocortisone 50µg PO alternate days if electrolytes deranged. If unwell, trauma or post-op double all steroid doses for at least 1wk. Replace oral dose with hydrocortisone 100mg IM if vomiting.
Addisonian crisis shock, reduced GCS or hypoglycaemia in a patient with Addison's disease or stopping long-term steroid therapy. Resuscitate according to p226, send bloods for cortisol and ACTH levels and give hydrocortisone 100mg IV stat followed by cefuroxime 1.5g IV.

Conn's syndrome (OHCM6 p314)

Excess of catecholamines (eg aldosterone) from adrenal cortex tumour.
Symptoms thirst, polyuria, weakness, muscle spasms
Signs hypertension
Investigations ↓K^+, normal or ↑Na^+, metabolic alkalosis, measure plasma renin and aldosterone together, consider CT abdo
Treatment Spironolactone 200–300mg/24h PO for 4wk followed by surgical removal of adrenal lesion.
Secondary hyperaldosteronism Diuretics, heart failure, liver failure and renal artery stenosis cause ↑renin and aldosterone, producing the features of Conn's. Spironolactone and ACEi combat this effect.

Phaeochromocytoma (OHCM6 p314)
Excess of catecholamines (eg adrenaline) from adrenal medulla tumour or ectopic source.
Symptoms episodes of anxiety, chest tightness, breathlessness, tremor, palpitations, headaches, sweating, abdo pain, vomiting
Signs episodic hypertension
Investigations glycosuria during attack, 24h urine for VMA/HMMA
Treatment phenoxybenzamine (α blocker), followed by propanolol (β blocker), followed by surgery

Hypopituitarism (OHCM6 p318)

Deficiency of one or more anterior pituitary hormones (ACTH, TSH, GH, FSH, LH, prolactin). Causes include iatrogenic, adenoma, trauma.
Symptoms headache, vomiting, blurred vision, oligomenorrhoea, galactorrhoea, impotence, lethargy
Signs bitemporal hemianopia, III, IV or VI nerve palsy
Investigations prolactin, TFT, short Synacthen® test (see Addison's opposite), testosterone, LH, FSH, pituitary MRI
Treatment hydrocortisone and thyroxine, testosterone/oestrogen according to sex, may need growth hormone and desmopressin (if the posterior pituitary has also been affected – see diabetes insipidus)

Acromegaly (OHCM6 p324)

Excess growth hormone from a pituitary tumour.
Symptoms headache, sleep apnoea, mood swings, depression, tingling fingers, weakness, joint pain, increasing shoe/ring size
Signs coarse skin, big hands, big tongue, deep voice, prominent jaw and brow, wide spaced teeth, heart failure, bitemporal hemianopia
Investigations random ↑growth hormone or ↑IGF-1, oral glucose tolerance test with GH measurement is definitive
Treatment trans-sphenoidal pituitary surgery, irradiation or octreotide
Complications diabetes, osteoarthritis, hypertension, heart failure, cardiomyopathy, hyperthyroid, colonic polyps

Diabetes insipidus (OHCM6 p326)

Deficiency of antidiuretic hormone (ADH).
Symptoms polyuria, thirst
Signs dilute urine, clinically dehydrated (p262)
Investigations ↓plasma osmolality and Na^+, ↓urine osmolality (<400mosmol/kg), 8h water deprivation test (measure urine and plasma osmolality, see OHCM6 p326 for details), use desmopressin (an ADH analogue) to determine if neurogenic (cranial defect – urine osmolality increases >50%) or nephrogenic (kidney defect – osmolality increase <45%)
Neurogenic treatment treat the cause, intranasal desmopressin
Nephrogenic treatment treat the cause, bendrofluazide and restrict salt and protein intake
Severe dehydration Rapid rehydration – match input to output, do not attempt to reverse hypernatraemia rapidly (see p243). Give desmopressin 1µg IM (neurogenic) or indomethacin 75mg PO (nephrogenic) or both if source unknown.

Multiple endocrine neoplasia syndromes (MEN)

Autosomal dominant genetic diseases causing tumours in endocrine tissue; MEN 1 is the most common and is often a new mutation.
MEN 1 parathyroid hyperplasia, pituitary adenoma, pancreatic tumour
MEN 2a phaeochromocytoma, medullary thyroid carcinoma, parathyroid hyperplasia
MEN 2b medullary thyroid carcinoma, phaeochromocytoma with multiple neuroma, especially on face, and Marfanoid appearance

Potassium emergencies

Airway	Check airway is patent; consider manoeuvres/adjuncts
Breathing	If no respiratory effort – **CALL ARREST TEAM**
Circulation	If no palpable pulse – **CALL ARREST TEAM**

Call for **senior help** early if patient deteriorating

Hyperkalaemia (↑K^+ ≥7mmol/l or >5.6mmol/l with ECG changes)

- **ECG changes:** arrhythmias, flat P waves, wide QRS, tall/tented T waves
- **High-flow oxygen** in all patients
- **Monitor** defibrillator's ECG leads, BP, pulse oximeter
- **Venous access**, take bloods for urgent repeat U+E
- If **ECG changes** seen or ↑K^+ ≥7mmol/l (arrhythmias, p134):
  - 10ml of 10% calcium gluconate IV over 2min, repeat every 15min up to 50ml (five doses) until ECG normalises
  - Salbutamol 5mg nebuliser and/or 10u Actrapid® in 50ml of 50% glucose over 20min
- **Arterial blood gas** to exclude severe acidosis
- Consider **calcium resonium** 15g PO or 30g PR
- Call for senior help
- Reassess, starting with A, B, C…

Hypokalaemia (↓K^+ <2.5mmol/l or <3.0mmol/l with ECG changes)

- **ECG changes**: arrhythmias, prolonged PR interval, ST depression, small/inverted T waves, U waves (after T wave)
- **High-flow oxygen** in all patients
- **Monitor** defibrillator's ECG leads, BP, pulse oximeter
- **Venous access**, take bloods for urgent repeat U+E and Mg^{2+}
- **Replace potassium**, 40mmol/l KCl in 1l 0.9% saline IV unless oliguric
  - Do not run fluids faster than 2hrly so that ≤20mmol KCl/h
  - Never give KCl stat
- **Arterial blood gas** to exclude severe alkalosis
- Call for senior help
- Reassess, starting with A, B, C…

Life-threatening causes

Hyperkalaemia

- Renal failure
- Acidosis
- Tissue necrosis

Hypokalaemia

- Hypovolaemia
- Alkalosis

Electrolyte imbalance

Hyperkalaemia (↑K^+ >5.3mmol/l)

Worrying symptoms ↓GCS, chest pain, palpitations, abnormal ECG

Causes excess potassium (oral or IV), renal failure, haemolysed blood samples, diuretics (spironolactone, amiloride), ACE inhibitors, trauma, burns, large blood transfusions, Addison's disease
Symptoms chest pain, palpitations, dizziness, sudden death
Signs bruises, burns, dark urine
Investigations ECG, urgent repeat U+E; if K^+ <7mmol/l with no new ECG changes or the sample is reported as haemolysed then await the repeat sample, otherwise follow the treatment plan opposite.
Treatment Calcium gluconate protects the heart against high potassium. Salbutamol and insulin move potassium into cells to reduce plasma levels in the short term (1–2h) after which a rebound increase may occur. Potassium is only excreted by the action of calcium resonium (takes 24h, give with lactulose 30ml/6h PO) or by dialysis (p268).

Hypokalaemia (↓K^+ <3.5mmol/l)

Worrying symptoms ↓GCS, chest pain, palpitations, abnormal ECG

Causes vomiting, diarrhoea, most diuretics, steroids and Cushing's, inadequate replacement in fluids, alkalosis, renal disease, Conn's
Symptoms weakness, cramps, spasms, chest pain, palpitations, dizziness
Signs muscle weakness, hypotonia, arrhythmias
Investigations ECG, Mg^{2+} (often low making hypokalaemia resistant to treatment), arterial blood gas if unwell, repeat U+E
Treatment If K^+ ≥2.5mmol/l with no ECG changes add 20–40mmol KCl to IV fluids or give Sando K 2 tablets/8h and monitor U+E, consider writing up Sando K® only for 3–5d to prevent continuous unmonitored treatment. If K^+ <2.5mmol/l or ECG changes see treatment plan opposite.

Hypernatraemia (↑Na^+ >145mmol/l)

Worrying symptoms ↓GCS, ↑pulse, ↓BP

Causes fluid loss (diarrhoea, burns, fever, glycosuria eg diabetes mellitus, diabetes insipidus) or excess sodium (excess 0.9% saline, Conn's)
Symptoms thirst, weakness, tiredness, confusion, coma
Signs assess fluid balance, urine output, volume status p262
Investigations plasma osmolality (this is likely to be raised for both causes), urine osmolality (>400mosmol/kg if fluid loss, <400mosmol/kg if excess sodium, normal range 350–1000mosmol/kg)
Treatment Fluid replacement with slow correction of Na^+. If hypovolaemic give 0.9% saline 1l/6h (prevents sudden Na^+ shifts) until normovolaemic; if normovolaemic encourage oral fluids or 5% glucose 1l/6h. Monitor fluid balance and plasma Na^+; consider a catheter.

Hyponatraemia (↓Na^+ <135mmol/l)

Worrying symptoms ↓GCS, irritable, seizures, ↑pulse, ↓BP

Hyponatraemia is usually asymptomatic initially. As plasma Na^+ falls below 120mmol/l the patient may become irritable or confused, below 110mmol/l there may be seizures or coma.

Causes

- ***Hypovolaemic*** diarrhoea, vomiting, burns, fluid sequestration (peritonitis/pancreatitis), insufficient fluid intake or due to renal loss (diuretics, Addison's, salt-losing nephropathy)
- ***Normovolaemic or mild overload*** excess 5% glucose or oral fluids, hypothyroidism, SIADH (malignancy, chest infections, stroke, trauma, opiates, antipsychotics), liver failure
- ***Oedematous*** heart failure, renal failure and nephrotic syndrome, liver failure

Ask about diarrhoea, vomiting, abdo pain, tiredness, urine frequency, quantity and colour, thirst, constipation, SOB, cough, chest pain, weakness, head trauma ***PMH*** heart, liver or kidney problems ***DH*** diuretics, opiates, antipsychotics

Look for assess fluid balance and volume status p262, air entry and basal creps, oedema (legs and sacrum), ascites, focal neurology

Investigations FBC, U+E, LFT, CRP, plasma osmolality, urine osmolality, Na^+ and dipstick, try to establish the underlying cause.

Spurious ↓Na^+ can be caused by taking blood from an arm with IV fluids running, a lipaemic sample (labs should detect this) or osmotically active substances in the blood, eg glucose. Discuss with lab if unsure.

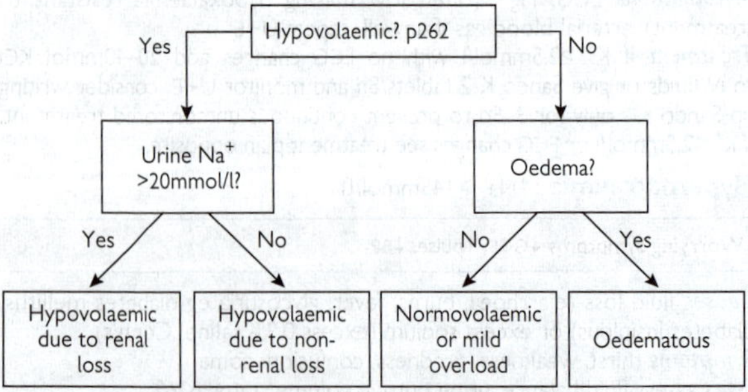

Treatment Get senior help if Na^+ <120mmol/l, seizures or coma; may need hypertonic saline. Chronic hyponatraemia should be corrected slowly to prevent fluid overload or osmotic demyelination (this is very rare). In all patients monitor fluid balance closely with catheter, regular obs and possibly CVP. Repeat U+E daily.

- ***Hypovolaemic*** replace lost fluid with 0.9% saline according to degree of dehydration, see p262; severe hypovolaemia should be corrected according to p151 and takes precedence over hyponatraemia. Try to establish the cause of fluid loss and treat accordingly. Stop diuretics.

- ***Normovolaemic or mild overload*** slow 0.9% saline IV eg 8–10h, sodium levels should rise over a few days. If urine osmolality >500mosmol/kg consider SIADH
- ***SIADH*** *plasma* Na^+ <125mmol/kg, osmolality <260mosmol/kg, *urine* Na^+ >20mmol/l, osmolality >500mosmol/kg in the absence of oedema, diuretics, hypovolaemia or abnormal thyroid/adrenal function. Fluid restrict to 500ml/24h and establish the cause, consider CXR, CT head.
- ***Oedematous*** urine Na^+ usually <10mmol/l, treat the underlying cause (see relevant chapter).

Hypercalcaemia (↑Ca^{2+} >2.65mmol/l)

Worrying symptoms ↓GCS, chest pain, palpitations, ↑pulse, ↓BP, abnormal ECG

Causes primary/tertiary hyperparathyroidism, malignancy (myeloma, bone metastases, PTH-related peptide secreting tumours), excess vitamin D supplements, sarcoidosis

Symptoms abdo pain, vomiting, constipation, bone pain, ±fractures, weakness, tiredness, renal stones, depression, thirst, polyuria, weight loss

Signs hypertension, arrhythmias, dehydrated (shock if severe), cachexia, bony tenderness secondary to a local lesion – especially along spine

Investigations ECG (short QT, arrhythmias), FBC, U+E, Mg^{2+}, Ca^{2+}, PO_4^{3-}, ALP, consider ESR, serum and urine electrophoresis, CXR, bone scan. Suspect malignancy if ↓albumin, ↓Cl^- and alkalosis.

Treatment continuous 0.9% saline 1l/4–8h for 4–5 days depending on degree of dehydration and coexistent heart disease. Consider catheterisation and CVP monitoring to assess fluid balance; monitor U+E, Ca^{2+} and Mg^{2+} daily. To further lower Ca^{2+} add furosemide 40mg PO or IV/12h in a well-hydrated patient (monitor fluid balance strictly; input = output) and pamidronate (see OHCM6 p437). Investigate and treat the cause of hypercalcaemia.

Complications renal failure, arrhythmias, osteopaenia, renal stones, peptic ulcers, pancreatitis

Primary hyperparathyroidism ↑PTH from parathyroid tumour

- *Investigations* ↑PTH, ↑Ca^{2+}, ↑ALP, ↓ PO_4^{3-}
- *Treatment* Correct hypercalcaemia then parathyroidectomy

Secondary hyperparathyroidism ↑PTH caused by ↓Ca^{2+}; treat the underlying cause of hypocalcaemia (p246)

Tertiary hyperparathyroidism Same presentation and treatment as primary, but caused by a parathyroid adenoma due to prolonged secondary hyperparathyroidsim. Consider if renal failure.

Myeloma plasma cell cancer secreting monoclonal immunoglobulins

- *Investigations* ↑ESR, ↑Ca^{2+}, normal ALP, often a degree of renal failure, monoclonal immunoglobulin band in urine or plasma
- *Treatment* Correct hypercalcaemia as above and with pamidronate IV; give adequate analgesia. Lesions can be treated palliatively with radiotherapy or chemotherapy
- *Complications* infection, renal failure, haemorrhage

Hypocalcaemia (↓Ca^{2+} <2.12mmol/l)

Worrying symptoms ↓GCS, chest pain, palpitations, ↓pulse, ↓BP, abnormal ECG

Causes vitamin D deficiency (asians, africans, chronic renal failure), hypoparathyroid, acute pancreatitis, alkalosis, magnesium deficiency
Symptoms spasm of hands and feet (carpopedal), twitching muscles, tingling around the mouth, bone fractures, depression
Signs hyperreflexia, tetany, Trousseau's (spasm of hand from inflated BP cuff) and Chvostek's (unilateral twitching of face from tapping facial nerve 2cm anterior to ear lobe), hypotension, bradycardia, arrhythmias
Investigations ECG (prolonged QT, arrhythmias), U+E, Ca^{2+}, PO_4^{3-}, Mg^{2+}, albumin, PTH
Treatment Treat arrhythmias according to p134. If tetany is severe give 10ml 10% calcium gluconate IV over 10min. Monitor if deficit is mild and the patient is asymptomatic. Prolonged hypocalcaemia will need vitamin D replacement and calcium supplements, eg Calcichew D3® one tablet/24h PO.
Complications arrhythmias, seizures, cataracts, bone fractures
Primary hypoparathyroidism ↓PTH, despite ↓Ca^{2+}

- *Causes* iatrogenic (neck surgery), infection, infiltration, idiopathic
- *Investigations* ↓Ca^{2+}, ↓PTH, ↑PO_4^{3-}
- *Treatment* vitamin D, eg calciferol 1–2.5mg/24h PO

Pseudohypoparathyroidism Genetic resistance to PTH, presents with hypocalcaemia, but ↑PTH, treat as hypoparathyroid
Pseudopseudohypoparathyroidism Patients with the morphological appearance of pseudohypoparathyroidism, but normal calcium and PTH.

Hypophosphataemia (↓PO_4^{3-}<0.75mmol/l)

Worrying symptoms severe co-morbid conditions

Causes vitamin D deficiency, hyperparathyroidism, diuretics, malabsorption, alcohol withdrawal, DKA treatment, liver failure, refeeding syndrome (high carbohydrate diet if malnourished)
Symptoms symptomatic ↓PO_4^{3-} occurs in very sick patients eg on ITU exacerbating CNS, respiratory, cardiac or renal failure
Investigations Ca^{2+}, PTH, LFT, blood gases if unwell
Treatment None required unless <0.4mmol/l, investigate and treat underlying cause. Senior help if severe.

Magnesium excess (↑Mg^{2+} >1.1mmol/l)

Worrying symptoms ↓GCS, ↓BP

Causes renal failure, excess antacids, excess magnesium replacement
Symptoms weakness, confusion, coma
Signs hypotension
Investigations ECG, U+E
Treatment If mild monitor magnesium levels and stop additives, treat any renal failure. If severe consider 10ml of 10% calcium gluconate IV over 2min.

Magnesium deficiency (↓Mg^{2+} <0.7mmol/l)

Worrying symptoms ↓GCS, chest pain, palpitations, dizziness, abnormal ECG

Causes diarrhoea, alcoholism, ketoacidosis, diuretics, total parenteral nutrition, ↓Ca^{2+}, ↓K^+, ↓PO_4^{3-}
Symptoms tingling, palpitations, dizziness, spasms, seizures
Signs arrhythmias, tetany
Investigations U+E, Ca^{2+}, PO_4^{3-}, ECG (prolonged PR, ST depression)
Treatment Slow IV infusion to correct deficit, eg 4–8g/8h (16–32mmol) IV; may need several days of therapy. May need oral replacement once deficit is corrected.
Complications arrhythmia, makes digitalis toxicity worse
Rapid IV infusions of magnesium may be used in severe asthma, torsades de pointes arrhythmias and eclampsia. Dose of 1.2–4g over 20min IV, get senior advice and help prior to giving. 10ml of 10% calcium gluconate IV over 2min acts as an antidote if excess is given.

Pyrexia

Worrying features ↑pulse, ↓BP, ↓GCS, ≥40°C, swinging fever, headache

Think about ***most likely*** focal or systemic infection including UTI, cellulitis, URTI/pneumonia, endocarditis, internal abscesses and septicaemia, meningitis ***other*** pulmonary embolism, iatrogenic (transfusion reaction/drug reaction, p280, infected lines), inflammatory conditions and malignancy ***rare*** malignant hyperpyrexia (OHA1 p199), neuroleptic malignant syndrome (OHCC2 p522)

Ask about urinary symptoms (frequency, dysuria, pyuria), respiratory/ENT symptoms (cough, sputum production and colour, haemoptysis, breathlessness, chest pain, sore throat/ear, coryza, contact and immunisation to TB), joints/skin (arthropathy, rash, erythema/breaks to skin and sores, eye symptoms), neurological (headache, photophobia, neck stiffness), general well-being (appetite, weight loss, night sweats) ***PMH*** previous UTI/URTI and previous TB, prosthetic heart valve or valvular lesion ***DH*** immunosuppressive agents (including steroids), blood transfusions or new drugs commenced (antipsychotic or anti-emetic), allergies ***SH*** any contacts with similar symptoms or known exposure to TB, smoking, recreational drug use (ecstasy)

Obs temp (?swinging), pulse, BP, RR, sats, cap refill, urine output

Look for pulse rate/rhythm/volume, warm peripheries, sweating, flushing, tachypnoea, tremor, splinter haemorrhages, break in skin, needle tracks in arms/feet/groin, focal skin infection, bronchial breathing/crackles/reduced air entry, heart murmur, suprapubic/loin tenderness, catheters/lines, joint swelling

Investigations septic screen (p253) ***urine dipstix*** and M,C+S (p504) ***blds*** FBC, ↑NØ (bacterial), ↑LØ (viral), ↑EØ (parasties/allergy), blood film (may suggest haematological malignancy), U+E, LFT, inflammatory markers (CRP, ESR/PV), D-dimer if PE suspected (but likely also to be positive in infection), bld cultures (p458) ***sputum*** M,C+S, if active TB suspected request urgent 'smear' microscopy for acid-fast bacilli (AFB) ***stool culture, skin swabs, sputum*** M,C+S ***ABGs*** respiratory failure or metabolic acidosis (p506) ***CXR*** pneumonia/effusion ***echo*** if you suspect bacterial endocarditis; transoesophageal is more sensitive than transthoracic (speak to cardiologist on call) ***LP*** if meningitis suspected (CT first)

Treatment

Assess the severity of illness, have a low threshold for treatment as septic shock (p153). Septic screen (p253) if new onset temp >38°C and treat with appropriate antibiotics (p254).

Symptom management paracetamol (1g/6h PO) and/or ibuprofen (400mg/8h PO) for pyrexia, analgesia for pain, ensure adequate hydration (consider IV fluids if nauseous or NBM), supplementary oxygen if O_2 sats <95%. An electric fan may produce symptomatic relief for the patient. Review patient with results of septic screen to form a management plan.

Request early ***senior review*** if in doubt of diagnosis or patient unwell.

Urinary tract infection, including pyelonephritis (OHCM6 p262)

Symptoms *cystitis* urinary frequency, dysuria, urgency, pyuria, haematuria, suprapubic pain *pyelonephritis* fever, rigors, vomiting, loin pain, pyuria, haematuria

Risk factors ♀, sexual intercourse, catheterisation, DM, immunosuppression, pregnancy, menopause, urinary tract strictures/stones, elderly

Signs warm peripheries, vasodilation, tachycardia, suprapubic/loin pain

Worrying signs ↓BP/shock (p153), temp >40°C, new renal impairment. Elderly patients can be afebrile but heavily bacteraemic.

Investigations *Urine dipstix* positive for two or more of blood, protein, leucocytes and nitrites suggests UTI (p504) *M,C+S* if high suspicion of UTI on dipstix and in all pyrexic/vomiting children *blds* FBC (↑WCC, ↑NØ), U+E (↑urea, ↑creatinine if outflow tract obstruction p452), ↑inflammatory markers, ↑BM (?DM/DKA) *bld cultures* if ↑temp (rigors) or systemically unwell *ultrasound/IVU/cystoscopy* if recurrent infections, evidence of renal impairment or male (p268)

Acute treatment If ↓BP/shock treat as septic shock (p153), otherwise paracetamol or ibuprofen (for fever), ensure investigations sent and consider commencing 'blind' antibiotic therapy (trimethoprim, amoxicillin or cephalosporin depending upon local guidelines) whilst awaiting sensitivities, ↑oral fluid intake, double voiding (half emptying bladder then emptying fully after 5min). Change to more appropriate antibiotic once sensitivity known and treat for 3–5/d for simple infections and 10d if complicated (♂, renal disease, systemically unwell). Repeat urine M,C+S post therapy to ensure resolution of infection.

Complications scarring of urinary tract including kidneys, CRF

Simple measures to treat urinary tract infections

- Drink >2l fluid day
- Voiding at 2–3h intervals
- Double voiding
- Voiding before bedtime and after sexual intercourse
- Wipe front to back after micturition (♀)

Recurrent urinary tract infections

- Avoidance of constipation which may impair bladder emptying
- Avoidance of bubble bath and other irritants in bathwater
- Antibiotic prophylaxis (trimethoprim, amoxicillin, quinolone)
- Drinking cranberry juice may have a protective action[1]

1 T Kontiokari 2001 *BMJ* **332** 1.

Endocarditis (OHAM2 p120)

Symptoms malaise, anorexia, weight loss, fever, rigors, night sweats, ±dyspnoea, oedema

Risk factors prosthetic valve, valvular lesion (aortic > mitral), congenital cardiac defect, pacemaker/central line, mural thrombus (post-MI), recurrent bacteraemia (IV drug users, severe dental disease), atrial myxoma

Signs new murmur, splinter haemorrhages, Janeway lesions, Roth spots, conjunctival haemorrhages, tachycardia, warm peripheries, CCF, poor teeth and oral hygiene

Investigations For diagnostic criteria see below *blds* FBC (↑WCC, ↑NØ, ↓Hb), U+E, LFT, ↑inflammatory markers *bld cultures* take 3–4 sets (prior to commencing ABx) from different sites at intervals of >1h *ECG* features of underlying valvular lesion, AV block, pericarditis, *CXR* pulmonary oedema, septic pulmonary emboli *echo* (transoesophageal more sensitive than transthoracic) valvular lesion/vegetation (normal does not exclude endocarditis) *V/Q scan* if pulmonary emboli suspected *urine dipstix* blood (often present in IE cases), ±protein

Acute treatment Try to obtain at least 3 sets of blood cultures prior to commencing antibiotics unless patient unwell. Blind treatment should include a penicillin (benzylpenicillin or flucloxacillin) and gentamicin, ±vancomycin if ?MRSA. O_2 if unwell, paracetamol or ibuprofen and other supportive measures (anti-emetics, IV fluids if dehydrated or NBM).

Chronic treatment Antibiotic therapy for at least 4–6wk. Surgical valve replacement indicated if heart failure evident or signs of aortic root abscess (lengthening PR interval, RBBB), prosthetic valve unstable, or infection uncontrolled.

Complications valve destruction → cardiac failure, AV-block, intra-cardiac abscess, embolism (to brain, limbs, lungs), septicaemia, death

Diagnostic criteria for infective endocarditis (IE) – Duke classification

Definite IE – 2 major, or 1 major and 3 minor, or 5 minor criteria

Possible IE – findings fall short of 'definite' but not 'rejected'

Rejected IE – firm alternative diagnosis or resolution within <4d of therapy

Major criteria

- Positive blood cultures

Typical micro-organisms for IE on three separate blood cultures[1] and/or persistently positive blood cultures

- Evidence of endocardial involvement

Positive echocardiogram (vegetation, abscess, new regurgitation, dehiscence of prosthetic valve)

Minor criteria

- Predisposing condition or drug use
- Fever >38°C
- Vascular phenomena (septic emboli anywhere)
- Immunologic phenomena (glomerulonephritis, rheumatoid factor)
- Microbiological evidence (non-major criteria positive blood cultures)
- Echo (positive for IE but not meeting major criteria)

1 Commonly Streptococci (esp *S. viridans*), Enterococci, Staphylococci (*S. aureus*, *S. epidermidis*), Gram negative bacilli, Diptheroids, fungi, multiple organisms.

Common fungal infections

Fungi are ubiquitous and infections are commonly superficial, though deeper infections by fungi are not uncommon in the immunocompromised (p256). Always confirm diagnosis microbiologically; consider why the patient has a fungal infection

Skin	*Tinea sp.* (*T. capitis, corporis, pedis*). Can appear dry and scaly or as moist indurated areas. Treat topically with clotrimazole (Canesten®). *Malassezia furfur*. Pityriasis versicolour, macular rash. Treat with ketoconazole.
Mouth	*Candida albicans*. White patches on tongue and inside mouth. Treat with nystatin suspension or pastilles (p570).
Vagina	*Candida albicans*. Creamy white discharge with adjacent erythema and fissuring. Treat with clotrimazole pessary/cream or oral fluconazole.
Chest	*Aspergillus fumigatus*. May precipitate asthma or cause an aspergilloma (usually patient very unwell). Discuss with microbiologist. *Pneumocystis jiroveci* (formerly *carinii*) (PCP), see p258.
Brain	*Cryptococcus neoformans*. Commonest in the immunocompromised and results in meningitis. Requires specialist treatment (OHCM6 p612).
Blood	In immunocompromised patients most of the fungi can cause a disseminated septicaemia. Patients likely to be very unwell. Seek expert advice (microbiologist).

Abscesses

Any pus-filled cavity is technically an abscess. Abscesses are commonly within the skin layers, but can develop anywhere in which case imaging with ultrasound or CT may be required. Abscesses within the body cavity commonly cause a swinging temperature; the patient may only have malaise, lethargy and anorexia.

Skin	Common sites: axilla, natal cleft (pilonidal abscess), groin (in IV drug users). May settle with antibiotics, may require surgical I+D.
Mouth	Dental abscesses are common. Often settle with antibiotics, may require tooth extraction and I+D (maxillofacial surgery).
GI tract	Peri-anal abscess associated with inflammatory bowel disease, Crohn's > ulcerative colitis. Often require surgical intervention. Uncommon in the liver, often related to tropical disease; seek expert infectious diseases advice. Pancreatic 'cyst' associated with pancreatitis – seek expert advice (upper GI surgeon).
GU tract	Vulval abscesses commonest including Bartholin's abscesses. Commonly treated with I+D (p358).
Chest	Pulmonary empyema (p171) common following pneumonia, requires chest drain and antibiotics. Focal 'abscesses' can occur in TB, aspergilloma, bronchial carcinoma, septic emboli, pulmonary infarction.
Brain	Intracranial abscesses can be difficult to detect. Suspect if patient has new seizure activity, signs of ↑ICP or focal neurology, following ENT/dental infections or ↑WCC/inflammatory markers; other risk factors include SBE, bronchiectasis and skull fracture, following pneumococcal meningitis. Image with CT/MRI. Seek expert advice (neurosurgeon/neurologist).
Heart	Intracardiac collections can occur in patients with bacterial endocarditis and can invade into the associated major vessels. Requires expert advice (cardiologist).

Pulmonary tuberculosis (TB) (OHCM6 p564)

Symptoms ***Primary*** fever, lassitude, anorexia, weight loss, cough, haemoptysis, erythema nodosum, exertional dyspnoea, ±pleuric chest pain ***Postprimary*** as for primary but with precipitant to cause immunocompromise (steroids, HIV, ↑age, DM, malignancy, chemotherapy)
Risk factors exposure to TB, immunocompromise, non-vaccination
Signs fever, tachycardia, dyspnoea, haemoptysis, weight loss (cachexia), lymphadenopathy; consolidation on examination, bronchial breath sounds in apices, ±pleural effusion
Investigations **CXR** consolidation (often apical), cavitation, fibrosis, calcification and hilar lymphadenopathy, ±pleural effusion ***sputum*** M,C+S acid-fast bacilli (AFB) on Ziehl-Neelsen (ZN) stain, traditional culture of mycobacteria is slow and can take up to 12wk; new liquid culture allows detection within 1–2wk. Presence of AFB in sputum implies patient is infectious and need to be barrier-nursed with masks ***histology*** typically caseating granuloma ***immunological*** (OHCM6 p566) tuberculin skin testing with Mantoux (positive indicates immunity, strong positive suggests active disease); Heaf test is used for screening and not for investigating active disease ***blds*** check base-line U+E, LFT, FBC
Acute treatment Resuscitate as necessary if dehydrated, hypoxic etc. *Antibiotics:* ***initial phase*** (8wk) rifampicin, isoniazid, pyrazinamide and either ethambutol or streptomycin if resistance suspected ***continuation phase*** (4mth) rifampicin and isoniazid, with ethambutol if resistance suspected. Give pyridoxine (vitamin B_6) throughout treatment to avoid neuropathy. Steroids may be employed if pericardial or meningeal disease. See *BNF* for doses. For MDR-TB see following page.
Chronic treatment Need for compliance must be stressed and side-effects of drugs discussed; consider HIV testing in anyone with TB (p260).
Contact tracing Individuals sharing kitchen and bathroom with someone who has active TB should have a CXR, ±tuberculin skin test performed.
Vaccination BCG (bacille Calmette-Guérin) has been used in the UK since 1954 and is routinely given to children aged 13; it is a live attenuated vaccine. It decreases the risk of developing TB by between 50–70%. Its cost-effectiveness is now questioned in low-risk areas/groups.

Non-pulmonary tuberculosis (OHCM6 p564)

Meningeal	Sub-acute meningitic symptoms; fever, headache, photophobia
Miliary	Haematological spread to all tissues; liver, spleen, lungs, marrow
Genitourinary	Frequency, dysuria, loin pain, haematuria
Bone	Vertebral collapse adjacent to paravertebral abscess
Skin	Jelly-like lesions on face and neck
Heart	Acute/chronic pericarditis, ±pericardial effusion

Malignancy	p173	Cellulitis	p295
Pneumonia	p168	Pulmonary embolism	p169
Septic shock	p153	Inflammatory/connective tissue disease	p417

Multi-drug-resistant tuberculosis (MDR-TB)

Strains of mycobacterium resistant to standard anti-tuberculosis drugs are becoming commoner; in these patients it is essential to minimise the risk of spread and to stress the importance of drug compliance. Isolation of patients with 'open' MDR-TB is crucial. Seek advice from microbiologist/infectious diseases consultant.

Septic screen

- Physical examination, CVS/RS/abdo/skin/ENT/wounds/catheters/lines
- Full blood count (repeat every 2d)
- Inflammatory markers, ESR/PV, CRP (repeat every 2–4d)
- Urine microscopy and culture
- Sputum microscopy and culture, if indicated
- Microbiology swabs of wounds/pressure areas/cannula or central line sites
- Blood cultures (3 sets at 6–8h intervals from different veins)
- CXR if productive cough or abnormal clinical signs present
- Echocardiogram if new murmur or new stigmata of bacterial endocarditis
- Lumbar puncture if CNS infection suspected or needs to be excluded (CT first)

Iatrogenic causes of pyrexia

Transfusion reactions (p280)

- Infected lines:
  - Cannula, central lines, arterial lines, urinary catheters, long-lines etc
- Malignant hyperthermia (OHA1 p199):
  - Muscle relaxants/volatile anaesthetic agents
- Neuroleptic malignant syndrome (OHCC2 p522):
  - Antipsychotic drugs
- Sulphonamides
- Isoniazid
- Aspirin
- Post-operative
  - Atelectasis (often 24h post-op)

Notifiable diseases

Inform microbiology/public health consultant

- Anthrax
- Cholera
- Diphtheria
- Dysentery (amoebic, typhoid, paratyphoid)
- Encephalitis
- Food poisoning
- Leprosy
- Leptospirosis
- Malaria
- Measles
- Meningitis (acute)
- Meningococcal septicaemia
- Mumps
- Plague
- Poliomyelitis
- Rabies
- Relapsing fever
- Rubella
- Scarlet fever
- Smallpox
- Tetanus
- Tuberculosis
- Typhus
- Viral haemorrhagic fevers, eg lassa and yellow fevers
- Viral hepatitis
- Whooping cough

Empirical antibiotic treatment

Choice of suitable antibiotic will depend upon many factors, including likely pathogen or known microbial sensitivity, patient factors such as age and coexisting disease, drug availability and local guidelines. Below are some common infections and a suggested antibiotic regimen (suitable for an otherwise healthy 70kg adult).

Local antibiotic guidelines should be available in every hospital, as organism sensitivity varies throughout the country as does drug availability. Do not hesitate to contact the on-call microbiologist if in doubt.

Taking cultures prior to commencing antibiotic therapy is very useful as it will allow subsequent therapy to be more specifically tailored. However, cultures should not delay treatment in the unwell patient.

Urinary tract	Trimethoprim 200mg/12h PO (or cefalexin 500mg/8h PO)
Cellulitis	Flucloxacillin 1g/6h IV + benzylpenicillin 1.2g/6h IV
Wound infection	Await wound swab, otherwise as for cellulitis
Meningitis	Ceftriaxone 2g/24h IV
Encephalitis	As for meningitis + aciclovir 10mg/kg/8h IV
Endocarditis (empirical therapy)	Benzylpenicillin 1.2 g/6h IV + gentamicin (p569) (take 3 sets of blood cultures first; d/w microbiology)
Septic arthritis	Flucloxacillin 2g/6h IV (or clindamycin)

Pneumonia	
Community acquired (CAP)	Amoxicillin 500mg/8h PO ±erythromycin 500mg/6h PO
Severe CAP	Cefuroxime 1.5g/8h IV + clarithromycin 500g/12h IV
Hospital acquired	Consult local guidelines – d/w microbiologist
Aspiration pneumonia	Consult local guidelines – d/w microbiologist
?MRSA pneumonia	Consult local guidelines – d/w microbiologist

Septicaemia	
Urinary tract sepsis	Cefuroxime 1.5g/8h IV, ±gentamicin (p569)
Intra-abdominal sepsis	Cefuroxime 1.5g/8h IV + metronidazole 500mg/8h IV
Meningococcal sepsis	Ceftriaxone 2g/12h IV
Neutropenic sepsis	Tazocin® [1] 4.5g/8h IV + gentamicin (p569)
Skin/bone source	Flucloxacillin 1g/6h IV – d/w microbiologist
Unknown source	d/w microbiologist

1 Tazocin® 4.5g = piperacillin 4g + tazobactam 500mg.

MRSA

Methicillin-resistant Staphylococcus aureus (MRSA) is just one of several multi-drug-resistant microbes which can result in disease; it is often referred to as the 'super-bug' in the media. MRSA does not always result in pathology and up to 10% of the 'healthy' population are believed to carry it in their naso-pharynx.

Transmission of MRSA is easy and can be greatly reduced by simple hygiene methods such as hand-washing, use of alcohol hand-gel and wearing plastic aprons when dealing with infected patients.

MRSA, like other *Staphylococci,* can result in cellulitis, pneumonia, septicaemia, wound infections and death. Most strains of MRSA remain sensitive to vancomycin or teicoplanin.

Measures to prevent spread include:

- isolation of known or suspected MRSA infected patients
- cohort MRSA infected patients together in one ward/bay
- wear protective clothing when handling MRSA infected patients
  - plastic aprons and gloves
  - dispose of these before exiting the side-room/bay
- hand-washing and alcohol-gel
- use of dedicated stethoscopes and other equipment
- eradication therapy
- rigorous hygiene for wounds, catheters and venous access
- surveillance swabs for patients and staff during outbreaks

MRSA screening is undertaken by nursing staff and involves swabbing the nose, perineum, any wounds (or inflamed skin-folds), plus culturing sputum and urine if symptomatic; this varies greatly between hospitals.

MRSA eradication regimen

Most patients on the wards will be eligible for eradication therapy. Some trusts limit eradication therapy to two courses due to increased risk of mupirocin resistance. The infection control team will usually notify the ward that the patient is colonised with MRSA and will recommend eradication therapy if appropriate.

Aquasept® (triclosan)	Used once daily for 5d. Used as a liquid soap for the body with particular attention paid to skin creases
Bactroban® (mupirocin)	Applied to the anterior nares every 8h for 5d. Comes in cream or ointment preparations

Remember – Trusts differ slightly in their approach to patients with MRSA, so check out the infection control file on your ward when you arrive and if you have any problems, contact the infection control nurse or microbiology department.

Immunocompromised patients

Worrying features ↑pulse, ↓BP, ↑temp, ↓GCS, neutropaenia, bleeding, ↑BM

Think about immune/marrow failure (congenital, marrow infiltration, HIV/AIDS, chemotherapy p379) and immune suppression (steroids p419, immunosuppressants, poorly controlled DM) and increasing age

Ask about previous (or recurrent) infections, childhood and developmental problems, symptoms of anaemia or thrombocytopenia (SOB on exertion, bruising/bleeding tendency) ***PMH*** malignancy, rheumatoid, skin or bowel disease requiring steroids or immunosuppressants, DM ***DH*** steroids (glucocorticoids), immunosuppressants (azathioprine, ciclosporin), chemotherapy, anti-retroviral agents, other drugs which may precipitate aplastic anaemia, herbal remedies/alternative medicines/plant extracts ***SH*** recreational drugs, participation in activities at high risk of transmission of blood-borne viruses (sex abroad, male sex with same sex partners, intravenous drug use, blood transfusions, operations/injections in developing world, unhygienic (prison) tattoos)

Obs pulse, BP, RR, sats, temp, GCS

Look for signs of sepsis (vasodilated, warm, tachycardic, sweaty, lethargy/malaise – though these can be subtle in the immunocompromised host), lymphadenopathy, signs of focal infections (skin, respiratory/ENT, cardiovascular (endocarditis), neurological (focal signs), intra-abdominal); signs of underlying disease process (steroid side-effects (striae, buffalo hump, moon-shaped face), diabetic neuropathy and retinopathy, skin or rheumatological disease)

Investigations ***blds*** FBC and differential (including CD4+ count if known HIV/AIDS), U+E, LFT, CRP, glucose, clotting if pancytopaenia suspected, blood cultures; consider HIV test only after discussing with senior and obtaining consent from patient (p261) ***sputum*** M,C+S, ±AFB (TB) ***urine*** blood, protein, leucocytes, nitrites, M,C+S ***CXR*** focal infection, heart size, evidence of malignancy ***skin swabs*** if ulcers or weeping erythema ***therapeutic drug levels*** of azathioprine, ciclosporin ***bone marrow biopsy*** if marrow failure suspected

Treatment

- Airway, breathing and adequate circulation
- IV access, take bloods and label samples as 'HIGH RISK' if unsure
- Identify likely cause and treat presenting complaint(s)
- Early input from senior, plus input from haematologist/immunologist
- Commence neutropaenic protocol if patient febrile and neutropenic

Immunocompromise – the first few steps

- Immunocompromise often needs no emergency treatment, though identify cause
- If neutropaenic (p257) ensure patient has a side-room; reverse barrier nursing
- Low threshold for starting treatment for sepsis (p153)
- If on steroids ensure patient is given steroid support (p419)
- Samples from patients with probable HIV must be labelled 'HIGH RISK'

Neutropenia (NØ <1.5 x 10^9/l, regardless of total WCC) management depends upon whether the patient is well and afebrile or sick/febrile (febrile neutropenia).

Causes of neutropenia requiring hospital admission are usually related to marrow suppression by chemotherapy (usually 7–10 days later) for an underlying malignancy. Other causes of neutropenia present less often to hospital, but include viral infections, brucellosis, TB, drugs (carbimazole, sulfonamides), hypersplenism or anti-neutrophil antibodies and marrow failure secondary to either infiltration or B_{12}/folate deficiency.

Well neutropenic patients clearly are immunocompromised so will be prone to infections; question if hospital is appropriate as the patient may be 'safer' at home. If admission is necessary ensure a clean side-room is used and the patient should have reverse barrier nursing to prevent health-care staff introducing infection to the patient (p25). Check cause of neutropenia and look at FBC and clotting to exclude a significant pancytopenia. Discuss with haematology and microbiology consultants if specialist prophylactic antibiotics or growth factors to encourage marrow activity should be given. Regularly change cannula sites (every 48h).

Febrile neutropenia requires prompt medical action. A trigger temperature of >38°C is usually taken as warranting urgent action, though severely ill or severely neutropenic patients may not be able to mount a febrile response to infection. The box below outlines assessment and management of febrile neutropenia.

Febrile neutropenia (OHAM2 p718)

Pre-conditions	• Neutropenia, usually <1.0 x 10^9/l • Pyrexia >38°C (though patient can be normo/hypothermic)
Source of infection	• Often not clear clinically; pyrexia of unknown origin (PUO) • Commonly: chest, Hickman/central line, urine, skin, perianal • Microbiological diagnosis made in only about 40% of cases
Investigations	• Monitor FBC and differential, ±clotting, U+E, LFT, glucose • Culture blood, urine, sputum, swab Hickman line and skin folds • CXR • Repetitive clinical examination
Treatment	• Manage underlying pathology as usual (eg O_2 for pneumonia) • Commence antibiotics early in accordance with local policy • Common empirical regimens are shown below • Two or more drugs are usually necessary • Early involvement with haematologist/microbiologist • Consider antifungal prophylaxis

Empirical antibiotic therapy for febrile neutropenia (OHAM2 p720)

Early discussion with microbiologist is advised (check your local policy guidelines)

1st line	Tazocin 4.5g/8h IV, plus gentamicin 5mg/kg/24h IV (monitor levels)
2nd line	Add in vancomycin 1g/12h IV or teicoplanin 400mg/24h IV
3rd line	Consider adding in amphotericin if fever not settling Rediscuss with haematologist/microbiologist

Recurrent/unusual infections

Patients reattending with recurrent infections are less likely to be identified in hospital than by the GP. In hospital, isolation of an unusual pathogen by microbiology staff will usually start alarm bells ringing, and a consultant microbiologist is likely to be the first to raise an eyebrow and initiate further investigations, as well as suggest appropriate treatment.

Opportunistic infections are commonly seen in HIV and other immunocompromised states, a list of some are shown below. Identification of an unusual pathogen doesn't infer immunocompromise, it merely makes it more likely. Equally, many immunocompromised patients develop 'standard' infections with 'standard' pathogens.

Causes of immunocompromise are diverse and diagnosis requires meticulous history taking, examination and investigation (mostly blood-based). Increasing age, steroids (p419) and immunosuppressants can cause a relative increase in susceptibility to infections, though less so than neutropenia (p257).

Common opportunistic pathogens in the immunocompromised (OHCM6 p581)

Candidiasis	Usually furry white oral plaques (thrush), though can form in skin folds, genitalia and oesophagus and in severe cases cause a septicaemia. Treated locally with nystatin or systemically with fluconazole or amphotericin B.
CMV retinitis	Most common in HIV patients. Reduction in visual acuity, ±blindness. 'Mozzarella pizza' appearance on fundoscopy. Treated with ganciclovir or foscarnet.
Cryptococcus	Can cause eye infections, but most commonly meningitis, often without neck stiffness. Amphotericin B and flucytosine are used.
Herpes virus	Cold sores, though more seriously CNS infections (meningitis/encephalitis). Requires high-dose intravenous aciclovir.
Pneumocystis jiroveci (formerly carinii)	Typically a severe pneumonia, most commonly in HIV, but also in patients with leukaemia and following bone marrow transplantation. Treat aggressively with co-trimoxazole (trimethoprim + sulfamethoxazole). HIV patients with low CD4+ counts should receive this in a lower dose as primary prophylaxis. Following PCP patients should remain on co-trimoxazole as secondary prophylaxis.
Tuberculosis (TB)	This is the commonest of the mycobacteria which present clinically. Frank pulmonary TB in the immunocompromised usually results from reactivation of a primary infection many years prior. Treatment should be aggressive and consist of triple or quadruple therapy (p252). Compliance is crucial and should be emphasised. Always consider MDR-TB.
Tinea	Fungal skin infections are common in the healthy, but more so in the immunocompromised. Treat with topical agents (nystatin, clotrimazole, terbinafine) unless more invasive disease.
Toxoplasmosis	Usually associated with HIV. Causes meningitis/encephalitis or serious intracerebral abscesses. Treat aggressively with sulphadiazine and pyrimethamine. Secondary prophylaxis required.
Varicella-zoster virus	Cutaneous manifestations (chicken pox and shingles) and more seriously pneumonitis/encephalitis. Requires high-dose intravenous aciclovir. Seek ophthalmology input if ophthalmic shingles.

Shingles (OHCM6 p568)

This disease presents at any age, but commonly in the elderly and immunocompromised. Varicella-zoster is the responsible agent and shingles only occurs in patients who have had chickenpox as it is viral reactivation which triggers the onset of the disease (like TB).

Clinical presentation initially pain in a dermatomal distribution together with malaise/fever and subsequent eruption of a rash consisting of macules, papules and vesicles along the same dermatomal distribution.

Distribution is commonly of the thorax, abdomen and ophthalmic division of the trigeminal nerve, though other areas can be affected.

Diagnosis is made clinically, as few other pathologies localise so precisely to a dermatomal distribution; seldom crosses the midline. Antibody titres (blood) and viral DNA (from vesicular fluid) can be assayed. Viral swabs can be cultured more easily than DNA analysis – consult with laboratory.

Treatment consists of analgesia (±low-dose amitriptyline), skin care and antiviral agents such as aciclovir (800mg/5h PO for 5–7d); if immunocompromised give aciclovir via IV route (see *BNF*). Steroids may reduce post-herpetic neuralgia. If ophthalmic division of CN V involved, apply 3% aciclovir ointment/5h to affected eye and seek ophthalmic opinion.

Complications include post-herpetic neuralgia (pain in original distribution of shingles for many years after) and damage to the cornea and iris.

The patient with an organ transplant (OHAM2 p724)

Kidneys, liver, heart, lungs, pancreas and small bowel transplants require subsequent immunosuppression to prevent rejection of the transplanted organ by the host; the commonly used agents are ciclosporin, azathioprine, steroids and less frequently tacrolimus and anti-T-cell antibodies.

Susceptibility to infection is increased in patients on immunosuppressants and mostly due to an inadequate T-cell response. Typical infections in such patients include skin infections (fungal, warts, herpes viruses, varicella-zoster) and opportunistic pathogens (TB, fungi, PCP, CMV).

Management of infections in patients with transplants depends on whether the patient is neutropenic or not; if so commence neutropenic regimen (p257), in addition to treatment for known or presumed infection. Ensure involvement of microbiologist and transplant consultant.

Malignancy is more common amongst transplant patients, especially the viral-related tumours (EBV, HBV, HHV-8) which include squamous cancers, lymphoma and anogenital carcinoma.

Lifestyle changes should be employed to maximise the life of the transplant and minimise the risk of infections and neoplasm in the host. These include: suitable healthy diet, smoking cessation, regular exercise, vaccination of cats and dogs, prophylactic antibiotics prior to dental treatment, suitable vaccination prior to foreign travel and protection from intense sunlight (skin malignancy).

The patient with a kidney transplant

Donor kidneys are often sited in the iliac fossa and this is a differential of an iliac fossa mass. Care must be taken not to expose the donor kidney to direct trauma or to accidental injection when tapping ascites, cannulating the femoral vessels or performing regional anaesthesia to the femoral nerve. Urinary tract infections must be treated aggressively as the consequences of ascending infection would be devastating.

HIV/AIDS (OHAM2 p337)

HIV infection results eventually in autoimmune deficiency syndrome (AIDS). Two forms of HIV exist, HIV-1 and HIV-2, though clinically no distinction can yet be made between these.

Transmission is mainly by sexual contact, both penile to vaginal and the reverse (with equal transmission rates) and penile to anus and the reverse (again with equal transmission rates); oral sex is now a recognised form of transmission. Increasingly seen in the developing world where transmission mainly occurs at birth; caesarian section and avoidance of breast-feeding reduces this risk. Needle sharing in drug users permits transmission, though needle-stick injuries (p34) and infection through blood products is now very rare, as is transmission via spray of infected bodily fluids to the eye (p34).

Presentation usually occurs with the onset of an opportunistic infection many years after initially contracting HIV; this generally marks the onset of **AIDS** (see below).

Acute seroconversion occurs at 2–6wk after primary infection with HIV, and may present as an influenza-like illness (fever, malaise, myalgia, pharyngitis, ±maculopapular rash).

Diagnosis is made in the laboratory. HIV antibody is still the commonest test, though HIV RNA can be identified by using PCR technology. The CD4+ sub-type of lymphocytes is usually assayed at this time too, as this, along with viral load, is used as a marker of disease progression.

Course Most cases of HIV undergo an asymptomatic, or latent, period which varies between months to over 10yr, though some infected patients have a persistent generalised lymphadenopathy. As the onset of AIDS approaches, minor opportunistic infections appear (candida, herpes zoster, tinea etc) and this is called the AIDS-related complex, probably a prodrome to AIDS.

AIDS occurs when HIV infection has resulted in immune deficiency sufficient to allow the establishment of an AIDS-defining disease; untreated patients die within 20mth, though can live for decades with treatment.

Treatment of HIV/AIDS involves drugs targeted at hindering retroviral replication and adherence to host cells. The three main classes are *nucleoside reverse-transcriptase inhibitors*, *non-nucleoside reverse transcriptase inhibitors* and *protease inhibitors*; *enfuvirtide* forms its own, fourth class and inhibits HIV from fusing to the host cell. It is unclear when therapy should be started or altered, but combination therapy or HAART (Highly Active Anti-Retroviral Therapy) and regular monitoring of viral load is common-place and appears to be the most effective means of delaying progression to AIDS. Check *BNF* for drug interactions.

Common AIDS-defining conditions

Cryptococcal meningitis	Progressive multifocal leukoencephalopathy
Chronic cryptosporidial diarrhoea	Recurrent non-typhi Salmonella septicaemia
CMV retinitis	Cerebral toxoplasmosis
Chronic mucocutaneous herpes	Kaposi's sarcoma
Mycobacterium avium intracellulare	Non-Hodgkin's lymphoma
Miliary or extrapulmonary TB	Primary cerebral lymphoma
Oesophageal candidiasis	HIV-associated wasting
Pneumocystis jiroveci	HIV-associated dementia

HIV testing (OHAM2 p342)

Results are often available within a week and sometimes within a day

Ideally performed in GUM/STI clinics or in primary care (by GP)

Occasionally needed in hospital when questioning HIV-related disease

Informed consent should always be obtained following a pre-test discussion

Very few instances when testing is permitted without consent (OHAM2 p342)

Patients with a positive test should have early access to an HIV clinician

Patients with a negative test should be counselled about risk reduction

Counselling for HIV test

This should be conducted by someone trained in GUM (usually specialist nurse)

Ascertain level of risk

Discuss benefits of testing (↓anxiety, protect partner and commence treatment)

Discuss difficulties (disclosure to family, effects upon job, finances, insurance)

Post-test discussion to plan for treatment or how to adjust risk factors

Treating patients with HIV

Patients with a new diagnosis of HIV can feel very lonely and isolated

Educate other staff that HIV is not transmissible by simply touching the patient

Patients with HIV can be nursed in normal hospital bays, unless they are lymphopenic

Use a private room to discuss their management to maintain confidentiality

Double glove to take blood samples and allow plenty of time and space

Ensure all samples are labelled with HIGH RISK stickers prior to sending to the lab

Needle-stick injuries should be managed as p34, but discuss with HIV consultant

Primary prevention of HIV transmission

Encourage safe sex (condoms, fewer partners)

Discourage needle sharing in drug users

Vigorous control of other STDs can reduce HIV incidence

Encourage antenatal screening of HIV (risk to unborn baby can be reduced)

Assessing volume status

Pulse, postural hypotension and low urine output (<0.5ml/kg/h) are sensitive signs of hypovolaemia while orthopnoea suggests overload.

Ask about ***hypovolaemia*** urine output, headache ***fluid overload*** shortness of breath, orthopnoea, cough, sputum (white/pink frothy), swelling

Obs ***early hypovolaemia*** fast pulse (including upper range of normal, ie >90/min – NB remains slow if taking β-blockers), postural BP (a drop of more than 20mmHg on standing is significant), urine output <0.5ml/kg/h ***late hypovolaemia*** urine output <17ml/h, low blood pressure ***fluid overload*** raised RR, low sats

Look for ***early hypovolaemia*** dry mucous membranes (lips, mouth, nose), prolonged central capillary refill (normal <2s), absent JVP on lying flat ***late hypovolaemia*** sunken eyes, increased skin turgor ***fluid overload*** raised JVP, bilateral basal crackles, pitting oedema (ankles if sitting, sacrum if in bed), gallop rhythm (3rd heart sound), cold hands and feet

Investigations ***early hypovolaemia*** *urine* dark, raised osmolality *blds* may be normal, ↑urea, ↑packed cell volume (PCV, also called haematocrit), ↑albumin, ↑osmolality, look for trends ***late hypovolaemia*** ↑creatinine ***fluid overload*** pulmonary oedema on CXR (p508), abnormal ECG (p514 – LVH, MI), ↑CVP

Fluid balance is calculated by measuring a patient's urine output and fluid input along with any losses from vomit, diarrhoea or drains. The patient must be catheterised for accurate measurement.

Insensible losses These are unrecordable fluid losses, eg sweating and breathing. 500–1,000ml is usually lost each day, but this increases with pyrexia (from sweating), breathing rapidly and burns; this loss will not be apparent from the fluid chart. Litres of fluid can be lost from burns and wound seepage which is missed unless the bandages are weighed.

Third space fluids Also called fluid sequestration; inflammation and injury causes capillary permeability to increase so that fluid and protein leak from the blood vessels (intravascular space) causing oedema. The patient is hypovolaemic despite normal fluid balance and fluid should be replaced according to clinical signs, especially urine output. It is common with sepsis, pancreatitis and after major operations.

CVP lines Central venous pressure measurements are used primarily in ITU and HDU since they require a central line (p476). By recording the pressure in the line at the level of the right atrium an estimate of blood volume is obtained. The normal range is 2–5mmHg (5–10cmH_2O); high pressure suggests fluid overload or heart failure while a low CVP suggests hypovolaemia. Trends are more important than absolute values; the CVP should rise with a fluid challenge and hypovolaemia has been corrected once this rise persists after the challenge has finished.

Simple fluids

Who needs fluids?

Hypovolaemic shock, dehydration, low urine output, excess fluid loss, third space losses (see opposite) ***Reduced intake*** nil-by-mouth (pre-op and post-op), reduced oral fluids, reduced consciousness, vomiting, acutely ill

Rate and type

Situation	Rate	Type of fluid
Resuscitation/acute shock	1l/stat–1h	Blood, 0.9% saline, Hartmann's, ±colloid
Hypovolaemic/acutely ill	1l/4–6h	0.9% saline, ±colloid
Maintenance	1l/8–10h	0.9% saline, glucose saline or 5% glucose
Elderly/mild overload	1l/10–18h	0.9% saline, glucose saline or 5% glucose

Maintenance fluids

The majority of hospital patients receive bags of fluid over 8h. A common regime, is shown below.

Date	Route	Fluid	Additives	Vol	Rate	Signature
19/08/05	IV	5% glucose	20mmol KCl	1l	8h	Dr CJFlint
19/08/05	IV	0.9% saline		1l	8h	Dr CJFlint
19/08/05	IV	5% glucose	20mmol KCl	1l	8h	Dr CJFlint

Fluid challenge

Patients with low blood pressure or low urine output are often prescribed a fluid challenge. A bolus of 500ml (250ml if frail or heart problems) colloid or 0.9% saline is infused over 30min. If the patient's urine output improves it suggests that hypovolaemia was the cause and the rate of IV infusion can be increased.

Date	Route	Fluid	Additives	Vol	Rate	Signature
19/08/05	IV	Gelofusine		500ml	30min	Dr CJFlint

Further fluids

Maintenance requirements On average adults require 30–35ml of water/kg/24h to cover their urine output and insensible losses (sweat, respiration, stool). This equals about 2–2.5l per day for a 70kg adult; paediatric fluid requirements are on p391.

Excess losses Illness may cause patients to lose excess fluid. This may be:
- *recordable* polyuria, NG aspirate, diarrhoea, vomiting, drains
- *insensible* wound leakage, pyrexia, tachypnoea, burns
- *third space* (p262), eg pancreatitis, post-op.

Fluid deficit Significant loss of fluid without adequate intake may be apparent on the fluid chart or from the history. The following table should act as a guide for fluid deficit in acute situations.

Fluid deficit	<750ml	750–1500ml	1500–2000l
Pulse	<100	>100	>120
Blood pressure	Normal	Normal	Reduced
Urine output	>30ml/h	<30ml/h	<17ml/h

Fluid requirements

No fluid chart The patient's 24h requirements are estimated from three components:
- estimate of maintenance requirement from weight (30ml/kg/24h)
- additional fluids if significant insensible losses are expected (0.5–1.5l/24h)
- estimate of fluid deficit (from history, examination, obs)

The following groups of patients may need less fluids than estimated:
- small/elderly/frail, heart problems, renal failure, partial oral intake

Fluid balance recorded The 24h requirement can be calculated more accurately if a patient's fluid balance has been recorded. This is especially important in patients at risk of fluid overload. Again three components need to be considered:
- recorded losses over last 24h (from fluid chart)
- estimate of insensible losses (usually 0.5–1.5l/24h)
- estimate of fluid deficit (from history, examination, obs and fluid chart)

Prescribing Once the 24h fluid requirement is known it can be converted into litre bags at appropriate rates. If there is a deficit the initial bags should be run more quickly to correct hypovolaemia. Prescribe the fluids so that they run out during the normal working day to reduce work for those on call and ensure continuity of care.

Electrolyte requirements

Estimation of electrolyte requirements should take into account U+E, medications (especially diuretics and supplements) and fluid loss. Average maintenance requirements are:
- ***sodium*** 2mmol/kg/24h – about 140mmol a day
- ***potassium*** 0.5–1mmol/kg/24h – about 40–60mmol a day

The table below shows the electrolyte content of the commonly used IV fluids. All of these are isotonic (the same osmolality as plasma).

Electrolyte constituents of common IV fluids

1l of:	Na^+ (mmol/l)	K^+ (mmol/l)	Cl^- (mmol/l)
5% Glucose	0	0/20/40	0
Glucose saline	30	0/20/40	30
0.9% Saline	150	0/20/40	150
Hartmann's	131	5	111
Gelofusine® (colloid)	154	0	120
Packed red cells			
Fresh	15	0.3	150
Expiry	10	6.0	?[1]

1 despite our best efforts we are unable to find this figure. If you know it see pvii at the front.

Special cases

Post-op Patients often leave surgery with hypovolaemia due to blood loss and oedema (third space); they may require more fluids to make up this deficit. Despite lysis of cells during surgery causing a release of potassium, most post-operative patients who remain NBM will still require supplementary KCl in their post-operative fluid replacement after 24h.

Intestinal fluid losses Most intestinal fluids have a composition similar to 0.9% saline with 20mmol/l of KCl and should be replaced with this. For the exact composition of different intestinal fluids see section 9.2 of the *BNF*.

Heart problems Patients with previous heart disease are more prone to fluid overload and pulmonary oedema. Simple attention to fluid balance prevents problems in the majority of patients. If fluid overload develops the patient may require a low sodium diet, daily weights and fluid restriction (eg 1.5l/24h). Try to avoid furosemide if possible.

Chronic liver failure Excess sodium causes ascites in chronic liver failure. Restrict sodium by using 5% glucose; fluid restriction is rarely required. If fluid resuscitation is required use salt-poor albumin (a blood product).

Acute renal failure Initially give rapid infusions of a colloid or 0.9% saline and avoid potassium. Further IV fluids should be determined by fluid balance and CVP in ITU or HDU.

Chronic renal failure A reduction in glomerular filtration rate (GFR) means that the kidney cannot excrete as much water, sodium or potassium. In mild renal failure excess fluids and sodium should be avoided though acute deterioration in renal function is usually a sign of hypovolaemia. In severe renal failure sodium, potassium and fluid restriction (eg 1.5l/24h) are required.

Low urine output

Worrying features prolonged low urine output <0.5ml/kg/h, ↑pulse, systolic BP <100mmHg, ↑K^+, ↑creatinine

Remember it is easier to treat fluid overload than acute renal failure.

	Volume in 24h	Volume in 1h
Normal urine output	>1,600ml	>60ml
Low urine output	<800ml	<30ml (0.5ml/kg)
Oliguria	<400ml	<17ml
Anuria	<100ml	<4ml
Absolute anuria	None	None

Think about ***severe*** acute renal failure, shock ***most likely*** hypovolaemia, urinary retention, blocked catheter, prostatic hypertrophy ***other*** rhabdomyolysis, chronic renal failure, renal vascular problems, urethral trauma, fluid overload

Ask about abdominal pain, hesitancy, poor stream, oral intake, vomiting, diarrhoea, stoma output, leaking wounds, sweating, breathlessness, orthopnoea, tiredness, recent falls/lying on floor ***PMH*** kidney disease, number of kidneys, prostate disease, hypertension, heart disease, diabetes ***DH*** nephrotoxic drugs (eg NSAIDs, gentamicin, ACEi)

Obs BP, pulse, fluid balance, CVP if possible

Look for volume status (p262), oedema, palpable bladder, suprapubic pain, evidence of infection or haemorrhage, unrecorded leakage from wounds, loin pain, enlarged prostate, extensive bruising

Investigations urine colour, dipstick, M,C+S. If not responding to fluid challenges send urine for osmolality (p504) and sodium ***blds*** FBC, U+E, CK, osmolality, CRP ***bladder scan*** if urinary retention or a blocked catheter is suspected; this may be available on the wards ***USS abdo*** if urine output is persistently low; request a Doppler USS if renal artery stenosis is suspected

Treatment

Insert a urinary catheter (most nurses are able to do this) and ask the nurses to keep an hourly fluid balance including any diarrhoea, vomiting and fluid loss from wounds. Consider asking for a catheter flush if already catheterised. Assess the patient and if in doubt treat as hypovolaemia (p267) and review in 1–2h.

If urine output is still low despite treatment It can take up to 2h for a fluid bolus to work. If there is still no improvement send a urine sample and bloods as described above. Ask for a bladder scan. Get senior advice. Do not ignore patients with very low urine output.

	History	Examination	Investigations
Hypovolaemia	Low fluid input, excess losses, post-op	Negative fluid balance, ↑pulse, absent JVP	↑urea, concentrated urine ↑osmolality
Shock	Feels ill, symptoms of infection, acute illness or blood loss	Tachycardia, hypotensive, may be septic, exclude haemorrhage	May have ↓Hb, ↑WCC and ↑CRP
Acute renal failure	Severe illness, untreated low urine output	May be dehydrated or shocked	New onset ↑urea and creatinine, ↑CK if rhabdomyolysis
Chronic renal failure	Diabetes, hypertension, tired, previous kidney problems	Pale, anaemic, oedema, bruising, peripheral neuropathy	Persistent ↑urea and creatinine, small kidneys on USS
Urinary retention	Lower abdominal pain, previous prostate problems	Palpable bladder, could be anuric, enlarged prostate	Full bladder on scan
Fluid overload	Cardiac history, excess fluids, SOB	↑JVP, basal creps, cold hands/feet, oedema	CXR shows pulmonary oedema

Hypovolaemia

This is by far the most common cause of low urine output.

Symptoms, signs, investigations see p262

Treatment Increase fluid input; the rate of rehydration depends on the patient. If urine output is >0.5ml/kg/h simply increase the rate of current IV fluids. If <0.5ml/kg/h consider a fluid challenge (p263) and prescribe some quick fluids to follow, eg 0.9% saline 1l/4h; review the patient in 2h.

Complications acute renal failure

Fluid overload

This is a rare cause of low urine output.

Symptoms, signs, investigations see p262

Treatment See p170 pulmonary oedema. For simple overload reduce the speed of IV fluids and review in a few hours; ask the nurses to weigh the patient, record hourly obs and contact you if the patient's respiratory rate rises. If you are certain they are overloaded try 20–40mg furosemide PO or IV. This will cause a diuresis in all patients and potentially cause acute renal failure if the patient was hypovolaemic.

Complications pulmonary oedema

Hypotension/shock	p149	Renal failure	p268
Urinary retention	p452	Pulmonary oedema	p170

Renal failure

There are two types of renal failure:

Acute renal failure usually caused by hypovolaemia or shock, it may be caused by primary renal disease and urinary obstruction.

Chronic renal failure usually caused by primary renal disease, diabetes or long-standing urinary obstruction. It is the end result if the following conditions progress:

- haematuria and/or proteinuria
- nephrotic syndrome
- nephritic syndrome

Acute renal failure (OHCM6 p272 or OHAM2 p378)

An acute rise in urea and creatinine over hours or days often with persistent oliguria. It has a poor prognosis if serum creatinine >400μmol/l, oliguria for >24h or anuria for >12h. There are two stages:

- ***Prerenal hypoperfusion*** this should be suspected if urine output is <0.5ml/kg/h for two consecutive hours. This stage is fully reversible if treated early, but otherwise progresses to acute tubular necrosis.
- ***Acute tubular necrosis*** usually caused by prolonged hypoperfusion; recovery takes days to weeks and there is often a polyuric phase.

Acute renal failure can also be caused by vasculitides, nephrotoxic drugs (eg NSAIDs, aminoglycosides, ACEi), rhabdomyolysis and urinary obstruction. For other causes see OHCM6 p272.

Investigations *urine* colour, dipstick, M,C+S, osmolality and Na^+(p504) *blds* FBC, U+E, LFT, CK, CRP, osmolality, ESR and clotting *ABG* expect acidosis *urgent ECG* hyperkalaemia causes flat P waves, wide QRS and tall, peaked T waves *CXR* and *renal USS*

Treatment Resuscitate (shock p148, ↑K^+ p242). Continue IV fluids without KCl, stop nephrotoxic drugs and get senior help. HDU or ITU with CVP monitoring (p262) is often required; acute tubular necrosis has a mortality of >50%. Try to distinguish between hypoperfusion (oliguria, urine osmolality >500mosmol/kg) and acute tubular necrosis (oliguria/normal/polyuria, urine osmolality <350mosmol/kg).

Complications hyperkalaemia, fluid overload, encephalopathy

> *Indications for urgent dialysis* persistent hyperkalaemia (>7mmol/l), severe metabolic acidosis (pH <7.2, BE <⁻10), unresolving pulmonary oedema, uraemic encephalopathy (falling GCS or seizures), uraemic pericarditis (chest pain)

Rhabdomyolysis (OHAM2 p392)

Symptoms lying on a hard floor for prolonged periods, crush injuries, strenuous exercise, burns

Signs extensive bruising or damaged tissue, dark urine

Investigations very raised CK with normal troponins; ↑urea, ±↑creatinine, ↑K^+, blood on urine dipstick, but not microscopy (myoglobin), ↑urate

Treatment Treat as for acute renal failure, may need sodium bicarbonate or surgical removal of damaged tissue.

Complications acute renal failure, hyperkalaemia

Chronic renal failure (OHCM6 p276)

Defined as a long-standing and irreversible rise in urea and creatinine. Patients are often asymptomatic or have non-specific symptoms such as tiredness and swollen ankles. There are many causes including diabetes, hypertension, glomerulonephritis, prostatic hypertrophy, polycystic kidneys, pyelonephritis, vasculitis, autoimmune disease and interstitial nephritis. The severity can be estimated by calculating the GFR. See OHCM6 p276 for investigations and long-term management.

Prescribing Use appendix 3 of the *BNF*. Try to avoid nephrotoxic drugs, eg NSAIDs, gentamicin and reduce doses of many others, eg opioids, benzodiazepines, cephalosporins and digoxin; do not prescribe metformin.

Fluid and electrolytes Fluid, Na^+ and K^+ restriction is required in severe renal failure. See p265.

Complications include hypertension, anaemia, weak bones and a tendency to infection and neuropathy. Fluid overload should be treated with furosemide and fluid restriction.

Radiology Avoid all types of contrast imaging, this is nephrotoxic.

Nephrotic syndrome Defined as oedema with proteinuria (>3g/24h) and hypoalbuminaemia (<30g/l), ±hypercholesterolaemia. There are many causes including several types of glomerulonephritis and diabetes. Patients have a high risk of infection and thromboembolism.

Treatment Monitor blood pressure, weight, fluid balance and U+E; restrict fluid (1–1.5l/24h), sodium (50mmol/24h) and protein. Use furosemide 80–250mg/24h PO and consider metolazone. Treat infections quickly and give prophylactic LMWH (p289). Refer to a renal specialist.

Nephritic syndrome This is the combination of haematuria with red cell casts and proteinuria often associated with hypertension, oedema, oliguria and uraemia. It is most commonly caused by glomerulonephritis (often post-infectious) or vasculitis.

Treatment If an infection is present prescribe antibiotics, but do not prescribe steroids. Refer to a renal specialist.

Haematuria and/or proteinuria Nephrotic and nephritic syndrome are the extremes of renal damage. Between these extremes patients may gradually develop asymptomatic renal failure with blood and/or protein in their urine, ±hypertension.

Haematuria Blood on a urine dipstick requires urine microscopy (unless menstruating); the causes of haematuria are shown in box overleaf. In the absence of infection the presence of persistent red cells should prompt a 24h urine collection for protein, estimation of the GFR and PSA (in men). If these tests are normal consider renal imaging (USS, IVU) and referral to a urologist, ±cystoscopy.

Macroscopic haematuria This is when the urine is bloodstained (pink, red or brown); also called gross haematuria. It is investigated in the same manner as microscopic haematuria. Rifampicin and beetroot also make the urine pink.

Causes of haematuria exercise, menstruation, recent intercourse, renal/urinary tract tumour, stones, stricture, trauma, infection, enlarged prostate, renal disease, vasculitis, hypertension, endocarditis, coagulopathies
Causes of haematuria without red cells exercise, trauma, myositis, ischaemia, alcohol, haemolysis, rhabdomyolysis, porphyria

Proteinuria Patients with persistent proteinuria on a morning dipstick (excludes orthostatic proteinuria) or a single dipstick and clinical suspicion of disease require investigation with a 24h urine collection (see p505). The causes of proteinuria are shown below. The type of protein can be determined by urine electrophoresis and this should guide investigations. If a renal cause is suspected a renal USS and nephrology referral will be required.

Causes of proteinuria exercise, prolonged standing (orthostatic), NSAIDs, infection, fever, pregnancy, diabetes, hypertension, heart failure, renal disease, vasculitis, myeloma, lymphoma, leukaemia

[illegible]

[illegible]

[illegible] (Crohn's disease), particularly [illegible]

[illegible]

[illegible]

[illegible]

[illegible] PR [illegible]

[illegible]

Treatment

[illegible]

- Confirm [illegible] and locate appropriate [illegible]
- [illegible] (refer to dietician?)
- Look for a cause; you need to exclude malignancy in patients [illegible] (p.[illegible])
- Note that Hb may [illegible] not [illegible] increase after a [illegible]

[illegible]

Consider blood transfusion (see p.[illegible])

Anaemia (↓Hb, ♂<13g/dl, ♀<11.5g/dl)

Worrying features Hb<8g/dl, SOB, ↑pulse, ↓BP, dizziness, fainting, lethargy, palpitations, weakness, chest pain, ↓GCS/restlessness

Think about ***most likely*** acute blood loss, iron-deficiency anaemia, anaemia of chronic disease, alcoholic liver disease, malignancy ***other*** folate/B_{12} deficiency, thalassaemia, haemoglobinopathy, haemolysis, inadequate dietary intake (elderly, alcoholism, vegan diet) ***medical*** hypothyroidism, coeliac disease, Crohn's disease, partial gastrectomy, pregnancy, lactation, diabetic enteropathy, lymphoma, rheumatoid arthritis, tropical sprue

Ask about any bleeding? (site (eg nose, rectum), quantity, frequency) SOB (exertional/at rest), tiredness, dizziness, lethargy, weight loss, tinnitus, chest pain, palpitations, abdominal cramps, reflux, change in bowel habit, blood in stool, menorrhagia, pregnancy, recent surgery, thalassaemia, haemoglobinopathy ***DH*** trimethoprim, anticonvulsants, NSAIDs ***SH*** alcohol, diet (vegan)

Obs pulse, BP, postural BP, sats, RR, GCS

Look for pallor, bruising, glossitis, mouth ulcers, hepatomegaly, splenomegaly, jaundice, ascites ***CVS*** palpitations, bruits, signs of active bleeding, signs of heart failure, new onset heart murmurs, lymphadenopathy ***PNS*** peripheral neuropathy ***CNS*** optic atrophy ***PR*** blood in stool

Investigations ***blds*** FBC (with MCV), blood film, iron, ferritin and TIBC, serum B_{12} and folate, reticulocyte count, Coombs' test, CRP, ESR, U+E, LFT, TFT ***ECG*** if CVS symptoms ***CXR*** if suspicion of cancer ***other*** LDH, Schilling test, osmolality, autoantibodies screen, bone marrow biopsy

Treatment

Asymptomatic anaemia

- Consider oral iron and folate supplements
- Assess diet (refer to dietician)
- Look for a cause; you need to exclude malignancy in patients >40yr (p179)
- Note that Hb may be normal immediately after a large acute bleed

Symptomatic anaemia or Hb <8g/dl

Consider blood transfusion (see p276).

Mean cell volume (MCV) in different forms of anaemia

MCV < 76fL	Normal MCV	MCV > 96fL
Iron deficiency	Pregnancy	B_{12}/folate deficiency
Thalassaemia	Haemorrhage	Alcohol
Haemoglobinopathy	Haemolysis	Liver disease
	Haemoglobinopathy	Thyroid disease
	Anaemia of chronic disease	Myelodysplasia
	Renal failure	Sideroblastic anaemia
	Malignancy	Anti-folate drugs (eg methotrexate)
	Bone marrow failure	

Laboratory findings in different forms of anaemia

	Iron	TIBC	Ferritin	MCV
Iron deficiency	↓	↑	↓	↓
Chronic disease	↓	↓	↑	↔
Haemolysis	↑	↓	↑	↔
Pregnancy	↑	↑	↔	↔

Abnormalities on the peripheral blood film (OHCM6 p628)

Acanthocytes	Spiculated RBCs (abetalipoproteinaemia)
Anisocytosis	RBCs of various sizes (megaloblastic anaemia/thalassaemia)
Blast cells	Nucleated precursor cells (myelofibrosis/leukaemia)
Burr cells	Irregularly shaped cells seen in uraemia
Howell-Jolly bodies	Nuclear remnants in RBCs (post-splenectomy)
Hypochromic	Pale RBCs (iron-deficiency anaemia)
Left shift	Immature white cells (infection)
Leukaemoid reaction	Reactive leucocytosis (infection/burns/haemolysis)
Poikilocytes	Variably shaped cells (iron deficiency/myelofibrosis)
Reticulocytes	Immature RBCs (haemorrhage/haemolysis)
Right shift	Hypersegmented polymorphs (megaloblastic anaemia/uraemia/liver disease)
Rouleaux	Clumping of RBCs (infection/inflammation)
Schistocytes	Fragmented RBCs (intravascular haemolysis)
Spherocytes	Spherical RBCs (familial)
Target cells	RBCs with central staining and outer pallor (liver disease/thalassaemia/sickle-cell disease)

Anaemia secondary to blood loss (p151)

Symptoms epistaxis, haematemesis, blood in stool (melaena), PV bleeding, chest pain, palpitations, gastroduodenal ulcer, recent surgery, trauma
Signs ↑pulse, ↓BP, postural BP drop, ↑RR, ↓GCS/restlessness, shock, pallor, sweating, cold, clammy; look at the wound site if post-op, PR
Investigations *acute* may be normal; repeat Hb, MCV, U+E, LFT, clotting, G+S/crossmatch, send stool sample for FOB *long-term* recheck Hb, reticulocytes, OGD/sigmoidoscopy if bleeding source not apparent
Acute treatment (p148)

- Lay flat, elevate legs if hypotensive; give O_2
- IV access, take bloods, give rapid IV infusion (500ml colloid stat)
- If bleeding site is obvious, apply firm pressure and elevate

Contact your senior – treat the cause (eg return to theatre if bleeding from operation site)

Acute blood loss

Measurement of haemoglobin does not accurately estimate the volume of blood loss in the first few hours after haemorrhage.

Acute	Hb concentration may be normal as volume of blood lost is compensated for by rise in heart rate and vasoconstriction. Only when IV fluids or normal haemodilution occurs will a fall in Hb become evident.
Intermediate	During IV fluid resuscitation Hb is diluted, unmasking loss of RBCs. Even in the absence of IV therapy the body retains salt and water in this circumstance, resulting in a natural haemodilution.
Late	Homeostasis regulates the volume of fluid in the intravascular compartment and the Hb often rises as the 'clear' fluid (colloids/crystalloids) is eliminated. Without IV therapy Hb may remain low and rise slowly over the following weeks as erythropoeisis generates more RBCs.

Anaemia of chronic disease

Causes infection (eg TB), rheumatoid arthritis, chronic renal failure, malignancy, collagen vasculitides, liver failure
Symptoms fatigue, SOBOE, lethargy; may have few symptoms/signs
Investigations ↓MCV, ↓TIBC/serum iron, ↑ferritin, ↓EPO levels
Treatment treat the underlying disease; consider EPO in CRF

Haemolytic anaemia

Causes *haematology* sickle-cell disease, thalassaemia, glucose-6-phosphate dehydrogenase deficiency *medical* malaria, lymphoma, rheumatoid arthritis, portal hypertension, artificial heart valves, renal/liver disease, infections *other* burns, chemicals, toxins, drugs, autoimmune haemolytic anaemias, blood transfusion incompatibility
Signs jaundice, murmurs, lymphadenopathy, hepatosplenomegaly
Investigations ↑unconjugated bilirubin, reticulocyte count >85 × 10^9/l, ↓haptoglobin, haemosiderin, urobilinogen; consider bone marrow aspirate
Treatment often steroids; splenectomy long-term

Iron-deficiency anaemia

Iron found in red meat, kidney beans, spinach
Causes GI loss (gastroduodenal ulcer, oesophageal varices, colitis, haemorrhoids, malignancy), menorrhagia, poor diet, malabsorption syndromes, tropical infections
Symptoms abdominal pain, blood in stool, dysphagia, haemoptysis, haematemesis, menorrhagia, pregnancy, diet, diarrhoea, epistaxis
Signs pallor, koilonychia, glossitis, angular stomatitis *PR* blood in stool
Investigations *blood* film (microcytic, hypochromic with anisocytosis and poikilocytosis), ↓serum iron, ↓ferritin, ↑TIBC *stool* check for FOB *other* sigmoidoscopy, endoscopy, barium enema
Treatment Treat the anaemia with oral iron supplements (ferrous sulphate 200mg/8h PO for 2wk, then 200mg/12h PO) though warn about side-effects: change in bowel habit, black stools, nausea, epigastric pain. Admit if anaemia is severe enough to warrant transfusion (p279), find and treat the cause. If the patient has been prescribed oral iron tablets, make sure they have been taking them.

> Treatment with oral iron raises the Hb by ~1g/dl per week at best

Folate deficiency

Folate found in liver, yeast, spinach, nuts, green vegetables
Causes *malabsorption* alcohol, coeliac disease, Crohn's disease, partial gastrectomy, tropical sprue ↑*requirement* pregnancy, DM, lymphoma, malignancy *drugs* anticonvulsants, trimethoprim, methotrexate
Symptoms changes in sensation, change in bowel habit, dementia
Signs peripheral neuropathy, Korsakoff's syndrome
Investigations check serum B_{12}, ↑MCV, investigate for malabsorption
Treatment treat the cause; folic acid 5mg/24h PO for 4mth. For chronic haemolysis give long-term, but always use vitamin B_{12} concurrently; folate alone in undiagnosed megaloblastic anaemia can precipitate neuropathy including sub-acute combined degeneration of the cord. If planning pregnancy, 0.4mg/24h until 12/40.

Vitamin B_{12} deficiency

Vitamin B_{12} found in liver, kidney, fish, chicken, dairy products
Causes poor dietary intake, pernicious anaemia, malabsorption (as for folate deficiency), ileal resection, Crohn's disease
Symptoms changes in sensation, autoimmune disorders (eg vitiligo, infectious mononucleosis, Addison's disease)
Signs sore mouth (glossitis, angular cheilosis, mouth ulcers), neurological defects (peripheral neuropathy, optic atrophy), jaundice
Investigations serum folate, ↑MCV, blood film, Schilling test (drink radioactive labelled B_{12} and measure its absorption by measuring urinary excretion; if malabsorption is corrected by adding intrinsic factor, the diagnosis is pernicious anaemia), bone marrow aspirate
Treatment dietary advice, hydroxycobalamine 1mg/72h IM for 2wk, then 1mg/2mth IM as maintenance dose

Transfusion of blood products

Blood product transfusions carry risks as well as benefits. Ensure the benefits outweigh the risks before commencing a transfusion. Risks and types of transfusion-related reactions are shown on p279 and p280.

When taking blood for blood bank samples it is essential to hand-label the blood bottle at the bedside and check them against the patient's identification wristband. Errors here would be disastrous.

Group and save (G+S) Blood is analysed for ABO and rhesus grouping (see table) and common 'atypical' antibodies which are documented in the notes and recorded on the pathology computer system.

Crossmatch (XM) blood is analysed in the laboratory to establish the patient's ABO and rhesus grouping and for common 'atypical' antibodies; it is mixed with donor blood to check compatibility prior to issuing.

Ordering blood products for *elective* use depend upon the type of surgery planned or the severity of anaemia. Most hospitals have guidelines instructing juniors on pre-operative blood bank requests to prevent excess crossmatching which results ultimately in products becoming out of date and being wasted. A G+S is sufficient for many procedures – check your local guidelines. Ensure blood bottle and form are labelled fully and clearly and indicate when the blood products are required.

Ordering blood products for emergency use is a daily occurrence in most hospitals. In extreme emergencies blood can be issued without a full crossmatch (p278), but this clearly carries greater risk of transfusion reactions. Ensure blood bottle and form are labelled fully and clearly, and indicate the quantity and type of blood product(s) needed as well as where they are needed. Speak to the haematology technician and arrange a porter to collect and deliver the blood products.

How many units to transfuse depends upon the clinical situation and following advice (where appropriate) from a haematologist. In adults it is seldom necessary to transfuse just one unit of packed red cells, even for elective transfusions for chronic anaemia as the risks in this situation would likely outweigh the benefits. Seek senior/specialist advice.

Checking blood products before they are given to a patient requires two people. Ask the patient their name, date of birth and check against the pink form supplied with the blood product. If the patient cannot offer this information check the form against their identification band. Next check the name, DoB, hospital number and blood product number, blood group and expiry date on each bag and the pink form; initial and time against each unit on the pink form once checked.

ABO blood groups

Blood group	Serum antibodies	UK frequency	Comment
O	Anti-A, anti-B	44%	Universal donor
A	Anti-B	45%	
B	Anti-A	8%	
AB	None	3%	Universal recipient

Packed red cells*

Indication	Symptomatic/severe anaemia or severe haemorrhage
Immunology	Needs ABO and rhesus compatibility between donor and recipient
Volume	220–320ml
Donor	Each unit from one donor
Shelf life	35d at 4°C; must be used within 4h once removed from fridge
Cost	~£120 per unit

* Whole blood seldom used and all blood is now leukocyte depleted

Platelets

Indication	Symptomatic thrombocytopenia, platelet dysfunction
Immunology	Rhesus compatibility more important than ABO, but not crucial[1]
Volume	300ml
Donor	Usually pooled from four donors
Shelf life	5d at room temperature – must be kept agitated
Cost	~£200 per unit

Fresh frozen plasma (FFP)

Indication	Replacement of coagulation factor deficiency (if no safe single factor concentrate available), multiple coagulation deficiencies (associated with severe bleeding), disseminated intravascular coagulation (DIC)
Immunology	Rhesus compatibility more important than ABO, but not crucial[1]
Volume	300ml (adult dose 600ml; two units)
Donor	Each unit from one donor
Shelf life	1–2yr at –30°C; must be used within 4h once thawed
Cost	~£30 per unit (~£60 per adult dose)

Cryoprecipitate (cryo)

Indication	Fibrinogen replacement and factors VIII, XIII, von Willibrand's factor
Immunology	Rhesus compatibility more important than ABO, but not crucial[1]
Volume	50ml (adult dose 500ml; 10 units/bags)
Donor	Each (50ml) unit from one donor
Shelf life	1–2yr at –30°C; must be used within 4h once thawed
Cost	~£33 per unit (~£330 per adult dose)

1 ABO compatibility is reversed for non-red cell blood products so AB becomes the universal donor and O the universal recipient. Rhesus status is unaffected, rhesus –ve recipients should receive rhesus –ve blood products if possible.

Red cell transfusion

Indications To correct symptomatic or severe anaemia, to replace blood loss in haemorrhage. Trigger factors for transfusion are illustrated opposite. Generally each unit of packed cells raises the Hb by 1g/dl.
Contraindications *absolute* patient refusal (eg Jehovah's witness) *relative* pernicious anaemia/macrocytic anaemia, CRF/fluid overload
Prescribing Blood should be prescribed on the fluid part of the drug chart. If the patient is hypovolaemic from haemorrhage then each unit of blood should be infused quickly (stat-30min), though for more elective transfusions each unit can be administered at 3–4h. In elective transfusions it may be necessary to give furosemide 20–40mg/stat PO/IV with alternate units (starting with the second unit) to prevent fluid overload in patients with LV dysfunction.
In acute haemorrhage it may be necessary to obtain blood quickly. The table below illustrates options available in this situation:

Options for crossmatching of packed red cells

O negative	Universal donor. Often stored in A+E/theatres/blood bank. Does not first require a specimen from patient.
Type-specific	ABO and rhesus status-specific. Takes ~15min.
Full crossmatch	ABO, rhesus status and antibody-tested. Takes ~45min.

Transfused blood should be given through at least a 18G cannula (green); larger bore cannula in the emergency setting. Blood should not be left unrefrigerated for more than 4h and cannot be returned to blood bank if it has been unrefrigerated for >30min.

Monitoring of the patient should be undertaken regularly in the initial stages of a transfusion, paying special attention to pulse rate, BP, RR and temperature. A small rise in temp and pulse rate are common. See p280 for transfusion reactions.

Example of an elective transfusion

Date	Route	Fluid	Additives	Vol	Rate	Signature
19/08/05	*IV*	*Blood*		*1 unit*	*4h*	*Dr CJFlint*
19/08/05	*IV*	*Blood*	*20mg furosemide PO*	*1 unit*	*4h*	*Dr CJFlint*
20/08/05	*IV*	*Blood*		*1 unit*	*4h*	*Dr CJFlint*
20/08/05	*IV*	*Blood*	*20mg furosemide PO*	*1 unit*	*4h*	*Dr CJFlint*

Example of an emergency transfusion

Date	Route	Fluid	Additives	Vol	Rate	Signature
19/08/05	*IV*	*Blood*		*1 unit*	*stat*	*Dr CJFlint*
19/08/05	*IV*	*Blood*		*1 unit*	*stat*	*Dr CJFlint*
19/08/05	*IV*	*Blood*		*1 unit*	*30min*	*Dr CJFlint*

When to transfuse

While consumption of blood products has remained pretty constant over the last few years, the size of the donor pool has shrunk, making blood and blood products more scarce. Up-to-date information on blood stocks in the UK can be viewed on the National Blood Service website.[1]

Why not transfuse? Besides the fact that blood products are expensive and have limited availability, they carry significant risks (see below).

Transfusion triggers have been used previously to aid doctors in deciding when to transfuse (Hb values of 8–9g/dl are commonly quoted as a transfusion trigger). The problem with these is that many patients are asymptomatic at these values and have sufficient haemoglobin to provide tissue oxygenation. In an otherwise fit and healthy patient (say a young man who has undergone repair of an open femoral fracture), transfusion is often not required for an Hb 8g/dl, though a frail arteriopath may suffer with SOB or anginal symptoms with a Hb of 9g/dl and require a slow transfusion to rectify this.

If in doubt speak to your senior or a haematologist after assessing the patient for signs or symptoms relating to anaemia.

Always ensure the cause for the anaemia is known and that appropriate treatment for this is being undertaken.

Complications of blood and blood product transfusion

Immunological	Non-immunological
Anaphylaxis	Transmission of infection:
Urticaria	• Viruses (HIV, HCV, CMV etc)
Alloimmunisation	• Parasites (malaria etc)
Incompatibility	• Bacteria (staph/strep)
Haemolytic transfusion reactions	• Prion (vCJD)
Non-haemolytic transfusion reactions	Fluid overload/heart failure
Transfusion-associated lung injury	Iron overload (repeated transfusions)
	Hypothermia

Massive blood transfusion

This is defined as replacement of one or more circulating volumes (usually >10units) within a 24h period.

Consider that platelets, clotting factors and fibrinogen will have been lost/diluted and that these should also be transfused, as well as electrolytes and minerals. Speak to a haematologist who will advise appropriately.

Ensure that steps are being taken to prevent further blood loss and that senior members of the team have a transfusion ceiling if appropriate.

Following a blood transfusion

It takes ~6–12h after a transfusion for the concentration of the RBCs to settle; measurement before this time is likely to give a falsely high value.

1 www.blood.co.uk

Transfusion reactions

- These are potentially fatal, so must be managed urgently
- ABO incompatibility is the most serious complication; reactions are seen within minutes of starting the transfusion
- Low-grade pyrexia is common during a transfusion, though a rapid rise in temp at the start is worrying

Signs ↑temp, ↑pulse, ↓BP, cyanosis, dyspnoea, pain, rigors, urticaria, signs of heart failure

Investigations ***blds*** FBC, U+E, blood film, regroup and save (check blood group), antibody screen, blood cultures (if pyrexia persists) ***ECG*** if signs of heart failure or chest pain ***CXR*** if signs of heart failure

Treatment

- As outlined below
- Inform senior/haematologist early
- If reaction serious, retain blood and giving set for later analysis in the laboratory

Acute transfusion reactions (OHCM6 p465)

Features	Management
≥2 of: • Temp >40°C • Chest/abdo pain • ↑Pulse/↓BP • Agitation • Flushing	Likely **acute haemolytic transfusion reaction** (OHCM6 p465) (ABO incompatibility – potentially life-threatening) Stop transfusion. **Call senior help**. 100% O_2, 1l 0.9% saline stat, hydrocortisone 200mg/stat IV, chlorpheniramine 10mg/stat IV. Monitor BP, urine output. Check ECG, U+E (↑K^+), clotting/fibrinogen.
• ↑Ⓣ<40°C • Shivering	Likely **non-haemolytic transfusion reaction** (OHCM6 p465) Slow transfusion. Give paracetamol 1g/6h PO Monitor obs (pulse, BP, temp) **Call senior help** if no improvement or worsening
• ↑Pulse/↓BP • Bronchospasm • Cyanosis • Oedema	Likely **anaphylaxis** (p156, OHCM6 p465) Stop transfusion. **Call senior help.** 100% O_2, 1l 0.9% saline stat, hydrocortisone 200mg/stat IV, chlorpheniramine 10mg/stat IV, epinephrine (adrenaline) 0.5mg (1:1000) IM if profoundly unwell
• Urticaria • ±itch • ±↑temp <40°C	Likely **allergic reaction** (OHCM6 p465) Slow transfusion. **Inform senior.** Monitor obs (pulse, BP, temp). Hydrocortisone 200mg/stat IV, chlorpheniramine 10mg/stat IV.
Fluid overload	Slow transfusion. 100% O_2 and sit upright. Consider furosemide 40mg/stat IV. Catheterise. See p170. **Call senior help** if no improvement or worsening

Pain

Worrying features ↑pulse, ↑↓BP, ↑↓RR, ↓GCS, sweating, vomiting, chest pain

Think about headache p210, chest pain p127, abdominal pain p183, back pain p223, limb pain p293, infection p248 *common* postoperative, musculoskeletal, chronic pain

Ask about site, onset, character, radiation, alleviating factors, timing (duration, frequency), exacerbating factors, severity, associated features (sweating, nausea, vomiting) ***PMH*** stomach problems, asthma, cardiac problems ***DH*** allergies, analgesia already taken and perceived benefit ***SH*** previous drug abuse

Ward round assess the effectiveness of analgesia daily and ask specifically about drowsiness, nausea, vomiting and constipation

Obs ↑pulse and ↑BP suggests pain; RR, pupil size and GCS if on opioids

Look for erythema, swelling, warmth, tenderness, distractability, sweating, bony deformity

Investigations These should be guided by your history and examination; none are specifically required for pain.

Treatment Use the steps of the WHO pain ladder. If a patient has moderate or severe pain start at step 3 or 4. Using paracetamol and NSAIDs reduces the dose of opioids required.

Strong opioids				✓
Weak opioids			✓	
NSAIDs		✓	✓	✓
Paracetamol	✓	✓	✓	✓
	Step 1	**Step 2**	**Step 3**	**Step 4**

Paracetamol ***contraindications*** moderate liver failure ***side-effects*** rare
- **Paracetamol** 1g/4h, max 4g/24h PO/PR/IV

NSAIDs Good for inflammatory pain, renal or biliary colic and bone pain ***contraindications*** (BARS) **B**leeding (pre-op, coagulopathy), **A**sthma, **R**enal disease (hypovolaemia), **S**tomach (peptic ulcer or gastritis). 10% of asthmatics are NSAID sensitive, try a low dose if they have never used them before. Use with caution in the elderly and prescribe with a PPI to protect the stomach ***side-effects*** GI upset, ulceration and bleeding, ↑BP
- ***Ibuprofen*** 400mg/8h, max 1.2g/24h PO, weaker anti-inflammatory action, but less risk of GI ulceration
- ***Diclofenac*** 50mg/8h, max 150mg/24h PO/PR (also IM/IV, see *BNF*)
- ***Naproxen*** 0.5g/12h or 1g/24h, max 1g/24h PO

COX-2 inhibitors These are similar to NSAIDs but with less risk of gastroduodenal ulceration. They have recently been shown to increase the risk of thromboembolic events (eg MI, CVA) and should be used with caution.

Weak opioids Dependence and tolerance to opioids do not occur with short-term use for acute pain. Consider prescribing regular laxatives and anti-emetics, use with ***caution*** if head injury, ↑ICP, respiratory depression, alcohol intoxication ***side-effects*** nausea, vomiting, constipation, drowsiness, hypotension ***toxicity*** ↓RR, ↓GCS, pinpoint pupils

- ***Codeine*** 30–60mg/4h, max 240mg/24h PO/IM, constipating
- ***Dihydrocodeine*** 30mg/4h, max 120mg/24h PO, constipating
- ***Tramadol*** 50–100mg/4h, max 400–600mg/24h PO/IM, stronger than others and less constipating for long-term use

Paracetamol and weak opioids combinations Useful for TTO analgesia; it is better to prescribe the components separately in hospital.

Co-codamol 30mg codeine and 500mg paracetamol

- ***Co-codamol 30/500*** two tablets/6h PO, nurses must give 8/500 dose if 30/500 not specified

Co-dydramol 10mg dihydrocodeine and 500mg paracetamol

- ***Co-dydramol*** two tablets/6h PO

Co-proxamol 32.5mg dextropropoxyphene (synthetic opioid, very toxic in overdose) and 325mg paracetamol and is being withdrawn

Strong opioids Morphine is used for severe pain; diamorphine is reserved for rapid action or palliative care. Use regular fast-acting opioids for acute pain with regular laxatives and PRN or regular anti-emetics. See 'weak opioids' for ***cautions, side effects*** and ***toxicity***. Use only one method of administration (ie PO, SC, IM, IV) to avoid overdose.

- ***Oral*** Sevredol® or Oramorph® 10mg/2–4h
- ***SC/IM*** morphine 10mg/2–4h or diamorphine 5mg/2–4h
- ***IV*** titrate to pain; dilute 10mg into 10ml H_2O for injections, give 2mg initially and wait 2min for response. Give 1mg/2min until pain settled.

Long-acting opioids These are used after major surgery or in chronic pain. Use standard opioids initially until morphine requirements known (p398) then prescribe a regular long-acting dose along with PRN fast-acting opioids to cover breakthrough pain (equivalent to 15% or one-sixth of daily requirements). Laxatives will be needed.

- ***Oral*** MST dose = half total daily oral morphine requirement (p398) given every 12h, usually 10–30mg/12h, max 400mg/24h
- ***Topical*** fentanyl patch lasts 72h, available in 25–100µg/h doses

Other options

Nefopam a non-opioid analgesia that can be given with paracetamol, NSAIDs and opioids ***contraindications*** epilepsy and convulsions ***side-effects*** urinary retention, pink urine, dry mouth, light-headed

- ***Nefopam*** 30–60mg/8h PO or 20mg/6h IM

Hyoscine gives good analgesia in colicky abdo pain ***contraindications*** paralytic ileus, ↑prostate, glaucoma, myasthenia gravis, porphyria ***side-effects*** constipation, dry mouth, confusion, urine retention

- ***Buscopan***® (hyoscine butylbromide) 20mg/6h PO/IM/IV

Diazepam acts as a muscle relaxant, eg spasm with back pain ***contraindications*** respiratory compromise, sleep apnoea ***side-effects*** drowsiness, confusion

- ***Diazepam*** 2mg/8h PO

Quinine used for nocturnal leg cramps ***contraindications*** haemoglobinuria, optic neuritis, arrhythmias ***side-effects*** abdo pain, tinnitus, confusion
- ***Quinine*** 200mg/24h PO – at night

Pain teams Many hospitals have specialists who help manage pain. They are excellent sources of help and can advise on complex patients.

Patient-controlled analgesia ***(PCA)*** A syringe driver that gives a bolus of IV morphine when the patient presses a button. The background infusion rate, bolus dose and maximum bolus frequency can be adjusted to prevent overdose/pain. The patient must be alert, sensible, have IV access and their pain under control before starting. Check hospital protocols.

Epidural These are often inserted by the anaesthetist in theatre prior to a major operation. The anaesthetist or pain team should also look after the epidural and dosing post-op. Complications include local haematoma and/or abscess (causes cord compression, p223) or local infection which requires epidural removal and aggressive treatment with IV antibiotics.

Syringe driver These are used mainly for palliative analgesia, see p399.

Neuropathic and chronic pain

Neuropathic pain is caused by damage to nerves, eg radiculopathy (nerve root pain), peripheral neuropathy, neuralgia and phantom limb pain. The pain tends to be difficult to describe or pinpoint; it is often hot, burning or shooting. Chronic conditions can cause significant pain, eg chronic pancreatitis, arthritis, post-traumatic; there is frequently a psychogenic component. Standard analgesia is often ineffective; try the following:

Tricyclic antidepressants given at a low dose ***contraindications*** recent MI, arrhythmias ***side-effects*** dry mouth, constipation, sedation
- ***Amitiptyline*** 10mg/24h PO – ideally at night

Gabapentin ***contraindications*** previous psychosis ***side-effects*** dizziness, tiredness, cerebellar signs **NB** do not stop suddenly, taper off the dose
- ***Gabapentin*** gradually build up dose by 300mg/day PO, see ***BNF***

Capsaicin a cream made from chillis ***side-effects*** burning sensation
- ***Capsaicin*** small amount every 6h topical

TENS Transcutaneous electrical nerve stimulation is believed to affect the gate mechanism of pain fibres in the spine and/or to stimulate the production of endorphins. Use at a high frequency for acute pain or slow frequency for chronic/neuropathic pain.

Steroids and nerve blocks Injections of steroids combined with local anaesthetic into joints or around nerves can reduce pain for long periods. This needs to be done by a specialist.

Sympathectomy The ablation of sympathetic nerves by surgery or injection; used as a last resort in chronic pelvic or abdominal pain.

Night sedation

Patients develop tolerance and dependence to hypnotics (sedating drugs) if they are prescribed long term. They are licensed for short-term use only and should be avoided if possible.

Causes of insomnia anxiety, stress, depression, mania, alcohol, pain, coughing, nocturia (diuretics, urge incontinence), restless leg syndrome, steroids, aminophylline, SSRIs, benzodiazepine withdrawal, sleep apnoea, poor sleep hygiene

Try to dose regular medications so that stimulants (steroids, SSRIs, aminophylline) are given early in the day, whilst sedatives (tricyclics, antihistamines) are at night. Encourage sleep hygiene (below), ear plugs (foam are best) and eye shades and treat any causes of insomnia.

Sleep hygiene *avoid* caffeine in evening (tea, coffee, chocolate), alcohol, nicotine, daytime naps, cerebral activity before sleep *encourage* exercise, light snack 1–2h before bed, comfortable + quiet location (ear plugs and eye shades), routine

If the patient is still unable to sleep and there is a temporary cause (eg post-op pain, noisy ward) then it is appropriate to prescribe a one-off or short course (≤5 day) of hypnotics. Some patients may be on long-term hypnotics; these are usually continued in hospital. If long-term hypnotics are stopped the dose should be weaned to minimise withdrawal.

Common oral hypnotics

Diazepam	5–10mg/24h	Significant hangover effect, useful for anxious patients
Temazepam	10–20mg/24h	Shorter action than diazepam, less hangover
Zopiclone	3.75–7.5mg/24h	Slightly less dependence and risk of withdrawal than diazepam, less hangover

Contraindications respiratory failure and sleep apnoea

Side-effects include *hangover* (morning drowsiness), *confusion*, *ataxia*, *falls*, *aggression* and a *withdrawal syndrome* similar to alcohol withdrawal if long-term hypnotics are stopped suddenly.

Discharge If a patient is not on hypnotics when they enter hospital they should not be on hypnotics when they leave. GPs get irritated if patients are discharged with supplies of addictive and unnecessary medications.

Violent/aggressive patients See p75 for emergency sedation.

Pre-op sedation Diazepam and temazepam can be used for sedation before a procedure or anaesthetic; this is usually prescribed by the anaesthetist 1–2h before hand. ***Midazolam*** is a rapidly acting IV sedative; it should only be used by experienced doctors under monitored conditions (sats, RR, BP and cardiac monitor) with a crash trolley present. Give 1–2mg boluses then wait 5min for the full response before repeating, >5mg is rarely needed.

Falls and collapse

Worrying features ↑pulse, ↓BP, chest pain, palpitations, head injury, loss of consciousness, recurrent vomiting, incomplete recovery, focal neurology

Think about ***serious*** MI, arrhythmias, shock, sepsis, CVA, seizure, hypoglycaemia, hypoxia, PE ***common*** postural hypotension, mechanical fall (eg tripping), syncope (vasovagal, situational, cardiac)

Ask about symptoms and activity before falling (aura, dizziness, chest pain, palpitations), speed of onset, visual changes, loss of consciousness (can you remember: falling, being on the floor, getting up), incontinence, recovery, head injury, other injuries ***PMH*** previous falls (and investigations), heart problems, diabetes, parkinsonism ***DH*** warfarin, antihypertensives, diuretics, nitrates ***SH*** usual mobility and aids, ability to eat and drink independently, alcohol

Obs temp, pulse, lying and standing BP, BM, GCS

Look for pulse volume, rate and regularity, carotid bruit, volume status (p262), heart murmurs (aortic stenosis), focal neurology, ability to stand, ability to walk, bruising, lacerations or haematomas on the head or body, movement of all limbs, sites of tenderness

Investigations Simple mechanical falls only need investigation for injuries, otherwise ***ECG*** arrhythmia or MI (consider cardiac monitor) ***blds*** FBC, U+E, CRP, cardiac markers (repeat at 12h, CK often raised if there is significant bruising) ***CT*** if focal neurology, persistent ↓GCS or post head injury (p308) ***X-ray*** clinical suspicion of a fracture

	History	Examination	Investigations
Vasovagal syncope	Onset in seconds, precipitated by fear, stress, pain or standing	±postural drop, otherwise normal	Normal
Cardiac syncope	Sudden onset and recovery, chest pain, palpitations, SOB	Fast, slow or irregular pulse	Arrhythmia or MI on ECG, raised cardiac markers
Neurological	Rapid onset, headache, ↓GCS, weakness, altered sensation	Focal neurology, persistent ↓GCS	CVA or intracranial haemorrhage on CT, check glucose
Seizure	±aura, no memory, limb movements, tongue biting, post ictal phase, incontinence	Drowsy, injuries, ±Todd's paralysis	Initial investigations often normal, check glucose

Treatment ABC. Give all patients 100% O_2 and lie flat or with legs up initially. Exclude serious conditions (pulse, ECG, BP, BM) and establish IV access. Treat according to diagnosis.

Please review this patient who has fallen...

If a patient falls whilst in hospital the nurses should fill out an incident form (p98) which requires the patient to have been reviewed by a doctor. You should exclude serious causes of falls (above) and post-fall injuries (particularly head and hip).

Ask the nurse for a **full set of obs** including BM, ±postural BP.

In the **notes** document the circumstances and symptoms, specifically mention chest pain, palpitations, head injury, loss of consciousness, vomiting and confusion.

Examination A brief cardiovascular and neurological examination is essential. Look over the head for signs of injury, feel for midline C-spine tenderness and check for reduced movement or pain in the shoulders, elbows, wrists, hips, knees and ankles.

Investigations Have a low threshold for an ECG. Consider X-raying painful joints (swelling, ↓range of movement, bony tenderness). Do not order skull X-rays, see p309 for the indications for a CT brain. Other investigations as indicated.

Review Ask the nurses to record regular neuro obs (pupils and GCS) and bleep you again if concerned.

Seizures	p215	Hypoglycaemia	p231
Focal neurology	p218	Pyrexia	p248
↓GCS + confusion	p228	Chest pain	p127
Head injuries	p308	Tachyarrhythmias	p135
Postural drop	p157	Bradyarrhythmias	p143
Joint examination	p440	Hypoxia	p165

Vasovagal syncope (faint)

Syncope is a transient loss of consciousness with complete recovery.
Symptoms brought on by stress, pain or fear, usually whilst standing, onset over seconds, feeling faint, nausea, blurred vision, spontaneous and full recovery within minutes, clammy, cold
Signs may have a postural drop (p157), pale, flushing, sweating, eyes rolling, twitching whilst unconscious, rapid recovery, otherwise well
Investigations normal ECG, consider a tilt table test if recurrent
Treatment 100% O_2 (until serious diagnoses excluded), lay flat with legs elevated, remove stimulus (eg needle, blood), gradually sit up once symptoms have passed

Situational syncope

Similar symptoms and signs to vasovagal syncope, but brought on by a specific action:

- ***micturation*** – middle-aged men; advise to sit down to urinate
- ***carotid sensitivity*** – can be brought on by shaving
- ***cough*** – brought on by coughing fits.

Causes of recurrent falls old age, confusion/dementia, inappropriate use of aids (sticks, frames), poor sight, peripheral neuropathy, Parkinson's, cerebellar disease, multiple sclerosis, alcoholism, foot drop, vertigo, incontinence/diuretics, arthritis

Clotting abnormality emergencies

Airway	Check airway is patent; consider manoeuvres/adjuncts
Breathing	If no respiratory effort – **CALL ARREST TEAM**
Circulation	If no palpable pulse – **CALL ARREST TEAM**

High INR (OHAM2 p694)

Most likely caused by over-anticoagulation with warfarin.

Patient not bleeding	Patient bleeding
INR 5–8 • Withhold warfarin until <5 • Identify cause of ↑INR **INR 8–12** • Withhold warfarin until <5 • Vitamin K 2mg/24h PO/IV • Admit for daily INR • Identify cause of ↑INR **INR >12** • Withhold warfarin until <5 • Vitamin K 5mg/24h PO/IV • Admit for daily INR • Identify cause of ↑INR	**Medical emergency** • Seek senior help • Give FFP 2–4 units IV stat • Vitamin K 5mg IV stat • Discuss with haematologist • Consider factors II, VII, IX or X • Withhold warfarin until INR <5 • Identify cause of ↑INR

Disseminated intravascular coagulation (OHAM2 p702)

Mechanism Clotting cascade triggered pathologically resulting in consumption of fibrinogen, platelets and clotting factors. Microthrombi form in small vessels; results in end-organ damage and RBCs lysed in the fibrin meshwork. Results in ↑bleeding tendency.

Signs bruising, bleeding, signs of triggering pathology (see below)

Investigations ↓platelets, ↑PT/INR, ↑APTT(r), ↓fibrinogen, ↑↑D-dimer

General treatment Request urgent senior help and discuss with haematologist. Treat underlying cause (most commonly sepsis), supportive measures for BP, acidosis, hypoxaemia and maintain normothermia. Blood transfusion to compensate for anaemia (may exacerbate coagulopathy).

Correction of coagulopathy Give FFP (15ml/kg, ie 4–5 units) if PT or APTT >1.5 x control (ie INR or APTTr >1.5). Platelets and cryoprecipitate (rich in fibrinogen) may be recommended by haematologist.

Complications massive haemorrhage, end-organ failure, death (severe DIC carries significant mortality)

Common precipitants of DIC

- Septicaemia (Gram –ve > Gram +ve)
- Disseminated malignancy
- Incompatible blood transfusion reactions
- Hypoxia
- Liver failure
- Severe trauma/burns

Anticoagulation

Anticoagulant drugs are used to prevent primary thrombotic events or to prevent clot propagation after a thrombotic event has occurred. The two main types of anticoagulants used are:

- **heparin** (low molecular weight or unfractionated) – used acutely or in the short term
- **warfarin** – used for long-term prophylaxis/treatment.

Indications and contraindications for anticoagulants

	Indications	Contraindications
Heparin	Venous thromboembolism (treatment and prophylaxis), PE, MI, ACS, unstable angina, acute peripheral arterial occlusion, haemodialysis, pre/post-op	Haemorrhage, haemophilia, active gastroduodenal ulcer, thrombocytopaenia, allergy, recent major trauma/haemorrhagic CVA
Warfarin	Venous thromboembolism, PE, prosthetic heart valves, AF (with a risk of embolism)	Recent haemorrhagic CVA, severely ↑BP, pregnancy, active gastroduodenal ulcer, cerebral artery thrombosis, endocarditis, liver failure, risk of falls or non-compliance

Thromboprophylaxis in *medical* patients

Consider if age >40yr, obese, known malignancy, prolonged immobility, oedema, inflammatory bowel disease, pregnant, on COC/HRT, recent surgery or trauma (within 2wk), long distance travel (within 1wk).

- Treat with LMWH, eg:
  - Enoxaparin® 20mg/24h SC for 6–14d or until mobile
  - Enoxaparin® 40mg/24h SC if **high risk,**[1] 6–14d or until mobile
- TED stockings (above knee)

If the patient has thromboembolic event whilst on anticoagulation:

- Contact haematologist
- Check clotting
- Check compliance with medication; review other medications

Thromboprophylaxis in pre-operative *surgical* patients

Generally, all surgical patients are given thromboprophylaxis unless they are day cases or actively bleeding. Those who are on long-term warfarin should stop taking this at least 3d pre-operatively. The INR should be <1.5 for most operations and lower if spinal or epidural anaesthetic techniques are to be employed; warn the anaesthetist. Patients who have prosthetic heart values will need IV heparin whilst warfarin is omitted (p290). See p291 for restarting warfarin post-operatively.

1 Previous DVT/PE, obesity, thrombophilia (OHCM6 p672).

Starting heparin (OHCM6 p648)

LMWH

DVT/PE prophylaxis or therapeutic for ACS/MI or DVT/PE.

- ***Prophylaxis*** eg Enoxaparin® 20–40mg/24h SC
- ***Therapeutic for ACS/MI*** eg Enoxaparin® 1mg/kg/12h SC
- ***Therapeutic for DVT/PE*** eg Enoxaparin® 1.5mg/kg/24h SC

Monitor platelets if long term (risk of heparin-induced thrombocytopenia).

Unfractionated heparin

Anticoagulation for prosthetic heart valves or in acute limb ischaemia.

- Check baseline clotting (INR and APTTr).
  - if APTTr <1.3 and patient weighs 50–100kg and <80yr give a bolus dose of heparin 5000iu IV. Start an infusion at 30,000iu/24h IV
  - if APTTr <1.3 and patient weighs <50kg or >100kg give a bolus of 80iu/kg and infuse at 25iu/kg/h IV
  - if APTTr <1.3 and patient aged >80 give an initial bolus dose of 2500iu/stat IV and infuse at 20,000iu/24h IV; if weight <50kg or >100kg d/w haematologist
  - if APTTr >1.3 omit bolus dose and commence infusion as above
- Check the APTT ratio 6h after starting treatment and then every 12–24h Adjust the dose according to the APTTr (see table below), rechecking the APTTr 6h after each dose change
- For heparin use in obstetric or paediatric patients discuss with the consultant obstetrician and haematologist
- If planning to discharge patient on anticoagulant therapy, start warfarin (see opposite) whilst still on heparin and monitor using the INR. Discontinue the heparin once the INR is therapeutic

Dose changes to unfractionated IV heparin

APTTr	Next dose	Retest time
<1.3	Bolus dose of 5000iu; ↑infusion by 5000iu/24h	6h
1.3–1.4	↑infusion by 5000iu/24h	6h
1.5–2.4	No change	12–24h
2.5–3.0	Stop infusion for 30min; ↓infusion by 5000iu/24h	6h
>3.0	Stop infusion for 60min; ↓infusion by 5000iu/24h	6h

Over-anticoagulation with unfractionated heparin

The elimination half-life of unfractionated heparin is 0.5–2.5h (longer in hypothermia), so stopping an infusion rapidly normalises the APTTr.

Reversal of anticoagulant effect can be achieved with protamine. Protamine 1mg/over 10min IV neutralises ~100iu unfractionated heparin within 15min. Maximum dose of 50mg; higher doses have anticoagulant effects.

Starting warfarin (OHCM6 p648)

Day 1 – give warfarin 9 or 10mg/PO at 1800h
Day 2 – measure INR at 0900h
- If INR <1.8 give warfarin 9 or 10mg/PO at 1800h
- If INR >1.8 give warfarin 5 or 6mg/PO at 1800h

Day 3 – measure INR at 0900h; use table below to guide further dosing

Warfarin dosing – can be written up for three days unless INR high or poor control

INR	<2.0	2.0–2.4	2.5–2.8	2.9–3.2	3.3–3.5	3.6–4.0	≥4.1
Day 3 dose	10mg	5mg	4mg	3mg	2mg	0.5mg	Omit[2]
Further doses[1]	≥6	5.5mg	4.5mg	4mg	3.5mg	3mg	Omit[2]

1 Day 4 dose and likely maintenance dose.
2 Omit this dose, give 1mg the next day at 1800h and recheck INR the following day.

Check INR daily for 5d, then alternate days until stable, then weekly if in-patient or hand care over to anticoagulation clinic or GP.

Target INR and duration of therapy for warfarinisation

Indication	Duration of therapy	Target INR range
DVT/PE prophylaxis	Whilst at high risk only	2–3
Treatment of DVT/PE	6mth (life if recurrent)	2–3
AF	Until in sinus rhythm	2–3
Prosthetic heart valve	Lifelong	3–4

Restarting warfarin post-operatively

Confirm with seniors that warfarin therapy is to be recommenced. Load with warfarin as described above.

Discharging patients on warfarin

- Explain to patient why compliance is crucial and need for INR checks
- Ensure suitable follow-up with either anticoagulation clinic or GP
  - speak to these directly and arrange patient's first appointment
- Issue yellow warfarin book
  - prescribe enough warfarin to last until next INR check
- Tablet colours – brown (1mg), blue (3mg), pink (5mg)

Drugs interacting with warfarin

Drugs which ↑INR	Alcohol, amiodarone, cimetidine, simvastatin, NSAIDs
Drugs which ↓INR	Carbamazepine, phenytoin, rifampacin, oestrogens

Over-anticoagulation with warfarin see p288

Acutely painful limb emergency

Airway	Check airway is patent; consider manoeuvres/adjuncts
Breathing	If no respiratory effort – **CALL ARREST TEAM**
Circulation	If no palpable pulse – **CALL ARREST TEAM**

Call for **senior help** early if patient deteriorating

- **Sit patient up**
- **High-flow oxygen** in *all* patients
- **Monitor** pulse oximeter, BP, defibrillator's ECG leads if unwell
- Obtain a full set of **observations**
- Take brief **history** if possible/check **notes**/ask ward staff
- **Examine patient**: condensed RS, CVS and abdo exam
- **Examine all limbs**: condensed vascular, neuro and joint exams
- Consider **serious causes** (below) and treat if present
- **Venous access**, take bloods:
  - FBC, ESR, U+E, CRP, ±cardiac markers, D-dimer, clotting, G+S
- **Ankle-brachial pressure index** if available
- **ECG** to exclude acute MI and pre-op
- **ABG** if systemically unwell
- Call for **senior help**
- **Reassess**, starting with A, B, C...

Life and limb-threatening causes

- Acute ischaemia
- Compartment syndrome
- Myocardial infarction (arm)
- Spinal cord compression
- Septic arthritis
- Necrotising fasciitis
- Gangrene

Limb pain

Worrying symptoms sudden onset, reduced sensation, pulselessness, cold, shock, pyrexia, recent surgery, concurrent chest pain

Think about ***serious*** acute ischaemia, septic arthritis, compartment syndrome, gangrene, necrotising fasciitis ***most likely*** muscular, joint or bone pain, DVT, cellulitis, thrombophlebitis, sciatica ***other*** osteomyelitis, Baker's cyst, vasculitidies, myositis, peripheral neuropathy ***chronic*** arthritis (osteo-, rheumatoid, gout), peripheral vascular disease, varicose veins, spinal stenosis, ulcers

Ask about location, trauma, speed of onset, change on moving and raising, recent surgery, back pain, chest pain, SOB, feeling unwell ***PMH*** previous limb pain, diabetes, MI, CVA, DVT, PE ***DH*** warfarin, heparin ***SH*** exercise tolerance

Obs temp, BP, pulse, sats, RR

Look for hot/cold, colour, mottling, skin trauma, swelling (distal, joint, calf), pulses (compare both sides), cap refill, power, sensation, reflexes, range of movement (active and passive), muscle, joint or bone tenderness, see p440 for specific joint examinations; resp exam if SOB

Investigations Most limb pain can be diagnosed from clinical examination; consider the following investigations ***blds*** FBC, U+E, ESR, CRP, D-dimer, blood cultures ***ankle-brachial pressure index (ABPI)*** for ischaemia ***ECG*** for AF ***X-rays*** for joint disease or bone fractures ***ABG*** if suspicion of PE

Treatment

Give everyone adequate analgesia, p282

- ***Acute ischaemia*** 100% O_2 , analgesia, heparin, (vascular) surgeons
- ***Compartment syndrome*** 100% O_2, remove plaster, orthopaedics
- ***Septic arthritis*** 100% O_2, joint aspiration, IV antibiotics, orthopaedics
- ***Necrotising fasciitis*** 100% O_2, fluids, IV antibiotics, surgeons
- ***Gangrene*** 100% O_2 , fluids, IV antibiotics, surgeons

	History	Examination	Investigations
Acute ischaemia	Rapid onset, distal>proximal, worse with legs raised	Pulseless, ↑cap refill, pale, cold, weak, reduced sensation	↓or absent Doppler pulse, obstruction on angiography
Infections	Gradual onset, feels unwell, history of trauma or bite	Pyrexia, red, tender, warm, swollen	↑WCC, ↑CRP, ↑ESR, D-dimer often ↑
DVT	Gradual onset, improved with legs raised	Red, swollen, hot, tender leg	↑D-dimer
Joint	Trauma, pain on movement, unable to bear load	Tender over joint, joint effusion, pain: active = passive	Arthritic changes on X-ray, abnormal synovial fluid
Muscle	Trauma, pain on movement	Tender, ±swelling on muscle/tendon insertion, pain: active>passive	Normal X-rays, may have a raised CK
Bone	Trauma, pain on movement and at rest	Bony tenderness with swelling and reduced range of movement	Abnormal X-ray

Acute limb ischaemia (OHCM6 p490)

This is an ***emergency***, ischaemia is irreversible after 6h.
Causes emboli, thrombosis, dissecting aneurysm, trauma
Symptoms unilateral painful, tingling, weak limb, worse on raising limb
Signs absent pulses, slow cap refill compared with opposite limb, cold and pale (can be red if limb below heart), reduced power and sensation
Worrying signs ↓sensation, purple mottling, non-blanching mottling
Risk factors AF, prosthetic heart valves, recent MI, arterial graft, peripheral vascular disease, previous thrombo-emboli, dehydration, malignancy
Investigations FBC, U+E, G+S, clotting, ±thrombophilia screen (if <40yr), ECG, Doppler
Treatment ABC, 100% O_2 and analgesia (morphine). IV access with IV fluids if dehydrated and call a senior surgeon since this needs urgent surgery (embolectomy, intra-arterial thrombolysis, bypass or amputation). May require heparinisation (p290) pre or post-op
Complications amputation, gangrene, hyperkalaemia, renal failure, sepsis

Dry gangrene (OHCM6 p486)

Ischaemic muscle necrosis without infection.
Signs well-defined, painless, shrivelled brown/black area
Treatment requires debridement or amputation to prevent infection, may autoamputate if not treated
Complications wet gangrene

Gas (wet) gangrene (OHCM6 p486)

This is an *emergency*, *Clostridium* infection causing necrosis and sepsis.
Symptoms unwell with painful extremities or wound
Signs pyrexia, shock, tender brown/black area with blistering and oedema, muscle necrosis, crepitus (from gas in tissue)
Risk factors ischaemia, diabetes, malignancy, surgery/trauma
Investigations FBC, U+E, LFT, CRP, CK, blood cultures, clotting, ABG (acidosis). Gram stain of pus or necrotic tissue. X-ray may show gas (dark patches in soft tissues).
Treatment ABC including 100% O_2 and fluids. Benzylpenicillin 2.4g/4h IV, clindamycin 600mg/6h IV, metronidazole 500mg/6–8h IV and surgical debridement. Consider hyperbaric O_2.
Complications amputation, sepsis, death

Necrotising fasciitis (OHCM6 p486)

This is an *emergency*, requires immediate surgery and antibiotics.
Symptoms unwell, painful red area, usually following trauma or surgery
Signs rapidly progressing tender erythema and necrosis with pyrexia
Investigations FBC, U+E, CRP and blood cultures, X-ray may show gas
Treatment ABC, 100% O_2 and fluids. Suspect in rapidly advancing cellulitis, requires IV clindamycin 600mg/6h, ciprofloxacin 400mg/12h and benzylpenicillin 2.4g/4h accompanied by urgent surgical debridement
Complications amputation, sepsis, death

Cellulitis

Infection of the skin, usually *staph* or *strep*.
Symptoms painful red limb or area of limb, feels unwell, may have a bite, local trauma, spot or cracked skin
Signs skin is warm, red, tender and swollen, may have blistering, look for tracking (red streaks radiating from the cellulitis – also called lymphangitis), local lymphadenopathy and systemic illness (pyrexia, tachycardia)
Investigations FBC, U+E, CRP and blood cultures, swab if pus present
Treatment Small areas in well patients can be treated with amoxicillin 500mg/8h PO. Any signs of tracking, systemic illness or underlying illness require flucloxacillin 1g/6h IV + benzylpenicillin 1.2g/6h IV with elevation. Use a marker pen to draw around the redness to monitor progress.
Complications abscesses, sepsis, necrotising fasciitis, ulcers

Superficial thrombophlebitis

Inflammation and thrombosis of a vein which can progress to DVT.
Symptoms gradual onset of tenderness over a vein
Signs red, tender area with hard palpable vein/varicosity
Risk factors IV cannulas, varicose veins, IVDU and DVT risk factors
Investigations No specific investigations but have a low threshold for blood and Doppler scans to exclude DVT which is common.
Treatment Resite/remove IV cannula, elevation, exercise, compression and NSAIDs eg ibuprofen, if suspicious of DVT start LMW heparin.
Complications deep vein thrombosis, pulmonary embolus
If thrombophlebitis recurs or affects other sites (migratory) suspect malignancy or vasculitis.

Deep vein thrombosis (OHCM6 p456)

Symptoms unilateral pain, worse when lowered, improved with elevation
Signs warm, red, tender, swollen limb (tape measure), pitting oedema
Risk factors age, obesity, recent surgery/immobility/travel, oestrogen (pregnancy, HRT, the pill), previous PE/DVT, malignancy, recent stroke or MI, thrombophilia
Investigations FBC, U+E, D-dimer, ECG, consider ABG. A negative D-dimer excludes DVT in 95% if there is low clinical risk, however a positive D-dimer is present with many conditions. Doppler USS of limb.
Treatment Treat PE if present (p169). Otherwise elevate affected limb, analgesia and LMW heparin, eg Enoxaparin® 1.5mg/kg/24h SC. Start warfarin at the same time (p291) for 3–6mth.
Complications pulmonary embolus

Baker's cyst

A swelling behind the knee common in osteoarthritis that can rupture to mimic DVT symptoms – can be distinguished by USS.

Compartment syndrome

This is an ***emergency***, measure compartment pressure if suspected.
Symptoms excessive pain following an injury or fracture, distal tingling, numbness or weakness
Signs pain at rest, worse on passive stretching of a muscle, reduced sensation (loss of two point discrimination), redness, swelling, slow cap refill; absent pulse and pallor are late signs
Risk factors long bone fractures and plaster casts, significant injury, crush injury, vascular injury, warfarin or heparin, burns
Investigations measure compartment pressure by inserting a manometer through the skin (eg Wick catheter), >30mmHg requires urgent treatment, check FBC, U+E, CK, clotting and urine dipstick
Treatment ABC, 100% O_2 and lie the patient flat. Give adequate analgesia; IV fluids if dehydrated and monitor urine output. Remove plaster cast if present and discuss with orthopaedics regarding urgent fasciotomy.
Complications hyperkalaemia, neurological damage, amputation

Osteomyelitis (OHCS6 p644)

Symptoms feels unwell, bone pain
Signs painful, tender, warm and erythematous with pyrexia
Risk factors diabetes, immunocompromise, open fractures, prostheses
Investigations FBC (↑WCC), U+E, ↑ESR, ↑CRP, blood cultures, X-ray
Treatment flucloxacillin 1g/6h IV for about 6wk with surgical drainage of abscess or prostheses if present
Complications septic arthritis, fracture

Initial investigations of monoarthritis (causes, p416)

FBC, ESR, U+E, CRP, rheumatoid factor and ANA (other autoantibodies, p418), urate, X-ray, joint aspiration, urine dipstick – exclude septic arthritis

Septic arthritis (OHCS6 p667)
Symptoms single painful and stiff joint, feels unwell
Signs pyrexia, warm and red joint with effusion, painful on passive and active movement, tender over joint
Risk factors arthritis, prosthesis, trauma, diabetes, septic source
Investigations FBC (↑WCC), U+E, ↑ESR, ↑CRP, blood cultures; joint aspiration shows white cells and bacteria; X-ray affected joint
Treatment Analgesia and refer to orthopaedics for joint aspiration; empirically treat with flucloxacillin 1g/6h IV and benzylpenicillin 1.2g/4h IV, consider gentamicin (discuss with microbiology). Splinting initially followed by physio. Requires at least 2wk IV antibiotics, may need lavage and removal of joint prosthesis.
Complications joint destruction, sepsis

Muscle pain (OHCS6 p663)
Causes trauma, strains, fibromyalgia, infection, rhabdomyolysis, drugs (statins, ACE inhibitors, steroids), inflammation (polymyalgia rheumatica, polymyositis, dermatomyositis, SLE), metabolic ↓Ca^{2+}, ↓K^{+}, ↓Na^{+}, alkalosis), endocrine (↓↑thyroid, Cushing's)
Investigations Often none; FBC, U+E, Ca^{2+}, CK, ESR, CRP, X-ray
Treatment Simple analgesia including NSAIDs, rest for first 24h then gradually exercise the joint, ice packs, compression (eg tubigrip) and elevation. Consider physiotherapy referral if persists.

Joint pain p304 Sciatica/radiculopathy p219

Other limb problems

Causes of swollen limbs

Bilateral	Venous insufficiency, heart failure, renal failure, nephrotic syndrome, cirrhosis, malnutrition, protein losing enteropathy, pre-eclampsia, myxoedema
Unilateral	DVT, cellulitis, Baker's cyst, trauma, compartment syndrome, lymphatic obstruction, thrombophlebitis, ischaemia
Non-pitting	Lymphoedema: congenital, lymph node excision, post-radiotherapy, malignancy, infection, filariasis

Causes of red limbs

• Venous eczema (venous insufficiency) • DVT • burns • cellulitis • ringworm • psoriasis • eczema • vasculitis • porphyria • erythema nodosum (Strep, fungi, TB, sarcoid, ulcerative colitis, OCP, antibiotics with sulphur) • pretibial myxoedema (hyperthyroid) • necrobiosis lipoidica (Type 1 DM) • skin cancer

Chronic limb pain

Peripheral vascular disease (PVD) (OHCM6 p490)
Chronic limb ischaemia causes intermittent claudication/critical ischaemia.
Intermittent claudication cramp in calf, thigh or buttock on walking a fixed distance, worse uphill, relieved by stopping or rest
Critical ischaemia pain in limb extremity at night, relieved by hanging legs out of bed, ulcers, dry gangrene
Signs *early* cool, hairless, pulseless limbs *late* pain and pallor on elevation
Investigations FBC, U+E, lipids, ESR, ECG, ankle brachial pressure index (<0.9 suggests disease, <0.6 is severe), arteriography
Treatment exercise, stop smoking, treat diabetes, BP and cholesterol, aspirin 75mg/24h PO, may need angioplasty, stent or bypass graft. Avoid β-blockers, GTN rarely helps.
Complications acute ischaemia, gangrene, rest pain, ulcers

Venous insufficiency
Symptoms bursting/throbbing leg pain, relieved by elevating legs, worse on standing, previous DVT or thrombophlebitis
Signs pain improved by lifting legs, red/dark red discolouration, swelling, varicose veins
Investigations Duplex ultrasound, D-dimer if DVT suspected
Treatment compression bandages (if ABPI >0.8), varicose vein surgery
Complications varicose veins, thrombophlebitis, ulcers, cellulitis

Lumbar spinal stenosis (spinal claudication) (OHCS6 p622)
Symptoms cramp in thigh or leg on walking, worse on walking downhill or standing, associated back pain
Signs pain on straight leg raise/back extension, often no neuro symptoms
Investigations lumbar spine X-ray and MRI spine
Treatment exercise, NSAIDs, steroid injections, spinal decompression
Complications cord compression, cauda equina syndrome (p223)

Nerve entrapment syndromes (OHCS6 p662)

Syndrome	Symptom
Carpal tunnel syndrome (Median)	Aching of wrist and forearm, tingling of thumb, index, middle, ±ring finger
Ulnar entrapment (wrist or elbow)	Tingling of ring and little fingers, ±forearm
Radial tunnel syndrome or posterior interosseous syndrome	Weak extension of fingers and thumb
Meralgia paresthetica	Tingling lateral thigh
Common peroneal compression	Weak dorsiflexion of foot

Other causes and relevant pages

Arthritis	p416	Sciatica/radiculopathy	p223
Peripheral neuropathy	p219	Analgesia in chronic pain	p284

Limb ulcers

Causes venous insufficiency, peripheral vascular disease, neuropathic (eg diabetes), pressure ulcers, trauma, infection, pyoderma gangrenosum (eg rheumatoid arthritis), vasculitidies, skin cancer, steroids
Ask about onset, duration, pain, trauma, claudication ***PMH*** peripheral vascular disease, hypertension, CVA, MI, angina, varicose veins, DVT, diabetes ***DH*** steroids ***SH*** smoking, alcohol
Look for number, site, size, base, edge, depth, sensation, shape, colour, discharge, lymphadenopathy, oedema, eczema, peripheral pulses
Investigations ankle brachial pressure index (ABPI), FBC, ESR and fasting glucose; consider duplex USS, wound swab, CRP, complement, RF, ANA, ANCA, serology, X-ray (if ulcer overlies bone), biopsy and histology

	Venous	**Arterial**	**Neuropathic**
History	Varicose veins, DVT	Intermittent claudication, MI, angina	Numbness, diabetes, family history
Leg	Pigmented, varicose veins, swollen, hot	Shiny, hairless, cold	Joint destruction
Site	Medial aspect of legs	Toes, bony prominences and pressure points	Heel, metatarsal head, lateral malleolus
Size	Can be very large	Usually small	Usually small
Base	Usually superficially with sloughy exudate	Deep with a dark, dry base, few signs of healing	Can be very deep and extend to bone
Edge	Irregular, areas of repeated healing and exacerbation	Well defined, often circular	Surrounded by thickened skin
Sensation	Painful	Painful	Relatively painless

Treatment Ensure good nutrition and treat the cause, 80% of leg ulcers are due to venous insufficiency. Healing often takes weeks to month and is commonly managed by community nurses:

- ***Venous*** So long as the ABPI is >0.8 compression bandaging should be used (eg 4 layer 'Charing Cross') with absorbable dressings to dry out the slough. Emollients and steroid creams also help; may need surgery
- ***Arterial*** As for peripheral vascular disease with referral to a vascular surgeon. Do not use compression bandages
- ***Neuropathic*** Avoid repeated injury, often needs surgical debridement and antibiotics, osteomyelitis is common
- ***Infection*** Ulcers usually have bacteria present; infection or cellulitis should be suspected if there is pus, excessive pain, surrounding erythema or pyrexia. Swab the ulcer and treat as for cellulitis (p295)

No improvement Consider other diagnoses (including TB and cancer) or dermatitis from therapeutic agents. Swab the ulcer and consider biopsy. Discuss with dermatology, may need curettage or skin grafting.

Chapter 8

Specialities

Accident and emergency

Starting in A+E can be a daunting experience due to the wide variety of presentations (eg sick children, foreign bodies in eyes) and severity of illness (paper cuts to cardiac arrests). Like any speciality you should ask a senior if you are at all unsure; remember that in your PRHO year you cannot discharge any patients from A+E without a senior review.

This chapter covers a few common A+E presentations; see the *Oxford Handbook of Accident and Emergency Medicine 2E* for more detail.

Main areas in an A+E department

- ***Triage*** ('sorting' in French) This is where experienced nurses take a full set of obs and assess how urgently patients need to be seen; relevant investigations may also be ordered (eg X-rays, bloods). Patients are often scored on a 1–5 scale with 1 being an emergency (eg cardiac arrest) and 5 being inappropriate attendance
- ***'See and treat'*** This is when a senior doctor (usually middle grade or consultant) sees uncomplicated patients before triage. Many can be treated and discharged at once
- ***Minors or ambulatory*** This is where minor injuries and the 'walking wounded' go, it often includes minor head injuries, cuts, fractures and sprains. This area can be especially scary when you start since it is so different from the conditions seen in other departments. The term 'minor' can be a misnomer since the injuries can be significant (eg multiple rib fractures with pneumothorax) or the patient may have been 'triaged' to the wrong area
- ***Majors or trolleys*** The medically unwell, seriously injured and those unable to walk tend to be seen in majors. These patients often require investigations and about 25% are admitted under specialist teams
- ***Resuscitation*** The sickest patients who need intense monitoring and nursing are brought into 'resus'. Includes all acute resuscitations and ambulance patients that have been phoned ahead (blue-calls)
- ***Paediatrics*** Most departments have a separate children's area with paediatric medical equipment and a separate toy-filled waiting room

Staff Many A+E nurses are able to do practical procedures including cannulas and taking bloods. Highly qualified nurses may be trained as Emergency Nurse Practitioners (ENPs) who see and treat patients with specific conditions (according to their training). They are often excellent at practical procedures (including suturing), very experienced and a good source of advice.

Four-hour target A+E departments are expected to discharge or admit 98% of patients within four hours of their arrival. While it is important not to let this target compromise your care, try to be efficient to avoid delays. Refer patients early if they clearly need admission regardless of investigation results and keep other staff informed of your management plan so that beds or transport can be arranged easily.

Minors

Clerking in minors should be brief and focused; concentrate on the presenting problem and the mechanism of injury. Always ask about:
- past medical history (if asthma are they NSAID sensitive?)
- drug history and allergies
- tetanus status if they have a cut
- occupation and L/R handed if arm/hand involved

If you find unrelated important findings (eg new orthopnoea) decide whether these need to be managed today in A+E or by referral back to the patient's GP. Try to avoid giving a second opinion on chronic problems.

Sprains and strains

A sprain is minor damage to a ligament while a strain is caused by minor damage to a muscle. Both are managed the same way (RICE):
- ***Rest*** initially, but weight bear or exercise as soon as symptoms allow
- ***Ice*** to reduce swelling over the first 48h; keep the ice away from the skin (eg use a tea towel) and apply for 10–15min at a time
- ***Compression*** with elasticised bandages though this makes little difference. Must be removed prior to going to bed
- ***Elevation*** reduces both swelling and pain

Prescribe adequate analgesia and give reassurance. Warn the patient that the symptoms may be worse the next morning and may take a few weeks to resolve completely. There should not be any long-term consequences, but they may need referral for physio.

Fractures

Fractures are treated in three ways:
- ***Analgesia only*** Fractures of single ribs or the coccyx are treated conservatively with analgesia. They do not need X-raying unless a complication is suspected (eg pneumothorax)
- ***Backslab/sling***, analgesia and fracture clinic follow-up for the majority of fractures that do not need an urgent orthopaedic review
- ***Orthopaedic referral*** if unstable, compound (open) or neurovascular involvement

Describing fractures

Side	Right or left, dominant or not
Bone	Clavicle, radius, tibia etc
Location	Proximal, midshaft, distal
Type	Simple (2 bits), comminuted (≥3 bits), oblique, spiral
Shape	Displaced, angulated, impacted, rotated
Joint surface	Intra-articular fracture or not, dislocation
Complications	Compound (open fracture, p312), neurovascular involvement

Specific joint problems (OHAEM2 p386)

As with any injury a good history and examination should dictate which investigations are ordered. Deciding which injuries require X-rays takes experience; suspect a fracture in the presence of bony tenderness, swelling and reduced range of movement (ROM) after trauma.

Hands Examination p446, common injuries include:

- ***Crushed fingertip*** (subungual haematoma) X-ray to identify a tuft fracture of the distal phalanx. If the haematoma covers <50% of the nail the pain can be improved by trephining the nail (rotate a green needle on the nail to 'drill' through). If >50% the nail should be removed for a nail bed repair (ask a senior, use absorbable sutures) Prescribe antibiotics after either procedure if a tuft fracture is present
- ***Dislocated finger*** The proximal interphalangeal joint often dislocates. X-ray and relocate with a digital nerve block or Entonox® by pulling the distal finger dorsally then straight. Repeat X-ray and neighbour strap
- ***Punch injury*** Often fractures the 4th or 5th metacarpal; check for rotational deformity by looking at the line of the nails (viewed end-on) both with the fingers fully extended and flexed to 90°. Analgesia, X-ray, volar slab and hand or fracture clinic follow-up. 'Bite' injuries in a fight (ie punching teeth) are often missed and can cause a septic joint

Wrist Examination p444, often injured by a fall on an outstretched hand (FOOSH). Common injuries include:

- ***Colles' fracture*** Distal radial, ±ulna fracture with dinner fork deformity and distal segment displaced dorsally. Manipulate under a Bier's block or haematoma block (ask a senior) and follow up in fracture clinic
- ***Smith's fracture*** Similar to a Colles fracture but with the distal segment displaced towards the palmar surface. Refer to orthopaedics
- ***Scaphoid fractures*** Suggested by tenderness over the anatomical snuff-box, palmar or dorsal aspect of scaphoid and pain on loading the thumb or stressing scaphoid by flexing and ulnar deviating the wrist. The fracture may show up on scaphoid views (scaphoid POP and hand/fracture clinic); if not give the patient a splint and reassess in 10–14 days

Forearm and elbow Examination p444, common injuries include:

- ***Radial head fractures*** May present with only reduced range of movement and pain at the extremes of supination and pronation. Look for raised anterior and posterior fat pads on X-ray
- ***Pulled elbow*** Suspect in children aged 1–4yr who are reluctant to use an arm after having their arm pulled with the elbow extended (eg swinging between parents or being pulled to stand up). Explain to the parents what you suspect has happened and what needs to be done. Flex the child's elbow to 90° with their hand supinated (palm up), hold their elbow and push down on radial head with your thumb whilst you pronate the wrist. You may feel a pop and the child will cry. If the symptoms do not resolve X-ray (depends on history) and apply a collar and cuff; discharge with analgesia and review in 24h if symptoms persist

Shoulder Examination p443, common injuries include:
- ***Clavicle fracture*** Tenderness over the clavicle, may feel crepitus or deformity. Listen to the chest to exclude pneumothorax. X-ray, broad arm sling and fracture clinic follow-up or refer to orthopaedics if the fracture fragment is causing skin tenting (?necrosis) or is compound
- ***Head of humerus fracture*** Usually elderly patients. Check they have normal axillary nerve sensation (50p-sized patch 5cm below the acromion) and radial nerve sensation. X-ray, broad arm sling and fracture clinic follow-up
- ***Anterior dislocation*** Bony deformity, anterior bulge of the humeral head and a gap below the acromion; unable to flex shoulder forwards. Check axillary nerve sensation and X-ray to exclude fracture. Discuss with a senior which of the many methods of reduction to use

Hip Examination p440, common injuries include:
- ***Hip fracture*** If the fracture is displaced the affected leg will be shortened and externally rotated; otherwise just pain on external and internal rotation and loading. X-ray and refer to orthopaedics

Knee Examination p440, common injuries include:
- ***Unable to weight bear*** If you are unable to examine a knee acutely then X-ray to exclude bony abnormality (check tibial plateau) and discharge with analgesia, Thackery splint and crutches. Review in 1–2wk
- ***Patella dislocation*** Use Entonox® for analgesia, gently straighten the knee and use your other hand to guide the patella back into place. Relief from pain is immediate on relocation

Ankles Examination p442, the Ottowa ankle rules are used to decide if an ankle X-ray is required (see below); common injuries include:
- ***Sprain*** This is the most common ankle injury. There may be significant swelling and tenderness. Use the Ottowa rules to differentiate from a fracture ankle. Treatment shown on p303
- ***Lateral malleoli fracture*** Check for medial malleoli tenderness and talar shift (on X-ray), refer to orthopaedics if the fracture is above the joint line or talar shift is present; otherwise backslab and fracture clinic
- ***Ankle dislocation*** The ankle may dislocate posteriorly following a fracture and this must be treated urgently. Discuss with your senior then use Entonox® and/or IV analgesia/sedation; pull the ankle forwards by gripping the toes with one hand and the heel with the other. Hold in place whilst plaster is applied. Check pulses, sensation and X-ray after relocation

Ottowa ankle rules

If all the following are present there is usually no need to X-ray an ankle:
- Can weight bear 2 steps or were able to weight bear immediately after injury
- No tenderness over the posterior surface or the tip of the lateral malleolus
- No tenderness over the posterior surface or the tip of the medial malleolus
- No tenderness over the calcaneum, navicular or base of 5th metatarsal
- No tenderness over the proximal fibula

Wounds (OHAEM2 p388)

History Get a clear idea of the mechanism of injury, paying particular attention to bites (animal or human), foreign bodies (broken glass), contamination with soil or manure and when the wound occurred. Always ask about and document tetanus status.

Examination Record the site, size (measure) and type of the wound, check distal sensation, pulse/cap refill and movement, look and feel inside the wound (possibly after anaesthetic) to assess depth, presence of foreign bodies and involvement of deep structures (eg tendons).

Types of wound

Puncture	A deep wound with a small skin defect, eg cat bite, nail
Incisional wound	A wound caused by sharp objects, eg knife/broken glass, often have straight edges and can be deep
Laceration	A wound following blunt trauma, eg banging head on pavement, edges are often ragged and bruised
Abrasion	Graze
Full thickness	A wound that fully penetrates the skin (epidermis and dermis) so that subcutaneous fat is visible
Superficial	A wound that does not fully penetrate the skin

Cleaning All wounds should be thoroughly cleaned with water or 0.9% saline. Abrasions may need to be scrubbed and deeper wounds may need cleaning with high pressure 0.9% saline (use a syringe and green needle with the needle broken off). Cleaning can be done under anaesthetic.

Important rules

- X-ray all wounds involving broken glass or metal foreign bodies
- Wounds should not be closed if:
  - Older than 12h (unless facial)
  - Very dirty or infected
  - Foreign bodies present
  - Bites
- Refer wounds that involve tendons, joints, arteries or nerves

Primary closure is closing the wound in A+E. There are several options:

- ***Glue*** For faces, children and small wounds (<2cm) if the edges are not gaping. The glue should just hold the edges together, not enter the wound
- ***Steristrips*** For fingertips, pretibial lacerations and small wounds
- ***Sutures*** (p494) For wounds which are large, deep or over joints. Simple, interrupted stitches of mono-filament, non-absorbable suture are used for the vast majority. A layered closure with absorbable sutures may be required if the wound is especially deep; seek senior help. Do not close wounds under tension unless under senior supervision

Delayed primary closure The wound is left open for 3–5 days then reviewed and closed if no infection is evident.

Secondary closure Allowing the wound to heal without intervention.

Tetanus status should be documented for all wounds. Ensure adequate prevention and remember that patients over 50yr and immigrants may have received no previous tetanus vaccinations.

Tetanus prophylaxis

Immunisation status	Clean wound	Tetanus prone wound[1]
Full course (5 injections) or booster <10yr ago	No prophylaxis needed	HATI[2] only if contaminated with manure
Partial course and booster ≥10yr ago	Tetanus booster	Tetanus booster and HATI[2]
Not immunised or unknown	Start tetanus course	Start tetanus course and give HATI[2]

1 Tetanus prone wounds:
- Heavy contamination especially with soil or manure (remember gardeners)
- Infection or wounds >6h old
- Puncture wounds (eg cat bites, nails)
- Devitalised tissue

2 HATI – human anti-tetanus immunoglobulin

Antibiotics should be prescribed for very dirty or infected wounds, puncture wounds, wounds involving bones (eg crushed fingertips) and patients with valvular heart disease; some departments also prescribe antibiotics for wounds >6h old. Amoxicillin 500mg/8h PO and flucloxacillin 500mg/6h PO for 5d are used in many departments. Animal bites should be treated with co-amoxiclav 625mg/8h PO for 5d.

Assaults The notes you make may be used in a legal case many years from now so think carefully about what you write. For example:
- Distinguish facts from hearsay; make it clear where information came from, eg 'Patient alleges assault with an iron bar, witnesses describe LOC for 3min.'
- Document injuries accurately including location, size (measure) and type of wound (see table opposite); use simple line diagrams. Do not interpret what caused the wound
- Write your notes imagining them being read out in public by someone wishing to make you appear stupid

Minor burns All burns (whether chemical or thermal) should be cooled with running cold water for 10–20min as soon as possible alongside adequate analgesia. Get a clear idea of the mechanism of injury including temperature and length of contact. Determine the depth:
- ***Superficial*** Tender, blanching red colour
- ***Partial dermal*** Tender, blanching red colour with blisters
- ***Deep dermal*** Tender, non-blanching red colour
- ***Full thickness*** Non-tender, white, brown or black and leathery

Refer burns to the face, hand or genitalia or deep dermal/full thickness burns to plastics and ask their advice on dressings; other burns should be cleaned and dressed (non-adherent dressing) and reviewed in 2–3d.

Head injuries (OHAEM2 p352)

Head injuries are very common and usually require minimal treatment, however it is important to distinguish those with intracranial injury from the rest. There are three treatment options:

- ***CT head*** and admit according to the NICE guidelines opposite
- ***Admit*** for 12h observation and regular neuro obs if patients are unwell but do not meet the NICE guideline criteria or if they live alone
- ***Discharge*** if they do not meet the NICE guideline CT criteria, are well with a GCS 15/15 and acting their normal selves so long as they have a responsible adult with them at home. Give a head injury advice sheet

Back pain see p223 or OHAEM2 p470

Musculoskeletal chest pain and rib fractures (OHAEM2 p322)

Mild trauma to the chest can cause pleuritic chest pain. Ask about the mechanism (±sharp objects eg knives), shortness of breath, previous breathing problems and smoking. Look carefully for flail segments and a pneumothorax (trachea, expansion, percussion, auscultation). Palpate the chest to distinguish between generalised tenderness, a single very tender rib or multiple very tender ribs. X-ray if you suspect multiple rib fractures or a pneumothorax; otherwise discharge with analgesia, advise to perform breathing exercises (regular deep breathes) and stop smoking.

Foreign bodies (FB) in the eye (OHAEM2 p516)

Distinguish between slow moving and fast moving FBs because hammering or grinding metal can cause the FB to penetrate the globe. Ask specifically about vision and where they feel the FB is. Check visual acuity and pupil reflexes. Examine with a slit lamp to identify the FB and check for blood in the anterior chamber.

- ***FB present*** Numb the eye with anaesthetic drops (eg proxymetacaine) and remove the FB with a cotton bud or green needle. Re-examine to check for complete removal, rust rings and that the anterior chamber is intact. Refer to ophthalmology clinic in 24h if any FB is still present, acuity is affected, FB was over the pupil or a rust ring is left. Discharge with chloramphenicol drops/ointment and advise to avoid driving; reattend if symptoms not improving in 48h or visual acuity deteriorates
- ***No FB*** Check throughout the conjunctiva and consider everting the upper eyelid. Use fluorescein drops to identify abrasions. Refer to ophthalmology clinic in 24h if abrasions are over the pupil or affect acuity:
    - ***Slow moving FBs*** Discharge with chloramphenicol drops/ointment and advise to avoid driving; eye patches may help symptoms. Reattend if symptoms not improving in 48h or visual acuity deteriorates
    - ***Fast moving FBs*** X-ray the eye to exclude intraocular FBs. Refer immediately if present; if absent treat as slow moving

NICE head guidance

Are any of the following present?

- GCS <13 at any point since the injury
- GCS 13 or 14 at 2h after the injury
- Focal neurological deficit
- Suspected open or depressed skull fracture
- Any sign of basal skull fracture (haemotympanum, 'panda' eyes, cerebrospinal fluid otorrhoea, battle's sign)
- Post-traumatic seizure
- >1 vomiting episode (clinical judgement on cause of vomiting and need for imaging should be used in children aged ≤12yr)

YES → Request CT imaging of the head immediately – imaging to be carried out within 1h of the request

NO ↓

Any loss of consciousness or amnesia since injury?

NO → No imaging required at present

YES ↓

Are any of the following present?

- Age ≥65yr
- Coagulopathy (history of bleeding, clotting disorders, current treatment with warfarin)

YES → Request CT imaging of the head immediately – imaging to be carried out within 1h of the request

NO ↓

Are any of the following present?

- Dangerous mechanism of injury (a pedestrian struck by a motor vehicle, an occupant ejected from a motor vehicle or a fall from a height of greater than 1m or 5 stairs)? A lower threshold for height of falls should be used when dealing with infants and young children (ie <5yr)
- Amnesia of greater than 30min for events before impact (the assessment of amnesia will not be possible in pre-verbal children and is unlikely to be possible in any child aged <5yr)

YES → Request CT imaging of the head immediately – imaging to be carried out within 8h of the injury, or immediately if the patient presents >8h post-injury

NO → No imaging required at present

Request CT imaging of the head immediately – imaging to be carried out within 1h of the request	Request CT imaging of the head immediately – imaging to be carried out within 8h of the injury, or immediately if the patient presents >8h post-injury	No imaging required at present

Adapted from Clinical Practice Algorithm no.4, June 2003
By kind permission of the National Institute of Clinical Excellence (NICE)

Majors

Clerking Requires more detail than a minors clerking but should still be focused. Aim to determine whether the patient requires admission and give a list of accurate differential diagnoses.

Notes You are not expected to provide a complete clerking; you should document the relevant positive (eg chest pain) and negative (eg no rash) features that show your thought processes as you try to distinguish between the possible diagnoses. Include your list of differential diagnoses, treatment and investigations. There should be a clear plan:

- ***Still in A+E*** – What results do you need to make a decision?
- ***Admission*** – Which team are they referred to and why (both investigations and treatment)?
- ***Discharge*** – Should they see their GP? What treatment was given? What should they look out for or reattend for?

Medical conditions are covered elsewhere in this book. Two presentations unique to A+E are described below.

Hypothermia (OHAEM2 p256)

Mild <35°C	Moderate <32°C	Severe <30°C

Young Usually due to falling into water or impaired conscious level (eg alcohol or drugs). ***Elderly*** usually due to immobility (CVA, acute illness or injury after falling). When severe it may mimic death.

Investigations FBC, U+E, TFT, cardiac markers, toxicology screen, clotting, amylase, ABG, ECG (look for prolonged P, QRS and T waves, arrhythmias, J waves), CXR and CT head if head injury or CVA suspected.

Treatment Monitor treatment with rectal thermometer. Use warming blankets (bear hugger) and warm fluids; if severe consider warm bladder washout and warm peritoneal lavage. Cardiopulmonary bypass may be required if very severe.

Complications ventricular fibrillation, respiratory depression

Overdose – OD (OHAEM2 p174 and *Toxbase*)

Overdoses are very common in A+E. The majority will be small overdoses of over-the-counter medicines. Large overdoses may present with ↓GCS; treat ABC first and involve a senior early.

History Try to determine exactly what was taken, how much and when. You should also assess suicidal intent, see p406.

Investigations Paracetamol and salicylate levels at 4h in all overdoses. If unwell consider BM, FBC, U+E, LFT, ECG and ABG

Treatments (OHAEM2 p174 and check *Toxbase*) Activated charcoal is indicated in the first 1h (2h for paracetamol) for some overdoses (check *Toxbase*). Severe overdoses may require supportive treatment with particular attention to GCS and respiration. The majority of overdoses can be discharged 4–6h after the overdose if their paracetamol and salicylate levels are normal. Discharge into the care of a responsible adult with appropriate psychiatric follow-up. If a patient is acutely suicidal refer to psychiatry as soon as medically well.

Paracetamol overdose

Take a blood sample 4h after the overdose to measure paracetamol and salicylate levels. If the level is above the relevant line then treat with N-acetylcysteine (Parvolex®). Give three doses to adults:

- 150mg/kg IV infusion in 200ml 5% glucose over 15min
- 50mg/kg IV infusion in 500ml 5% glucose over 4h
- 100mg/kg IV infusion in 1000ml 5% glucose over 16h

High-risk line Use if malnourished, HIV +ve, eating disorder, excess alcohol intake or if regularly taking carbamazepine, phenytoin, phenobarbitone, primidone, St John's Wort or rifampicin.

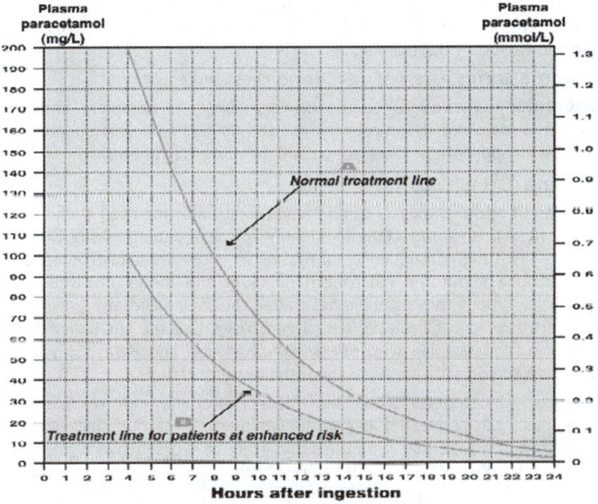

National Poisons Information Service guidelines 2003
Reproduced by kind permission of the Paracetamol Information Centre.

Features of common overdoses

Features	Obs	Likely drug
↓GCS, dilated pupils, ↑tone and reflexes, seizures	↑pulse	Tricyclic antidepressants (TCA)
↓GCS, ↓tone and reflexes	↓BP, ↓RR	Benzodiazepines, barbiturates, alcohol, severe tricyclic OD
↓GCS, pinpoint pupils	↓RR	Opiates
Agitation, tremor, dilated pupils	↑pulse	Ecstacy (±↑temp), amphetamines, cocaine
Nausea, sweating, tinnitus, ±deafness	↑pulse, ↑RR	Salicylate poisoning

Trauma (OHAEM2 p312)

The treatment of the major trauma victim follows the principles of Advanced Trauma and Life Support (ATLS®). You may have the opportunity to attend the three-day course that teaches these principles.

Primary survey Performed immediately with C-spine protection and immediate treatment of life-threatening problems as they are identified:

- ***Airway*** with C-spine control
- ***Breathing*** or ventilation with 100% O_2
- ***Circulation*** with haemorrhage control and good IV access
- ***Disability*** Rapid AVPU; can all 4 limbs move?
- ***Exposure*** Fully undress and log-roll to ensure no injury is missed

If you do not have ATLS training then you should only undertake tasks allotted to you by the team leader.

Trauma series X-rays of the C-spine, chest and pelvis.

Secondary survey Once the primary survey is complete and the patient is stabilised a comprehensive head to toe survey is undertaken along with appropriate investigation and definitive treatment.

C-spine (OHAEM2 p370)

Patients often have their C-spine immobilised following road traffic accidents (RTA). It is important to identify the few patients with C-spine injuries since the consequences of missing an injury are catastrophic. Get a clear idea about the mechanism of injury and forces involved. Ask specifically about moving their neck after the injury and any tingling of their arms or legs. Check peripheral neurology. Use the NICE guidelines opposite to determine who needs immobilisation and X-ray. Show the films to a senior if at all unsure about their interpretation.

Whiplash Once concerns over bony/neurological injury are resolved the neck injury can be treated as a sprain (whiplash). Prescribe analgesia and NSAIDs and advise that symptoms are likely to worsen overnight. Recommend GP follow-up if pain is not resolving

Important questions to assess RTAs

Speed, seatbelt, airbag, driver/passenger, front/back, type of impact, what stopped the car, was the car written off, was the car drivable, did the doors open

Open fractures (OHAEM2 p408)

Do not be distracted by gruesome injuries, start with ABC. Once the patient is stable then assess fractures and injuries. Check distal sensation and circulation (pulses and cap refill); if abnormal or joint clearly dislocated then involve a senior early. Give analgesia (eg IV morphine). If a digital camera is available take photos to show orthopaedics then cover the wound with saline soaked swabs and backslab under gentle traction. Start IV antibiotics (often cefuroxime, ±metronidazole) and review tetanus status. X-ray and refer to orthopaedics

NICE neck guidance

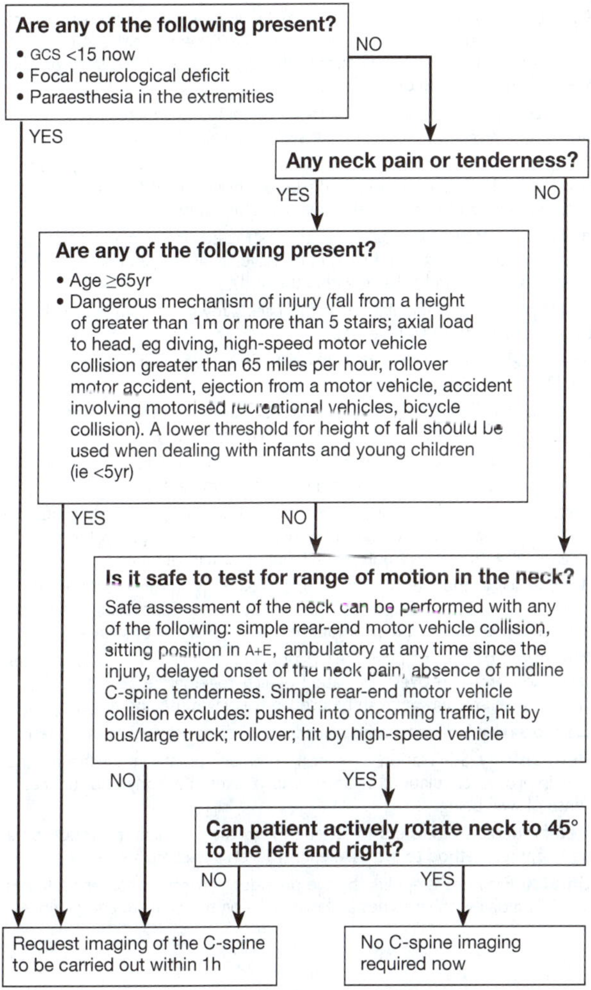

Adapted from Clinical Practice Algorithm no.4, 2003
By kind permission of the National Institute of Clinical Excellence (NICE)

Alternative/complementary medicine

A wide variety of alternative and complementary medicines exist, overseen by numerous associations.[1] Patients access them as either an adjunct to, or a substitute for, 'conventional' therapy. Some are available on the NHS; the majority are only offered privately.

Evidence supporting the use of these therapies is limited, though it is clear that many people obtain great symptom relief by using them.

Acupuncture This stems from Chinese medicine. 'Qi' flows around the body in health but in disease is disrupted. Insertion of fine needles into certain points on the body helps restore natural flow.

Aromatherapy Essential oils are extracted from plants (flowers, leaves, roots, bark etc) and used in massage, inhalation and baths to help restore harmony and balance within the body.

Chiropractice Manipulation of the back allows harmony and balance to be restored to the whole body.

'Healing' Various forms used, including Reiki (see below), Crystal Healing, Distant Healing and Sound Healing.

Herbal medicine Extracts of medicinal plants are used to treat illness, in a similar fashion to that of conventional drug therapy.

Homeopathy Extracts of plant, animal and mineral are diluted to infinitesimal doses and used to stimulate the immune system.

Hypnotherapy Combining elements of counselling and psychotherapy with hypnosis, an altered state of consciousness is induced in the patient to give relaxation and symptomatic relief of certain ailments.

Kinesiology Muscle testing is undertaken by tensing, and used in conjunction with massage, touch, nutrition and counselling. Used to balance the emotions and promote health, which fights off disease.

Massage Stroking, tapping, light friction and kneading of the skin induces relaxation and improves circulation, which together lessen tension and can aid in self-healing and can be used in treating musculoskeletal injuries.

Osteopathy Similar to chiropractic but whole musculoskeletal system.

Reflexology Stimulation of specific pressure points in the hands and feet improves circulation, balances and relaxes the body and induces a sense of well-being.

Reiki Therapist transfers Reiki energy to the recipient by touch or a non-contact method to increase energy levels and stimulate healing.

Shiatsu Pressure is applied by the provider's fingers, hands, arms, knees and feet along with stretches and manipulation to stimulate energy flow.

1 http://www.bcma.co.uk/
http://www.the-cma.org.uk/

Herbal remedies

Over 2000 different plants and plant extracts are used worldwide in the treatment of illness and prevention of disease. Below are the most popular single-herb preparations sold in the United Kingdom.

Aloe vera ***(Aloe barbadensis)*** Commonly used to treat burns and soothe irritated skin. Found in many cosmetics and toiletries. Side-effects are uncommon.

Echinacea ***(Echinacea angustifolio)*** Believed to act like an antibiotic and aids in reducing fever, infections, bad breath and mucous build-up. Side-effects have been reported and include hepatotoxicity, nephrotoxicity and its use is discouraged in pregnancy and the very young (<2yr).

Ephedra ***(Ephedra sinica)*** Used to treat asthma and aid in decongestion. Side-effects include increased heart rate and blood pressure; can cause insomnia and nervousness. Ephedra should not be used in patients taking MAOI and used with caution in patients with IHD.

Garlic ***(Allium sativum)*** Most often used to balance gut flora and also to treat chest infections. Side-effects include cutaneous reaction to the raw vegetable and potentiation of anticoagulation effects of warfarin.

Ginger ***(Zangiber officinale)*** Aids in normal digestion and useful for nausea and indigestion. Also used to treat asthma and colds. Side-effects include dyspepsia and potentiation of anticoagulation effects of warfarin.

Gingko biloba Believed to improve the circulatory system, particularly in the elderly where it is used to treat short-term memory loss, headache and tinnitus. Side-effects include dyspepsia, headache and potentiation of anticoagulation effects of warfarin and aspirin.

Ginseng ***(Panax ginseng)*** Used to enhance physical and mental endurance and to boost the immune system. Side-effects include headaches, insomnia, anxiety, skin reactions and rise in blood pressure; may interfere with warfarin and digoxin.

Kava Kava ***(Piper methysticum)*** At low doses is believed to stimulate the body, but at higher doses reduce stress and anxiety. Side-effects include hypertension, muscle weakness and dizziness. Sale of Kava Kava is now banned in the UK due to concerns over safety.

St John's wort ***(Hypericum perforatum)*** Used to treat mild depression and symptoms of nervousness and low self-esteem. Side-effects include photosensitivity of the skin, nausea and hypertension.

Does St John's wort relieve mild depression?

Numerous clinical trails have been undertaken to investigate this and while St John's wort appears to be better than placebo, it is unknown if it is at least comparable to conventional antidepressants (see Cochrane Review; Linde *et al*, St John's wort for depression. In: The Cochrane Library, Issue 4, 2004).

Anaesthetics/ICU

Role of the anaesthetist in hospital The anaesthetist has many roles: providing anaesthesia and analgesia for surgical procedures and obstetrics, caring for patients on ITU and in other high dependency areas, part of the trauma, cardiac- and paediatric-arrest teams, in-patient and out-patient pain management and in the teaching of medical and nursing staff. The anaesthetist is also frequently asked to site central lines and to help with patients who have difficult venous access.

Anaesthetic history The purpose of the anaesthetic history and examination is to identify potential/actual risks and to determine the safest and most appropriate anaesthetic technique (OHCS6 p761).

- Previous anaesthetics – ask the patient if they recall any problems and check old anaesthetic charts to see if any were documented
- Past medical history – asthma/COPD, IHD, diabetes, rheumatoid arthritis; how well controlled are these?
- Indigestion/reflux – are they being treated for this or do they suffer with acid regurgitation or reflux after meals or lying flat?
- General health – exercise tolerance; can they climb a flight of stairs?
- Current health – do they have a cold or a chest infection?
- Drug history – anticoagulants, cardiac medications
- Allergy – document allergy and reaction encountered
- Family history – have other family members had problems with either general or local anaesthetics?
- Social history – smoking, alcohol and recreational drugs
- Teeth – document site of caps, crowns, false or loose teeth
- Fasted – when was their last meal and last drink?
- Consent – see p94

Pre-op examination Cardiorespiratory examination by the anaesthetist is not always necessary unless pathology is known or suspected. Pre-op assessment usually includes cardiac and respiratory examination (p116).

- CVS – evidence of heart failure or a sinister murmur
- RS – bronchospasm, focal infection, pleural effusions, pneumothorax
- Airway – limited mouth opening, limitation of neck movement, prominent upper teeth and small chins are potential markers of 'the difficult airway' and/or difficult intubation
- Weight – document this, especially for children

Pre-op investigations[1] Most hospitals will have specific guidelines on this (OHCS6 p762), common indications are shown below; serious pathology needs to be assessed and treated before elective surgery:

- FBC – age >60yr, anaemia suspected or transfusion anticipated
- Sickle-cell trait – African, Caribbean, Middle Eastern or Mediterranean
- Group and save/crossmatch – depends on type of surgery, see p421
- U+E – age >60yr, diabetes or other chronic disease, diuretic therapy
- Clotting – anticoagulation therapy, liver disease or bleeding tendency
- ECG – age >60yr, suspected or known IHD, diabetes, obesity
- Echo – history suggests cardiac failure, sinister murmur
- CXR – unexplained breathlessness or abnormal physical findings
- Respiratory function tests – severe asthma, severe COPD/emphysema

1 NICE guidelines: http://www.nice.org.uk/page.aspx?o=CG003

ASA classification (American Society of Anesthesiologists)
1. Normally healthy
2. Mild systemic disease, but with no limitation on activity
3. Severe systemic disease that limits activity; not incapacitating
4. Incapacitating systemic disease which poses a threat to life
5. Moribund. Not expected to survive 24h even with operation

CEPOD The **C**onfidential **E**nquiry into **P**eri**o**perative **D**eaths is an on-going study which helps to stratify the urgency for surgery for any given patient based on extensive retrospective analysis of perioperative deaths. A CEPOD scoring system is used in most hospitals, but as yet a national standardised system has not been formulated. Below is an example:
- CEPOD 1 – Surgery needed immediately or ≤1h
- CEPOD 2 – Surgery needed within 24h
- CEPOD 3 – Surgery needed within 72h
- CEPOD 4 – Surgery needs to be scheduled
- CEPOD 5 – Elective surgery

Special circumstances Some patients need extra consideration and are admitted a day or more pre-operatively to stabilise a chronic disease:
- insulin; often switched to an insulin sliding scale (p235)
- warfarin; if anticoagulation is crucial consider IV heparin (p290)
- steroids; patients often admitted on the day of surgery (OHCM6 p472)

Premedication This was once routine for all patients, but is now reserved for select individuals (OHCS6 p763). Benzodiazepines are used as anxiolytics in the over-anxious; drugs acting to raise gastric pH are used when risk of aspiration is increased; topical anaesthetics (EMLA® and Ametop®) are used to anaesthetise the skin prior to cannulation; antibiotics, bronchodilators, steroids and anticholinergic agents are also used.

Giving an anaesthetic The steps involved in checking anaesthetic equipment and giving a safe anaesthetic are complex and require specialist training (OHCS6 p764). Anaesthesia is broadly divided into *general anaesthesia*, where the patient is unconscious, and *regional anaesthesia*, where specific nerves or groups of nerves are anaesthetised and the patient remains awake, though usually offered light sedation (OHA1 p996).

Postoperative complications Immediate complications are common, the most frequent are nausea and vomiting (OHA1 p923), though others will be encountered by the anaesthetist before the patient leaves the recovery room (OHCS6 p772). Subsequent problems on the ward include pain (p282), low urine output (p266), hypotension (p149), hypoxia (p165), pyrexia (p248), confusion (p229), bleeding (p151) and inadvertent nerve injury (OHA1 p948). A sore throat following intubation is common and resolves within a few days.

Post-regional anaesthesia Following regional anaesthesia the patient often returns to the ward with residual sensory and motor blockade. Care must be taken to avoid damage to the anaesthetised area and special attention should be paid to pressure areas; compartment syndrome (p296) can be masked by regional anaesthesia and this should be considered in all susceptible patients. Bleeding, systemic toxicity of local anaesthetics (p492) and headache can also occur (OHA1 p996).

Intensive/high dependency units

The setting Intensive care and high dependency care are wards like any other, though the ratio of nursing staff to patients is often greater and 1:1 on most ITUs. Consultant intensivists run ITU, whereas patients on HDU remain under the care of either a surgical or medical consultant, though they may also receive regular intensivist input.

Patients Most have multi-organ failure requiring drug and/or mechanical support, intensive nursing care and close observation. Many are sedated (usually with continuous infusions of morphine and midazolam) and have assisted ventilation either through an endotracheal tube or tracheostomy; patients who require assisted ventilation for long periods of time often have tracheostomy tubes sited (OHCC2 p38) as these are tolerated well in conscious patients, whereas endotracheal tubes are not.

Admission/discharge Patients are admitted from A+E, theatre or wards (following deterioration); referral is usually made between consultants. Most patients are discharged onto general wards before going home.

Monitoring Most patients will have several invasive and non-invasive monitoring modalities, including:

- *ECG* Rate and rhythm
- *Pulse oximetry* Delivery of oxygen to the peripheries
- *BP* Often invasive via an arterial line or non-invasive via a BP cuff
- *Temperature* Either cutaneous or oesophageal probes
- *CVP* Either internal jugular vein or subclavian vein; aids assessment of fluid balance
- *Urine output* Helps determine fluid balance and renal perfusion
- *ICP* Intracranial bolts are often sited following head injury or after neurosurgery; allows cerebral perfusion pressure to be calculated
- *Capnography* The concentration of gases in the inspiratory and expiratory phases are measured in patients whose ventilation is assisted
- *Pulmonary artery wedge pressure* Indirect and often criticised for being an inaccurate measurement of left atrial filling/pre-load
- *Cardiac output* Various invasive and non-invasive methods looking at left ventricular ejection fraction (OHCC2 p122)
- *EEG* Neurological activity is sometimes recorded

Drugs Besides the drugs used to treat the underlying condition many patients will require circulatory support in the form of IV drug infusions:

- epinephrine (adrenaline) and isoprenaline: positive inotropes
- dobutamine: positive inotrope
- norepinephrine (noradrenaline): vasopressor, increases SVR

Nutrition This can be either enteral (gut) or parenteral (IV), see p485. Enteral feeding via NG tubes is common since parenteral feeding relies on central venous access and carries the risks of infection/sepsis.

Infection control Immunocompromise is common in HDU/ITU (secondary to underlying pathology and drugs) so hand-washing and other precautions should always be taken. White coats should be taken off.

ITU scoring systems Scoring systems are used to predict patient outcome and progress in response to treatment (OHCC2 p572).

Dermatology

The skin is allegedly the largest organ of the body. There are countless primary pathologies affecting the skin, but many medical, surgical and psychiatric diseases also have cutaneous manifestations (p323).

Dermatology history taking complements a good general history; here are a few specific questions which are essential in dermatology:

- site of onset, spread and distribution
- symptoms (itch, pain)
- medical history/systemic disease
- previous treatments
- occupation (chemical exposure)
- duration
- aggravating factors (light, heat)
- drug history/allergy
- family history (atopy, psoriasis)
- pets

Physical examination may be appropriate if systemic disease is suspected; all the skin, hair and nails should be inspected where appropriate.

Distribution of rashes often aids diagnosis:

- symmetrical flexural (atopic eczema)
- symmetrical extensor surfaces (psoriasis)
- contact with jewelry or cosmetics (allergic contact dermatitis)
- areas exposed to sun (photosensitivity)
- grouped lesions (eg herpes virus in a dermatomal distribution)

Describing rashes accurately, including their nature, distribution and history, is often sufficient to allow the diagnosis to be made. Some of the commoner and more useful terms are explained opposite. When describing a lesion mention:

- site (where is it on the body)
- size (measure with a tape measure)
- shape (round, linear)
- borders (well demarcated, adjacent erythema)
- surface (scaly, crusted, flat, raised)

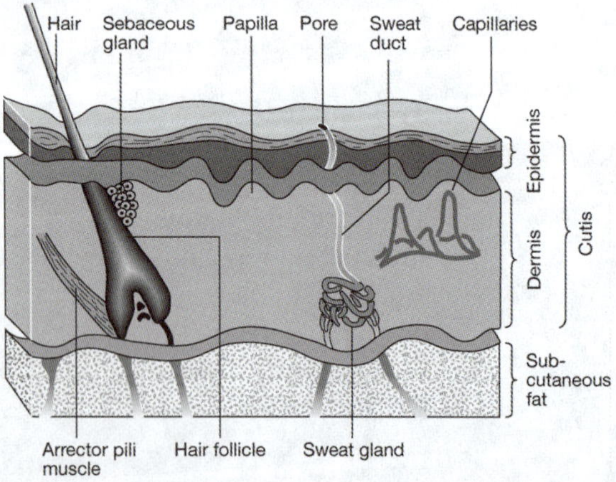

Structure of the skin

Dermatology terms (OHCS6 p576)

Non-palpable	
Ecchymosis	Bruising; discolouration from blood leaking into the skin
Macule	Flat well-defined area of altered skin pigmentation
Petechia	Non-blanching pinpoint-sized purple macule
Purpura	Purple lesion resulting from free red blood cells in the skin non-blanching
Telangiectasia	Abnormal visible dilatation of blood vessels (spider naevi)
Palpable	
Nodule	Solid, mostly subcutaneous lesion (>0.5cm diameter)
Papule	Raised well-defined lesion (<0.5cm diameter)
Plaque	Raised flat-topped lesion, usually >2cm diameter
Weal	Transient raised lesion with pink margin
Urticaria	Weals with pale centres and well-defined pink margins
Blisters	
Abscess	Fluctuant swelling containing pus beneath the epidermis
Bulla	Fluid filled blister larger than a vesicle (>0.5cm diameter)
Pustule	Well-defined pus-filled lesion
Vesicle	Fluid filled blister (<0.5cm diameter)
Skin defects	
Excoriation	Linear break in the skin surface (a scratch)
Atrophy	Thinning and loss of skin substance
Crust	Dried brownish/yellow exudates
Cut	Break to the skin by sharp object
Erosion	Superficial break in the continuity of the epidermis
Abrasion	Scraping off superficial layers of the skin (a graze)
Fissure	Crack, often through keratin
Incisional wound	Break to the skin by sharp object
Laceration	Break to the skin caused by blunt trauma/tearing injury
Lichenification	Skin thickening with exaggerated skin markings
Scale	Fragment of dry skin
Ulcer	Loss of epidermis and dermis resulting in scar

Dermatology presentations

Psoriasis is a common and chronic inflammatory condition affecting about 2% of Caucasians with peak incidence in the 20s and 50s. Classical features are silvery scaly plaques over the extensor aspects of knees, elbows, scalp and sacrum. *Tx* emollients, tar, salicylic acid, topical corticosteroids, UVB/PUVA, retinoids and systemic cytotoxics (OHCS6 p586).

Eczema can be atopic, allergic or caused by irritants. Always ask about employment, hobbies and pets. Common in children; classically involves face, trunk and limb (flexor > extensor surfaces). *Tx* emollients, topical corticosteroids, antihistamines, tar, UVB/PUVA, dietary and environmental modification and immunosuppressive agents (OHCS6 p588).

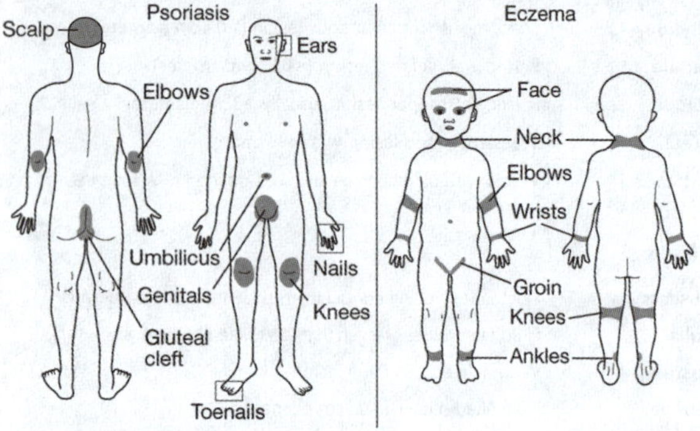

Typical cutaneous distributions of psoriasis and eczema

Skin cancer Basal cell carcinomas (BCC) and squamous cell carcinomas (SCC) are often easier to identify than melanomas. For melanomas refer if ≥3 of ABCD: asymmetric lesions, border irregularity, colour irregularity, diameter >6mm or if bleeding, pain or itching (OHCS6 p584).

Purpuric rash in the acute setting should be presumed to be meningococcal septicaemia (p212), especially if the patient is systemically unwell. Purpuric rashes are non-blanching and can be petechial or form larger macules or papules. Other causes include idiopathic thrombocytopenic purpura (OHCS6 p275) and Henoch–Schönlein purpura (OHCS6 p584).

Drugs applied to the skin *Ointments* are oil-based and most often used for areas of dry skin; *creams* are emulsions of oil in water and used for moist areas (OHCS6 p577). *Lotions* are generally water-based and have a limited range of uses in dermatology. *Collodions* are painted onto the skin and dry to form a flexible film. *Gels* generally have a high water content and *pastes* are stiff preparations containing a high proportion of powdered material suspended in an ointment.

Topical corticosteroids

Topical steroids are used in the treatment of many inflammatory skin diseases, other than those due to infection. As with corticosteroids given orally or intravenously the mechanism of action is complex; arachidonic acid mobilisation is inhibited (the first step in prostaglandin synthesis) and the expression of various genes involved in pro-inflammatory mechanisms is altered. Corticosteroids offer symptomatic relief and are seldom curative. The least potent preparation (see table below) should be used to control symptoms. Withdrawal of topical steroids often causes a rebound worsening of symptoms and the patient should be warned about this.

Side-effects of topical steroids are predominantly related to skin atrophy (especially on face and flexures) although excessive or prolonged use can result in systemic effects (Cushingoid features, p239).

Topical corticosteroid potencies

Potency	Example
Mild	Hydrocortisone 1%
Moderately potent	Clobetasone butyrate 0.05%
Potent	Betamethasone 0.1%, hydrocortisone butyrate 0.1%
Very potent	Clobetasol propionate 0.05%

Common skin manifestations in systemic disease

(OHCS6 p580)

Diabetes mellitus	Candidiasis, necrobiosis lipoidica, folliculitis, skin infections
Coeliac disease	Dermatitis herpetiformis
IBD	Erythema nodosum, pyoderma gangrenosum
Rheumatoid arthritis	Rheumatoid nodules, vasculitis, pyoderma gangrenosum
SLE	Facial butterfly rash, photosensitivity, red scaly rashes, diffuse alopecia
Hyperthyroidism	Pre-tibial myxoedema, clubbing, diffuse alopecia
Hypothyroidism	Sparse coarse hair, dry skin, eczema craquelé (asteatotic)
Neoplasia	Acanthosis nigricans, dermatomyositis, ichthyosis, pruritus
Drug eruptions (OHCS6 p593)	Erythema multiforme (target lesions, Stevens-Johnson syndrome), urticaria, exfoliative dermatitis, toxic epidermal necrolysis
HIV	Infections (thrush, molluscum contagiosum, herpes simplex, varicella-zoster), inflammatory conditions

Stridor in a conscious adult patient

Airway	Acute stridor: bleep anaesthetist and ENT urgently
Breathing	If no respiratory effort – **CALL ARREST TEAM**
Circulation	If no palpable pulse – **CALL ARREST TEAM**

Call for **senior anaesthetics and ENT help** immediately

- **Do not** attempt to look in the mouth/examine the neck
- Avoid **disturbing/upseting** the patient in any way
- Let the **patient sit** in whatever position they choose
- Offer **high-flow oxygen** to all patients
- **Fast bleep** a registrar anaesthetist
- **Fast bleep** a registrar ENT surgeon
- **Epinephrine (adrenaline) nebs** (1ml of 1:1000 with O_2)
- **Monitor** pulse oximeter, ±defibrillator's ECG leads if unwell
- Check **temp**
- Take brief **history** from relatives/ward staff or check **notes**
- **Look for** swelling, rashes, itching (?anaphylaxis)
- Consider **serious causes** (below)
- Await **anaesthetic** and **ENT** input
- Request urgent portable **CXR**
- Call for **senior help**
- **Reassess**, starting with A, B, C...

Life-threatening causes

- Infection (epiglottitis, abscess)
- Tumour
- Trauma
- Foreign body
- Post-op
- Anaphylaxis

Ear, nose and throat (ENT)

ENT is a separate surgical subspeciality which covers a wide range of common complaints seen in A+E and by the GP.

History taking

As well as a good general history, specific symptoms to note include:

- ***Ears*** pain, blocked ears, discharge, tinnitus, deafness, unilateral/bilateral features, vertigo, trauma, itching, foreign bodies (FB), noise exposure
- ***Nose*** blocked nose, watery discharge, sneezing, itching, coughing, change in voice, altered sensation of smell/taste, external deformity/recent trauma, epistaxis, sinusitis; ask about daytime variation in symptom severity, pattern of obstruction, effects on speech and sleep
- ***Throat*** dysphagia, pain on swallowing (odynophagia), hoarseness, difficulty opening jaw (trismus), stridor, sleep apnoea/snoring; ask about neck lumps

Examination

- ***Ears*** inspect the pinna, auditory meatus (pull the pinna upwards and back), tragal, pinna or mastoid tenderness; otoscopy examine all 4 quadrants of the eardrum (colour, translucency, bulging/retraction, perforation, exudate); test hearing (see below)
- ***Nose*** look for obvious scars, deviations/deformities, tilt the head back and look down each nostril; rhinoscopy (administer lidocaine spray first), look for polyps, inflamed turbinates, pus
- ***Throat*** inspect the lips, around and inside the mouth, examine the tongue and tonsils using a torch and tongue depressor, check palate movements by asking the patient to say 'ah'
- ***Neck*** look for swellings, asymmetry, scars; ask the patient to swallow and protrude the tongue; palpate the neck from behind and ask the patient to take a sip of water; feel for tracheal deviation, lymphadenopathy, tenderness; auscultate for a bruit; examine any lumps (see p333)

Hearing tests (adults) (OHCS6 p532)

- *Whisper* a different number into each ear, standing 1 foot away whilst blocking the other ear. Ask the patient to repeat it in turn
- *Tuning fork tests:* ***Rinne's test*** place the tuning fork on the patient's mastoid bone until it is no longer heard; the tuning fork is then placed near the external auditory meatus where it is still heard in the normal ear and in sensorineural deafness, but not in conductive deafness. ***Weber's test*** place the tuning fork in the middle of the forehead and ask which side the sound is loudest; in nerve deafness the sound is loudest in the normal ear, in conductive deafness the sound is loudest in the abnormal ear. The sound is equal if both ears are normal or equally affected
- *Audiometry* usually done in out-patients by a specialist; assesses hearing threshold at various sound frequencies

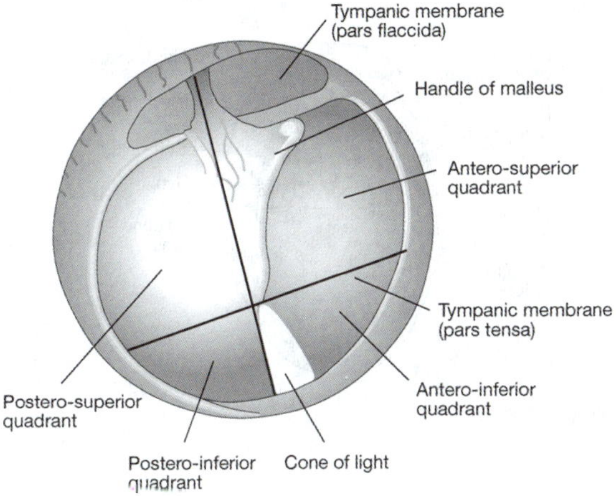

Structures and quadrants of the right tympanic membrane (ear drum) as seen on otoscopy.

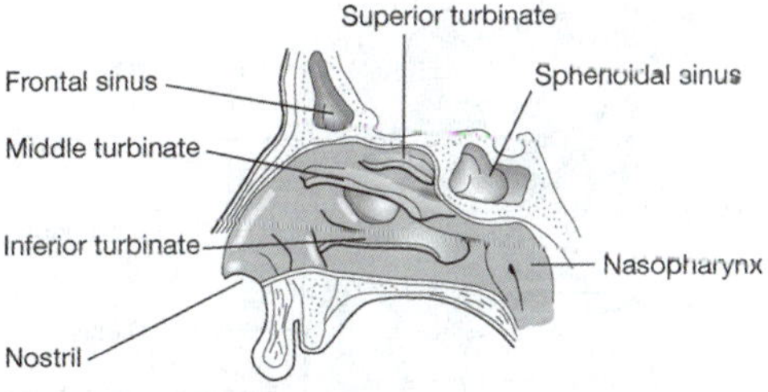

Anatomy of the nose

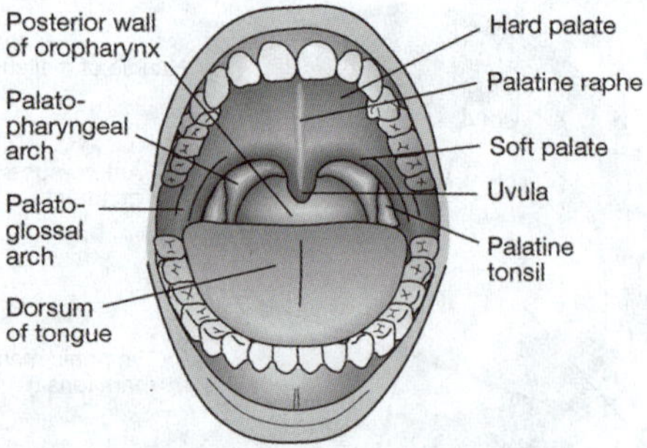

Mouth and oropharynx

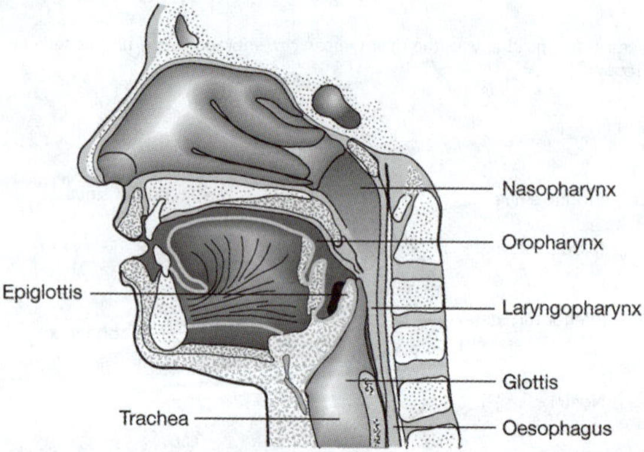

Pharynx and major structures within

Common ENT terms

Adenoid	Lymphatic tissues in the nasopharynx
Arytenoids	Cartilage which support the vocal cords in the larynx
Cerumen	Earwax, material secreted by sebaceous glands of ear canal
Cholesteatoma	Benign growth of eardrum which can cause local invasion and introduce infection into the CNS
Croup	Laryngotracheobronchitis, commonly viral
Epiglottitis	Infection/inflammation of the epiglottis and local structures
Epistaxis	Nosebleed
Eustachian tube	Tube connecting middle ear to pharynx
Glottis	Space between two vocal folds/cords
Glue ear	Accumulation of fluid in middle ear causing deafness
Laryngitis	Inflammation of the larynx
Laryngomalacia	Floppy ary-epiglottic folds
Larynx	Organ responsible for vocal sounds
Mastoiditis	Inflammation of the mastoid
Mastoid process	Bony prominence of the temporal bone behind ear
Ménière's disease	Disease of the inner ear characterised by episodes of deafness, tinnitus and vertigo
Myringoplasty	Surgical repair of a perforated eardrum
Myringotomy	Incision of the eardrum
Nasopharynx	Part of the pharynx which lies above the soft palate
Oropharynx	Part of pharynx which lies between soft palate and hyoid
Otalgia	Earache
Otitis externa	Inflammation/infection of the external auditory canal
Otitis media	Inflammation/infection of the middle ear
Otoplasty	Surgical repair or reconstruction of the pinna (pinnaplasty)
Otosclerosis	Overgrowth of bone around stapes causing deafness
Pinna	Fleshy (cartilaginous) part of the ear
Presbyacusis	Sensorineural deafness associated with increasing age
Rhinitis	Inflammation of the mucous membranes of the nose
Rhinoplasty	Surgery to alter the shape of the nose
Rhinorrhoea	Watery mucous discharge from the nose
Septoplasty	Surgical procedure to reshape the nasal septum
Tinnitus	Sensation of sound in the absence of external stimulus
Tracheostomy	Surgical opening (hole) in the neck into the trachea
Vertigo	Hallucination of movement even whilst stationary

Ears

Otitis externa

Ask about pain, discharge, history of trauma, unilateral/bilateral, recent infections, itching
Look for tenderness, erythema, discharge
Management aural toilet, ear drops (steroid, ±antibiotic if infective cause); send exudate for M,C+S

Otitis media

Type	Features and management
Acute	Rapid onset, pain, fever, irritability, anorexia, vomiting *Examination* bulging eardrums, discharge if perforation *Treatment* analgesia, antibiotics if indicated
Chronic	Inflammation, discharge, painless, ↓hearing *Examination* exudate, thickened eardrum *Investigations* test hearing, swab discharge if possible *Treatment* lavage, antibiotics, steroid drops; refer to senior to assess if appropriate for surgery
Glue ear (otitis media with an effusion)	May cause painless hearing loss, ↓speech and language development in children *Examination* retracted/bulging eardrum, opaque, fluid level present *Investigations* test hearing, swab discharge *Treatment* review in outpatients regularly, may need myringotomy, grommet insertion, ±adenoidectomy; give antibiotics with steroid ear drops if indicated

Perforated eardrum

Ask about discharge, pain, changes in hearing, unilateral/bilateral symptoms, recent flights, trauma, diving

Look for discharge; no eardrum or tympanic perforation seen
Investigation swab if pus present
Management usually conservative, antibiotics if signs of infection

Adult deafness

- ***Conductive deafness*** ↓sound transmission through the external canal/ossicles, eg perforation, wax, foreign body in the ear canal, cholesteatoma

Management aural toilet, remove FB etc

- ***Sensorineural deafness*** affecting cochlea, eg presbyacusis (age-related deafness with loss of high-frequency hearing), infection (meningitis), Ménière's disease, ototoxic drugs (aminoglycosides), congenital, acoustic neuroma

Management assess severity; hearing aid, cochlear implant/other surgery

Tinnitus see p208

Vertigo see p209

Nose

Epistaxis

Ask about onset, duration, severity, previous episodes, frequency, trauma, ↑BP, NSAID/anticoagulation therapy, bleeding tendency, alcohol

Investigations stabilise first, postural BP, FBC, clotting/INR, LFT, E+S

Management put on gloves, apron and eye protection

- Sit patient up, tilt head down and apply pressure to the nasal cartilage.
- Pack the nostril with ribbon gauze soaked in Otrivine® for 5min
- If you can see the source of the bleeding apply silver nitrate sticks
- Pack with nasal tampons for 48h. Make sure you leave the attached string/ribbon hanging, so that they can be removed with ease
- If bleeding persists or severe, seek senior advice as they may need ligation/examination under anaesthetic

Nasal polyps

Ask about sex (♂>♀), watery discharge, postnasal drip, anosmia, taste disturbance, allergic rhinitis, chronic sinusitis, nasal blockage, voice changes, asthma, cystic fibrosis, snoring

Investigation rhinoscopy

Management steroid nasal drops, antibiotics if indicated, polypectomy

Allergic rhinitis

Ask about bilateral intermittent nasal blockage, itchy nose/eyes, sneezing, watery nasal discharge, precipitating factors, asthma

Look for swollen turbinates, discharge

Investigations *blds* RAST, allergy testing

Management ↓allergen exposure, steam inhalation, topical drugs (beclomethasone 2 puff/12h, sodium cromoglycate), drugs (eg loratidine 10mg/24h PO), refer to allergy clinic, desensitisation

Sinusitis

- ***Acute:*** frontal headache, facial pain (worse on moving/bending), URTI
- ***Chronic:*** postnasal drip, cough, frontal headache, facial pain, blocked nose, nasal polyps, history of allergic rhinitis

Look for clear fluid dripping from nose; tenderness around nasal bridge, cheeks and forehead

Management antibiotics, steam inhalation, steroid nasal spray, surgery

Nasal fractures

These do not require an X-ray as the nose is composed mostly of cartilage which is radio-translucent.

Symptoms/signs pain over nasal bridge, swelling, trauma; check for septal haematoma (cherry in septum); if present, contact your seniors urgently as needs draining

- ***Undisplaced*** analgesia and conservative management
- ***Visible deformity*** analgese and aim to reduce in 1–2wk

Throat

Tonsillitis

Think about EBV, URTI, agranulocytosis, leukaemia
Ask about pain (onset, duration), discharge, dysphagia, pain on swallowing, tender neck lumps, abdominal pain, anorexia, headache, fever, malaise, drugs, recurrent episodes
Look for inflamed, red tonsils, ±exudate, tender cervical lymphadenopathy
Investigations throat swab, FBC, CRP, ESR, Monospot/Paul Burnell antibodies (to exclude glandular fever)
Management rehydration, analgesia, gargle with salt water; *viral* conservative; *bacterial* penicillin V 500mg/6h PO (avoid amoxicillin/ampicillin); if unilateral consider excision biopsy
Tonsillectomy is becoming less popular due to the risk of CJD. Undertaken when recurrent episodes of tonsillitis are resulting in repeated school absence, where there is airway compromise (eg with sleep apnoea), where tonsils are chronically infected (>3mth with halitosis), quinsy or suspicion of malignancy.

Glandular fever (infectious mononucleosis, Epstein–Barr virus, EBV)
Ask about age, speed of onset, persistent sore throat, rash, lethargy, similar symptoms in friends/family
Look for malaise, fatigue, lymphadenopathy, splenomegaly, petechiae, rash
Investigations throat swab, FBC, LFT, CRP, ESR, Monospot/Paul Burnell
Management rest, rehydration, analgesia, gargle with warm saline/aspirin, avoid amoxicillin/ampicillin and avoid alcohol, treat secondary infection; consider short course of oral steroids

Dysphagia

Think about malignancy, lymphadenopathy, myasthenia gravis, stricture, pharyngeal pouch, achalasia, systemic sclerosis, oesophagitis, iron-deficiency anaemia
Ask about difficulty swallowing solids/liquids, onset, duration, worsening throughout the day, constant/intermittent, pain (odynophagia), neck bulging/gurgling, weight loss, vomiting, aspiration, choking
Investigations *blds* FBC, LFT, U+E, ESR *imaging* CXR, barium swallow, OGD ±biopsy, oesophageal motility studies
Management treat malnutrition (refer to dietician) and treat the cause

Hoarseness investigate urgently if duration ≥3wk
Think about laryngitis, URTI, trauma, malignancy, hypothyroidism, motor neurone disease, myasathenia gravis, laryngeal nerve palsy, smoking
Ask about weight loss, dysphagia, haemoptysis, change in voice, neck lumps, cough, smoking history, general malaise, weakness, lethargy, poor appetite
Look for neck lumps, cachexia, cranial nerve palsies
Investigations laryngoscopy, biopsy
Management treat the cause (OHCS6 p560)

Neck lumps

Think about see table below

Ask about age, unilateral/bilateral, onset, size (is it growing?), location, duration, pain, discharge, isolated/multiple

Look for scars, lumps, asymmetry, erythema; ask patient to protrude tongue and swallow; palpate neck from behind, feeling for masses and asymmetry, ask patient to take a sip of water; assess mass (see p434)

Investigations do not biopsy; refer for urgent USS, ±fine-needle aspiration cytology *blds* FBC, TFT, CRP, ESR *imaging* CT/MRI/CXR

Management treat the cause

Common neck lumps

Location	Differential diagnoses
Midline	Dermoid cyst, thyroglossal cyst, thyroid masses
Anterior triangle	Lymph nodes, branchial cyst, cystic hygroma, carotid body tumours, parotid tumours
Posterior triangle	Lymph nodes (TB, HIV), lymphoma, metastases, cervical rib

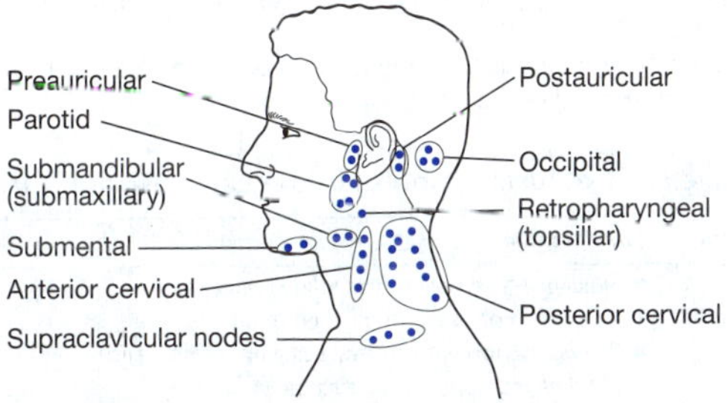

Lymph nodes of the head and neck

ENT tumours

Investigation by MRI/CT is essential.

Nasopharyngeal cancer

Symptoms epistaxis, diplopia, conductive deafness, blocked nose, neck lumps, difficulty breathing, change in smell, previous EBV infection, smoking/chewing tobacco
Investigations OGD, ±biopsy
Management radiotherapy, ±chemotherapy, ±surgery

Pharyngeal cancer

Symptoms sex (♂>♀), elderly, sore throat, sensation of lump at the back of throat, change in voice, dysphagia, intolerance to hot/cold foods, earache, difficulty breathing ***PMH*** Plummer-Vinson syndrome, smoking
Signs lymphadenopathy, trismus, angular stomatitis, glossitis, cachexia
Management surgery, radiotherapy

Acoustic neuroma benign space occupying lesion
Symptoms ipsilateral tinnitus, change in hearing/balance, facial numbness, or weakness
Signs signs of ↑ICP, cerebellar signs, multiple CN palsies
Management surgical excision

Foreign bodies (see table below)

- Establish what foreign body has been inserted and when; ask about its size and consistency
- Find out what symptoms the patient has in order to establish how urgent the removal of the object is

Management of foreign bodies in the ear, nose and throat

Location	Management
Ear	• *Small objects* syringe/warm saline lavage • *Insects* immobilise with oil, then remove • *Soft objects* forceps retrieval using magnifying lens • *Hard objects* apply gentle suction • If unsuccessful, book theatre for removal under GA
Nose	• Apply 2% lidocaine spray to vasoconstrict the mucosa • Use forceps/gentle suction to remove object • Consider using a Foley catheter to remove the object • May need exploration under GA; do not remove unless superficial
Throat	• May lead to acute airway obstruction • Attempt to dislodge using backslaps and abdominal thrusts • Visualise airway and remove obvious FB if possible • Consider intubation/cricothyrotomy

General practice

This chapter covers the most common GP consultations; the *Oxford Handbook of General Practice* (OHGP) covers a wider range in greater detail.

What you can do

Your GP is responsible for your clinical actions in the same way a consultant is responsible for you in hospital. You should agree clear boundaries with your GP and review these as you progress. You are allowed to:

- see patients alone, so long as they are reviewed by the GP in person or over the phone
- perform home visits alone, so long as you review the patient with the GP by phone or when you return. **NB** the GP needs to sign any prescriptions
- suggest management plans, investigations, prescriptions and referrals, but these should be reviewed by the GP before being acted upon

What you cannot do

- Send patients home without a review (unless the GP has specifically given you permission to do so for that particular consultation type)
- Prescribe – this should always be signed by the GP
- Order investigations without GP review
- Refer patients without GP review

The GP consultation

The widely read book *The Inner Consultation* (2nd edition, 2005) written by Roger Neighbour suggests a five-stage model for a GP consultation:

- ***Connecting*** Building rapport, 'getting on the patient's wavelength'
- ***Summarising*** Taking a focused history and showing you understand the patient's chief concerns
- ***Handing over*** Securing the patient's cooperation in a plan of action you are both happy with
- ***Safety netting*** Anticipating and planning for unexpected, serious or unlikely developments; examples are given throughout this chapter.
- ***Housekeeping*** Keeping oneself in good mental condition for each successive patient: 'The consultation's not over till you're ready for the next one'

A further useful concept in GP consultations is:

- ***Red flags*** Symptoms suggesting serious pathology that must be drawn to the GP's attention, examples are given throughout this chapter

Investigations GPs have immediate access to far fewer investigations than in a hospital. The following are usually available:

- ***Home visit*** pulse, BP, RR, cap refill, urine dipstick, BM, PEFR, $\pm O_2$ sats
- ***GP consultation*** pulse, BP, RR, cap refill, urine dipstick, BM, PEFR, O_2 sats, cervical swabs, ±ECG, phlebotomy (1–3d for results), spirometry
- ***Hospital*** X-rays, USS, ±CT, ±MRI, microbiology, histology, ABG, respiratory function, echo, ECG, phlebotomy

When ordering investigations write more clinical details on the forms than usual since it is difficult for the laboratories to contact you

Referrals GPs are the gatekeepers to the NHS, accordingly there are many referral and review options available. Hospital admission can often be avoided by considering alternative routes of referral. Options include:

Some referral options

Accident and emergency (dial 999)	Midwife
GP admission (ambulance, taxi, own car)	Health visitor
Acute psychiatry team	School nurse
Acute social services	Practice nurse
Hospital speciality 2wk wait (cancer)	Asthma nurse
Hospital speciality normal referral	Diabetic nurse
Yourself eg review in a week	Community nurse
Another member of your practice	Counsellor
Family planning clinic	Occupational health
GUM clinic	Complementary therapy
COPD home service	Social services

GP targets A large proportion of a GP's salary is derived from meeting government targets for specific diseases and risk factors. Many of these are simply educating patients, assessing risk factors, checking simple measurements and updating records. You should use the extra time allotted to your consultation to pursue these. Useful checks include:

- Check BP and weight
- Smoking/intent to stop/advice
- Alcohol intake/advice
- Exercise advice
- Diet advice
- Contraception and Smear tests
- Cholesterol check
- Vaccinations (children and flu)
- Asthma/diabetes review
- Chronic disease surveillance

Education A patient who understands their condition is much more likely to comply with treatment and take appropriate steps if their condition changes. Taking 5min to explain what hypertension is and why it needs treating can have a life-saving effect. Take every opportunity to empower patients to understand and treat their own problems.

Leaflets and further information Patients will remember only a fraction of what you have said. Writing down important points (eg changes in doses) and giving information leaflets will improve compliance and recall. The internet offers a wealth of information on different conditions – guide your patients towards some of the better sites (see p525).

Clinical generalism General practice requires more than a working knowledge of all the clinical specialities. GPs have to deal with undifferentiated illness, atypical presentations, multiple pathologies and inconsistent findings whilst making decisions in the absence of reliable evidence. Along with diagnosis and treatment they must consider how the disease affects individual patients and how individuals deal with their diseases.

Respiratory

Coughs and colds (SOB p165 and Paeds respiratory p393)

Red flag very unwell, unable to swallow, drooling, stridor, night sweats, weight loss, haemoptysis, SOB, chest pain

Acute causes *serious* epiglottitis, foreign body, PE, pulmonary oedema *common* URTI, croup, pneumonia, asthma, exacerbation of COPD, postnasal drip
Chronic causes (>2wk) *serious* lung cancer, cystic fibrosis, TB *common* postviral, postnasal drip, asthma, smoker's cough, COPD, bronchiectasis, oesophageal reflux, heart failure, ACE inhibitors, restrictive lung disease
Ask about duration, time of day, sputum quantity and colour (?bld), shortness of breath, chest pain, malaise, runny nose, ability to eat and drink, night sweats, weight loss, calf pain
Look for pyrexia, RR, O_2 sats, tonsils, lymphadenopathy, air entry, creps, bronchial breathing, ↑JVP, heart murmur, swollen calves or ankles
Management Most coughs and colds require minimal treatment; paracetamol can help. Consider PEFR. Specific treatments include:

- ***Postnasal drip*** beclomethasone 2puffs/12h intranasal or antihistamines
- ***Asthma*** and ***COPD*** see below; ***croup*** see p393
- ***Pneumonia*** amoxicillin 500mg/8h PO, refer if unwell (p168)

Persistent Consider FBC, U+E, CRP, CXR and respiratory function tests. Advice about reducing smoking.

Safety net reattend if no better in 1wk or feeling unwell, A+E if severely SOB

Asthma (OHGP1 p310)

Red flag low sats, PEFR <50%, incomplete sentences, recession, tachypnoea/cardia

Symptoms chronic cough, night/morning cough, poor exercise tolerance, short of breath, tight chest, atopy (hayfever, eczema), family history
338
Signs reduced PEFR, wheeze, Harrison's sulcus, barrel chest
Diagnosis symptom diary, PEFR diary (pre and post-inhaler), spirometry
Exacerbation regular salbutamol inhalers, ±oral steroids, ±amoxicillin
Chronic Use the treatment steps below, the aim is for no symptoms with minimal treatment. Practices often have asthma nurses who can monitor, check inhaler technique and recommend therapy.

	Step 1	Step 2	Step 3*		Step 4	Step 5
Oral steroids						✓
High-dose steroid inhaler				✓	✓	✓
Long-acting β-agonist			✓		✓	✓
Low-dose steroid inhaler		✓	✓			
Salbutamol/terbutaline	✓	✓	✓	✓	✓	✓

* Either low-dose steroid inhaler and long-acting β-agonist or high-dose steroid inhaler

Safety net asthma nurse if symptoms worsen, A+E if severely SOB

COPD (OHGP1 p316)

Red flag ↓GCS, cyanosis, tachypnoea, haemoptysis, night sweats, weight loss

Symptoms chronic cough, ±productive (?colour/bld), shortness of breath, recurrent resp infection, wheeze, reduced exercise tolerance, weight loss
Signs ↑RR, ↓O_2 sats, reduced PEFR, wheeze, creps, pursed lips
Diagnosis CXR, spirometry (with reversibility), trial of steroids
Exacerbation regular inhalers, ±oral steroids, ±amoxicillin, consider involving COPD home service to prevent unnecessary admission
Management Encourage to stop smoking and start exercising, inhalers as guided by spirometry; anticholinergic (ipratropium) and inhaled steroids are especially effective. May need home nebulisers or home O_2.

Safety net Attend if symptoms worsen, A+E if severely SOB

Common inhalers for asthma and COPD

Type of drug	Colour	Medication	Trade
Short-acting β-agonist	Blue	Salbutamol	Ventolin
	Blue	Terbutaline	Bricanyl
Inhaled steroids	Brown	Beclometasone	Becotide
	Brown	Budesonide	Pulmicort
	Orange	Fluticasone	Flixotide
Short-acting anticholinergic	White + green	Ipratropium	Atrovent
Short-acting β-agonist and anticholinergic	White + orange	Salbutamol and ipratropium	Combivent
Inhaled steroids with long-acting β-agonist	Red	Budesonide and formoterol	Symbicort
	Purple	Fluticasone and salmeterol	Seretide
Long-acting β-agonist	Green	Salmeterol	Serevent
Long-acting anticholinergic	Grey	Spiriva	Tiotropium

Hayfever and atopy (OHGP1 p780)

Red flag tachycardia, hypotension, stridor, tachypnoea, perioral oedema

Symptoms runny nose, recurrent blocked nose, cough, headaches, itchy and watering eyes, sneezing, rash, allergens (pollen, animals, nuts)
Signs clear nasal discharge, red/swollen nostrils
Management Allergen avoidance. Antihistamines are especially useful for hayfever (eg loratadine, cetirizine). Try intranasal steroid sprays or drops; decongestants can be tried short term (≤1wk). Patients with severe atopy or previous anaphylaxis should be prescribed two epinephrine pens (>12yr 0.3ml 1:1000 IM, ≤12yr see *BNF* 3.4.3) for home and school/work.

Safety net A+E if swelling, itching and SOB; prescribe epinephrine pens

Anaphylaxis 0.5ml 1:1000 IM epinephrine (adrenaline) can be repeated at 5min intervals whilst waiting for ambulance.

Cardiology and diabetes

Cardiac problems often require many drugs, be careful not to prescribe:

- β-blockers in patients with asthma
- β-blockers with Ca^{2+} channel blockers (verapamil and diltiazem)
- aspirin with warfarin

Cardiac risk factors (OHGP1 p232)

Many causes of coronary heart disease are reversible. The OHGP and the back of *BNF* have Framingham charts to estimate a well patient's 10yr risk. All patients should be encouraged to exercise, stop smoking and improve their diet (↓salt). As risk increases the reversible risk factors should be targeted (cholesterol, smoking, BP, diabetic control, weight).

Hypertension (p159 or OHGP1 p220)

Red flag BP ≥200/110, headache, ↓GCS, visual problems, pregnancy (cf booking BP)

Causes essential (95%), alcohol, renal disease, diabetes, steroids, Conn's, phaeochromocytoma, acromegaly, pregnancy, aortic coarctation
Symptoms usually asymptomatic, eye, kidney, heart or renal problems
Signs BP>140/90mmHg, displaced apex, heart failure, retinopathy
GP monitoring Hypertension should be recorded on ≥3 occasions before starting treatment unless worrying signs are present. Checks should take place over weeks if BP is 199/109 to 160/100 or months if 159/99 to 140/90. Consider 24h ambulatory monitoring if anxious or in doubt.
Investigations FBC, U+E, fasting glucose, lipids, urine dipstick, ECG, consider echo if LVH suspected (p163)
Management education, exercise, stop smoking, reduce alcohol, restrict salt, diet, relaxation. Aspirin 75–150mg/24h PO if ≥50yr. Antihypertensive medications include thiazides, ACEi, β-blockers, α-blockers, Ca^{2+} blockers. β-blockers and bendrofluazide are common 1st line treatments. Warn patients about side-effects (eg cold hands, erectile dysfunction).

Safety net reattend if visual problems, medication side-effects, regular monitoring

Angina (Chest pain p127 or OHGP1 p240)

Red flag pain at rest or minimal exertion, increasing frequency/severity of attacks

Symptoms central/left chest pain or tightness, radiating to left arm or jaw, brought on by exertion/cold/emotion, improved with rest/GTN
Signs often normal, may have displaced apex, exclude arrhythmias
Investigations FBC, ESR, TFT, fasting glucose, lipids, ECG (p514), exercise ECG, may need angiography (referral)
Acute see p126, sit up, O_2, GTN, aspirin, urgent referral (dial 999)
Management Control risk factors (see above), start aspirin 75–150mg/24h PO and prescribe a GTN spray. Medications to improve symptoms: nitrates (eg ISMN), β-blockers, Ca^{2+} channel blockers. Many districts have rapid access chest pain clinics if symptoms are escalating.

Safety net reattend if frequent attacks, A+E if acutely SOB or chest pain >20min

Post MI (OHGP1 p244)

Educate regarding need to continue meds, check U+E (ACEi and statin).

Heart failure (OHGP1 p246)

Red flag chest pain, arrhythmia, tachypnoea, swelling above the ankle

LVF symptoms short of breath, reduced exercise tolerance, tiredness, orthopnoea, cough worse at night, pink/frothy sputum
RVF symptoms swollen ankles, tiredness, nausea
Signs ↑JVP, 3rd heart sound, displaced apex, symmetrical basal creps, wheeze, pleural effusions, ascites, tender hepatomegaly, pitting oedema
Investigations FBC, U+E, LFT, TFT, glucose, cholesterol and lipids, ECG (p514), CXR (enlarged heart, p508), echo
Acute see p170, sit up, 100% O_2, urgent referral (dial 999)
Management Stop smoking, exercise, adequate diet (↓salt), control BP. Drugs with a life-prolonging effect: β-blockers, ACEi (see starting an ACEi, p163), spironolactone, nitrates; other drugs with only symptomatic improvement: diuretics and digoxin. Review regularly.

Safety net reattend early if swelling or SOB worsens, A+E if acutely SOB/chest pain

High cholesterol (OHGP1 p226)

Management Low cholesterol diet (fish, vegetables, margarine) can lower cholesterol by 10%. Statins improves prognosis if total cholesterol is ≥5mmol/l but are usually only prescribed if risk ≥30% or post MI/CVA.

Aspirin (OHGP1 p230)

Prescribed to patients with ↑BP and age ≥50yr, previous angina, MI, stroke, intermittent claudication, atrial fibrillation (unless on warfarin).

Diabetes (p236 and OHGP1 p284)

Red flag weight loss, polyuria, thirst, vomiting, ketones

See p236 for presentation and diagnosis.
Monitoring urine dipsticks, BM, HbA_{1C}, BP, cholesterol
Acute management Refer new type 1 diabetics to exclude DKA and start an insulin regime. Start treatment and monitoring in type 2 (p237).
Chronic management Education and regular reviews are essential. Aim for rigorous control of cardiac risk factors (opposite) and encourage self-monitoring and treatment to reduce complications. Ensure the patient is familiar with the 'sick day rules', ie what to do if feeling ill:

- never stop taking your insulin or tablets (may need to increase dose)
- test your blood for glucose ≥4 times a day
- test your urine for glucose (and ketones if on insulin)
- drink plenty of liquids
- if not eating try milk, soup, cereals, fruit juice or fizzy drinks instead
- contact your GP or diabetes team if you cannot keep fluids down

Diabetic review check for chest pain, leg pain, numbness/tingling, erectile problems; review foot care and problems, inspect feet and pulses; check visual acuity and retina; check urine dipstick; discuss cardiac risk factors and their treatment/prevention, check BP; discuss other reviews and appointments

Safety net reattend if feeling acutely unwell or losing weight

Other medical problems

Headache	p210/OHGP1 p826	**Abdo pain**	p183/OHGP1 p488

Fatigue and tiredness (OHGP1 p888)

Red flag weight loss, polyuria, bone pain, haemoptysis, melaena, suicidal

Causes *serious* diabetes, cancer *common* depression, anxiety, alcohol, recreational drugs, anaemia, hypothyroid, infections (EBV, CMV), menopause, insomnia (p285), heart/renal failure, antihistamines, sedatives, chronic fatigue

Ask about duration, onset, exacerbating factors (exertion suggests physical illness), change through day (worst in morning suggests depression), sleep quality and hygiene, early morning waking (depression), snoring, weight loss, urinary frequency, thirst, swelling, recent colds or sore throat, SOB, cough, worries, anorexia, anhedonia

Look for pyrexia, lymphadenopathy, tonsils, CVS, resp, abdo and neuro for physical disease, consider depression scoring (p407)

Management Investigate physical illnesses suggested by history and/or examination; consider FBC, U+E, ESR, TFT, fasting glucose and EBV serology. Low threshold for urine dipstick or BM if diabetes is possible, further investigations rarely help. Sleep hygiene advice p285.

Chronic fatigue Acute onset, often following a viral infection, fatigue is worse after exertion and accompanied by muscle/joint pain, headaches, sore throat or poor concentration. Treat with reassurance, cognitive behavioural therapy and antidepressants. See OHGP1 p374.

Safety net reattend if feeling acutely unwell or losing weight

Health promotion

Smoking (OHGP1 p170) Repeated advice will help 5% people give up per year. Encourage picking a day to throw all the cigarettes and lighters away. Nicotine gum, patches and sprays are prescribable. Repeated reviews and support groups help to prevent and limit relapses.

Alcohol (see p24 and OHGP1 p172) Targets are: <21u/wk for men (>50u is high intake) and <14u for women (>35u). Monitor FBC (↑MCV) and LFT (↑γGT). Strategies include drink diaries, Alcoholics Anonymous, community alcohol teams. Chlordiazepoxide for withdrawal is rarely prescribed by GPs, refer to psychiatry.

Exercise (OHGP1 p168) Aim for at least 30min of exercise twice a week at a level that induces slight breathlessness. Walking, cycling and swimming are all good low impact sports.

Diet and obesity (OHGP1 p162) Encourage patients to eat fresh vegetables and fruit with less fat, sugar and salt. Exercise, low calorie healthy diets and encouragement all help weight loss. Dieting medications (eg orlistat and phenteramine) are controversial, consider discussing with a specialist. Low carbohydrate diets (eg Atkins) do promote weight loss, but their long-term effects are currently unknown.

Psychiatry

See p400, includes psychiatric history, mental state examination, suicidal risk factors, depression scoring and numerous diseases.

Depression (see p404 or OHGP1 p870)

Red flag anhedonia, suicidal intent and plans, previous DSH, psychosis

Common and underdiagnosed, especially in the elderly and adolescents.
Symptoms low mood, lack of pleasure (anhedonia), suicidal, early morning waking, insomnia, tiredness, lack of energy, poor concentration, agitated, feeling worthless/guilty, anorexia, weight change, stressful events
Signs self-neglect, poor eye contact, objectively low mood
Treatment Acute psychiatric review if suicidal or psychotic. Treatment options include: education, problem-solving strategies, self-help groups, exercise, counselling, cognitive behavioural therapy (CBT), other psychological therapies. Refer if not improving despite ≥2 attempts at treatment.
Antidepressants should be prescribed for persistent or moderate/severe depression, eg tricyclics (dangerous in overdose), SSRIs and MAOIs. Tell the patient that they take 2–6wk to have an effect and that stopping them suddenly can cause withdrawal. Monitor regularly.

Safety net monitor regularly (1–2wk), reattend or A+E if feeling suicidal/harmful

Anxiety (see p408 of OHGP1 p864)

Red flag recurrent sudden headaches, weight loss, severe chest pain

Anxiety can be psychological (fearful, restless, poor concentration, obsessions) or physical (tingling, chest discomfort, fluttering heart). There are several types of anxiety disorder:

- Simple phobias (eg jellyfish)
- Social phobias (eg agoraphobia)
- Post-traumatic stress disorder
- Obsessive-compulsive disorder
- Panic
- Somatization ('hypochondria')

Differentials physical illness can cause anxiety: hyperthyroid, hypoglycaemia, phaechromocytoma, Cushing's, stoke/TIAs, chronic fatigue
Physical illness be open to the possibility of new physical illness, eg MI
Treatment explore beliefs, reassurance, education, avoid phobias, ↓caffeine, counselling, self-help groups, CBT, antidepressants, refer if diagnostic doubt or uncontrollable anxiety, try to avoid benzodiazepines

Safety net monitor regularly (1–2wk), reattend or A+E if acutely unwell

Dementia (see p410 or OHGP1 p880)

Red flag acute onset, weakness, headache, confusion, slurred speech

Symptoms forgetful, neglect, unable to cope, altered personality
Signs self-neglect, falls, check mini-mental state (p403)
Investigations FBC, U+E, LFT, Ca^{2+}, TFT, glucose, ESR, B_{12}, folate, CXR, MSU, consider VDRL (syphilis) and HIV. Consider depression.
Treatment Refer to a psychogeriatrican to confirm diagnosis, social services, benefits, check vision, hearing and exclude UTI. Use anticholinesterase inhibitors for Alzheimer's and aspirin/BP control if vascular.

Safety net Reattend/home visit if acute deterioration/new symptoms

Orthopaedics

Back pain (p223 or OHGP1 p340)

Red flag bilateral leg pain, bladder/bowel changes, progressive/night pain, weight loss, age <20yr or >55yr, steroids, thoracic or non-mechanical pain, previous Ca

Causes serious cauda equina, cancer, myeloma *common* mechanical pain, Paget's, ankylosing spondylitis, vertebral collapse
Ask about trauma, onset, duration, leg pain, numbness, weakness, location, bladder and bowel changes, weight loss, worse at night
Look for back movements whilst standing, tenderness, leg power, sensation and reflexes, straight leg raise (mechanical if pain at <45°)
Investigations if red flag symptoms FBC, ESR, Ca^{2+}, PO_4^{3-}, ALP, lumbar spine and pelvic X-rays
Management Prescribe adequate analgesia:

- ***Mechanical*** Reassure and educate regarding posture, weight, lifting. Analgesia and diazepam 2mg/8h PO for muscle spasm. Suggest/refer to a chiropractor. If no improvement by 4wk refer to orthopaedics if sciatica is present or a back pain team (OT, physio and psych) if not
- ***Red flag symptoms*** refer and perform investigations above
- ***Cauda equina*** see p223, admit urgently to orthopaedics

Safety net reattend if no change, A+E if bladder/bowel problems or bilateral neuro

Osteoarthritis (see p416 or OHGP1 p358)

Red flag pyrexia, hot and swollen joint

Symptoms joint pain and stiffness, clicking, deformity
Signs effusion, pain on moving, reduced movement, crepitus
Investigations X-rays show ↓joint space, cysts, osteophytes and sclerosis
Management Exercise and muscle strengthening, stop smoking, weight reduction, walking stick, hot/cold pads may help. Pain relief (p282), creams eg capsaicin and deep heat, steroid injections. Refer if diagnosis in doubt or symptoms uncontrolled (wash out, joint replacement).

Safety net reattend if acute worsening of symptoms or unable to cope at home

Osteoporosis (OHGP1 p360)

Aim to prevent prior to a fracture or treat aggressively afterwards. Risk factors include early menopause, age, female, low BMI (especially previous eating disorder), family history, dairy intolerance, steroids, alcohol. Screen those at risk by DXA scan to check bone mineral density (BMD).
Management stop smoking, regular weight-bearing exercise, reducing falls, calcium and vitamin D supplements, bisphosphonates (especially if on steroids), Protelos® (strontium ranelate). HRT should only be used for short term relief of menopausal symptoms (<5yr).

Minor injuries

See p306 for treatment of common injuries and p440 or OHGP1 p336 for specific joint examinations and problems. Referral options include A+E, X-ray or review after treatment with NSAIDs. Most cuts can be treated with simple cleaning, glue or steristrips. Check tetanus status.

Ears and throats

See p326 for examination and treatment of common ENT conditions.

Earache and deafness (OHGP1 p782)

Red flag very unwell, unilateral hearing loss, peripheral perforation, mastoid pain

Acute causes *serious* mastoiditis, foreign body *common* URTI, otitis media, otitis externa, earwax

Chronic causes *serious* cholesteatoma, acoustic neuroma *common* glue ear, chronic suppurative otitis media (CSOM), earwax, presbyacusis

Ask about onset, duration, discharge, itching, hearing loss, speech problems, runny nose, sore throat, trauma, malaise

Look for pyrexia, appearance of eardrum (?perforated), effusion, colour of canal, discharge, tonsils, lymphadenopathy, sinus pain, teeth, mastoid

Management Most earache simply requires analgesia, consider:

- ***Otitis media*** pus/bloody discharge if drum perforated, red, bulging drum, ±effusion; analgesia, amoxicillin if ≥3d, perforated or unilateral
- ***Otitis externa*** itching, tender, discharge, ±pus; clean canal and keep dry (may need oral toilet by ENT), give gentamicin + steroid ear drops

Persistent Consider hearing tests:

- ***Ear wax*** olive oil, ±syringing so long as drum not perforated
- ***Presbyacusis*** bilateral hearing loss with age, consider hearing aid
- ***Glue ear*** persistent middle ear effusion with deafness usually lasts 3–6mth; a 2–6wk course of amoxicillin may help. ENT referral for grommets is only required if persistent and falling behind at school
- ***CSOM*** central perforation of drum, treat as for otitis externa

Peripheral perforations (***cholesteatoma***) and unilateral deafness (***acoustic neuroma***) require ENT referral

Safety net reattend if persistent discharge or hearing/speech problems

Sore throats (OHGP1 p774)

Red flag unilateral tonsillar enlargement, unable to swallow, tonsils meeting in midline, very unwell, night sweats, weight loss

Causes *serious* quinsy (peritonsillar abscess – seen in adults), retropharyngeal abscess (children), leukaemia *common* viral sore throat, tonsillitis, glandular fever

Ask about duration, cough, malaise, runny nose, ability to eat and drink, night sweats, weight loss

Look for pyrexia, enlarged tonsils, red throat, pus, lymphadenopathy

Management Reassurance, gargle with salt water, regular analgesia (paracetamol and ibuprofen), hot drinks, over-the-counter medications (Difflam, Lemsip, Strepsils, see *BNF*). Consider antibiotics (penicillin V 500mg/6h PO or erythromycin 500mg/6h PO) if persistent or pus seen.

Persistent Consider alternative diagnosis including FBC and EBV serology. May need referral to ENT for tonsillectomy if:

- ≥5 sore throats needing time off each year for two years
- ≥3mth sore throat
- sleep apnoea or unilateral enlargement

Safety net reattend if no improvement in 3–5d or feeling unwell

Obstetrics and gynaecology

See p350, includes history and examinations, contraception, pregnancy problems, period/bleeding problems and gynae infections.

Pill checks (OHGP1 p616)

Women taking the COC or POP need a review 3mth after starting and then every 6mth. This review should cover:

- ***Problems*** headaches, weight gain, bloating, breakthrough bleeding, depression, acne, breast tenderness
- Check ***blood pressure***
- ***Education*** stop smoking, DVT risks, missed pill rules (if >12h take next pill at normal time, use alternative contraception for 7d, start another pack without a break if due to finish pack within 7d), similar precautions if vomiting, severe diarrhoea or some drugs (eg ABx)

NB The OCP should not be prescribed to women ≥35yr who smoke.

Safety net reattend in 6mth, immediately if painful, ±swollen leg

Smear test (OHGP1 p580)

Screening for cervical cancer should be offered to all women aged 25–64yr (or younger if sexually active for >3yr). The test is often performed by the practice nurse and should be repeated every 3yr unless previous tests were abnormal and frequent monitoring is required.

Pregnancy (see p368 and OHGP1 p630)

Pre-pregnancy Folic acid 400μg/24h PO and review regular medications.

Pregnant If a women suspects she is pregnant check her urine for β-HCG (+ve from day 10 to week 20) and refer to the midwives. Check the following at presentation (booking) and further consultations:

- Oedema
- Blood pressure (cf booking BP)
- Urine dipstick (protein/glucose)
- Bump size (see p370)
- Foetal heart beat after 12wk
- Foetal movements after 20wk

Post-pregnancy consider contraception, breast problems, depression and pelvic floor exercises. By the 6wk postnatal check the uterus should not be palpable and bleeding should have stopped.

Heavy and painful periods (see p357 and OHGP1 p588)

Red flag intermenstrual bleeding (p357), weight loss, tachycardia, hypotension

Heavy if large clots or requiring >5 tampons/towels a day.

Causes dysfunctional uterine bleeding (50%), fibroids, infection, congenital abnormality, endometriosis, polyps, IUCD, cancer, coagulopathy

Investigations usually none: FBC, clotting, TFT, smear, swabs, USS

Treatment exercise, stop smoking, paracetamol, mefenamic acid, tranexamic acid, oral contraceptive pill, refer if no improvement after 3–6mth

Safety net reattend in 3–6mth if no improvement, sooner if feeling unwell

Menopause and HRT (see p365 and OHGP1 p596)

HRT should only be prescribed for 5yr to treat acute symptoms unless menopause/ovarian failure is premature (eg age 35–40yr).

Paediatrics

See p386, includes recognising sick children, vaccination schedule, history, examination, developmental stages, resp and abdo problems.

Child health check-ups (OHGP1 p680)

Children are seen routinely 6 times between birth and starting school: neonatal (<48h), 6wk, 8mth, 18mth, 3yr and preschool (4yr). These checks are to address parental concerns, ensure normal development, growth, vision and hearing, check vaccinations and offer health promotion advice.

Rashes (OHGP1 p734)

Red flag unwell, headache, not acting normal self, non-blanching

Causes *serious* meningitis, HSP, ITP *common* viral rash, eczema, nappy rash, seborrhoeic eczema (including cradle cap)

Ask about onset, location, spread, itching, painful, trauma, malaise, urine output, eating and drinking

Look for location, distribution, character (p320), red ears/throat

Management Urgent referral for non-blanching rashes, give benzylpenicillin if unwell, for other rashes:

- ***Nappy rash*** caused by contact with urine/faeces, use absorbent nappies, regular changing and time without nappies; zinc barrier creams and aqueous cream instead of soap; antifungal cream if not clearing
- ***Seborrhoeic eczema*** shiny red rash in groin/axilla (treat with aqueous cream and 1% hydrocortisone) or yellow crusting to scalp or neck (treat with 2% salicyclic acid and zinc paste, wash out after application)
- ***Eczema*** aqueous cream, bath emollients, topical steroids, antibiotics if signs of infection, antihistamines if itching is a problem
- ***Viral rash*** try to identify the source (eyes, ears, urine), if well discharge with safety netting, if unwell consider referring

Safety net reattend if rash not improving or becomes unwell

Warts and verrucas (OHGP1 p478)

Symptoms warty lesions on hands or feet, usually resolve in <6mth, can be painful, especially on feet

Treatment spontaneous resolution (ie watch and wait), topical salicylic acid, cryotherapy (painful), curettage (single warts)

Acne (OHGP1 p466)

Red flag hypertension, diabetes, weight gain, vasculitis

Symptoms spots over head, neck and back, otherwise well

Signs whiteheads, blackheads, pustules, scars and sinuses

Treatment Ask if bothered by spots (may be embarrassed), reassurance, wash twice daily with soap, moisturisers, topical benzoyl peroxide, retinoids (topical or oral – Roaccutane® requires dermatology referral), antibiotics (topical or oral). NB if prescribing females tetracycline give contraception as well (teratogenic) – Dianette® may also help the acne

Safety net reattend if not improving – there are other treatments

Haematology

Leukaemia (OHCM6 p650–7)

Type		Patient	Prognosis
Acute	Lymphoblastic (ALL)	2–4yr or >60yr	Children 80% cure Elderly <20% cure
	Myeloid (AML)	Old>young, post-chemo	20% 3yr survival
Chronic	Lymphocytic (CLL)	>40yr, often male	60% 5yr survival
	Myeloid (CML)	Middle aged	50% 5yr survival

Symptoms recurrent/unusual infection, easy bruising, bleeding, joint pain, bone pain, malaise, weakness, abdo pain, weight loss, sweats
Signs pale, petechiae, bruises, bleeding (check gums), lymphadenopathy, signs of infection, hepatosplenomegaly, focal neurology
Investigations FBC (anaemia, ↑WCC, look at differential), blood film, U+E, LFT, LDH, urate, ESR, clotting, bone marrow biopsy
Treatment *acute* antibiotics, blood and platelet transfusions *chronic* chemotherapy, radiotherapy, bone marrow transplant
Complications infection, bleeding (DIC), hyperviscosity, cell lysis

Lymphoma (OHCM6 p658–60)

Type	Patient	Prognosis
Hodgkin's	Young adults or elderly, often male	60–90% 5yr survival
Non-Hodgkin's	Low grade >50yr, high grade <35yr	40% 5yr survival

Symptoms enlarged non-tender lumps, fever, night sweats, infection, itching, tiredness, weight loss, malaise, weakness, rarely pain with alcohol
Signs pale, lymphadenopathy, hepatosplenomegaly
Investigations FBC, blood film, U+E, LFT, Ca^{2+}, LDH, urate, ESR, CXR, CT/MRI of thorax, abdo and pelvis, lymph node and bone marrow biopsy
Treatment chemotherapy, radiotherapy
Complications infection, bone marrow failure, SVC obstruction

Paraproteinaemia Several diseases can cause an excess of a single (clonal) immunoglobulin including **myeloma** (see p245). Elderly patients may get a benign monoclonal gammopathy that causes a mild but stable increase in IgG, IgM or IgA, often mistaken for myeloma. A raised IgM can also be caused by the malignant Waldenström's macroglobulinaemia.

Myeloproliferative disease (OHCM6 p664)

A group of neoplastic diseases including:

- polycythaemia rubra vera (↑RBCs – angina, focal neurology)
- essential thrombocythaemia (↑platelets – bleeding, thrombosis)
- myelofibrosis (↑fibroblasts – bone marrow failure, splenomegaly)

Causes of lymphadenopathy

Infection local infection, EBV, CMV, hepatitis, HIV, TB, syphilis, toxoplasmosis, bartonella 'cat-scratch', fungal **malignancy** lymphoma, leukaemia, metastases **autoimmune** SLE, rheumatoid **other** sarcoidosis, amyloidosis, drugs

Pancytopenia – ↓Hb, ↓plts and ↓WCC (OHCM6 p662)
Marrow failure aplastic anaemia, malignancy, myelodysplasia, fibrosis
Non-marrow hypersplenism, SLE, infection (eg TB, AIDS)
Investigations FBC, blood film, bone marrow biopsy
Treatment treat the underlying cause, blood and platelet transfusions

Sickle-cell disease and trait (OHCM6 p640)
Common genetic disease in African and Caribbean populations; all patients with an Afro-Caribbean background must be tested pre-op.
Homozygote haemolytic anaemia (Hb 6–8g/dl), ↑reticulocytes, ↑bilirubin
Complications thrombosis, aplastic anaemia, severe haemolysis, cerebral infarction, priaprism, gallstones, avascular necrosis, sickle crisis
Heterozygote (trait) normal Hb, healthy; can get sickle-cell crises from hypoxia eg surgery, severe disease, strenuous exercise, high altitude, cold
Sickle crisis Thrombosis secondary to hypoxia or infection can cause infarctions and severe pain (long bones, back, ribs, sternum, chest). Chest symptoms (pleuritic pain and SOB) are serious and may need ITU.
Treatment Warmth, O_2, IV fluids, analgesia (often IV opioids), folic acid, ±antibiotics, avoid acidosis. May need an exchange transfusion.

Thalassaemia (OHCM6 p642)
These are common genetic diseases in Mediterranean, Arabian and Asian populations. ***β thalassaemia major*** (homozygote) and ***α thalassaemia*** cause severe anaemia that requires treatment (see below). ***β thalassaemia minor*** (heterozygote) causes a mild anaemia (>9g/dl, MCV<75fl) that rarely requires treatment.
Treatment repeated transfusions, desferrioxamine (protection against iron overload), folate, ascorbic acid, may need splenectomy

Causes of splenomegaly

Massive CML, myelofibrosis, malaria, leishmaniasis **moderate** EBV, HIV, endocarditis, TB, leukaemia, lymphoma, malignancy, autoimmune, sarcoidosis, amyloidosis, portal hypertension, haemolysis, sickle cell, thalassaemia, paraproteinaemia

Splenectomy Performed after trauma, cysts, tumours and the treatment of some haematological disease. Patients are immunocompromised by the operation so should have pneumococcal, haemophilus type B and meningitis A+C vaccines (ideally before splenectomy) and yearly flu vaccine. They should take penicillin V for 2yr post-splenectomy (or until age 16yr) and start amoxicillin at the first sign of infection.

Bone marrow aspiration and biopsy This is a common investigation of haematological disease. The sample is taken from the iliac crest or sternum via a small incision made under local anaesthetic. The needle is gently drilled through the bone cortex and 2–3ml of marrow is aspirated; a marrow biopsy may be taken with another needle. Complications include bleeding, infection and pain.

Graft vs host disease Rashes, vomiting, diarrhoea and deranged LFT following bone marrow transplants in immunocompromised patients. Discuss with transplant centre and treat with high-dose steroids.

Obstetrics and gynaecology

As well as taking a good general history (p114) you also need to ask some specific questions:

Gynaecological history

- ***Menstrual history*** cycle length and regularity, duration of periods, age at menarche/menopause
- ***PV bleeding*** intermenstrual bleeding, postcoital bleeding, post-menopausal. Ask about menorrhagia (clots, flooding). How many pads/tampons are needed per day?
- ***Sexual history*** age at first intercourse, dyspareunia (deep or superficial), type of intercourse, travel abroad, history of STIs (specifically PID)
- ***Contraception*** barrier methods, oral, depo, intrauterine devices
- ***Cervical smear history*** always normal? Last smear date? Ever been seen in colposcopy clinic?
- ***Previous gynaecological operations*** or problems
- ***Family history*** of malignancy (reproductive tract, breast or bowel)
- ***Other*** urinary symptoms (p366), prolapse, history of breast/thyroid problems, medications eg use of HRT

Obstetric history

- ***Gravida*** total number of pregnancies, including current pregnancy, terminations, miscarriages and stillbirths
- ***Parity*** number of pregnancies ≥20wk (includes stillbirths)
- ***Terminations and miscarriages*** at what gestation, why and how?
- ***Last menstrual period*** (LMP) and length of gestation
- ***Problems conceiving*** history of subfertility, IVF
- ***Symptoms during pregnancy*** hyperemesis, PV bleeding, discharge
- ***Delivery history*** normal vaginal deliveries, instrumental (forceps, ventouse). Previous Caesarean sections: elective or emergency? Why? Birthweight and sex of the baby. Did baby spend time on the SCBU?
- ***Complications of pregnancy*** gestational diabetes, hypertension, pre-eclampsia, anaemia, bleeding, concerns about fetal growth. Any hospital admissions during pregnancy?
- ***Family history*** multiple pregnancies, hypertension, DM, pre-eclampsia

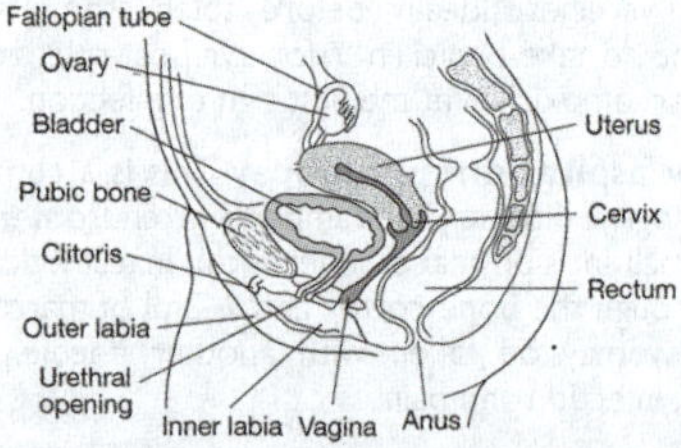

Structure of the female genitourinary system

Examination

This involves three parts: abdominal, vaginal and speculum examination. Always have a chaperone (who can also guard the door) and interview the patient without other family members present as they may inhibit the patient's responses.

- ***Abdominal examination*** *inspect* for scars, striae, hernias, distribution of body hair, tense abdomen, everted umbilicus *palpate* for masses, tenderness *percuss* to check for solid masses, shifting dullness
- ***Per vaginal examination*** *inspect* vulva and vagina for ulcers, lumps, prolapse, discharge, bleeding, swelling, erythema *palpate* the cervix (texture, consistency, cervical excitation), uterus bimanually (size, shape, consistency, regularity, mobility, tenderness, position: anteverted/retroverted), adnexae (look for tenderness, masses)
- ***Speculum examination*** *Cuscoe's* ask the patient to lie flat on her back (supine) with knees bent and flopped apart. Look at the cervix (ulceration, bleeding, cysts, irregularities) and the cervical os (open in multiparous women), take swabs/cervical smear *Sim's* position the patient as for PR and use the speculum to pull back each vaginal wall in turn (used to examine prolapses)
- ***Per rectal examination*** helps distinguish an enterocele and rectocele, assess cervical cancer spread/presence of endometriosis

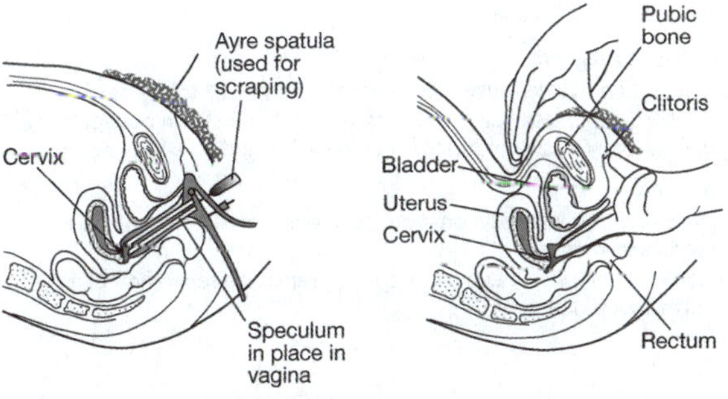

Speculum (left) and bimanual examination (right)

Common investigations

- ***β-HCG (serum or urine)*** serum levels double every 48h in the first trimester of pregnancy, reaching a peak at 12wk
- ***Triple swabs*** high vaginal, endocervical, chlamydial, ±urethral
- ***Tumour markers*** CA 125 (see p378)
- ***Pelvic USS (vaginal or abdominal)*** to exclude pelvic masses
- ***Pipelle biopsy*** endometrial sampling without visualisation (outpatients)
- ***Hysteroscopy*** endometrial visualisation and sampling; may be therapeutic, eg polypectomy, curettage
- ***Laparoscopy*** for diagnostic and therapeutic purposes

Useful definitions in obstetrics and gynaecology

Periods

- *Primary amenorrhoea* failure to start menstruating by 16yr
- *Secondary amenorrhoea* lack of menstruation for >6mth (not due to pregnancy)
- *Oligomenorrhoea* infrequent periods, >42d cycle
- *Menorrhagia* excessive blood loss during periods, >80ml
- *Menopause* the last menstruation
- *Climacteric* transition period occurring prior to menopause

Pain

- *Dysmenorrhoea* painful periods
- *Dyspareunia* pain associated with sexual intercourse

Pregnancy

- *Termination of pregnancy (TOP)* removal of an unwanted pregnancy <24/40
- *Miscarriage* delivery/loss of pregnancy with no signs of life <24/40
- *Stillbirth* delivery of a fetus showing no signs of life >24/40
- *Pre-term delivery* delivery between 24–37/40 gestation
- *Trimester* pregnancy is divided into three periods according to gestation; first trimester is ≤14/40; second trimester is 15–28/40; third trimester is beyond this

Bleeding in pregnancy

- *Antepartum haemorrhage* bleeding from the genital tract >24/40
- *Postpartum haemorrhage* blood loss >500ml in first 24h post-delivery (primary); excessive blood loss between 24h and 6wk (secondary)

Placenta

- *Placenta praevia* partial/complete positioning of placenta in lower uterine segment
- *Placental abruption* bleeding following premature separation of a normally sited placenta

β-HCG measurements

- Detected in maternal serum within 7d of conception
- Detected in maternal urine by the time of next period
- –ve urine β-HCG test excludes 97% of pregnancies; –ve serum β-HCG excludes 100%
- Serum β-HCG doubles every 48h in first trimester; a suboptimal rise may indicate an ectopic pregnancy
- β-HCG >1000iu/ml should result in a visible fetal sac on transvaginal USS, otherwise exclude ectopic pregnancy
- Not detected reliably after 20/40

Gynaecology

Emergencies

Ectopic pregnancy usually presents at 6–9wk
Symptoms abdominal pain, shoulder tip/back pain, PV bleeding, history of amenorrhoea, dizziness *ruptured ectopic*: collapse, shock, peritonism
Risk factors ↑maternal age, previous ectopic, tubal surgery, previous STIs/PID, IUCD, assisted conception techniques
Signs unilateral iliac fossa tenderness, guarding *PV* extreme tenderness on touching cervix
Investigations β-HCG (serum and urine), FBC, G+S/crossmatch, transvaginal ultrasound (look for fetal sac/pole in the adnexae, free fluid in Pouch of Douglas)
Differentials miscarriage, appendicitis, pelvic infection, ovarian cyst accident
Management IV access (14–16G) and fluids *conservative* (if haemodynamically stable, monitor β-HCG; if doubling every 48h, likely IUP) *Surgical* (laparoscopic/open salpingectomy/salpingostomy or oophorectomy; send sample for histology) *medical* (methotrexate sometimes used for small <3.5mm early ectopics in stable patients)
Giving methotrexate: this is a cytotoxic agent and should not be administered without senior advice or following local protocols.

Ovarian cysts 2 main acute presentations: haemorrhage or torsion
Symptoms lower abdominal pain (acute onset), vomiting
Signs pyrexia, unilateral iliac fossa tenderness (±rebound/guarding), ±palpable mass *PV* adnexal tenderness and palpable mass, may have features of shock
Haemorrhage usually resolves in 2–4wk; check CA 125 and USS pelvis; organise USS in 6wk to review cyst size. If haemodynamically unstable, prepare for laparoscopic or open cystectomy/oophorectomy.

Torsion severe abdo pain with vomiting, usually patient fails to settle. USS shows a mass, requires urgent oophorectomy.
Non-acute presentation pelvic mass, dull abdominal pain/discomfort, ↑abdominal girth, urinary symptoms, change in bowel habit, leg oedema

Toxic shock syndrome *Staph. aureus* associated with tampon use
Symptoms fever, headache, lower abdominal pain, vomiting, diarrhoea, muscle pain, dizziness
Signs pyrexia, hypotension, macular rash *PV* tenderness, palpable tampon *speculum* visible tampon
Investigations MSU *blds* FBC, U+E, clotting, LFT, blood cultures *other* vaginal swabs for M,C+S, ECG, CXR
Management IV access for fluids and antibiotics, keep NBM, remove tampon, may need ITU if not managed aggressively

Problems in early pregnancy

Acute presentations in pregnancies <20/40 gestation are usually seen by the gynaecological team.

Miscarriage loss of pregnancy <24/40 gestation
Symptoms lower abdominal crampy pain (↑severity as ↑gestation), PV bleeding, nausea, vomiting, weakness, dizziness
Signs ↑pulse, ±↓BP, pallor, abdominal tenderness *speculum* open cervical os, clots, ±products of conception in vagina/coming through cervical os
Investigations *blds* FBC, G+S, β-HCG *swabs* endocervical, high vaginal and urethral swabs for M,C+S and chlamydia, USS
Differentials ectopic pregnancy, UTI, placenta praevia (usually presents later in pregnancy)

Type of miscarriage	Description	USS finding
Threatened	Pain, PV bleeding/discharge; os closed	IUP with FH
Incomplete	Pain, PV bleeding ++; open os	PoC; no FH
Inevitable	Pain, PV bleeding ++; open os	IUP, ±FH
Complete	Pain, settling PV bleeding	Empty uterus
Missed	Asymptomatic or PV bleeding	IUP; no FH

IUP intrauterine pregnancy; FH fetal heart; PoC products of conception

Management

- After diagnosing a miscarriage counsel the patient and provide written information on miscarriage (~25% of pregnancies end in miscarriage).
- Miscarriages cannot be prevented by bedrest, so reassure the mother, who is often anxious
  - *<6/40*, repeat ultrasound (fetal pole/heart may not be visible if earlier gestation)
  - ***Inevitable miscarriage*** conservative management, fluid replacement, analgesia
  - ***Incomplete miscarriage*** monitor β-HCG levels and USS to see endometrial thickness; may proceed to complete miscarriage. Observe, ERPC* if unstable/heavy bleeding
  - ***Missed miscarriage*** *medical* mifepristone and misoprostol *surgery* ERPC* (formal ultrasound report confirming miscarriage first; send products of conception for histological analysis)
  - ***Complete miscarriage*** counsel and reassure
- Refer patients with >3 miscarriages to a specialist recurrent miscarriage clinic for further investigation. If these patients undergo an ERPC*, send the products of conception for histology and cytogenetics and take blood for parental karyotype (both parents) and maternal antiphospholipid antibodies
- Advise the patient to wait until she and her partner both feel ready to try and conceive again

* Evacuation of Retained Products of Conception

Hyperemesis gravidarum (excessive vomiting in pregnancy)

Be aware that the risk of hyperemesis is increased in multiple and molar pregnancies.

Symptoms recurrent and prolonged vomiting (frequency, onset), unable to eat/drink, anorexia, tiredness, lethargy, weight loss, ↓ADL, vomiting with previous pregnancy, dysuria, ↓urine output

Signs ↑pulse, ±↓BP, low volume status (p262)

Investigations MSU (ketones in urine), FBC, U+E, LFT, TFT (if severe/ second admission), USS to confirm viable intrauterine pregnancy

Management

- Admit if ketonuria/severe recurrent vomiting/signs of dehydration
- IV access for fluids and replace K^+ if necessary (daily U+E)
- Keep NBM for first 24h, then start on sips – if able to tolerate, light diet otherwise refer to dietician
- On the drug chart:
  - cyclizine 50mg/8h IM/IV
  - metoclopramide 10mg/8h IV
  - vitamins B_1, B_6, B_{12}
  - consider ranitidine 50mg/8h IV and Gaviscon® 10ml/8h PO (if second trimester)

Giving anti-D to rhesus-negative mothers in early pregnancy

Administer 250iu IM if:

- Ectopic pregnancy
- Spontaneous miscarriage <12/40 with instrumentation
- Spontaneous miscarriage >12/40
- Threatened miscarriage >12/40. If bleeding persists, repeat anti-D every 6wk throughout the pregnancy
- In threatened miscarriage <12/40, anti-D is required if the pregnancy seems viable or in the presence of ongoing bleeding/abdominal pain

Gynaecology presentations

Menorrhagia

Symptoms heavy bleeding during periods (may restrict daily activities), tiredness, SOB, dizziness (2° anaemia); often long-lasting, ±clots/flooding *FH* fibroids

Signs often normal *PV* enlarged uterus if fibroids present

Differential diagnosis dysfunctional uterine bleeding (no organic pathology), fibroids, IUCDs, endometriosis, polyps, endometrial malignancy, bleeding disorders

Investigations FBC, endometrial sampling and hysteroscopy if >40yr

Management treat any underlying cause *medical* tranexamic acid 1g/6h PO, mefanamic acid 500mg/8h PO (both during periods), consider COC, progestogens, Mirena® coil *surgery* endometrial ablation/resection, hysterectomy (if severe)

Abnormal vaginal bleeding

Think about intermenstrual, postmenopausal and postcoital bleeding The differential diagnosis varies with age: *young* pregnancy-related disorders and dysfunctional uterine bleeding; *perimenopausal* endometrial Ca, HRT related problems, dysfunctional uterine bleeding

Symptoms bleeding heaviness, colour, frequency, duration, onset/timing, relation to periods/intercourse (also check the bleeding is PV, not rectal or urethral), pain, discharge, odour, dyspareunia

History pregnancy, STIs, recent infections/pyrexia *PGH* polyps, IUCD, smear history, menstrual and sexual history, *POH* parity *PMH* breast/GI cancer *DH* COC, HRT *SH* smoking

Signs pyrexia, abdominal mass/tenderness/distension, PV enlarged uterus, palpable cervical mass/adnexal tenderness

Investigations *blds* FBC *PV* HVS, ECS, urethral swabs for M,C+S and Chlamydia, endometrial biopsy *surgery* EUA (hysteroscopy, cystoscopy, laparoscopy)

Management treat the cause

Types and causes of abnormal PV bleeding

Type	Causes
Intermenstrual bleeding	Cervical polyp/ectropion, cervicitis/vaginitis, IUCD/other foreign body (FB), pregnancy, cancer
Postcoital bleeding	Cervical trauma/polyp/ectropion/cancer, STIs
Postmenopausal bleeding (bleeding >1 yr after LMP)	Atrophic vaginitis, polyps, cervicitis, oestrogen withdrawal, cervical/endometrial cancer

Amenorrhoea OHCS6 p12 Oligomenorrhoea OHCS6 p10, 13

Dysmenorrhoea

Symptoms cyclical pain associated with periods (ask about onset, severity, radiation, relieving factors), dyspareunia, rectal pain, change in bowel habit during periods, urinary symptoms, affecting lifestyle *PMH*, STIs, fibroids, endometriosis
Signs abdominal tenderness
Investigations FBC, ESR, triple swabs, USS, laparoscopy
Differential diagnosis infection, endometriosis
Management treat the cause; mefenamic acid 500mg/8h PO during bleeding for analgesia, antibiotics if evidence of infection, COC, Mirena® coil

Pelvic pain (abdo pain p183)

Symptoms pain (location, mode of onset, nature, radiation and relation to menstrual cycle), associated PV bleeding/discharge, LMP, contraception, bowel or urinary symptoms
Signs pyrexia, ↑pulse, abdominal tenderness/rebound/guarding/masses, hernias *PV* tenderness/mass, cervical excitation
Causes endometriosis, Mittelschmerz, pelvic inflammatory disease, ovarian cyst torsion/haemorrhage, pelvic adhesions *acute early pregnancy problems* ectopic pregnancy, miscarriage *bowel-related* inflammatory bowel disease, constipation *urinary problems* cystitis, urinary calculi, bladder tumours, *neuropathic pain, psychological*

Vaginal/vulval lumps

Think about Bartholin's abscess, infected sebaceous cysts, prolapse
Ask about location, unilateral/bilateral, discharge, ↑pain, duration of onset, ↑size, history of previous lumps, STIs, systemic symptoms (fevers/rigors)
Look for give analgesia prior to examining if in pain; compare both sides, size, consistency, fluctuance, colour, discharge, if suspecting Bartholin's look for tender red lump at 5/7 o'clock from the vaginal introitus, with a punctum (similar to a golf ball)
Investigation M,C+S if pus present
Management *Bartholin's* incision, drainage and marsupialisation (keep NBM, IV access for bloods and fluids, senior review and book theatre) *infected sebaceous cyst* excision

Vaginal discharge

Ask about colour, nature (mucoid, serous, bloody, purulent), consistency (watery, viscid), duration (continuous, intermittent), irritation, smell, itch, foreign bodies, last intercourse, dyspareunia, contraception, sexual contacts/practices/orientation, menstrual history and relation to periods, previous STIs or urinary tract infections, recent pregnancies and outcomes, hygiene practices (vaginal douching, tampons)

Symptoms purulent/bloody/odorous vaginal discharge, pyrexia, general malaise, intermenstrual bleeding, lower abdominal pain, dysuria, urethral discharge, genital lesions

Risk factors for STIs age 15–34yr, multiple sexual partners, previous STIs, IUCD, post-partum sepsis, recent termination/miscarriage

Signs abdominal/PV tenderness, speculum (cervical erythema, swelling, exudates)

Investigations *triple swabs* high vaginal, endocervical and urethral swabs for M,C+S and chlamdyia, vaginal pH, Gram stain, colposcopy *surgery* biopsy if age >40yr and Ca suspected

Differentials physiological discharge, infection (see table next page), cervical ectropion, polyps, foreign bodies (eg tampon, condom), malignancy

Treatment *infection* empirical treatment with doxycycline 100mg/12h PO, metronidazole 500mg/8h IV/PO/PR for shortest possible course. Discuss barrier contraception, organise GU clinic follow-up and contact tracing.

Pelvic inflammatory disease (PID)

Infection of the upper genital tract commonly with *Chlamydia trachomatis* or *Neisseria gonorrhoeae*

Symptoms pyrexia, vaginal discharge (may be foul-smelling), intermenstrual/postcoital bleeding, dysuria, dyspareunia, lower abdominal pain, nausea, vomiting, infertility, general malaise

Signs *abdomen* tenderness *PV* adnexal tenderness, cervical excitation

Risk factors young age at first intercourse, multiple sexual partners, no barrier contraception, smoking

Differential diagnosis appendicitis, endometriosis, ovarian cysts, ectopic pregnancy, other STIs, HIV, urinary tract infection

Investigations MSU *triple swab* for M,C+S (high vaginal, endocervical, chlamydial, ±urethral) *blds* FBC, CRP, cultures, USS (to exclude ovarian cyst)

Management IV access for fluids, analgesia, broad-spectrum antibiotics eg metronidazole and doxycycline, refer to GUM for contact tracing

Complications tubo-ovarian abscess, septicaemia, recurrence, secondary infertility, ectopic pregnancy, chronic pelvic pain

Causes, investigations and treatment of vaginal discharge

Infection	Symptoms/signs	Investigation	Treatment
Infective causes			
Bacterial vaginosis	Fishy-smelling vaginal discharge	HVS M,C+S (look for clue cells); ↑vaginal pH	Metronidazole 1g PO stat; clindamycin 2% vaginal cream
Candidiasis (thrush)	White curd-like discharge, painful vulva/vagina, dyspareunia, dysuria, itching; O/E red vulva/vagina	Vaginal swab for M,C+S	Topical imidazole (eg Canesten®), oral fluconazole; vaginal hygiene
Chlamydia trachomatis	Often no symptoms, may have fever, IMB, pelvic pain	ECS for M,C+S Chlamydial culture medium	Azithromycin 1g PO (stat)/doxycycline 100mg/12h PO for 14d
Neisseria gonorrhoea	Often no symptoms, urethritis, cervicitis, monoarticular septic arthritis	Urethral swab for M,C+S	Ceftriaxone 250mg IM stat
Trichomonas vaginalis	Profuse grey/yellow discharge, dyspareunia, vulval irritation; PV 'strawberry' cervix	Wet film microscopy, HVS M,C+S	Metronidazole 200mg/8h PO for up to 7d
Non-infective causes			
Physiological	Mucoid, cyclical white discharge; may be pregnant	Nil	Nil required
Cervical ectropion	Clear discharge; speculum-erythema around cervix	Negative swabs	Conservative/ cryotherapy
Malignancy	Red/brown discharge, may have odour, IMB, PCB, dyspareunia, history of HPV	EUA and biopsy	Colposcopy/ sugery/radiotherapy

HVS high vaginal swab; ECS endocervical swab; IMB intermenstrual bleeding; PCB postcoital bleeding; EUA examination under anaesthetic.

Fibroids benign tumours of the myometrium found in 40% >40yr
Ask about pain, abdominal fullness/distension, menstrual problems (menorrhagia, dysmenorrhoea, intermenstrual bleeding), urinary symptoms (frequency, urinary retention, incontinence), changes in bowel habit
Risk factors Afro-Caribbean origin, +ve FH, nulliparous
Investigations FBC, USS
Treatment nil if asymptomatic *medical* tranexamic acid 1g/6h PO during bleeding, mefenamic acid 500mg/8h PO *surgery* myomectomy, hysterectomy (consider a course of goserelin (GnRH analogue) pre-op to shrink the fibroids)

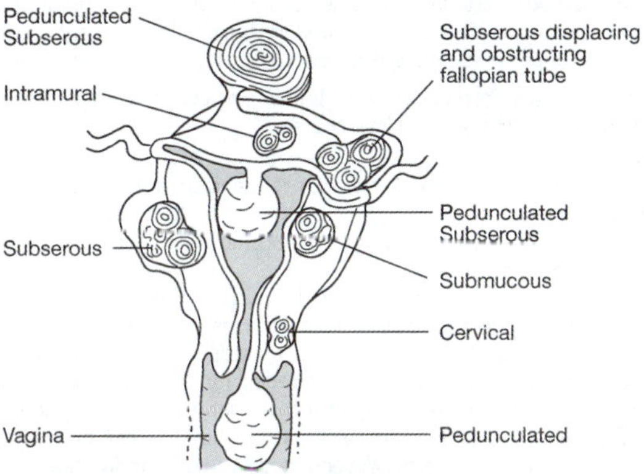

Common sites for fibroids and their classification

Endometriosis endometrial tissue outside the uterus found in 10%
Symptoms commonly asymptomatic: may be incidental finding at laparoscopy, pelvic pain associated before/with periods, menorrhagia, deep dyspareunia, infertility, rectal pain, change in bowel habit, difficulty urinating
Signs *PV* palpable nodule in pouch of Douglas, uterine/adnexal tenderness
Investigation laparoscopy and biopsy (gold standard)
Treatment *medical* COC, norethisterone 5–10mg/12h PO continuously for 6–9mth *surgery* laser ablation to remove abnormal ectopic tissue

Contraception

Ideally, this should be discussed with both partners present in the consultation. Provide advice on:

- the benefits and side-effects of each method
- the effectiveness in preventing pregnancy

Take the couple's views into consideration, giving written information/leaflets if possible. Allow the couple time to discuss and think things over before coming to a decision.

Methods

Barrier methods include condoms, caps, diaphragm, femidoms and sponges used at the time of intercourse in conjunction with spermicides; discard after intercourse. Noted to reduce transmission of most STIs.

IUCD local progesterone-releasing (Mirena®) or copper-containing plastic device inserted >48h prior to intercourse

Insertion

- Check the patient is β-HCG –ve prior to insertion and that the patient is not menstruating
- Assess the patient's cervix and uterine position and sound the uterus to ascertain its depth
- Insert the IUCD up to the fundus with care (using the depth noted on the uterine sounding device), withdraw the inserting device (this also releases the IUCD 'wings') and cut the threads 2–3cm from the cervix
- Patients should document their PV bleeding for 3mth and palpate the threads after each period. This initial check should be done by the GP

Side-effects bleeding, pain, risk of ectopics (if they become pregnant despite IUCD), risk of infertility/infection, expulsion, perforation. If the pain/bleeding become unbearable, advise them to go to their GP or local A+E to have the IUCD removed.

Contraindications PID, pregnancy, congenital uterine abnormalities, abnormal genital tract bleeding

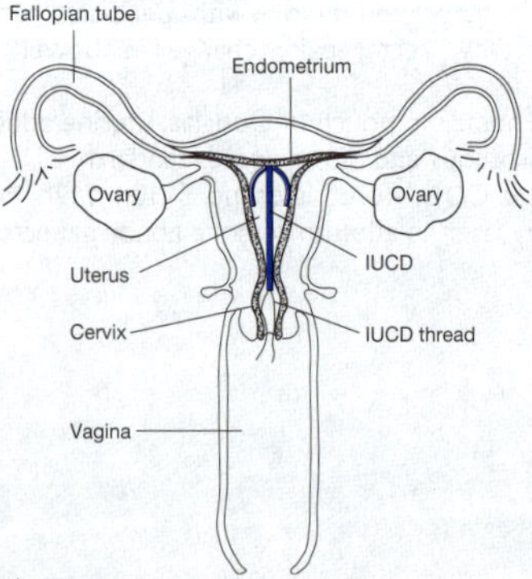

An IUCD *in situ* in the uterus

Oral contraceptive pill may contain oestrogen and progesterone (combined oral contraceptive pill, COC) or progesterone alone (POP, progesterone only pill). Advise patients to use barrier methods in conjunction with the contraceptive pill.
Ask about age, history of thrombosis, hypertension/MI, liver problems, SLE, breast problems, drugs, smoking. If older/smoker, consider progesterone only pill.

Contraindications: combined oral contraceptive pill

Absolute	History of thrombosis, IHD, previous CVA, TIAs, focal migraine, hyperlipidaemia, chronic liver disease, breast Ca, pemphigoid
Relative	Smoker, age >35yr, DM, □BP, cholelithiasis, obesity, Crohn's disease, sickle-cell disease, FH of breast/cervical problems

Practical advice preparations are either 28d or 21d packets.
- Packets with 28 days' worth of pills usually include 7d of placebo tablets ('sugar pills'), during which time the patient will experience a withdrawal bleed
- If the patient is taking a 21d packet preparation they can continue this 'back-to-back' with another 21d packet or have a 7d break at the end of each packet before starting another 21d packet. If they choose to continue 'back-to-back', this can be done continuously for 3–4 months after which they should consider a 7d break for a withdrawal 'period'. This prevents endometrial thickening
- Patients on the progesterone only pill must take this at the same time every day ±3h
- If one pill is missed, it should be taken as soon as possible and the next pill taken at the regular time, even if this means taking two tablets on the same day. Use additional contraception for the next 7d

Reduced effectiveness if patient is on rifampicin, carbemazepine, phenytoin, griseofulvin, phenobarbitone, antibiotics (advise patient to take additional contraceptive precautions whilst on these medications)
Side-effects acne, breakthrough bleeding, breast tenderness, bloating, weight gain, mood changes, nausea and vomiting
Warning signs new onset chest pain/SOB/calf pain, changes in vision, prolonged unusual headache
Patients on the oral contraceptive pill should be reviewed by the GP every 6mth (p346).
Other hormonal preparations subdermal implants (last 3yr) and long-acting injectable preparations
Female sterilisation Suitable for older women who have completed their family. Discuss with patient and partner; note that the failure rate for female sterilisation is 10 times greater than that of vasectomies.
Effectiveness of contraceptive methods Male sterilisation (>99% success), female sterilisation/Mirena® coil (99.7%), COC (99.7%), IUCD (98%), barrier methods (97%), coitus interruptus (60%), postcoital douche/breast-feeding (55%)

Emergency contraception

Ask about time since unprotected intercourse, LMP, history of PE/focal migraine, social situation (long-term relationship, previous contraception used). Discuss future contraception and STI testing

- COC *Levonelle-2*® available over the counter; 1.5mg (two 750µg tablets) asap within 72h of intercourse. Use barrier contraception until the next period
- *Copper* IUCD (unlicensed use) can be inserted within 5d of unprotected intercourse; more effective but infection is a risk. Use prophylactic antibiotic cover (azithromycin 1g/PO as a single dose)

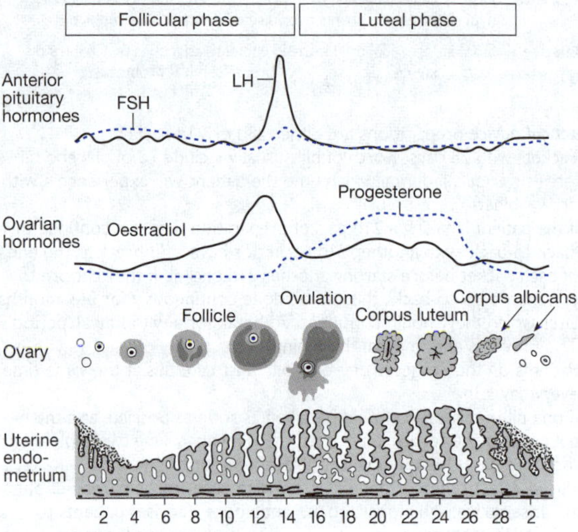

The menstrual cycle

Termination of pregnancy (TOP)

To decide whether a patient is eligible for TOP, two doctors are required (eg GP and gynaecologist) and patients must be referred for TOP by their GP or a family planning centre. No doctors are obliged to participate in TOP and patients are often seen in dedicated clinics, separated from patients with infertility/miscarriage. Confidentiality is paramount and future contraception should also be discussed.

Methods Medical (<9wk) mifepristone 600mg PO, then 1mg gemeprost PV 36–48h later. Surgery will still be required in approximately 5%. *Surgical* vacuum aspiration, dilatation and evacuation (a vaginal prostaglandin pessary should be given 1–2h pre-operatively to soften the cervix). Check rhesus status in every patient – if rhesus negative give anti-D post-operatively, p356.

Complications haemorrhage, infection, retained products of conception, uterine perforation, feelings of guilt, depression

Menopause average age 51yr in UK

Symptoms most women have minimal symptoms: amenorrhoea, vasomotor (hot flushes, sweats, blushes), skin (dry, atrophic vaginitis leading to dyspareunia), urinary (urgency, frequency, incontinence, UTIs), cardiovascular (↑risk of CVA/MI), bone (osteoporosis, fractures), psychological (insomnia, inability to concentrate, anxiety, ↓libido, lethargy), ↓breast size

Investigations ↓serum FSH, LH

Management consider HRT in symptomatic patients, those with premature menopause (eg following hysterectomy and removal of ovaries), osteoporosis. Counsel on routes of administration and regimes available (see below) and allow the patient to decide whether HRT will benefit them. Those on HRT should have annual check-ups to review symptoms, BP and the need for HRT; stop after 5yr.

HRT *regimens*

- ***Combined oestrogen/progesterone*** most common form of HRT; continuous oestrogen and progestogen
- ***Sequential*** cyclical oestrogen and progesterone taken like the COC causing regular periods
- ***Oestrogen only*** for women who have had hysterectomies

HRT *preparations*

- Tablets
- Implants, last 6mth; inserted subcut under local anaesthetic into the abdominal wall. May need progesterone if uterus still intact
- Transdermal patch, self-adhesive oestrogen-containing patches (may include progestogen)

Contraindications oestrogen-dependent tumours, unexplained PV bleeding, active/previous thrombosis, breast-feeding, pregnancy

Benefits and risks of hormone replacement therapy

Benefits	Risks
• Vasomotor symptom relief	• Thrombosis
• ↓ risk of fractures	• Breast cancer (prolonged use)
• ↓ risk of colon cancer	• Vascular disease

Urogynaecology

Incontinence

- ***Stress incontinence*** rises in intra-abdominal pressure without bladder contraction causing leakage on exercise/coughing/laughing
- ***Detrusor instability/urge incontinence*** spontaneous bladder contraction (detrusor contractions noted on cystometry) causing urgency

Ask about fluid intake, urgency, frequency, dysuria, poor stream, haematuria, leg weakness, urine leakage, dribbling, faecal incontinence, effects on ADL *POH* parity, delivery type, birthweight of children *PMH/PSH* spinal surgery, stroke, pelvic trauma, DM, chest problems (eg chronic cough)

Look for weight, abdo/pelvic masses, bladder distension *PV* (Sim's speculum ?prolapse, ?urethrocele/cystocele), ask the patient to cough with a full bladder; check perineal skin for soreness/irritation

Investigations MSU, BM, frequency and volume chart (urinary diary), urodynamics studies

Treatment *general* weight loss, reduce caffeine intake, stop smoking *stress incontinence* fluid restriction, pelvic floor exercises (physio) *surgery* trans-vaginal tape *detrusor instability* behavioural therapy (bladder drill), tolterodine 2mg/12h PO

NB Stress incontinence, detrusor instability and prolapse can coexist.

Prolapse

Ask about dragging sensation, vaginal lumps, urinary symptoms, recurrent UTIs, pain, PV bleeding/discharge, bowel problems, intercourse problems, *POH* parity, type of delivery, menopause, previous repairs

Look for *PV* exclude any masses *Sim's speculum* (left lateral position) to assess prolapse type (see table)

Risk factors obesity, childbirth, multiparous, oestrogen deficiency, chronic cough, pelvic mass, constipation (similar to risk factors for hernias)

Investigations MSU, urodynamics if incontinence

Treatment weight loss, stop smoking, treat constipation, physio, topical oestrogen if post menopausal *interventional* ring pessaries or shelf pessaries (less common) *surgery* hysterectomy, pelvic floor repair

Ring pessary Review every 6mth to replace, check for bleeding/ulceration and symptoms. Prescribe topical oestrogen to reduce the risk of ulceration.

Types of gynaecological prolapse

Type	Description
Uterine prolapse	• **First degree** cervix remains within vagina • **Second degree** cervix visible at introitus • **Third degree** (procidentia) uterus protruding from vagina
Vault prolapse	Prolapse of the vaginal wall after hysterectomy; may contain small intestine or omentum
Urethrocele	Urethra bulges onto the lower anterior vaginal wall
Cystocele	Bladder wall bulges on the anterior vaginal wall
Rectocele	Rectal wall bulges into the middle posterior vaginal wall
Enterocele	Intestinal loops herniate into the upper posterior vaginal wall

Gynaecological malignancy

Ovarian (>55yr)

Risk factors early menarche, late menopause, +ve FH, nulliparity
History and examination abdominal distension, PV bleeding, SOB, ascites, urinary/bowel symptoms, leg oedema, pain (rarely)
Investigations CA 125, USS, CT abdomen/pelvis
Treatment removal of all visible tissues (uterus, ovaries, omentum) ascitic/peritoneal washings, chemotherapy

Uterine (>40yr)

Risk factors obesity, polycystic ovarian syndrome, nulliparity, late menopause, tamoxifen, breast Ca
History and examination menorrhagia, abnormal PV bleeding (intermenstrual, postcoital, postmenopausal)
Investigations hysteroscopy, D+C, CXR, CT
Treatment total abdominal hysterectomy and bilateral salpingo-oophrectomy/radiotherapy

Cervix (30–55yr)

Risk factors early age of first intercourse, human papilloma virus (HPV)/other STIs, multiple partners, smoking, immunosuppression
History and examination postcoital/intermenstrual bleeding, discharge, irregular cervix
Investigations cone biopsy, EUA, cystoscopy, MRI abdomen/pelvis
Treatment IB_1 Wertheim's hysterectomy/radiotherapy, IB_2 chemoradiotherapy only

Vulva (rare)

Risk factors VIN, human papilloma virus
History and examination pruritus, bleeding, discharge, mass, lichen sclerosis
Investigations biopsy
Treatment radical vulvectomy, bilateral groin node dissection

Cervical screening

- Offered to all sexually active women aged 25–64yr
- Used to detect pre-cancerous cells in the cervix
- Performed at family planning clinics/GP/gynaecology out-patient clinic

Ask about abnormal bleeding (postcoital or intermenstrual bleeding), menstrual history, sexual history, previous smear results/colposcopy, number of pregnancies
Method Obtain consent and ensure a quiet room with a chaperone; perform a PV examination to assess the position of the cervix. Scrape an Ayre's (or Aylesbury's) spatula gently on the inner aspect of the cervix to pick up transformation zone cells. Smear onto a microscope slide and fix with solution immediately. Label the slide using a pencil.
Treatment mild/repeat smear in 6mth; moderate/severe dyskaryosis refer to colposcopy (may require LLETZ/cone biopsy)

Obstetrics

Obstetrics involves:

- risk assessment and counselling on perceived risks for mother/fetus
- education and guidance about pregnancy, problems and childbirth
- identification and treatment of maternal and fetal problems in pregnancy

Pregnancy

Symptoms amenorrhoea, nausea and vomiting, ↑urinary frequency, breast tenderness, food cravings, ↑abdominal girth
Signs abdominal distension/mass *PV* ↑uterus size
Investigations β-HCG (urine or serum), urinary β-HCG detects levels >50iu/ml, present 1/52 after a missed period
Dating pregnancy Gestation by dates calculated from the first day of the last period, so the length of the menstrual cycle is important. Check contraception used prior to pregnancy *Ultrasound dating* as indicated below. Expected date of delivery (EDD) is obtained using Naegele's formula: LMP+1yr 7d–3mth (see obstetric table on opposite).

Gestational age (wk)	Measuring parameter
<6	Gestational sac
6–12	Crown–rump length
>12	Biparietal diameter and head circumference

Always check what the patient would like to do with the pregnancy; never assume she wants to continue with it. If she does, hospital antenatal care should be arranged via the GP; if not, discuss options (eg TOP, adoption).

Abdominal examination in pregnancy

- ***Inspection*** look for striae, linea nigra, venous distension, scars
- ***Measure*** the fundal height in cm from the top of the fundus to the symphysis pubis (36cm at 36wk; 2cm either way of the gestation is acceptable up to 35wk; this becomes 4cm after 35wk)
- After 24wk, palpate for ***fetal lie***; longitudinal if head/breech is felt over the pelvic inlet, oblique if felt in the iliac fossa, transverse if the fetus lies horizontally
- Feel for ***presentation and engagement*** using Pawlik's grip (palpate with two hands over the lower uterine pole for presentation and degree of engagement); if only 2/5 of the presenting part is palpable, the fetus is engaged

Imaging in pregnancy

- Avoid X-rays and CT if possible
- Use USS or MRI if necessary

OBSTETRICAL TABLE

January	1	2	3	4	5	6	7	8	9	10	11	12	13	14	15	16	17	18	19	20	21	22	23	24	25	26	27	28	29	30	31	January
October	**8**	**9**	**10**	**11**	**12**	**13**	**14**	**15**	**16**	**17**	**18**	**19**	**20**	**21**	**22**	**23**	**24**	**25**	**26**	**27**	**28**	**29**	**30**	**31**	**1**	**2**	**3**	**4**	**5**	**6**	**7**	**November**
February	1	2	3	4	5	6	7	8	9	10	11	12	13	14	15	16	17	18	19	20	21	22	23	24	25	26	27	28	—	—	—	February
November	**8**	**9**	**10**	**11**	**12**	**13**	**14**	**15**	**16**	**17**	**18**	**19**	**20**	**21**	**22**	**23**	**24**	**25**	**26**	**27**	**28**	**29**	**30**	**1**	**2**	**3**	**4**	**5**	—	—	—	**December**
March	1	2	3	4	5	6	7	8	9	10	11	12	13	14	15	16	17	18	19	20	21	22	23	24	25	26	27	28	29	30	31	March
December	**6**	**7**	**8**	**9**	**10**	**11**	**12**	**13**	**14**	**15**	**16**	**17**	**18**	**19**	**20**	**21**	**22**	**23**	**24**	**25**	**26**	**27**	**28**	**29**	**30**	**31**	**1**	**2**	**3**	**4**	**5**	**January**
April	1	2	3	4	5	6	7	8	9	10	11	12	13	14	15	16	17	18	19	20	21	22	23	24	25	26	27	28	29	30	—	April
January	**6**	**7**	**8**	**9**	**10**	**11**	**12**	**13**	**14**	**15**	**16**	**17**	**18**	**19**	**20**	**21**	**22**	**23**	**24**	**25**	**26**	**27**	**28**	**29**	**30**	**31**	**1**	**2**	**3**	**4**	—	**February**
May	1	2	3	4	5	6	7	8	9	10	11	12	13	14	15	16	17	18	19	20	21	22	23	24	25	26	27	28	29	30	31	May
February	**5**	**6**	**7**	**8**	**9**	**10**	**11**	**12**	**13**	**14**	**15**	**16**	**17**	**18**	**19**	**20**	**21**	**22**	**23**	**24**	**25**	**26**	**27**	**28**	**1**	**2**	**3**	**4**	**5**	**6**	**7**	**March**
June	1	2	3	4	5	6	7	8	9	10	11	12	13	14	15	16	17	18	19	20	21	22	23	24	25	26	27	28	29	30	—	June
March	**8**	**9**	**10**	**11**	**12**	**13**	**14**	**15**	**16**	**17**	**18**	**19**	**20**	**21**	**22**	**23**	**24**	**25**	**26**	**27**	**28**	**29**	**30**	**31**	**1**	**2**	**3**	**4**	**5**	**6**	—	**April**
July	1	2	3	4	5	6	7	8	9	10	11	12	13	14	15	16	17	18	19	20	21	22	23	24	25	26	27	28	29	30	31	July
April	**7**	**8**	**9**	**10**	**11**	**12**	**13**	**14**	**15**	**16**	**17**	**18**	**19**	**20**	**21**	**22**	**23**	**24**	**25**	**26**	**27**	**28**	**29**	**30**	**1**	**2**	**3**	**4**	**5**	**6**	**7**	**May**
August	1	2	3	4	5	6	7	8	9	10	11	12	13	14	15	16	17	18	19	20	21	22	23	24	25	26	27	28	29	30	31	August
May	**8**	**9**	**10**	**11**	**12**	**13**	**14**	**15**	**16**	**17**	**18**	**19**	**20**	**21**	**22**	**23**	**24**	**25**	**26**	**27**	**28**	**29**	**30**	**31**	**1**	**2**	**3**	**4**	**5**	**6**	**7**	**June**
September	1	2	3	4	5	6	7	8	9	10	11	12	13	14	15	16	17	18	19	20	21	22	23	24	25	26	27	28	29	30	—	September
June	**8**	**9**	**10**	**11**	**12**	**13**	**14**	**15**	**16**	**17**	**18**	**19**	**20**	**21**	**22**	**23**	**24**	**25**	**26**	**27**	**28**	**29**	**30**	**1**	**2**	**3**	**4**	**5**	**6**	**7**	—	**July**
October	1	2	3	4	5	6	7	8	9	10	11	12	13	14	15	16	17	18	19	20	21	22	23	24	25	26	27	28	29	30	31	October
July	**8**	**9**	**10**	**11**	**12**	**13**	**14**	**15**	**16**	**17**	**18**	**19**	**20**	**21**	**22**	**23**	**24**	**25**	**26**	**27**	**28**	**29**	**30**	**31**	**1**	**2**	**3**	**4**	**5**	**6**	**7**	**August**
November	1	2	3	4	5	6	7	8	9	10	11	12	13	14	15	16	17	18	19	20	21	22	23	24	25	26	27	28	29	30	—	November
August	**8**	**9**	**10**	**11**	**12**	**13**	**14**	**15**	**16**	**17**	**18**	**19**	**20**	**21**	**22**	**23**	**24**	**25**	**26**	**27**	**28**	**29**	**30**	**31**	**1**	**2**	**3**	**4**	**5**	**6**	—	**September**
December	1	2	3	4	5	6	7	8	9	10	11	12	13	14	15	16	17	18	19	20	21	22	23	24	25	26	27	28	29	30	31	December
September	**7**	**8**	**9**	**10**	**11**	**12**	**13**	**14**	**15**	**16**	**17**	**18**	**19**	**20**	**21**	**22**	**23**	**24**	**25**	**26**	**27**	**28**	**29**	**30**	**1**	**2**	**3**	**4**	**5**	**6**	**7**	**October**

Obstetric table showing LMP dates and their corresponding estimated delivery dates

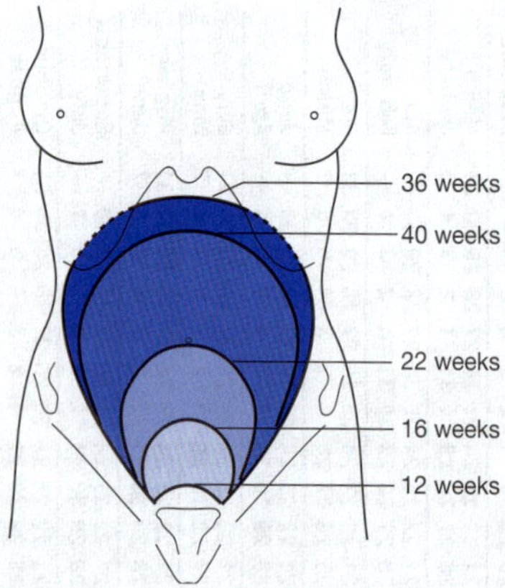

Uterine size in pregnancy

Normal ranges in pregnancy

Feature	Range
Haematocrit	No change
Haemoglobin	11–15g/dl
WCC	5–16 x 10^9/l
Platelets	No change
ESR	44–114mm/h
Fibrinogen	400–600mg/dl

Feature	Range
Albumin	28–40mmol/l
Urea	1.6–6μmol/l
Creatinine	No change
$PaCO_2$	3.6–4.2kPa
PaO_2	No change
HCO_3^-	18–23mmol/l

Antenatal care: timetable of events

Gestation/wk	Assessment
8–12	Booking visit, dating scan and blds (FBC, G+S, antibody screen, rubella, syphilis, hepatitis B, HIV serology, sickle-cell disease)
15–16	Serum screening for anencephaly
20	Anomaly scan
26–28	Fetal growth
36	Assess presentation/lie
40	Pre-delivery

Prescribing in pregnancy Check *BNF* Appendix 4

- When prescribing, make sure the benefits to the mother are greater than the risk to the fetus
- Use the smallest effective dose for the shortest period of time possible
- Try and avoid all drugs in the first trimester

Acceptable drugs penicillins, cephalosporins, nystatin, heparin, cimetidine, ranitidine, paracetamol, phenytoin, vitamin A

Drugs to avoid tetracyclines, streptomycin, quinolones, warfarin, thiazide diuretics, ACEi, lithium carbonate, NSAIDs, alcohol, retinoids, barbiturates, opioids, cytotoxic drugs, phenytoin, vitmain A

Prenatal testing

- Take a careful history, noting risk factors such as maternal age >35yr, previous fetal abnormality, FH of inherited conditions
- Make sure the patient understands that ultrasound cannot provide a definite diagnosis of Down's syndrome, but assesses the risk
- When considering invasive tests such as chorionic villus sampling go through the procedure and why it is necessary, outline the risks and benefits to the patient and obtain consent

Prenatal testing

Method and timing	Use
Ultrasound (11–14wk and 20wk)	Detects external structural abnormalities, eg spina bifida, nuchal translucency (risk of Down's syndrome)
Chorionic villus sampling (10–12wk)	Karyotyping, DNA analysis
maternal αFP (17wk)	↑in neuronal tube defects, exomphalos, nephrosis, GI obstruction, Turner's; ↓in Down's syndrome
Amniocentesis (16wk)	Obtain amniotic fluid for chromosomal analysis, enzyme assays, αFP, fetal infection
Antenatal fetal blood sampling (>17wk)	To confirm fetal infection, fetal hydrops, rhesus/other blood group antibody problems

Cardiac arrest in pregnancy

Follow the resuscitation guidelines for adults (p122), the same principles apply in pregnancy. However, certain important points should be noted:

- the arrest team includes an obstetrician and a paediatrician
- the life of the mother is the first priority
- CPR should be performed as normal, but this can be very difficult due to increased breast size and splinting of the diaphragm by the uterus
- early intubation is preferable, high risk of gastric aspiration in pregnancy
- the uterus exerts pressure on the aorta and inferior vena cava, reducing venous return and cardiac output. Move the uterus with:
  - sandbags, pillows or a Cardiff wedge under the patient's right flank
  - manually shifting the uterus to the left or using the left lateral position
- an emergency caesarean section offers the best chance of survival to both mother and baby if arrest lasts longer than 5min in patients >26/40

Normal vaginal delivery

Onset of labour painful uterine contractions, 'show' of mucous discharge and blood, cervical dilatation
Look for feel the abdomen, listen for fetal heart with Pinard/Doppler *PV* inspect the perineum and palpate to assess cervical dilatation

Stages of labour

- *First stage* defined as the time between onset of labour and the attainment of full dilatation (10–12h in primips, 6–8h in multips), ↑frequency and duration of contractions
- *Second stage* from full dilatation to delivery of baby (1–2h in primips, less than 1h in multips)
- *Third stage* delivery of placenta, membranes and retraction of uterus (~15min)

Management of a normal vaginal delivery (NVD)

- Call the obstetric SHO on-call
- Reassure the patient and make sure she is comfortable (avoid the supine position)
- Assess basic observations: maternal pulse, BP, temp, urine output, and fetal heart rate (either continuous monitoring or intermittent auscultation every 15min)
- Entonox® (50:50 nitrous oxide and O_2)
- Stand on the patient's right with sterile gloves on
- Once the head crowns, advise the mother to take rapid shallow breaths and resist pushing
- Control the rate at which the head appears with your left hand and hold the perineum in place with the flat of your right hand
- Once the head is delivered, allow it to extend
- Feel for the cord around the neck and slip it over the head if present
- Deliver the anterior shoulder first (mother pushing if necessary)
- 5u oxytocin and 500μg ergometrine IM (one syntometrine ampoule)
- Deliver the baby, wrap it and resuscitate it as required
- Note the time of delivery
- Clamp the cord twice 15cm from the umbilicus and cut the cord in between the clamps
- Put a plastic clamp 1–2cm from the umbilicus and cut 1cm distally
- Check 2 arteries are present in the cord and send off fetal arterial blood gases

Third stage

- Feel for the placenta in the vagina as regular contractions start again
- If necessary, apply gentle traction to the cord whilst putting pressure on the uterus (to prevent inversion)
- Examine the placenta and give anti-D if rhesus –ve mother

What about...

If baby isn't coming out Get senior help; instrumental delivery (forceps/ventouse) may be warranted; failing this, an emergency LSCS must be performed.

Episiotomies These are required if the baby's head is bigger than the vaginal outlet. Infiltrate 5–10ml 1% lidocaine at 7 o'clock from the posterior fourchette. Cut the perineal tissues posterolaterally using straight scissors; do not cut directly down towards the anus, as this encourages a full-length tear, which may involve the anal sphincter.

Shoulder dystocia (the heartsink scenario) Remember **HELP:** call for senior **h**elp, perform an **e**pisiotomy, hyperextend the **l**egs onto the abdomen (McRobert's manoeuvre) and apply suprapubic **p**ressure.

Meconium-stained liquor Deliver the head, call the paediatrician. If there is meconium in the mouth and the baby is not breathing, perform neonatal resuscitation. Otherwise wait for the paediatrician.

Massive post-partum haemorrhage Deliver the placenta and call for help. Lie the patient flat with legs elevated, give O_2, insert 2 large-bore IV cannulae, take blds (FBC, clotting, crossmatch) and give rapid colloid/ O –ve blood. Compress the uterus bimanually, review delivery. Check obs (pulse rate, BP) and look for pallor, assess uterine size, check for abdominal tenderness and vaginal tears. Suture tears, give Syntocinon® 40u/6h in 500ml 0.9% saline to contract the uterus; if bleeding persists may need Hemabate®/EUA/laparotomy for hysterectomy *Think about* the four T's: Tone (uterus), Trauma (vagina/cervix), Tissue (retained placenta), Thrombus.

Breech delivery

If noted antenatally, offer the patient the following options

- Watch and wait, to review in 2wk
- Undergo external cephalic version at 37/40 (remember to give anti-D to rhesus –ve mothers)
- Elective Caesarian section
- Normal vaginal delivery regardless

If noted at time of delivery

- Contact the obstetrician on-call
- Once fully dilated, get the mother to push until the baby's buttocks and anus are visible
- Perform an episiotomy and deliver the baby up to its umbilicus without traction
- Abduct the baby's hip and flex the knees to deliver the legs
- Deliver the arms by adducting the shoulders and flexing the elbows
- Once the nape of the neck is visible, swing the baby up through 180° until you can see the mouth
- Put 2 fingers over the maxillae to flex and deliver the head. Alternatively, the head is delivered using forceps – this is performed routinely by some obstetricians

Pre-term labour (PTL) ie onset of labour between 24–37wk

Symptoms regular contractions, ±pain, ruptured membranes

Think about polyhydramnios, placental abruption, UTI, appendicitis, infection, DM, pyelonephritis, cervical incompetence, multiple pregnancies, congenital uterine anomaly, intrauterine growth restriction (the cause remains unknown in ~40%)

Ask about pyrexia, previous pre-term labour, dysuria, PV bleeding, UTI, recent infections

Look for cervical shortening, dilatation

Investigation fibronectin test

Management alert paediatricians, consider short-term steroids (if <34wk) and tocolysis (GTN patches, β-agonists, nifedipine, magnesium sulphate); if delivery is required, aim for NVD if cephalic presentation; avoid ventouse if <34wk

Fetal monitoring always check maternal pulse

- *Doppler probe* make sure you are listening to fetal heart
- *Cardiotocography* normal features include:
  - rate 110–160bpm
  - baseline variability >5bpm
  - minimal variation in rate during contractions
  - accelerations (transient ↑FH >15bpm lasting 15s is normal)

Worrying features call your senior for advice if there is:

- ***Loss of baseline variability <5bpm*** (think about fetal hypoxia, opiate drugs; check fetal scalp pH if persistent)
- ***Baseline bradycardia <110bpm/tachycardia >160bpm*** (think about fetal hypoxia; turn patient to side, give O_2 and check fetal scalp pH
- ***Decelerations*** slowing of FH below the baseline level of >15bpm, lasting >15s (think about head/cord compression or hypoxia; consider fetal pH)

Think DR C BRaVADO: Define Risk, look for Contractions, Baseline Rate, Variability, Accelerations, Decelerations, Overall: reassuring or not

Giving anti-D to rhesus-negative mothers in later pregnancy

- Administer 500iu IM routinely at 28/40 and 34/40
- Give 250iu IM <20/40 or 500iu IM >20/40 after any potentially sensitising event:
  - amniocentesis
  - chorionic villus sampling
  - antepartum haemorrhage
  - ECV (external cephalic version) attempts
  - abdominal trauma
- Administer 500iu IM post-partum if baby rhesus positive

Medical problems in pregnancy

Pre-eclampsia (PET) pregnancy-induced hypertension (>140/90mmHg) with proteinuria (>300mg/24h), ±oedema, >20/40 (eclampsia refers to the occurrence of seizures in a patient with pre-eclampsia)

Symptoms headache, epigastric pain, visual disturbances

Risk factors age <20yr or >35yr, BMI >34, first pregnancy, multiple pregnancy, hydatidiform mole, +ve FH, fetal hydrops, known DM/↑BP, past history of pre-eclampsia

Obs BP (check correct cuff size)

Signs epigastric/hepatic tenderness, ankle oedema, renal bruits, papilloedema, radio-femoral delay, hyperreflexia with ankle clonus, focal neurology

Investigations MSU *blds* FBC, U+E, uric acid, LFT, clotting, G+S *USS* ECG

Assess the fetus USS (fetal growth, size, presentation, liquor volume, fetal movements), umbilical artery dopplers

Management refer to antenatal medical clinic; may need antihypertensive therapy. If there is evidence of eclampsia follow department protocol or:

- Call obstetrician and anaesthetist, check airway and BM, gain IV access for blds and IV diazepam
- Give IV loading dose of 4g magnesium sulphate over 20min; continue at maintenance dose of 2g/h
- Repeat BP. If diastolic >105mmHg IV hydralazine/labetalol (p161)
- Consider urgent delivery

After delivery treat BP >160/110mmHg; strict fluid balance (may need urinary catheter); take FBC, U+E, LFT; keep in hospital for 5d and organise medical review

Note:

- Avoid ergometrine/syntometrine in the third stage as this may cause a hypertensive CVA; use oxytocin
- Check for signs of magnesium sulphate toxicity patellar/biceps reflexes, diplopia, slurred speech, flushing. Stop infusion if respiratory rate <14/min

Gestational diabetes (OGTT, glucose ≥7.8mmol/l)

Think about polyhydramnios, ↑perinatal mortality and morbidity

Ask about previous gestational diabetes, FH, previous macrosomia (large babies)/stillbirths

Look for abdominal tenderness, large for dates

Investigations urine dipstick (glycosuria), 24h urinary protein excretion/creatinine clearance; U+E, GTT, HbA_{1C}; regular USS to assess fetal growth

Management diet changes, consider insulin if BMs remain uncontrolled. Consider sliding scale if necessary during labour; check glucose tolerance test (p237) at 6wk post-partum

Anaemia in pregnancy (Hb <11g/dl)

Ask about PV bleeding, SOB, malaria, previous pregnancies, diet, history of anaemia, drugs eg anticonvulsants
Antenatal screening FBC at 12, 28 and 36wk, sickle-cell screen, if high risk *thick film* for malaria parasites, Hb electrophoresis
Treatment *iron-deficiency anaemia* ferrous sulphate 200mg/24h PO, aim for a rise in Hb levels of 1g/dl per week. Avoid transfusion if possible *folate deficiency* folate 0.4mg/24h PO preconception (5mg/24h PO if patient is on anticonvulsants)

Thromboembolic disease (p296)

Risk factors obesity, ↑age, LSCS, previous DVT/PE, bed rest, clotting abnormalities
Management *prophylaxis* regular Clexane® 20–40mg/24h SC *treatment* p290, avoid warfarin

Pregnancy >41wk

- Recheck gestation and lie
- Consider induction of labour; discuss with a senior obstetrician

Other problems

Antepartum haemorrhage *bleeding >20/40*

Think about placenta praevia, placental abruption, infection
Risk factors pre-eclampsia, previous abruption, trauma, smoking, high parity
Look for ↑pulse, ±↓BP, pallor; abdomen tenderness, uterine size, presentation, engagement; avoid PV until placenta praevia is excluded
Investigations *blds* FBC, U+E, glucose, crossmatch, Kleihauer, clotting *cardiotocogram, USS*
Management resuscitate and call obstetrician if acute. Give O_2, insert 2 large-bore IV cannulae for IV fluids/O –ve blood. May need emergency LSCS, steroids if <34/40 and anti-D immunoglobulin if Rhesus –ve

Abdominal pain in pregnancy

- ***Obstetric causes*** labour (p372), ectopic pregnancy (p354), fibroid degeneration (p361), pre-eclampsia (p375), placental abruption (p374), ovarian cyst accidents (p354)
- ***Other common causes*** UTI (p249; avoid trimethoprim; use amoxycillin or augmentin), appendicitis (p187), gallstones (p197), acute pancreatitis (p198), pyelonephritis (p249), intestinal obstruction (p186)

For other medical problems in pregnancy refer to OHCS6 p152.

Post-partum complications

Pyrexia

Think about pelvic infection, UTI, mastitis, URTI, DVT, wound infection (episiotomy/LSCS)
Ask about mode of delivery, prolonged ruptured membranes, pyrexia in labour, pain, cough/SOB, PV bleeding/discharge, dysuria
Look for ↑pulse, abdominal/loin tenderness *PV* uterine/adnexal tenderness, lochia (period-like discharge) *CVS* murmur (think of endocarditis) *RS* PE, pneumonia
Investigations MSU and M,C+S *blds* FBC, clotting, CRP, G+S *swabs* high vaginal swab, sputum, wound *imaging* CXR *Doppler USS* of limbs
Management resuscitate; give O_2, gain IV access for fluids/antibiotics if indicated (review with culture sensitivities); treat the cause

Mastitis/breast abscess

Ask about breast-feeding, infection, tenderness, swelling, exudate, colour of milk
Look for erythema, tenderness, swelling, abscess, ulceration
Investigations *blds* FBC, G+S, CRP; swab any pus (M,C+S)
Management abscess incision and drainage; express and discard milk from affected breast; advise patient to continue breast-feeding from other breast

Psychiatric problems see p400

- ***Postnatal depression*** affects <10% of women and is more common in socially/emotionally isolated women. If severe, consider psychiatric input
- ***Puerperal psychosis*** affects 0.2% of women, with acute onset of psychotic symptoms 3–7d post-partum. More common after first pregnancy with a +ve FH. May require admission and antipsychotic therapy

Prescribing in breast-feeding check *BNF* Appendix 5

- ***Safe drugs*** warfarin, aminoglycosides, NSAIDs, penicillins, cephalosporins, antihypertensive drugs, salbutamol, anticonvulsants
- ***Drugs to avoid*** benzodiazepines, barbiturates, amiodarone, COC, cytotoxics, aspirin

Oncology

Raised ICP	p212	Febrile neutropenia	p257
Seizures	p215	Infection	p248
Cord compression	p223	Hypercalcaemia	p245
DVT	p296	SIADH	p245
Bleeding	p148	Nausea and vomiting	p206

Hyperviscosity An excess of cells or proteins in blood; acute leukaemia and myeloma can raise the blood viscosity and impair the circulation. This presents with headaches, confusion, visual impairment and/or heart failure and is treated with venesection or plasmaphoresis.

Tumour lysis The destruction of malignant cells during chemotherapy can cause metabolic derangement and acute renal failure; haematological malignancy is particularly prone. Allopurinol limits this effect if given 24–48h before chemotherapy; IV fluids (3–5l/day) also help. It is important to monitor for ↑K^+, ↑ PO_4^{3-}, ↓Ca^{2+} and ↑urate very frequently.

SVC obstruction Thoracic tumours can gradually compress the superior vena cava, eg lung cancer, mediastinal metastases and lymphoma. *Symptoms* headache (worse on bending over), cough, SOB *Signs* raised JVP, head/arms swollen and red with distended veins. The diagnosis can be confirmed by CXR, CT and venography. The obstruction is relieved by tumour shrinkage (eg radiotherapy) or SVC stenting, otherwise it can lead to raised ICP and potentially airway obstruction.

Airway obstruction Tumours can also compress the trachea causing severe SOB, cough and stridor. SVC obstruction is a warning sign. If the obstruction is severe the patient may need intubation, otherwise O_2 and steroids followed by tumour shrinkage.

Tumour markers These are used to monitor treatment and assess severity; except for PSA, they are rarely used for diagnosis.

Tumour marker	Cancer	Non-cancer
α-fetoprotein (αFP)	Liver, testes, ovaries	Hepatitis, cirrhosis, pregnancy
CA 125	Ovary, breast, GI, uterus, liver	Ascites, peritonitis, pregnancy, menstruation
CA 15.3	Breast	Benign breast disease
CA 19.9	Pancreatic, GI	Pancreatitis, gallstones
Carcino-embryonic antigen (CEA)	GI, lung	Smoking, COPD, IBD, pancreatitis, cirrhosis
Human chorionic gonadotrophin (hCG)	Testes, ovaries, hydatidiform mole	Pregnancy, cannabis use
Prostate-specific antigen (PSA)	Prostate	Old age, benign prostatic hypertrophy

Cancer chemotherapy (OHCM6 p440)

The range of drugs used to treat malignant disease is ever increasing and the indications and side-effects below do not apply to *all* drugs within this group.

Groups and mode of action	DNA damaging – alkylating agents, platinum compounds Antimetabolites – folic acid, pyrimidine and purine antagonists DNA repair inhibitors – cytotoxic antibiotics, eg doxorubicin Antitubulin agents – vinca alkaloids, taxanes
Indications	Neoadjuvant – to shrink tumour prior to surgery Primary therapy – as a curative treatment (eg leukaemia) Adjuvant – to reduce chance of relapse Palliative – to aid symptom relief
Side-effects	Nausea and vomiting – common, often requires multiple anti-emetics Hair loss – common, but hair growth returns once therapy stops Marrow suppression – common, see below Sterility – common, sperm or oocyte storage advised Mucositis – common, use antiseptic/anticandidal mouthwash Secondary malignancy – chemotherapy can cause leukaemia Cardio-, neuro- and nephrotoxicity – incidence varies with agent used

Bone marrow suppression following chemotherapy

Bone marrow suppression is an unavoidable consequence of chemotherapy and is dose related; all cell lineages are suppressed (RBC, platelets and WCC) and neutropaenia is most evident 10–14d post-chemotherapy (p257). Whole blood and platelet transfusions can be used as required and peripheral blood stem cell harvesting is evolving to allow autologous WCC transfusions post-chemotherapy.

Radiotherapy (OHCM6 p442)

Targeted ionising radiation induces cell death within malignant cells of several tumours, which need to be localised and have known sensitivity to such therapy.

Indications	Neoadjuvant – to shrink tumour prior to surgery Primary therapy – primary treatment (eg retina, CNS, cervix/vagina) Palliative – symptom relief (bone pain, SVC obstruction, haemoptysis)	
Side-effects	**Acute (within days)**	**Late (weeks to years)**
	Anorexia, nausea, malaise Mucositis; oesophagitis, diarrhoea Skin reactions; erythema/dryness Alopecia Myelosuppression	CNS – somnolence, myelopathy Lung – pneumonitis, fibrosis GI – dry mouth, bowel strictures GU – cystitis, fibrosed bladder Skin – ulceration, fibrosis Vagina – dyspareunia, bleeding Heart – pericarditis, myopathy Bone – necrosis, fracture Gonads – infertility, menopause

Ophthalmology

Although local ocular problems are common, pathology in the eye often reflects systemic disease. Therefore it is important to interpret your findings in the context of any systemic illnesses that the patient is known to have. As with any other speciality, a good history and examination helps narrow the differential diagnoses. It is also helpful if you need to refer the patient for an ophthalmological review.

History taking

As well as a good general history, specific factors to note include:
Symptoms change in eye appearance (eg redness), associated symptoms (eg itching, photophobia, gritty feeling), changes in vision (gradual/sudden visual loss, diplopia), flashing lights, floaters, eyelid changes (eg ptosis), squint, refractive error; are the changes unilateral/bilateral? *Relevant medical history* DM, hypertension, vascular disease, RA, SLE, thyroid disease *Previous ophthalmic disease* glaucoma, myopia *Family history* glaucoma, retinoblastoma *Social* functional impact of changes in vision

Examination

Inspection exophthalmos, proptosis, jaundice, pallor, xanthelasma, oedematous eyelids, redness, corneal arcus
Visual Acuity this *must* be tested in *all* patients with eye problems

- Use a Snellen chart at 6m to test visual acuity
- Use a newspaper if a Snellen chart is not available
- Make sure the patient is using the correct glasses for the test (reading vs distance) if in doubt use a pin-hole in a piece of card
- If visual acuity is very bad assess ability to *count fingers, awareness to movement* (waving hand) or *perception to light* (pen torch)

Pupillary response and reflexes check the pupils are equal, reacting to light and accommodation (PERLA) and for a relative afferent papillary defect. Look for the red reflex (absent in dense cataracts).

Visual fields confrontation testing to identify any visual field loss and to establish if the defect is unilateral or bilateral
Ocular movements look for loss of conjugate gaze or nystagmus
Ophthalmoscopy Allows examination of anterior structures and retina:

- With the ophthalmoscope set on +10 the cornea and anterior chambers can be examined. Adding 1 or 2 drops of fluorescein (1% or 2%) highlights corneal ulcers, abrasions and foreign bodies, especially under the blue light which most ophthalmoscopes have
- With the ophthalmoscope set on 0 the user can visualise the retina. It is important to dilate the pupil with 1 or 2 drops of a weak mydriatic (eg 0.5% or 1% tropicamide) to allow full visualisation of the retina. The risk of causing acute glaucoma with mydriatics is small

Slit lamp examination usually undertaken by ophthalmologists to examine the anterior structures of the eye and with a lens to view the retina. Often used to remove foreign bodies and to measure intraocular pressure; ensure adequate training before undertaking this alone.

Common ophthalmology terms (OHCS6 p475)

Accommodation	Alteration in lens (and pupil) to focus on near objects
Acuity	Ability of the eye to discriminate fine detail
Anterior chamber	Chamber anterior to the lens, containing aqueous
Aqueous	Fluid-like jelly in the anterior chamber of the eye
Blepharitis	Inflammation/infection of eyelids
Canthus	Medial or lateral junction of the upper and lower eyelids
Chemosis	Conjunctival oedema
Choroid	Layer sandwiched between retina and sclera
Ciliary body	Structure posterior to iris, containing ciliary muscle
Conjunctiva	Mucous membrane covering sclera and cornea anteriorly
Cycloplegia	Ciliary muscle paralysis preventing accommodation
Dacryocystitis	Inflammation of the lachrymal sac
Ectropion	Eyelids evert outwards (away from the cornea)
Entropion	Eyelids invert towards the cornea (lashes irritate cornea)
Fornix	Junction of sclera and lid conjunctiva
Fovea	Highly cone-rich area of the macula (yellow-spot)
Fundus	Area of the retina visible with the ophthalmoscope
Hyphaema	Blood in the anterior chamber seen as a red fluid level
Hypopyon	Pus in the anterior chamber seen as a white fluid level
Limbus	Border between cornea and sclera
Macula	Rim around the fovea, rich in cone cells
Miotic	Agent resulting in pupillary constriction (eg pilocarpine)
Mydriatic	Agents resulting in pupillary dilatation (eg tropicamide)
Papillitis	Inflammation of the optic nerve head (optic disc)
Optic cup	Depression in the centre of the optic disc
Optic disc	Optic nerve head seen as white opacity on fundoscopy
Posterior chamber	Chamber behind the lens, containing vitreous
Presbyopia	Age-related reduction in near acuity (long-sightedness)
Ptosis	Drooping eyelid(s)
Sclera	The visible white fibrous layer of the eye
Scotoma	Defect resulting in loss of a specific area of vision
Strabismus	Squint, loss of conjugate gaze
Tonometer	Apparatus for indirectly measuring intraocular pressure
Uvea	Iris, ciliary body and choroids
Vitrectomy	Surgical removal of the vitreous
Vitreous	Jelly-like matter which occupies the globe behind the lens

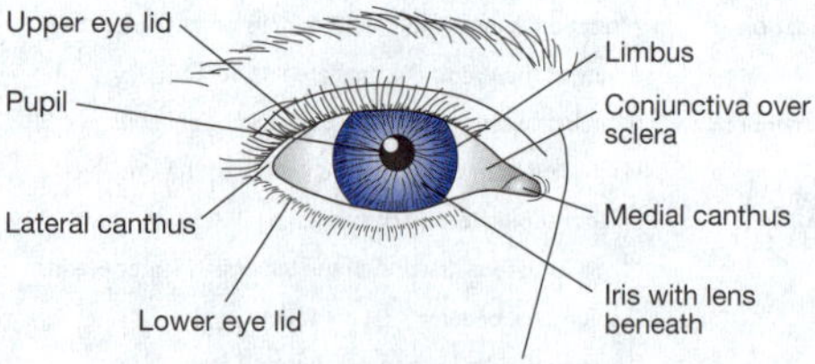

Surface anatomy of the right eye

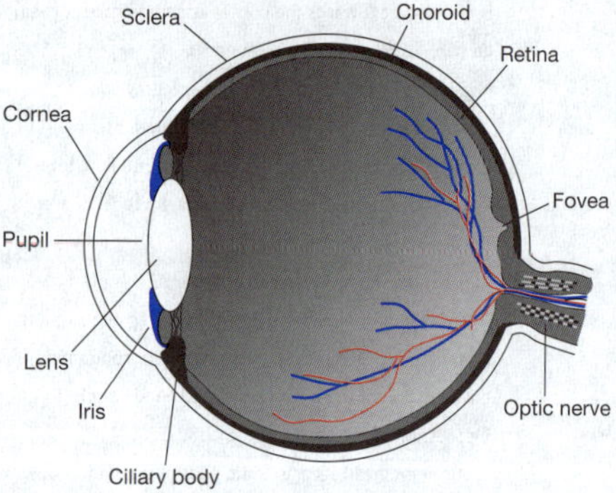

Cross-sectional anatomy of the eye

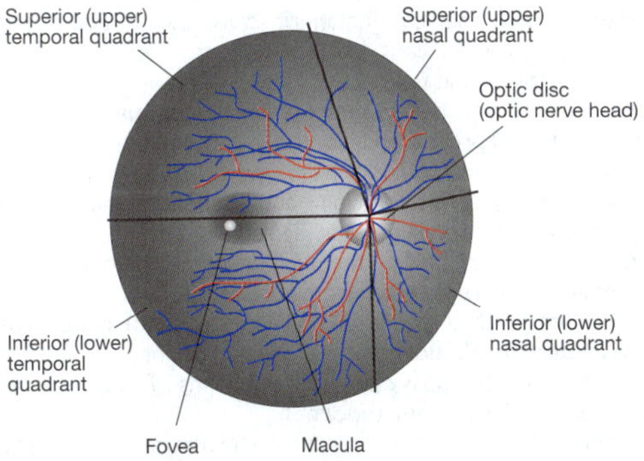

View of the right retina at fundoscopy

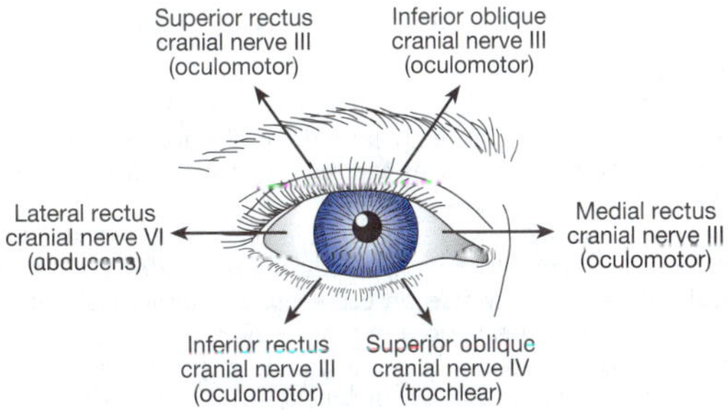

Muscles of eye movement and their innervation of the right eye

Drugs used in ophthalmology

- ***Antibiotics*** chloramphenicol, gentamicin, ciprofloxacin, neomycin, fusidic acid, aciclovir
- ***Antivirals*** aciclovir, ganciclovir
- ***Steroids*** prednisolone, betamethasone, dexamethasone (check with your seniors first; if prescribed incorrectly they could exacerbate the condition)
- ***Anti-inflammatory*** agents containing antihistamines (eg antazoline) and agents for allergic conjunctivitis (eg sodium chromoglicate)
- ***Mydriatics*** agents which dilate the pupil (atropine, cyclopentolate, tropicamide) – they relieve pain from abrasions
- ***Miotics*** agents which constrict the pupil (eg carbachol, pilocarpine)
- ***Topical local anaesthetics*** lidocaine, oxybuprocaine (Minims® Benoxinate), proxymethacaine (Minims® Proxymetacaine) and tetracaine (Minims® Amethocaine)
- ***Glaucoma*** β-blockers (timolol, betaxolol), prostaglandin analogues (latanoprost, travoprost), sympathomimetic agents (α-agonists such as brimonidine or apraclonidine), parasympathetic agents (pilocarpine) and the carbonic anhydrase inhibitors (dorzolamide or acetazolamide given orally)
- ***Dry eye*** carbomers (Viscotears®), hypromellose, polyvinyl alcohol (Hypotears®), hydroxyethylcellulose (Minims® Artificial Tears)

Cataracts (OHCS6 p504)

Causes congenital, diabetes, steroids, trauma, eye surgery

Symptoms blurred vision (bilateral), poor distance judgement (unilateral)

Signs cataract visible in lens; retina and red reflex visible unless cataract is dense

Management Cataract surgery is performed on a single eye at a time if the cataract(s) are interfering with lifestyle (eg reading or driving). They are usually done as a day-case procedure under local anaesthetic; the lens is removed (phacoemulsion) and an artificial lens implanted. The posterior capsule commonly becomes cloudy after the operation and may require laser treatment as an out-patient.

Ophthalmic presentations and their causes

Sudden visual loss (OHCS6 p498)	Retinal vein/artery occlusion, ischaemia/embolic (transient), acute glaucoma (painful), giant cell arteritis (pain in temporal area), vitreous haemorrhage, retinal detachment, optic neuritis Rapid assessment and referral is required, with prompt treatment
Gradual visual loss (OHCS6 p500)	Local cataract, refractive error, macular disease, tumour, glaucoma (open angle), DM, optic nerve compression
Diplopia	Local trauma, CN palsy, orbital fracture, thyroid dysfunction, myasthenia gravis, ↑ICP

Causes of the red eye or painful eye

Cause	Features	Treatment
Conjunctivitis	Pain/gritty feeling, swelling, sticky/ watery discharge	Topical antibiotics even if viral. Avoid contact as it is contagious. Check acuity is normal and that cornea is clear – senior help if not
Episcleritis	Inflamed nodule under conjunctiva, dull ache	Oral NSAIDs; topical steroid if no improvement. Check acuity is normal and that cornea is clear – senior help if not
Foreign body (FB)	Pain/gritty feeling or sensation of foreign body, watery discharge	Anaesthetise cornea, use fluorescein and evert lids to identify FB. Remove with cotton wool bud or irrigate away. May need removing with a needle – seek senior help
Acute iritis	Photophobia, blurred vision, watering, ↓VA	Topical steroids, analgesia, refer to ophthalmologist
Acute closed angle glaucoma	Blurred vision, haloes, N+V, tender and hard globe, semi-dilated pupil	Urgent referral to ophthalmologist; consider topical 2% pilocarpine eye drops every 15min bilaterally
Corneal ulcer (ulcerative keratitis)	Corneal ulceration, photophobia, ±herpetic vesicles around the eyes	Refer to ophthalmalogist
Orbital cellulitis	Pyrexia, swelling, redness, proptosis	Potential medical emergency. Refer to ophthalmologist. X-ray and IV antibiotics
Stye	Eyelash follicle infection; eyelid red and swollen	Topical antibiotics, warm compress
Chalazion	Granuloma of meibomian glands; eyelid swollen, hot and tender	Conservative – topical antibiotics and warm compress; may require incision and curettage

The eye in systemic disease

- ***Vascular disease*** patients with previous vasular disease (eg MI, CVA) are at high risk of retinal artery/vein occlusion
- ***Diabetes*** (OHCS6 p508) cataracts, background retinopathy (microaneurysms, haemorrhages, yellow exudates), proliferative retinopathy (cotton wool spots, new vessels), vitreous haemorrhage
- ***Hypertensive retinopathy*** haemorrhages, exudates, AV nipping, papilloedema (p161)
- ***Metabolic disease*** hyperthyroid exophthalmos (OHCM6 p305)
- ***Granulomatous disorders*** TB, sarcoidosis, leprosy, syphilis, brucellosis
- ***Collagen disease*** Reiter's disease, PAN, SLE, ankylosing spondylitis
- ***Systemic infection*** eg syphilis

Paediatrics emergency

Airway	Check airway is patent; consider manoeuvres/adjuncts
Breathing	If poor respiratory effort – **CALL ARREST TEAM**
Circulation	If pulse rate <60 – **CALL ARREST TEAM**
Disability	If unresponsive to voice – **CALL ARREST TEAM**

Call the **arrest team** if severely unwell; call **senior help** early

Airway – if irreversibly obstructed CALL ARREST TEAM

- Airway manoeuvres: (**head tilt**), **chin lift, jaw thrust** (see table opposite)
- **Oropharyngeal** or **nasopharyngeal** airway if responding only to pain
- If still impaired CALL ARREST TEAM

If you suspect **epiglottitis** (stridor, drooling, septic) do not look in the mouth, but give O_2 and call an anaesthetist and ENT surgeon

Breathing – if poor or absent respiratory effort CALL ARREST TEAM

- Bag and mask with high-flow O_2 if poor or absent breathing effort
- Non-rebreath mask and 15l O_2 in all other patients
- **Monitor** pulse oximeter
- **Effort** stridor, wheeze, rate, recession, grunting, accessory muscle use (head bobbing in infants), nasal flaring
- **Efficacy** chest expansion, air entry (does R=L?), O_2 sats
- **Effects** heart rate, pallor, cyanosis (late sign), agitation, drowsiness

Circulation – if pulse rate <60 or absent CALL ARREST TEAM

- Start **CPR** if pulse rate <60 or absent
- **Monitor** defibrillator ECG leads
- **Status** heart rate + rhythm, pulse volume, cap refill (≤2s normal), BP
- **Effects** RR, mottled/pale/cold skin, urine output, agitation, drowsiness
- **Venous access** (may need intraosseous) check BM and send bloods
- Consider **fluid bolus** (20ml/kg IV 0.9% saline stat) if shocked
- **Exclude heart failure** JVP, gallop rhythm, crepitations, large liver

Disability – if unresponsive to voice CALL ARREST TEAM

- Assess **AVPU** (**A**lert, responds to **V**oice, responds to **P**ain, **U**nresponsive); check **BM** if not already done
- **Look** for pupil size and reflexes; assess posture and tone

Exposure

- **Look** all over body for rashes, check **temp**, **cover** with a blanket

Life-threatening conditions

- Croup (exclude epiglottitis)
- Inhaled foreign body
- Bronchiolitis
- Asthma
- Dehydration
- Sepsis, meningitis, pneumonia
- Anaphylaxis
- Heart failure (especially infants)

Basic paediatric life support

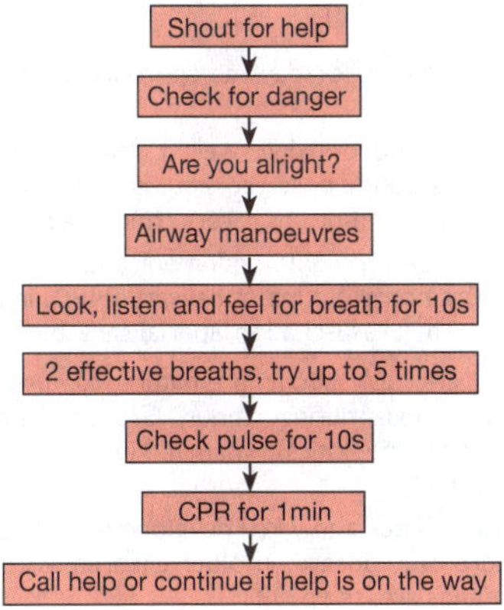

Main age-related differences in paediatric life support

Feature	Infant	Child <8yr	≥8yr or adult
Airway position	Neutral	Slightly extended	Slightly extended
Breaths	Mouth and nose	Mouth, ±nose	Mouth only
Pulse	Brachial	Carotid/femoral	Carotid/femoral
CPR position	1 finger below nipple line	1 finger above xiphisternum	2 fingers above xiphisternum
For CPR use	Two fingers	One hand	Two hands
Chest:breaths	5:1	5:1	15:2

Common emergency drug doses

- **Fluid bolus** 20ml/kg 0.9% saline IV
- **Glucose** 5ml/kg 10% glucose IV
- **Epinephrine (arrest)** 0.1ml/kg 1:10,000 IV
- **Epinephrine (anaphylaxis)** 0.1ml/kg 1:1000 IM
- **Diazepam** 0.5mg/kg PR
- **Lorazepam** 0.1mg/kg IV
- **Ceftriaxone** 100mg/kg IV

Normal range for observations by age

Age	RR (/min)	Pulse (/min)	Systolic BP (mmHg)
<1yr	30–40	110–160	70–90
2–5yr	20–30	95–140	80–100
6–12yr	12–20	80–120	90–110
>12yr	12–16	60–100	100–120

Paediatrics

History

Basics age in years, months or days as appropriate, sex, who gave the history, who was present

Current state feeding and drinking, weight gain, wetting nappies/urine output, bowels, crying, runny nose (coryza), cough, pulling ears, drawing up legs, fever, rash, other symptoms carers concerned about

Birth history pregnancy problems and medications, how many weeks gestation (37–42/40 is normal), type of delivery (NVD, induced, ventouse, forceps, if LSCS ask why), resuscitation, special care, birth weight

If less than 6mth also ask about premature rupture of membranes (PROM), maternal pyrexia during labour, Group B *Strep* (if so were mother or child given antibiotics), vitamin K (two oral doses a week apart or one IM dose).

Development history Check a few key developmental targets as a screening test unless there is a concern; in older children ask if they are doing everything their friends are, see p392.

Immunisation history Check the child is up to date with vaccinations. Jabs will be postponed if the child is unwell or febrile beforehand and children often get a slight fever for <24h afterwards.

Birth	BCG (if baby, parents or grandparents born in an area with high incidence), Hepatitis B (if maternal infection, rpt @ 1 + 2mth)
2, 3 + 4mth	Diphtheria, tetanus, pertussis, Haemophilus influenzae type B (DTwP-Hib), polio, meningitis C (MCC)
12–18mth	Measles, mumps, rubella (MMR)
4–5yr	Diphtheria, tetanus, pertussis (DTaP), polio, MMR
15–18yr	Diphtheria, tetanus, polio

- ***Others*** single pneumococcal and yearly influenza if diabetic, severe chronic illness (heart, liver, lungs, GI), immunodeficient, splenectomy
- ***Live vaccines*** oral polio, MMR, BCG, yellow fever, oral typhoid – avoid if immunodeficient

Social history *home* who does the child live with, who has parental responsibility, who looks after the child, if parents separated who has access, parental jobs and smoking (in house or outside) *nursery/school* attendance, type of school (mainstream vs special needs), academic ability, sporting ability, friends at school, enjoyment of school

Family history family tree with parents and siblings, ask diplomatically about consanguinity if relevant, any illnesses in the family, how are their parents and siblings at the moment, asthma, eczema, hayfever, diabetes, epilepsy, other diseases specific to presenting complaint

Examination

The art of paediatric examination is to gather most of your information from simply observing. The child is likely to cry at some point during your examination which can make it more difficult. Try to keep young children on their parent's knees and feeling secure. Follow the routines of examining adults with the extras shown below.

ABC if unwell (p386)

Chaperone Ask a nurse to accompany you if the child is older than 10yr of either sex, there is a child protection issue or you feel it is necessary.

Hydration fontanelle, capillary refill (≤2s), mucous membranes, skin turgor, sunken eyes, tachycardia, lethargic

Respiratory grunting, head bobbing, nasal flaring, tracheal tug, sternal, subcostal and intercostal recession, cervical lymphadenopathy, wheeze, air entry, crackles

Cardiovascular cyanosis (check mouth), clubbing, mottled skin, murmurs (see box) and listen at the back (PDA, coarctation, atrial septal defect) brachial and femoral pulses (coarctation), radio-femoral delay, dextrocardia, hepatomegaly

Innocent murmur • asymptomatic • quiet • systolic (short) • does not radiate • may vary with position • any cardiac investigations are normal

Suspicious murmur • symptomatic • loud • pansystolic (long) • diastolic • radiating

Abdominal feel for organomegaly including kidneys, tenderness and masses, check the external genitalia if young, relevant or boys with abdominal pain (torsion) and never do a PR (this is for seniors to consider)

Neuro observation is the key, AVPU (**A**lert, responds to **V**oice, responds to **P**ain, **U**nresponsive), check tone, moving all limbs, normal gait, able to use both hands, reflexes, head circumference (growth chart)

ENT Always check the ears and throat. Get the child sitting on their parent's lap facing to the side. Ask the parent to hug the child towards them with one arm round their chest and the other hand holding the top of the child's head against them so that the child cannot move their head.

- ***Ears*** Describe the colour of the each canal (normal, pink or red) and the appearance of each eardrum (clear, dull, effusion, perforated)

Now get the child to face towards you with one parental arm right around their chest and the other hand on the child's forehead hugging their head towards them. You may need a wooden spatula:

- ***Throat*** Describe any gross abnormalities, look at the tonsils' colour (normal, pink, red), size (normal, enlarged, meeting in midline) and if pus is present (swab and give ABx if pus seen)

Spine Look for straight spine and whether there is a sacral dimple (if so can you see its base, looking for spina bifida).

Weight and length should be plotted on a sex-specific growth chart.

Baby check

• parental concerns • jaundice • cyanosis • dysmorphology • hands • brachial pulses • fontanelles • ears • eyes • red reflex • mouth • cleft (look and feel) • moro reflex • clavicles • heart and rate • lungs and rate • abdomen • femoral pulses • hips • external genitalia • testes • passed urine? • spine and dimples • limb tone and movements • patent anus • truncal tone

Observations

Observations are performed on children in a similar manner to adults. The normal values are different in children according to their age (see p387). Blood pressure is performed infrequently (except in renal disease or sepsis) since it is inaccurate and difficult; cap refill and food intake charts are commonly recorded.

Common investigations

Urine Often sent for dipstick and M,C+S in any kid who is pyrexial or vomiting. A clean catch (holding a sterile pot under the child) is the equivalent of a MSU. Urine can also be used for a toxicology screen or various metabolic tests.

Suprapubic aspirate Only performed if <1yr and with senior supervision until competent. Clean with an alcohol swab then insert a blue (23G) needle vertically 1–2cm into the abdomen right above the pubic symphysis. Aspirate as you advance and abandon if no urine is obtained on the first pass.

Stool sent for M,C+S and viruses or for metabolic/absorption tests

Nasopharyngeal aspirate (NPA) This is a sample of mucous obtained by sucking through a small tube inserted a few cm up each nostril. It is used to detect upper respiratory tract viruses.

Bloods Use a topical anaesthetic covered with a venflon dressing unless acutely unwell:

- ***EMLA*** >1yr, takes about 1h
- ***Ametop*** >1mth, takes 30–40min

Once the cream has 'cooked' ask a nurse to hold and squeeze the arm (no tourniquet) and ideally involve a play specialist to distract the child. Blood is often obtained drop by drop either by skin prick (diabetic lancet with Vaseline®) or a small needle; cut-off butterflies are especially good. Paediatric bloods go in smaller bottles that hold between 0.5 and 1.5ml.

Capillary blood gas for severely unwell children, especially suspected DKA, pyloric stenosis, sepsis and deteriorating respiratory distress.

- **ABG** are rarely performed on the wards

CXR These are done much less frequently than in adults; they should only be requested if there is good clinical suspicion of pneumonia or other chest pathology.

ECG Check for prolonged 'corrected QT' (QTc); this is usually calculated by the ECG machine, normal = 0.35–0.45s (p140).

CSF Lumbar punctures are frequently performed on <1yr-olds as part of a septic screen and on older kids if meningitis/encephalitis suspected.

Cranial USS If the child still has a fontanelle this can be used to check for intracranial haemorrhage.

Electroencephalogram (EEG) Used to investigate epilepsy and encephalitis. Recorded by attaching electrodes to the scalp.

Metabolic investigations

Metabolic disease can cause a wide range of paediatric symptoms. A baseline set of investigations is often performed to exclude common metabolic diseases or guide further investigation.

Metabolic screen

• **Urine** amino acids and organic acids • **Stool** sugars • **NPA** • **Bloods** FBC, U+E, LFT, TFT, glucose, ammonia, HCO_3^-, lactate, venous blood gas • **Sweat test**

Features failure to thrive, hypoglycaemia (metabolic screen should be within 30min of episode), apnoea, lethargy, hypotonia, seizures

NB Labs need to be alerted prior to taking an ammonia or lactate sample and receive the sample within 15min. Check which bottles are needed.

Prescribing

The vast majority of paediatric medicine is prescribed according to weight. Use *Medicines for Children* (published by the RCPCH) or new children's *BNF*. Always look up a dose if you are not 100% certain and use a calculator. If the dose looks wrong it probably is. Two doses worth remembering:

• paracetamol (Calpol®) – 15mg/kg/4h (prescribe to nearest 60mg)
• ibuprofen (Neurofen®) – 5mg/kg/8h (prescribe to nearest 50mg)

Feeds and fluids

Milk volume Babies require 150ml/kg milk each day (1oz = 30ml).
Maintenance Calculate daily fluid (oral or IV) requirements from the table below. Add 10mmol KCl to each 500ml bag unless there is a potassium deficit or excess.

Weight	Fluids/kg/24h	Fluids/kg/h	Expected 24h volume
first 10kg	100ml/kg/24h	4ml/kg/h	0–1000ml
10–20kg	50ml/kg/24h	2ml/kg/h	1000–1500ml
above 20kg	20ml/kg/24h	1ml/kg/h	1500–3000ml

Example 23kg child 10 x 100ml + 10 x 50ml + 3 x 20ml = 1560ml/24h

Resuscitation Fluid bolus of 20ml/kg 0.9% saline stat

Paediatric development

Paediatric wards should have a chart that allows accurate assessment of a child's development in four areas • fine motor • gross motor • language • social. A full assessment is only required if a problem is suspected. When taking a history it is worth checking that the child acts appropriately for their age as a screening tool.

	Motor	Speech	Social
2mth	Lifts head when prone, eyes follow objects	Laughing	Smiles
4mth	Supports head as sat up, holds toy	Squealing	Spontaneous smiling
6mth	Turning over, sitting against wall, transferring objects between hands	Puts vowel sounds together	Objects to mouth
9mth	Sitting unsupported, crawling	Babbling (dada)	Responds to name
12mth	Cruising, pincer grip	First words	Waving
18mth	Climbs stairs, scribbling	>5 words	Pointing, uses cup
2yr	Walking backwards, turning single pages	Puts words together	Asking, undressing
3yr	Jumping, draws a circle	Knows full name, likes stories	Helps with dressing
4yr	Hopping, draws a stick man	Uses sentences, knows colours	Dressing

Common causes of developmental delay

• ***Global*** cerebral palsy, learning difficulties • ***Motor*** cerebral palsy, congenital dislocation of the hip, muscular dystrophy • ***Speech*** deafness, autism • ***Social*** autism, ADHD

Apnoeic attacks

An apnoea is when an infant does not breath for >20s (or less if associated with bradycardia). It is common in premature neonates but suggests pathology in full-term infants. It is normal for infants to breath hold before crying. Ask about central cyanosis (blue gums or tongue).

Common causes prematurity, reflux, RSV infection, sepsis, cardiac abnormalities, metabolic disease, seizures, CNS abnormality

Management If the baby is not breathing ***call the arrest team*** and resuscitate according to p386. Usually require septic, ±metabolic screen and broad-spectrum antibiotics according to local policy, eg cefotaxime and gentamicin.

Coughing and wheezing

Respiratory diseases can rapidly worsen. Admit children who are dehydrated, exhausted or have respiratory distress (recession, tachypnoea, sats ≤92%). Monitor sats, review frequently and consider ITU admission.

Epiglottitis ***age and sex*** 2–3yr ♂=♀ ***pathology*** cellulitis of epiglottis by *Haemophilis* (rare since HiB vaccine) ***clinical picture*** rapid, severe stridor, unwell and febrile, ±septic, drooling, unable to eat, resp distress ***management*** do not look in the mouth or upset child, get an anaesthetist and ENT surgeon urgently for intubation, ±tracheostomy.

Croup ***age and sex*** <4yr ♂=♀ ***pathology*** inflammation of upper respiratory tract, often viral (laryngotracheobronchitis) ***clinical picture*** gradual onset mild stridor and barking cough, able to swallow fluids, ±resp distress ***investigations*** usually none ***management*** if severe do not upset the child and give 1ml of 1:1000 epinephrine (adrenaline) added to 4ml of 0.9% saline via nebuliser; may need ITU. Give one-off oral dexamethasone (0.3–0.6mg/kg) or prednisolone (1–2mg/kg) in all children. Admit and give steroids for 48h if moderate resp distress or persistent stridor at rest.

Bronchiolitis ***age and sex*** <2yr, ♂>♀ 1.5:1, winter epidemics ***pathology*** mucosal oedema from RSV/parainfluenza in small airways ***clinical picture*** coryza, cough, fever, wheeze, resp distress, apnoea, poor feeding – examine CVS carefully to exclude cardiac abnormality ***investigations*** NPA, CXR only if pneumonia suspected ***management*** O_2, may need NG tube, bronchodilators (poor response <1yr), treat for reflux if suspected.

Asthma ***age and sex*** >2yr, ♂>♀ 3:1 ***pathology*** reversible airway obstruction ***clinical picture*** cough, wheeze, chest tightness, triggers (smoking, pets, cold, exercise), resp distress ***investigations*** PEFR not possible in <5yr, CXR only if pneumonia suspected ***management*** O_2, bronchodilators, steroids, discharge if comfortable with 4hrly inhalers and off O_2.

Pneumonia ***age and sex*** any, ♂=♀ ***pathology*** bacterial infection of the lungs, often *Strep. pneumoniae* ***clinical picture*** fever, unwell, cough, chest pain, tachypnoea, resp distress, creps, uneven air entry, bronchial breathing ***investigations*** CXR, FBC, U+E, CRP, viral serology, bld cultures ***management*** O_2, oral amoxicillin or IV benzylpenicillin if vomiting or pleural effusion. Add oral erythromycin if *Mycoplasma* suspected.

URTI ***age and sex*** any, ♂=♀ ***pathology*** infection ***clinical picture*** coryzal, cough (±sputum), wheeze, sore throat, ear pain, fever, red ears, red throat ***investigations*** usually none ***management*** regular paracetamol and ibuprofen, antibiotics if pus on tonsils (penicillin V, 10d) or bulging red eardrum with pain for >3d (amoxicillin/co-amoxiclav 5d).

Also think about cystic fibrosis, TB, whooping cough (*Bordetella*), autoimmune diseases

Meningitis and rashes

Any child with a non-blanching rash, headache, altered consciousness or fits has meningitis until proven otherwise. If a diagnosis of meningitis is likely give ceftriaxone 100mg/kg IV immediately.

Meningococcal septicaemia and meningitis

- ***Features*** fever, unwell, shock, cap refill >2s, vomiting, non-blanching rash in 20% (petechiae, purpura) ***if meningitis*** headache, photophobia, neck stiffness, altered behaviour, ↓GCS, seizures
- ***Treatment*** O_2, ***contact a senior urgently***, ceftriaxone 100mg/kg IV or cefotaxime 50mg/kg, large-bore IV access, consider fluid bolus and ITU
- ***Investigation*** FBC, U+E, glucose, Ca^{2+}, Mg^{2+}, PO_4^{3-} CRP, clotting, blood cultures, venous gas, G+S, throat swab, lumbar puncture
- ***If in doubt*** treat for 48h until blood culture results available

Other non-blanching rashes idiopathic thrombocytopaenic purpura (ITP), Henoch Schönlein purpura (HSP), leukaemia, petechiae over head, neck and arms (SVC distribution) following screaming or coughing

Viral rash children often develop a fever and blanching maculopapular rash when they have a viral illness, eg URTI. See also p320.

Seizures and febrile convulsions

If in doubt presume meningitis, encephalitis or raised intracranial pressure.

Febrile convulsions ***age and sex*** 6mth–5yr, ♂=♀ ***pathology*** viral URTI, UTI, pneumonia, meningitis ***clinical picture*** ≤2 symmetrical tonic-clonic seizures lasting <5min associated with a fever, look for source (ears and throat) ***investigations*** urine dipstick ***management*** O_2, treat seizure if >5min, regular paracetamol and ibuprofen, 30% chance of recurrence.

Epilepsy ***age and sex*** any, ♂=♀ ***pathology*** abnormal and excessive neuronal discharge ***clinical picture*** any type of partial or generalised seizure, absence seizures are particularly common ***investigations*** none if single seizure and no signs of meningitis, otherwise consider EEG, cranial USS, CT/MRI, cardiac investigations, UV light examination (ash leaf spots) ***management*** treat the seizure with lorazepam if >5min, try to establish cause of seizure prior to starting long-term treatment.

Raised ICP ***age and sex*** >2yr, ♂>♀ 3:1 ***pathology*** meningitis, space occupying lesion, hydrocephalus, trauma ***clinical picture*** altered behaviour, ↓GCS, vomiting, headache, diplopia, papilloedema, tense fontanelle ***investigations*** CT ***management*** get senior help and urgent neurosurgical opinion.

Infant sepsis and irritability

Like the elderly, young children can develop sepsis without specific signs of infection. Clinical management relies heavily on investigations so there is a low threshold for performing a full septic screen on ill children <12mth and a very low threshold <3mth.

Worrying features inconsolable crying, unusual crying sound, irritable, lethargic, apnoeas, rashes (especially non-blanching), tachy or bradycardia, slow cap refill (>2s), mottled skin, resp distress, hypotonic

Common causes • *neonate* pneumonia, meningitis and septicaemia (group B *Strep*, coliforms, *Staph. aureus*, *Haemophilus*, *Listeria*, *Candida*) • *infant* meningitis, pneumonia, UTI (*Strep. pneumoniae*, *Neisseria*, *Haemophilus*, *Listeria*)

Management Involve a senior early if you suspect sepsis. Resuscitate according to p386 and perform a full septic screen. Start broad-spectrum antibiotics according to local policy, eg cefotaxime and gentamicin.

Septic screen

• **Urine** microscopy, culture • **Stool** culture and virology • **Swabs** eyes, ears, throat, sites of infection • **NPA** • **Bloods** FBC, CRP, HCO_3^- glucose, blood cultures, virology • **CSF** for microscopy, culture, biochemistry and virology • **CXR**

Neonatal jaundice

Normal 2–5d after birth, especially if mother breast-feeding

Abnormal • *neonatal* <24h after birth • *prolonged* >14d (>21d if premature) after birth

Causes • *neonatal* haemolysis (rhesus, ABO), polycythaemia, bruising, prematurity, infection, metabolic • *prolonged* idiopathic, infectious, endocrine, metabolic, genetic (CF, α1-antitrypsin, Alagille), structural

Prolonged jaundice screen

• **Urine** microscopy, culture, bilirubin, non-glucose reducing substances • **Stool** examine (?pale) • **Bloods** conjugated and unconjugated bilirubin, LFT, prothrombin time, Gal-1-PUT, blood group, Coombs, serum save for TFT and TORCH and hep B screen if other tests abnormal

Further investigations • **Genetic** α1-antitrypsin, cystic fibrosis • **USS liver** • **HIDA scan** • **Liver biopsy**

Abdo pain, vomiting and diarrhoea

Posseting ***age and sex*** 0–4mth, ♂=♀ ***pathology*** relaxation of gastro-oesophageal sphincter ***clinical picture*** normal regurgitation of small amounts of feed with normal growth and no pain or distress

Reflux ***age and sex*** 0–4mth, ♂=♀ ***pathology*** significant reflux of stomach contents into the oesophagus ***clinical picture*** recurrent vomiting, drawing up legs after feeds, worse on lying flat, wheeze, apnoeas, pneumonia, failure to thrive ***investigations*** oesophageal pH study ***management*** avoid over-feeding, hold upright after feeds, Infant Gaviscon® with feeds; usually resolves by 9mth

Pyloric stenosis ***age and sex*** 2–10wk, ♂>♀ 4:1 ***pathology*** blockage of the stomach outlet ***clinical picture*** hungry baby with projectile (>1m) vomiting soon after feeds, no bile in vomit, constipation, failure to thrive, palpable mass in epigastrium or RUQ with peristaltic waves – seen best during a feed: look and feel ***investigations*** urine, bloods: venous gas, U+E, Cl^- (↓K^+, ↓Cl^-, alkalosis), abdo USS ***management*** resuscitate (p386), refer to surgeons, wide-bore NG tube, surgical pyloromyotomy

Infantile colic ***age and sex*** 1–4mth, ♂=♀ ***pathology*** unknown ***clinical picture*** episodes of inconsolable crying and drawing up legs, normal weight gain ***management*** reassure parents, no specific treatment though simethicone drops (Infacol®) are commonly used, a trial of hypoallergenic milk may help, usually resolves by 3–4mth

Intussusception ***age and sex*** 4–12mth, ♂>♀ 3:1 ***pathology*** segment of bowel is drawn into the neighbouring section (invaginated or telescoped) ***clinical picture*** classically severe colicky abdo pain, child quiet between episodes, vomiting, pr bleeding (redcurrant jelly) and abdo mass; features are often less specific, high clinical suspicion in unwell children ***investigations*** abdo USS ***management*** resuscitate (p386), refer to surgeons, NBM, often relieved with an air enema, otherwise surgery

Appendicitis ***age and sex*** rare <2yr, ♂>♀ 2:1 ***pathology*** acute inflammation of the appendix ***clinical picture*** unwell, fever, vomiting, unable to hop, peritonism, absent bowel sounds ***investigations*** urine, bloods and IV access (FBC, U+E, CRP, G+S), AXR (exclude volvulus) ***management*** resuscitate (p386), refer to surgeons, NBM

Gastroenteritis ***age and sex*** any, ♂=♀ ***pathology*** infectious ***clinical picture*** acute onset vomiting and/or diarrhoea, may have a fever, abdo pain and tenderness ***investigations*** urine, may need bloods if dehydrated ***management*** Calpol®, rehydration sachets, admit if unable to keep fluids down or severely dehydrated, try NG feeding if young

Also think about constipation, UTI, diabetes, volvulus, inflammatory bowel disease, pancreatitis (mumps), Meckel's diverticulum, gynae cause, renal cause, HSP

Failure to thrive

This is when a child is gaining weight more slowly than expected and dropping between centiles on the appropriate growth chart. Initial investigation is clinic based with repeated weighing. If no improvement is seen the child may be admitted for a feeding trial and further investigation.

Common causes • ***Non-organic*** insufficient food, infrequent food, improper food, poor feeding, dysfunctional family, neglect • ***Intrauterine*** prematurity, infection, toxins, placental abnormalities, genetic abnormalities • ***Inadequate intake*** poor appetite, structural abnormalities, recurrent vomiting (eg pyloric stenosis, reflux) • ***Malabsorption*** coeliac disease, cystic fibrosis, chronic diarrhoea • ***Metabolic*** diabetes, endocrine disease, genetic abnormality • ***Excess expenditure*** hyperthyroidism, heart failure, renal failure, respiratory failure, chronic infection

Child abuse

There are four patterns of child abuse, they can occur together:

- ***Physical*** hand-shaped bruises (slaps), ring-shaped bruises (bites), cigarette burns, bruises in unusual places, subdural haematoma (shaking injuries), parents unable to account for injuries, mechanism inappropriate to age or injury, vague description of mechanism, inappropriate reaction from parent, recurrent injuries
- ***Emotional*** domestic violence, child rapidly forms attachment with strangers, urinary or faecal incontinence in older children
- ***Neglect*** failure to thrive, late disease presentation, dirty child, ±clothing, bad nappy rash
- ***Sexual*** allegation from child, trauma to genitalia, vaginal discharge or bleeding, sexually transmitted infection

If you suspect child abuse refer to SpR or above immediately:

- fully document any history and examination findings including who was present, ages of other children, where they are, bone or clotting problems in the family and who chaperoned you during the examination
- do not accuse parents of child abuse at this stage
- if the parents attempt to leave do not stop them, inform social services who will contact the police

An SpR or consultant will take a full history and examination then:

- treat the medical problems and injuries first
- alert social services immediately
- leave examination of the genitalia for a consultant paediatrician and police surgeon if sexual abuse is suspected

Further action may include:

- checking old notes and X-rays, discussion with health visitor and GP
- skeletal survey (X-rays of whole body), FBC, clotting, CT head or cranial USS

Palliative care

Palliative care is the non-curative treatment of a disease; originally focused towards terminal cancer, but now covers other disorders. In practice cancer patients are still able to access more services, including the excellent Macmillan nurses who should be involved as early as possible. The aim is to provide the best quality of life for as long as possible – this may include admission to a hospice (usually temporarily).

Pain is a common problem in palliative care and opioids are the main treatment. It is important to be imaginative in treating pain, consider:

- treating the source (urinary retention, bowel spasm, bony mets)
- non-opioid analgesia (nerve blocks, TENS, neuropathic pain)
- alternative routes (intranasal, PR, transdermal, SC, IM, IV).

The table below is a guide to converting between opioids, it is not an exact science and changes need to be monitored for over or underdosing.

Opioid	Route	Typical dose	24h max	Relative[1]
Codeine	PO	60mg/4h	240mg	0.1
Dihydrocodeine	PO	30mg/4h	120mg	0.1
Tramadol	PO	50mg/4h	600mg	0.2
Sevredol/oramorph/MST	PO	10mg/1–4h	N/A	1
Oxycodone	PO	5mg/4h	400mg	2
Morphine	SC/IM/IV	5mg/1–4h	N/A	2
Diamorphine	SC	2.5mg/1–4h	N/A	3
Fentanyl	Topical	25µg/h	2400µg	100–150

1 multiply current 24hr dose by this number to get equivalent 24h oral morphine dose

Other symptoms Many of the treatments listed below can be used in non-palliative patients. For further information on prescribing in palliative problems see *BNF* and OHCM6 p438.

Symptom	Treatments
Breathlessness	Oxygen, open windows, fans, diamorphine, benzodiazepines, steroids, heliox (helium and oxygen for stridor)
Constipation	See p204, also bisacodyl
Cough	Saline nebs, antihistamines, simple/codeine linctus, morphine
Dry mouth	Chlorhexadine, sucking ice or pineapple chunks, consider Candida (thrush) infection, synthetic saliva
Hiccups	Antacids eg Maalox®, Gaviscon®, chlorpromazine, haloperidol
Itching	Emollients, chlorphenamine, cetirizine, colestyramine (obstructive jaundice), ondansetron
Nausea/vomiting	See p206, also levomepromazine and haloperidol

The dying patient

If a patient is very ill and unexpected to survive the decision may be taken by a senior doctor to withdraw active treatment and simply keep the patient comfortable. The patient will often (but not always) be bed bound with minimal oral intake and reduced GCS.

- Document what the patient and the family have been told and the reasons if they have not been informed (eg unconscious)
- Ask a senior doctor to sign a 'not for resuscitation' form
- Stop unnecessary medications (including anti-arrhythmics, anticoagulants, antibiotics, steroids, insulin); anticonvulsants should be converted to a suitable route or a midazolam infusion used instead
- Stop blood tests, IV fluids, O_2 except for symptomatic improvement

Pain Exclude a treatable cause of pain, eg urinary retention, constipation, and prescribe adequate analgesia. If the patient is currently in pain give an immediate diamorphine bolus at the PRN dose:

On opioids Use the table opposite to convert oral opioids to equivalent 24h SC diamorphine dose and prescribe a PRN bolus dose.

- **Syringe driver** diamorphine infusion SC at rate calculated
- **PRN** diamorphine dose equivalent to $1/6^{th}$ of 24h dose SC max 1hrly

Not on opioids Prescribe a PRN dose.

- **PRN** diamorphine 2.5–5mg SC max 1hrly

Agitation This may be a sign of pain. Try PRN doses initially; add a syringe driver (with additional PRN dose) if regular doses are required:

- **PRN** levomepromazine 6.25mg SC max 4hrly
- **PRN** midazolam 5mg SC max 4hrly
- **Syringe driver** levomepromazine 12.5mg and midazolam 10mg SC

Nausea + vomiting Continue existing antiemetics in a syringe driver if they are controlling the symptoms; if there is no nausea then prescribe PRN levomepromazine and add a syringe driver if it is needed regularly. If further antiemetics are required use a 5-HT antagonist (eg ondansetron).

- **PRN** levomepromazine 6.25mg SC 4hrly
- **Syringe driver** levomepromazine 12.5–25mg SC

Secretions The patient's breathing may become rattley due to the build-up of secretions with a poor cough/swallow reflex. Sitting the patient up slightly may help; medication improves the symptoms in about 50%. Start with a PRN dose and add a syringe driver if regular doses are required.

- **PRN** hyoscine butylbromide 20mg SC
- **Syringe driver** hyoscine butylbromide 40–80mg SC

Hyoscine will also improve pain from bowel colic. Hyoscine hydrobromide has a similar effect but a much lower dose is used (0.3mg SC PRN).

Further care Monitor the patient regularly and include them on your daily ward round. Ask the patient and/or relatives if there are any new symptoms and adjust syringe driver doses accordingly. If you are unable to control symptoms ask for palliative care review.

Psychiatry

The 'medical profession' is very good at caring for physical illness, eg fixing broken bones and diagnosing and treating diabetes. What the profession as a whole is less good at is identifying and treating psychiatric illness. Many patients presenting to general practitioners (up to a quarter) and hospital specialities will have a mental health problem, which complicates or mimics physical illness.

Patients with psychiatric disease deserve as much respect and dignity as patients with medical or surgical conditions. Ask new patients how they wish to be referred to (Mr Brown or Mick), ensure your identification is on display, always explain who you are and what you would like to do (take a history, ask how treatment is progressing etc).

Listening to what patients say not only allows the history to be taken, but it also shows the patient that you are interested in them and will, in time, allow them to trust you more. Listening to what patients say or don't say (non-verbal communication), as well as how they say it, also gives information needed in the mental state examination (p402). Listen actively by reflecting back to the patient; they are likely to expand upon issues or explore them further, whilst yielding further information.

Safety on psychiatric wards is paramount for both staff and patients. Very few patients are ever physically violent to staff. Patients who have a history of being physically abusive should not be clerked alone; an accompanying ward nurse should be used as a chaperone. Avoid situations where you could get 'cornered' in by staying close to doors and consider leaving doors open as long as this doesn't compromise patient confidentiality. Patients who are at risk to themselves or other patients need to be under close supervision and should have any potentially dangerous objects (belts, pens, glass etc) taken away.

Classification of psychiatric disease is difficult mainly due to the overlap. Depression (affective disorder) can have features of neurosis and even psychosis; pure psychotic disease equally often has neurotic components and overlaps with some of the personality disorders.

The International Classification of Diseases recognises the following as major psychiatric disease (OHCS6 p313):

- Affective (mood) disorders
  - Depression
  - Mania
- Neurosis
  - Anxiety neurosis
  - Obsessional neurosis
  - Depersonalisation/phobias
  - Hysteria
  - Sexual disorders
- Organic reactions
  - Acute
  - Chronic (dementia)
- Schizophrenia
- Paranoid and other psychoses
- Mental retardation
- Personality disorder
- Alcoholism
- Drug addiction

Psychiatrists should be good at eliciting the history (good listeners, good reflectors), good at putting the patient at ease and remain non-judgemental and non-accusatory. To impart one's moral values onto a patient will simply distress and maybe even aggravate the patient, limiting the amount and quality of information they divulge.

Psychiatric history (OHCS6 p322)

As always, ensure you and the patient are comfortable and are not going to be disturbed (consider leaving your bleep with someone else). Use a chaperone if the patient is aggressive or has the potential to be so. Introduce yourself and ensure you have plenty of time. Explain that anything the patient says will remain confidential and that the consultation can be stopped at any time if they feel uncomfortable. Spend time listening to the patient and watching them, as you may be able to elicit much of the mental state examination during this time. Try not to write too much down during the consultation; this could distract the patient. Have some tissues available as the patient may cry.

Presenting symptoms Ask about what symptoms or 'problems' the patient has; for each of these assess their severity, intensity and effects upon the patient's life. When did they start and have they changed over time? What triggered them initially and what triggers them now? Have these problems ever been treated and if so how and with what effects?

Past psychiatric history Previous informal/formal admissions. Does the patient have a community psychiatric nurse (CPN)? Any previous DSH? What treatments have been tried, and with what effects?

Past medical history Ask about all medical/surgical complaints and their treatment and course.

Drug history Ask about all current and previous medications and allergy.

Family history Ask about family members, their ages, occupations and personal relationships, especially with mother, father and siblings.

Personal history Ask about early development (if known), memories of school and childhood friends, qualifications obtained and occupations since school. Enquire about a sexual history, noting any abuse, sexual orientation and sexual relationships (see below). What are the current and previous social circumstances; where do they live, with whom, what condition is the property in, are there concerns over money and finances and have they ever been in contact with the police or the legal system?

Personality How would the patient describe their personality now? How was it before this illness? What is their current main mood? Have they ever had thoughts about self-harm, if so have they ever made plans or steps towards undertaking this? What hobbies do they have and who are their friends? Do they smoke, drink alcohol or use recreational drugs (now and previously)? What is their reaction to stresses and what is their relationship like with others?

Talking about sex, sexual history and sexual abuse

Be open and not embarrassed about talking about these issues yourself.
Avoid medical terms such as 'coitus'. Use terms the patient will understand.
Remain non-judgemental and ask the patient to describe words you are unsure of.
'Do you have/have you had a sexual partner?' is a good opening question.
'Have you ever slept with another man?' is a way of asking a man about his sexuality.
'Has anyone ever touched you in a way that hurt or embarrassed you sexually?'

Mental state examination (OHCS6 p324)

This is an examination of the mind of a patient with a potential psychiatric illness, just as one would examine the chest for a patient with shortness of breath. It can, in part, be undertaken during the history taking, as much of it is based on appearance, actions, mood, speech and thought processes. A few components need to be asked about specifically, namely perception and general intellect.

Appearance How does the patient dress (bright or clashing colours might suggest mania, poor interest in clothes may suggest low mood, tin foil wrapped over the chest may suggest a psychosis)? Do they take care of themselves (shave, combed hair, body odour etc)? Do they look overly anxious (neurosis), irritable/twitchy (mania), nervous/paranoid (psychosis) or withdrawn and uninterested (depression)

Behaviour Do they act appropriately or are they jumping around (mania), peering through windows and doors or acting as though they can see or hear things which are invisible/inaudible to you (psychosis), or totally withdrawn and barely allowing eye contact (depression)?

Speech Note the qualities of speech: rate, tone, form, quality and content. Depressed patients may have very little to say and say it quietly. The manic patient will speak very quickly, loudly and be very flamboyant with language and descriptions (flight of ideas etc).

Mood and affect What is the overall mood of the patient: are they anxious, depressed or elated? How does the patient feel (their *mood*). Does this match up with your assessment of their mood (their *affect*)? Are they depersonalised (lacking in normal human emotion/mood)?

Thought Is the stream of thought process normal or are there jumps between ideas/conversations (eg knight's move)? Are the thoughts and ideas normal in form or distorted? Is the content suitable and truthful? Are there any delusions (an erroneous belief that is held in the face of evidence to the contrary)? Are some ideas overvalued or have too much emphasis placed upon them? Does the patient have any obsessions or compulsions (rituals or behaviour which the patient cannot break away from)? Does the patient believe that they are not in control of their own thoughts (does someone or something 'insert' thoughts into them or control their thought processes)?

Perception Does the patient have illusions (a misinterpretation) or hallucinations (perceptions of a visual, auditory or tactile stimulus which does not exist)?

Cognition Does the patient remain concentrated on the task in hand or are they easily distracted? Are they able to concentrate on a task or have no ability/desire to do so? Are they orientated in time, place and person? Can they remember things which happened 20min ago, last week, 20yr ago?

General intellect Do they have a normal awareness of events and the world around them? Do they know who the Prime Minister is?

Insight Does the patient appreciate they have an illness? Do they think that everyone else is crazy for keeping them in hospital?

Mini-mental state examination (MMSE) (OHCM6 p59)

This is a standardised means of assessing the memory and cognition of a patient and can be used over time to monitor changes. Results are unreliable if the patient is delirious or has an affective disorder. An abbreviated (10 point) version is often used (p229).

The maximum score is 30, though ≥28 is regarded as 'normal'. Scores of 25–27 are borderline and <25 suggests dementia.

What day of the week is it?	1 point
What is the date today?	1 point
What is the month?	1 point
What is the year?	1 point
Which season of the year is it?	1 point
What country are we in?	1 point
What town/city are we in?	1 point
What are the two main streets nearby?	1 point
What floor of the building are we on?	1 point
What is the name of this place?	1 point
Read the following. Then offer the paper: 'I am going to give you a piece of paper. Take it in your right hand, fold it in half and place it on your lap.'	1 point for each of three actions
Show a pencil and ask what it is called	1 point
Show a wrist-watch and ask what it is called	1 point
Say: 'Repeat after me. No ifs, ands, or buts.'	1 point
Say: 'Read what is written here and do as it says.' Show them a card which reads 'CLOSE YOUR EYES'	1 point
Say: 'Write a complete sentence on this sheet of paper.'	1 point
Say: 'Here is a drawing, please copy it.' [See drawing at bottom of page]	1 point
Say: 'I am going to name three objects. When I have finished repeat them back to me, and remember them as I am going to ask you to say them again in a few minutes. Apple, penny, table.'	1 point for each object repeated
Say: 'I want you to take 7 away from 100. Take 7 away from that number and keep subtracting until I say stop.' [100, 93, 86, 79, 72, 65]	1 point for each of 5 subtractions
What were the objects I asked you to remember? [Apple, penny, table]	1 point for each object

Close your eyes

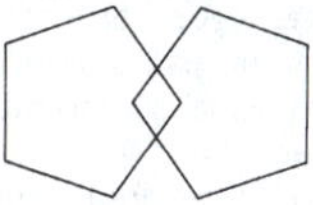

Affective disorder (depression, mania)

(OHCS6 p324) Normal mood is referred to as euthymia; this can become lowered (depression) or elevated (mania) and can fluctuate (bipolar disorder or manic-depression); postnatal depression is also an affective disorder, though with a clear precipitant (p377).

Symptoms are divided up into psychological (anhedonia, reduced concentration, reduced self-esteem and confidence, negative memories and thoughts, suicidal thoughts (ideation/intent), psychomotor retardation and psychosis) and biological (disturbed sleep (early morning wakening and nocturnal insomnia), loss of appetite and weight, loss of libido, constipation and amenorrhoea). Other symptoms include low mood, fatigue, anxiety and tearfulness.

Classification is as difficult for affective disorder as it is for psychiatric illnesses in general, though groups of symptoms and their severity can be 'pigeon-holed' as follows: depressive disorder (mild, moderate, severe, psychotic), bipolar disorder, mixed anxiety–depression.

Organic causes of depression (use investigations appropriately to exclude these)

Endocrine	Neurological	Drug-associated
Cushing's disease	Cerebrovascular disease	β-blockers
Addison's disease	Epilepsy	Digoxin
Hypothyroidism	Brain tumour	Anti-epileptics
Hypercalcaemia	Head injury	
Folate deficiency	Parkinson's disease	

Epidemiology Women are more prone to affective disorders than men are and the reasons for this remain unclear (eg genetic, hormonal, social pressures (environmental), greater willingness to admit to symptoms, depressed men given alternative diagnosis, eg alcoholism).

Management is multi-focal. General measures include discussion (counselling) of issues which *predispose*, *precipitate* and *maintain* depression. Therapeutic methods of controlling disease severity (antidepressants) are indicated in certain patients (see opposite) and should be continued until a response is seen and then for a further 6mth. Selective serotonin reuptake inhibitors are the most common group of antidepressants used while the older tricyclics and monoamine oxidase inhibitors (MAOI) are less frequently employed. ECT can be used (see opposite). Mania is usually controlled by lithium or sodium valproate (OHCS6 p354). Psychological intervention can be used alongside other means, commonly cognitive-behavioural therapy (p414).

Prognosis depends upon the aetiology. Reactive depression (secondary to a life-event) has a good prognosis, though other forms are more refractory and 50% of patients will have recurrent depressive episodes; attempted and actual suicide rates are about 8 times more common in this latter group.

Admission may be required if suicide risk is high (p407) or if the patient has social isolation or other mental health issues.

Patients who are likely to benefit from antidepressant therapy

Patients who have had persistent low mood or anhedonia for >2wk
Patients who have >4 of the following:
- Suicidal ideation or intent
- Unexplained feelings of worthlessness or guilt
- Inability to function – psychomotor retardation
- Concentration impaired
- Impaired appetite
- Decreased sleep
- Low energy, fatigue

Electroconvulsive therapy (ECT)

ECT is used in the management of refractory depression, when psychotic features are present and when symptoms need to be controlled fast (risk of complications of depression, such as alcoholism, suicide risk etc, are great).
Avoid if recent sub-arachnoid/intracranial bleed and caution if cardiovascular or other cerebrovascular disease.
Seizure activity precipitated by passing small currents across the brain are believed to increase/restore the levels of neurotransmitters in the brain and help alleviate the symptoms of profound depression.
Patients must be starved as they require a short general anaesthetic for the procedure to be undertaken.

Commoner drugs used to treat depression

Selective serotonin-reuptake inhibitors	**Tricyclic antidepressants**
Fluoxetine (Prozac®)	Amitryptyline
Paroxetine (Seroxat®)	Imipramine
Citalopram (Cipramil®)	Lofepramine
Setraline (Lustal®)	Dosulepin
Venlafaxine (Efexor®, an SNRI)	
Monoamine oxidase inhibitors	**Others**
Phenelzine	Trazodone
Moclobemide	Lithium

Suicide and deliberate self-harm (DSH)

(OHCS6 p338, OHAEM2 p586) Suicidal ideation is when one has thought about committing suicide transiently. Suicidal intent is when one makes plans, thinks about the means of committing the act and makes preparations, writes a note etc.

Assessing suicidal risk is difficult and far from foolproof. Several factors give patients a high risk of attempted or actual suicide and are usually related to the social situation and build up to an acute presentation (opposite).

Scoring an individual's risk can be undertaken, but again is not fool-proof. A modified 'sad person scale' is often used in A+E and in admission units to decide on the safest means of patient disposal. A modified scoring system is illustrated opposite.

Suicide and DSH are precipitated by many reasons. Suicide is often the final step in patients with severe mental illness who feel hopeless and cannot see any other option/way out. Suicide can also be part of a more sudden grief/stress response to a major life-event (more spontaneous). Attempted suicide and DSH can equally occur for other reasons – classically the patient who 'cuts' is seeking help, either as part of a genuine call for help or as part of a personality disorder.

Question the patient as to the reasons behind their actions, whether they had planned to undertake this or if it was spontaneous and whether they were under the influence of drugs or alcohol at the time. It is often useful to know if they have attempted suicide/DSH previously and if they plan to attempt it again. Assessing their social network is important, as this will help to decide if the patient can be discharged or not.

Look for signs of underlying psychiatric and physical illness and especially consider mood; a withdrawn depressed patient (low affect, poor eye contact, poverty of speech) is likely to be at higher risk than a patient who is laughing and free from psychiatric symptoms.

Investigations will be determined by the nature of any physical injuries (eg overdose or cuts). All patients with potential drug/substance overdose should have paracetamol and salicylate levels taken, even if the patient denies taking them (as many over-the-counter drugs contain paracetamol and salicylates and patients may lie). Paracetamol and salicylate overdoses can kill and cause end-organ damage, yet if identified early these can be prevented (p310). An internet toxicology resource called Toxbase® should be accessed if an overdose of any drug is known or suspected and most A+E departments have access to this. **The Poisons Information Service can always offer 24h advice (0870 600 6266).**

Management should initially concentrate on treating the injuries or overdose appropriately. As this is being undertaken, the level of risk needs to be assessed (opposite) and, if appropriate, referral made to the emergency psychiatric services for immediate or subsequent assessment.

Acutely suicidal patients must not be allowed to leave the hospital until they have been assessed by psychiatric services. They can be restrained or sedated if need be (p75) under common law. Always seek senior help in this circumstance.

Factors associated with high risk of actual or attempted suicide

S	**Sex:** women attempt suicide more often, but men are much more successful **Spouse:** single, divorced or widowed people more likely to commit suicide **Stressful** life-events make suicide more common
U	**Unemployment** and retirement raise risk of suicide **Unsuccessful attempts** previously increase risk of future suicide attempts
I	**Identification** with others who have committed suicide is high-risk behaviour
CI	**Chronic illness** (medical or psychological) is associated with high risk
D	**Depression** is associated with high risk of suicide
A	**Age:** the older the patient, the greater the risk of suicide **Alcohol** or drug abuse makes suicide more likely **Availability** of lethal weapons is associated with increased risk of suicide
L	**Lethality** of previous attempts (using guns, hanging) carries increased risk compared with drug overdose or wrist cutting

A modified sad person score

Means of assessing an individual's risk of suicide	
Male	Score 1
Age <19yr or >45yr	Score 1
Depression or hopelessness	Score 1 or 2
Previous suicide attempts	Score 1
Excessive alcohol or drug use	Score 1
Loss of rational thinking (psychotic or organic illness)	Score 1 or 2
Separated, widowed or divorced	Score 1
Organised or serious attempt	Score 1 or 2
No social support	Score 1
State future intent (determined to repeat or ambivalent)	Score 1 or 2

Interpretation of total score:
Score <6; may be safe to discharge, depending upon circumstances
Score 6–8; probably requires psychiatric services assessment
Score >8; likely to need hospital admission and urgent psychiatric services assessment

Neurosis

Anxiety neurosis (OHCS6 p344)

Neuroses are very common with up to 15% of the population suffering with them at some stage; ♀>♂.

Common symptoms include: emotional/mood (anxiety and irritability), cognition (exaggerated worries and fears), behavioural (avoidance of feared situations, checking and seeking reassurance), bodily symptoms (tight chest, shortness of breath, palpitations, 'butterflies', tremor, tingling of fingers, aches and pains, frequent desire to pass urine and motions).

Phobic anxiety, eg spiders, refers to situational anxiety, with avoidance behaviour which is counter-productive and reinforces phobia. *Management* depends upon behavioural and cognitive therapy, anxiolytics and antidepressants. *Agoraphobia* is a fear of open spaces or crowds and individuals often describe panic attacks or an impending sense of doom/demise. *Social phobia* is more than just shyness and individuals have an overwhelming fear of embarrassing themselves in front of others.

Panic disorder often propagates from phobic anxiety, with panic attacks arising through fear of having a panic episode. *Management* relies on CBT and sometimes antidepressants.

Generalised anxiety disorder covers the remaining neuroses which are not situational, episodic or lifelong. *Management* as for other neuroses.

Non-therapeutic means of relaxation to help break acute and chronic anxiety

Breathing exercises (count to 10 silently as one breathes in and out)
Tensing and relaxing muscle groups in turn, starting at the toes
Relaxation CDs
Yoga
Hypnosis; must be undertaken by expert initially, though many patients can induce self-hypnosis after prolonged teaching

Obsessive-compulsive disorder (OHCS6 p346)

Obsessions (eg thought that hands are dirty or door is unlocked) and compulsions (eg repeated hand-washing or repeated door-checking) are very common, though only a small percentage ever present to psychiatric services.

Common symptoms include: emotional (anxiety about the topic of obsessional thought), cognition (preoccupation with obsessions), behavioural (tension, especially if prevented from doing a compulsive act and associations with depression).

Management relies on cognitive-behavioural therapy to identify obsessions and rationalise compulsions; antidepressants may have a role.

Eating disorders

Anorexia nervosa (OHCS6 p348)

Anorexia occurs when the patient believes they are excessively overweight, while their BMI is usually very low. Carries high mortality.

Defining features usually consist of: deliberate weight loss (primarily by restriction of food intake), weight >15% below normal (ie BMI <17.5), dread of fatness and disturbance in perception of body weight (overvalued idea rather than delusion), amenorrhoea.

Clinical features are diverse. Range of bodily signs (gaunt face, lanugo hair (very fine body hair), poorly developed/atrophic breasts, scanty pubic hair, peripheral oedema, slow pulse), depressive and obsessional symptoms, delay in secondary sexual characteristics if before puberty, preoccupation with food and enjoyment of cooking for others, fatigue, irritability and coldness, social withdrawal and narrowing interests, use of diuretics, laxatives and excessive exercise.

Aetiology Much commoner in females than males (10:1), average age of onset 15–16yr, about 1% prevalence in UK 12–18 year-olds.

Management relies on developing a good rapport with the patient. Encourage weight gain and consider low-dose antidepressant or antipsychotic. Psychotherapy and CBT to help explore underlying issues and monitor physical status with weight charts.

Prognosis depends upon time of presentation to psychiatric services. Long duration pre-presentation carries a poorer prognosis and anorexia can develop into bulimia (below). Mortality remains at 20%.

Admission may be required if severe or intractable anorexia or if episode is life-threatening.

Bulimia (OHCS6 p349)

Defining features usually consist of: recurrent binge-eating, feeling of lack of control during binging episodes, regular use of mechanisms to overcome the fattening effects of binging (eg vomiting, laxatives, excessive exercise), persistent over-concern with weight, does not meet criteria for anorexia (BMI>17.5).

Clinical features include painless enlargement of salivary glands, tetany, Russell's sign (calluses on the back of the hand from repeated self-induced vomiting), acid erosion of teeth.

Aetiology Much commoner in females than males. Affects 2% of women aged 16–35yr. Only 10% of patients with bulimia present to health professionals.

Management relies on behavioural or cognitive techniques and encouraging a healthy, non-binging attitude towards food. Self-help groups are nationwide. Antidepressants may have a role to play, though evidence is minimal.

Prognosis is better than for anorexia, though some patients do go on to develop anorexia.

Dementia (OHCS6 p352)

Dementia can be considered as chronic brain failure, resulting in impaired memory, but in the presence of normal consciousness (cf delirium).

Clinical features include memory impairment, short term > long term (which should be present for >6mth to secure diagnosis and severe enough to affect normal social functioning), behavioural and personality changes (wandering, aggression, disinhibition). Other features may be present such as dysphasias, dyspraxias and focal neurological signs, psychotic symptoms and unawareness of deficits. Inevitable progression.

Aetiology Dementia is the end-point of several disease processes (Alzheimer's disease, vascular dementia, Lewy body dementia and rarer causes eg degenerative causes, normal pressure hydrocephalus, space-occupying lesion (SOL), head injury), though differentiation is seldom helpful in management; the most important consideration is to exclude reversible causes and other differential diagnoses (see below). Pre-senile dementia accounts for ~5% of cases of dementia and occurs in patients <65yr whereas 20% of all patients >80yr have features of dementia.

Pathology to exclude prior to diagnosing dementia

Depression	Poor concentration and impaired memory – pseudodementia
Delirium	Check level of consciousness and duration of history
Deafness	Check patient can hear you
Dysphasia	Check the patient can respond to your questions
Amnesia syndrome	A purer short-term memory deficit
Paraphrenia	Check for features of psychosis

Investigations Patients with suspected pre-senile dementia need neurologist assessment and investigation. Patients with rapid onset symptoms may need head CT to exclude subdural haematoma and other investigations as appropriate.

Management relies on confirming the diagnosis and excluding other differentials. Rarely a reversible cause is identified and treatment resolves memory symptoms. Anticholinesterase drugs such as donepezil may slow disease progression by increasing acetylcholine within the brain.

Prognosis depends upon cause. Most patients' symptoms progress and death usually occurs within 10yr of presentation.

Delirium (p229, **OHCS6** p350)

Clinical features include: clouding of consciousness (drowsiness, decreased awareness of surroundings, disorientation, distractibility), together with visual hallucinations, irritability and sometimes aggression, impaired concentration and memory, fluctuating course (often worse at night).

Causes include: hypoxia, hypoglycaemia, toxic (alcohol/alcohol withdrawal), drugs (opiates, steroids, digoxin), metabolic (liver/renal failure, nutritional deficiencies), infections, trauma (head injury), post-ictal.

Management relies on identifying the precipitant and treating this, whilst supporting the patient and treating any other symptoms as they arise.

Substance misuse (OHCS6 p362)

A substance is misused if it produces physical, psychological or social harm to the individual or to others.

'Street' names for commonly misused drugs

Amphetamines	Speed, Whizz, Billy, Uppers
Cannabis	Weed, Dope, Ganja, Hash, Grass, Pot, Marijuana, Wacky Backy
Cocaine	Coke, Snow, Dust, Charlie, C
Crack cocaine	Crack, Rock, Base
Ecstasy	'E', Pills, Doves, MDMA
Heroin	Smack, Junk, Skag, Brown
Ketamine	'K', Special K, Ket, Vitamin K, Horse
LSD	Acid, Trips, Tabs (LSD stands for Lysergic acid diethylamide)
Magic mushrooms	'Shrooms, Mushies, Psilocybe mushrooms
Poppers	Nitrites, Liquid Gold, Amyl/butyl nitrite

Alcohol (OHCS6 p363/p24)

Dependence Individual feels compelled to drink and there is a preference for drinking over other activities. Tolerance to alcohol increases and drinks in response to stress. Usually aware of harmful significance to drinking and gets withdrawal if stops.

Withdrawal occurs 24–72h after stopping drinking. Become tremulous (the shakes) and agitated. Nausea and vomiting common, together with sweating and overwhelming desire to drink.

Delirium tremens occurs 24–48h after drinking cessation. Delirious, visual hallucinations, delusions and fear/agitation. Tremor usually coarse and seizures can occur. Insomnia is prominent. Can result in death if unrecognised/untreated. *Management* is supportive, with reducing dose of benzodiazepines (usually chlordiazepoxide) and vitamin supplementation (p24) and long-term programmes to address dependence and associated issues.

Opiates (OHCS6 p362)

Dependence Individuals vary in the amount of opiate they consume per day. Most 'serious' drug users inject heroin 3–4 times per day, costing between £10–100 per day. After a dose the individual relaxes and, depending upon the amount taken, may sleep. Intravenous access is often a problem in these patients (p25).

Withdrawal occurs 8–12h after last dose. Patients usually have a craving for opiates and become very restless and agitated, sometimes aggressive. Insomnia, myalgia and sweating are common, as are abdominal pains, vomiting and diarrhoea. Many patients are observed to yawn and have 'goose bumps' which is where the term 'cold turkey' comes from. *Management* relies on either replacement of opiate with methadone or benzodiazepine and appropriate referral to specialist services for a withdrawal programme, which can usually be undertaken in the community.

Psychosis

Schizophrenia (OHCS6 p356)

Psychotic disorders consist of delusions, passivity phenomena, abnormal perceptions (hallucinations), disordered thought processes and changes in behaviour. Schizophrenia is just one type of psychosis, the others being psychosis in affective disorder, organic or drug-induced psychosis and delusional disorder.

Aetiology of schizophrenia is unclear; may be genetic, developmental, brain abnormality, neurotransmitter abnormality, related to life event(s).

Epidemiology Lifetime risk about 1%, ♂=♀. Men often present earlier (15–25yr) than females (25–35yr) and onset of symptoms >45yr is referred to as paraphrenia. Schizophrenia appears to be more common amongst the lower social classes, though this could be due to social downward drift.

Acute presentation of a patient who is acting oddly is usually the initial step to making a diagnosis. On probing deeper the positive symptoms appear to predominate (cf chronic schizophrenia) and many of the first-rank symptoms can be identified (see below). Most patients lack insight into their illness and retrospectively have had a prodromal period of decline in performance and social withdrawal.

First-rank symptoms

Delusions	**Passivity**
Delusional perception	Passivity of thought, feelings or actions
Hallucinations	**Thought flow and possession**
Thought echo (audible thoughts)	Thought withdrawal
Third person auditory hallucinations	Thought insertion
Running commentary	Thought broadcasting

Chronic presentation is unlike the acute, new presentation since the negative symptoms predominate: flattened (blunted mood), apathy and loss of drive, social isolation, poverty of speech, poor self-care, cognitive impairment of varying degrees.

Investigations are used, as in other mental illness, to exclude potential reversible causes (mostly organic ones). Concurrent physical disease is also common, so a thorough physical examination is required.

Management aims to prevent relapses and optimising level of functioning at all levels. The classes of therapeutic agents are shown opposite. Besides drugs, ECT has been used (only in catatonic stupor) and all patients should undergo some form of cognitive-behavioural therapy, ±family therapy.

Prognosis varies. Good prognostic factors include: female sex, older age at onset, married, good pre-morbid personality and social functioning, absence of other psychiatric illness, acute onset, short episode, onset precipitated by life-event, good response to medication.

Drugs used in the treatment of schizophrenia

Antipsychotics (neuroleptics)	Dopamine antagonists Sedating Need therapy for 12–24mth following episode Persistent negative symptoms not relieved by antipsychotics **Chlorpromazine, flupenthixol, thioridazine – typical** **Clozapine, olanzapine, risperidone – atypicals**
Anticholinergic	Address imbalance between dopamine and acetylcholine Limit extra-pyramidal side-effects **Procyclidine**
Benzodiazepines	Short-term sedation in acute setting **Lorazepam, diazepam, temazepam**
Antidepressants	If depression also problematic **SSRIs, SNRIs, tricyclic, MAOI**

Monitoring atypical antipsychotic agents

Some of the atypical antipsychotic drugs are associated with agranulocytosis, and monitoring of the full blood count is needed on a weekly basis for up to 18wk after commencing treatment, then every 2wk. Check with pharmacist first before commencing an atypical antipsychotic.

Personality disorders (OHCS6 p364)

Personality describes characteristic behavioural, emotional and cognitive attributes of an individual. Personality traits which are excessive and dysfunctional constitute a personality disorder.

Classification varies, depending who you ask, though the ICD-10 scheme is a commonly used one and relies on three cluster classifications.

Cluster A or the *eccentric* group consists of odd, aloof or suspicious behaviours. Includes paranoid and schizoid personalities. *Treatment* relies on antipsychotic therapy; psychotherapy is contraindicated.

Cluster B or the *dramatic* group consist of emotionally labile, intense or erratic behaviours. These include dissocial, emotionally unstable and histrionic personalities. *Treatment* relies on cognitive-behavioural therapy and antidepressants for impulsive behaviour.

Cluster C or the *anxious* group comprise constitutionally timid or worried behaviours and include avoidant, dependent and anancastic personality disorders. *Treatment* relies on identifying and treating underlying neurosis or mood disorder and avoidance of escalating contact which fosters dependency.

Non-drug therapies in psychiatry (OHCS6 p368)

'Psychotherapy' is a term that the lay-person often associates with leather couches and mind-probing analysts, though this is far from reality. Many forms of psychotherapy exist and very few fit this stereotype.

Behavioural therapy identifies abnormal (pathological) behaviour and attempts to address and correct this. For example, for a patient with agoraphobia (fear of crowded environments) the symptoms precipitated by such environments are discussed along with the various environments in which this occurs. The individual is then encouraged to rank various situations in which symptoms would be least/most likely. Between sessions of therapy the patient desensitises themselves by increasing their exposure to such environments and employs strategies to cope with symptoms (management of panic for example). *Suitable for*: phobias, obsessions, eating disorders, sexual disorders, generalised anxiety disorder and mild depression. *Not suitable for*: psychosis (unless with other therapies), severe depression or dementia.

Cognitive therapy identifies abnormal (pathological) behaviour and attempts to address and correct this. For example, for a patient with agoraphobia (fear of crowded environments) the symptoms precipitated by such environments are discussed and the logical reasons for these explored. Some patients may fear that they will stand out in a crowd and the therapist will explore why this would happen, and if it did, what would be the deleterious effects of it. The individual would then be able to rationally discuss the irrational fears they hold and consider strategies to compensate, as well as methods to control, somatic manifestations (such as panic episodes). *Suitable for*: depression, neurosis, chronic fatigue, alcohol abuse, smoking cessation, insomnia, bulimia, chronic pain disorders. *Not suitable for*: severe psychosis, dementia.

Psychoanalysis uses a therapist who acts as a catalyst, encouraging the individual to think aloud and reflecting ideas and statements back which further promotes verbal analysis within the individual. Very little material originates from the therapist and most stems from within the individual themselves.

Counselling is an 'informal' form of psychotherapy, often using the techniques of psychoanalysis.

Group therapy, as its name implies, uses a group setting where individuals are encouraged to openly discuss and debate issues, utilising aspects of behavioural, cognitive and psychoanalytical skills (unknown to them) to help individuals arrive at solutions to problems. *Suitable for*: addictions and major physical illness such as cancer.

Family therapy is similar to group therapy, though the group consists of a family unit and a therapist who keeps the discussion going.

Sex therapy utilises the principles of family therapy, but involves just a sexual couple and again encourages issues/problems to be discussed openly and solutions to be reached.

The Mental Health Act

Formal admission (OHCS6 p398)

Psychiatry in-patients can be either *informal* (stay in hospital of their own accord) or *formal* (are held in hospital under a section of the Mental Health Act). The Mental Health Act is complex, though below is a summary of the commoner sections used in daily practice. Always seek senior advice if unsure or inexperienced with the legality and formalities of this Act.

Restraint and emergency pharmacological sedation for patients at immediate high risk to themselves or others is a topic often debated and should be discussed locally before starting a psychiatric attachment. Generally restraint should not harm the individual and should be viewed by others as appropriate to the situation in hand.

Section 2 (admission for assessment) is used to undertake only an assessment of a patient and expires after 28d. A close relative or social worker can make the application on the recommendation of two doctors (one should be a psychiatrist and the other, ideally, a doctor who knows the patient).

Section 3 (admission for treatment) is used to undertake treatment for a diagnosed mental health condition and expires after 6mth. The act needs to be signed by two doctors who appreciate that the illness cannot be treated in the community (due to risk to self or others or likely/previous non-compliance with treatment regimen).

Section 4 (emergency treatment) is used to admit a patient to hospital as a matter of urgency for initial treatment of a crisis. On arrival, and once emergency treatment is given, the section is usually converted to a section 2 to allow full assessment prior to conversion to a section 3 to initiate definite treatment. Expires after 72h.

Section 5(2) (detention of a patient already in hospital) is used by the doctor in charge of a ward (or his representative eg SHO) to prevent a patient from leaving the ward when they are at imminent risk to themselves or others; they can be restrained by reasonable force. The section expires after 72h, and the patient has to be an in-patient; A+E and outpatients departments are not covered by this section so patients must be held there by common law. Conversion to another section must occur before 72h or the section expires and the patient must be allowed to leave.

Section 5(4) (nurses' holding powers) is used by trained psychiatric nurses to restrain a psychiatric patient admitted informally for up to 6h until personnel and paperwork can be found to section the patient under a longer component of the Mental Health Act as appropriate.

Section 136 can be used by the police to arrest and detain a person they perceive to be at risk to themselves or others due to mental illness and transfer them to a place of safety (usually A+E or a police station) where the individual can be assessed formally by psychiatric services.

Rheumatology

Arthropathy is a term used to describe any pathology of joints, commonly 'arthritis' (inflammation). Joint disease is usually classified into acute and chronic and either monoarthritis or polyarthritis.

Monoarthritis causes include: septic arthritis, psoriatic and reactive arthritides, trauma (haemarthrosis), pseudo-gout (calcium pyrophosphate dihydrate crystal arthropathy), gout (uric acid crystal arthropathy), osteoarthritis, monoarthritic presentation of a polyarticular disease.

Polyarthritis causes include: viral infections (reactive arthropathy), rheumatoid arthritis and osteoarthritis, spondylarthritides, connective tissue disease (SLE), crystal arthropathy (gout and pseudo-gout), post-streptococcal reactive arthritis, sarcoidosis.

Rheumatoid arthritis (RA) is the commonest inflammatory polyarthritis, it is symmetrical, destructive and often results in deformity; small and large synovial joints are affected (OHCM6 p414). Inflammatory markers are usually raised, with positive rheumatoid factor (RF) in 50–90%; radiographs show destructive arthropathy. *Tx*: anti-inflammatory and analgesic drugs. Consider DMARD therapy (disease-modifying antirheumatic drugs), corticosteroids, surgery (joint replacement/fusion).

Classical clinical hand signs in rheumatoid arthritis (p446)

Swan neck deformity of fingers	Ulnar deviation of fingers
Z-deformity of the thumb	Dinner-fork deformity of the wrist
Boutonnière's deformity of distal IPJ	Wasting of instrinsic muscles of the hand

Osteoarthritis (OA) results from degeneration of articular cartilage and simultaneous proliferation of new bone, cartilage and connective tissue. OA arises for many reasons and is usually secondary to other disease processes such as trauma, developmental abnormality or following a primary inflammatory arthropathy. Hips and knees are most commonly affected. Radiographs show loss of joint space, osteophytes, subchondral bone sclerosis and bone cyst formation. Inflammatory markers will be normal in pure OA. *Tx*: weight loss and maintenance of exercise with oral analgesia or steroid joint injections. Physiotherapy and protection of further joint damage with rubber shoe heels may delay progression. Arthroscopy and wash-out may offer some symptomatic relief. Severe disease may require joint replacement or joint fusion (OHCM6 p416).

Seronegative arthropathies are diseases which affect the joints, but are generally RF negative and include: Lyme disease, Behçet's, leukaemia, pulmonary osteoarthropathy, endocarditis, acromegaly, Wilson's disease, familial Mediterranean fever, sarcoid, haemophilia, sickle-cell, haemochromatosis and infections.

Septic arthritis is a medical emergency, even more so in a prosthetic joint. Typically the joint is acutely painful, warm, red and swollen. Inflammatory markers and WCC will be raised and synovial fluid will be rich in WCCs and protein *Tx*: adequate analgesia, joint aspiration (p490) followed by IV antibiotics (p297), and early involvement of a specialist, either rheumatologist or orthopaedic surgeon (OHAM1 p740).

Systemic lupus erythematosus (SLE) is a multi-system connective tissue disease, most prevalent in USA and Far East, with 9♀:1♂. Commonly affects: joints (either acute or chronic), skin (in 2/3 of patients, often photosensitive; alopecia less common), cardiopulmonary (pericarditis, alveolitis), renal (haematuria, nephrotic syndrome, CRF), CNS (mild psychiatric disturbance, epilepsy) and other systems (abdo pains, GI ulcers, lymphadenopathy, ocular findings). Investigations show typical autoantibody pattern (ANA, dsDNA, RF). *Tx*: steroids, NSAIDs, DMARDs, immunosuppressive drugs for severe disease; aspirin and anticoagulation in antiphospholipid syndrome (OHCM6 p422).

Vasculitis is inflammation of blood vessels. It is either occlusive (as in SLE) or non-occlusive (as in Henoch-Schönlein purpura). It can be precipitated *de novo* (eg polyarteritis, Churg-Strauss, giant cell arteritis, Takayasu's and Wegner's), by drugs, by infection or by autoimmune complexes and complement activation (SLE and RA). Signs and symptoms depend upon system and organs involved: general – fever, malaise, arthralgia, myalgia; skin – purpura, ulcers, livedo reticularis, nailbed infarcts, digital gangrene; eyes – episcleritis, ulceration, visual loss; ENT – epistaxis, nasal crusting, stridor, deafness; pulmonary – haemoptysis, dyspnoea; cardiac – loss of pulses, heart failure, MI, angina; GI – abdo pain, malabsorption; renal – hypertension, haematuria, casts, ARF/CRF; CNS – mononeuritis multiplex, neuropathy, fits, hemiplegia, confusion. Diagnosis is made on clinical findings supported by histological features. *Tx*: specialist opinion required; steroids and cyclophosphamide.

Crystal arthropathies often present as an acute monoarthropathy, though can affect several joints. Gout often affects the first metatarsophalangeal joint whereas pseudo-gout often affects the wrist or knee. Diagnosis is confirmed by synovial fluid examination and crystal identification. Tx: NSAIDs, treat underlying of crystal formation (OHCM6 p416).

Ankylosing spondylitis occurs most often in young men, presenting with low back pain and early morning stiffness. Diagnosis is clinical supported by radiological features of abnormal sacroiliac joints, squaring of vertebrae and eventually bamboo spine; often HLA B27 positive. *Tx*: exercise with analgesia (NSAIDs); surgery in severe disease (OHCM6 p418).

Polymyalgia rheumatica (PMR) occurs mostly in elderly patients (>70yr), usually symmetrical in distribution with early morning stiffness of shoulders and proximal limb muscles. Associated with depression, fatigue, fever, weight loss and anorexia. Similar to giant cell arteritis. ESR and ALP are usually raised. *Tx*: prednisolone with bone protection.

Giant cell (temporal) arteritis (GCA) is associated with PMR in about 25% of cases. Commoner in the elderly; rare <55yr. Headaches (p210), scalp and temporal tenderness, jaw claudication, amaurosis fugax or sudden blindness in one eye are classical symptoms. Inflammatory markers are elevated, an ESR >100mm/h is pathognomic. Classified as a medical emergency due to high risk of blindness and stroke and requires immediate steroid therapy (p213 or OHCM6, p424). Diagnosis confirmed by temporal artery biopsy.

Autoantibodies

Common autoantibodies and the diseases in which they are present

Autoantibody	Disease (% frequency where known)
Acetylcholine receptor	Myasthenia gravis (80)
Antinuclear (ANA)	SLE (95), RA (32), JIA (76), chronic active hepatitis (75), Sjörgen's syndrome (70), systemic sclerosis (64), normal 'controls' (0–2)
Anticardiolipin	Primary antiphospholipid syndrome
Anticentromere	CREST variant systemic sclerosis
Anti-Ro	Sjörgen's syndrome, sub-acute cutaneous lupus, SLE (30), systemic sclerosis (60), interstitial pneumonitis
Anti-La	Sjörgen's syndrome (65), SLE (15)
C-ANCA	Wegener's granulomatosis (90), MPA (11), Churg-Strauss syndrome
P-ANCA	Churg-Strauss syndrome (60)
dsDNA	SLE (60)
ssDNA	SLE (70), autoimmune rheumatic disease, inflammation
ENA	Includes: Anti-Ro, Anti-LA, Jo-1, RNP, Scl-70, Anti-Sm
Gastric parietal cell	Autoimmune gastritis, pernicious anaemia
Glycolipid	Multi-focal motor neuropathy, Guillain-Barré syndrome, Miller-Fisher syndrome
Glomerular basement membrane	Goodpasture's syndrome
IgA-endomysial	Coeliac disease
Anti-Jo-1	Myositis
Mitochondrial (AMA)	Primary biliary cirrhosis (>95)
Rheumatoid factor	RA (50–90), SLE (15–35), systemic sclerosis (20–30), juvenile RA (7–10), polymyositis (5–10), infection (0–50)
RNP	SLE and MCTD
Anti-Scl-70	Systemic sclerosis
Anti-Sm	SLE
Smooth muscle (SMA)	Chronic active hepatitis (40–90), primary biliary cirrhosis (30–70), idiopathic cirrhosis (25–30), viral infections (80), 'controls' (3–12), autoimmune sclerosing cholangitis
Thyroid peroxidase	Hashimoto's thryoiditis (>80), Graves' disease (50)
Thyrotopin receptor	Graves' disease (50–80)

Steroid therapy

This is common in patients with skin, joint and bowel disease. Steroids given for >14d should never be abruptly discontinued as this can precipitate an Addisonian crisis (p240). Patients can need >60mg prednisolone per day for severe disease and this must be converted to an appropriate intravenous corticosteroid dose if they are NBM, eg surgery.

Conversion table of oral prednisolone dosing into IV hydrocortisone requirements

Prednisolone/24h PO	Hydrocortisone/6h IV
60mg	240mg
50mg	200mg
40mg	160mg
30mg	120mg
20mg	80mg
10mg	40mg

Steroid conversion (See *BNF* 6.3.2)

These are equivalent corticosteroid doses compared to 5mg prednisolone, but do not take into account dosing frequencies or mineralocorticoid effects

- Hydrocortisone 20mg – usually given IV 6–8h
- Dexamethasone 750μg – usually given once daily
- Methylprednisolone 4mg – usually given once daily

Steroid side-effects

GI ulceration	Consider PPI or H_2-receptor antagonist
Infections and reactivation of TB	Low threshold for culturing samples or CXR
Skin thinning/poor wound healing	Pressure care and wound care
Sodium and fluid retention	Twice-daily BPs
Hyperglycaemia	Twice-daily BMs if taking high-dose steroids
Osteoporosis	Bone protection (calcium + bisphosphonate)
Hypertension	Twice-daily BPs

Withdrawing steroid therapy is an art and must be performed gradually if steroids have been used for >14d. Large doses (>20mg prednisolone or equivalent) can be reduced by 5–10mg/wk until dose is 10mg prednisolone/d. Thereafter the doses must be reduced more slowly, by 2.5mg/wk until the dose is 5mg/d. Thereafter reduce the dose by 1mg/wk down to zero.

Surgery

Pre-op assessment

Elective patients generally attend pre-admission clinics a few weeks before their operation. This enables you to:

- assess the patient's problem (ie does it still warrant an operation?)
- gauge their medical fitness for an anaesthetic and for surgery
- request any pre-operative investigations (see NICE guidelines[1])
- check consent (this should be obtained by the surgeon performing the procedure or a person competent to undertake it – p94)
- answer any queries the patient may have
- also allows you to develop a rapport with the patient, prior to their admission

Clerking

- ***History*** note initial presentation, proposed operation, risk factors and systemic symptoms (if suspected malignant lesion) ***PMH*** previous operations ***DH*** allergies, previous reactions to general anaesthetic and CASES (Contraception, Anticoagulation, Steroids, ETOH, Smoking) ***SH*** mobility, home help ***systems review*** CVS, resp, GI, neuro, musculoskeletal. If the patient is seen on the day of the operation, document the time of their last meal
- ***Examination*** area of operation, CVS and resp; others will depend upon history/presentation/planned surgery
- ***Investigations*** see table below

Pre-op investigations[1] (p316)

Investigation	Indication
FBC	To exclude infection or anaemia
Sickle-cell screen	African/Mediterranean patients, +ve FH
U+E	Age >60yr, cardiovascular or renal disease, patients on steroids, diuretics, ACEi
LFT	Previous or suspected abnormal liver function, biliary surgery
Clotting	Established or suspected abnormal liver function
Urine β-HCG (pregnancy test)	Women of child-bearing age
CXR	Age >60yr, cardiovascular or respiratory disease, malignancy, major thoracic and upper abdominal surgery, unexplained SOB
ECG	Age >50yr, cardiovascular disease, DM, smokers

1 NICE guidelines: http://www.nice.org.uk/page.aspx?o=CG003

Requesting blood pre-op

Each hospital will have guidelines on the transfusion requirements for most elective operations – become familiar with these.

Blood for transfusion is in limited supply and should only be cross matched when necessary. The table below shows commonly accepted blood bank requests for elective surgery.

Summary of operations and blood requirements

Blood bank request	Operation
No request	Minor day-case surgery (in-growing toe nails, carpel tunnel syndrome, peripheral lipoma excision etc)
Group and save	Laparoscopy, appendicectomy, cholecystectomy, hernia repair, simple hysterectomy, hepatic biopsy, mastectomy, varicose veins
Crossmatch 2units	Colectomy, hemiarthroplasty, laparotomy, TURP, thyroidectomy, THR
Crossmatch 4units	AP excision, hepatic/pancreatic surgery
Crossmatch 6units	Aneurysm repair (book ITU bed post-op)

Patients with medical problems

- ***DM*** see p236, make sure the patient is early on the operating list
- ***CVS*** inform the anaesthetist if patients have had recent chest pains or symptoms of LV dysfunction. The anaesthetist may want you to request an echo or see the patient themselves
- ***Obstructive jaundice*** check clotting, WCC, CRP, U+E and hydration

Contacting the anaesthetist/ITU

Find out who the anaesthetist is for your theatre list and inform them as soon as possible about any patients who may need further investigations or senior review prior to surgery.

If a patient needs an ITU bed post-op, inform ITU well in advance with the date the bed is required. Phone to confirm that the bed is still available on the day of the operation; if it is not the patient may be cancelled.

Special circumstances

- ***Steroids*** (p419) patients taking regular steroids must have extra steroid cover during surgery and be converted to IV preparations if NBM. Discuss each patient's need with your team and the anaesthetist
- ***Warfarin*** this should be stopped at least 3d pre-operatively. The INR should be <1.5 for most operations and lower if spinal or epidural anaesthic techniques are to be employed; warn the anaesthetist. Patients who have prosthetic heart values will need IV heparin whilst warfarin is omitted (p290)
- ***Aspirin and clopidogrel*** should be stopped 7d prior to surgery
- ***Oestrogens and progestogens*** HRT can be continued as long as DVT/PE prophylaxis is undertaken. Progestogen-only contraceptives can be continued, but combined oral contraceptives should be stopped 4wk prior to surgery and alternative means of contraception used
- ***Bowel preparation for GI surgery*** see opposite

Writing the drug chart

Try and do this at pre-admission clinic to save yourself time later. Document any allergies. Things to check include:

- ***Prophylactic anticoagulation*** check the hospital policy (usually clexane 20mg/24h SC; more if obese and high risk of DVT/PE). Discuss with haematology for advice on patients with prosthetic heart valves (see p290 for APPT checks)
- ***Antibiotics*** consider pre-operative antibiotics if indicated (check local guidelines)
- ***Bowel preparation and IV fluid*** see opposite
- ***Regular drugs*** review these and write up those which should be continued in hospital (stop COC, aspirin etc)
- ***TED stockings*** prescribe these under the regular medications
- ***Analgesia and anti-emetics*** (p282 and p206) the anaesthetist will usually write these up during the operation

Instructions for the patient

- Make sure you tell them where and when to go for admission and write this down for them
- If they are to have bowel prep, they should be on clear fluids at least 24h before the operation (opposite)
- Tell the patient about any drains, NG tubes or catheters which may be inserted during the operation
- Tell them if they are being admitted to ITU post-op

Nil by mouth Patients should not eat 6h pre-operatively and they should stop clear fluids 2h before the operation. They can take their medication with up to 60ml fluid.

Booking theatre lists

Elective lists

Discuss the order of the list with your consultant/SpR (you may need to obtain the operating list from the booking officer).

The list usually must be submitted by the afternoon before the operating day. You should include:

- Theatre number
- Name of the consultant surgeon
- Name, sex, age, hospital number and location of each patient
  - Special patient requirements (eg DM, ITU bed booked, crossmatch requested, obese, etc)
- Operation and side (eg open left inguinal hernia repair with mesh)
- Sign and leave your bleep number

If the order of the list needs to be changed, contact theatres and inform them as soon as possible.

Booking emergency operations

- Make sure the case is discussed with the SHO and SpR on call and that they have agreed to put the patient on the list
- Enter the patient's details as outlined above, noting the time at which the patient last ate
- Inform the on-call anaesthetic SHO/SpR about the patient
- Check the patient has been consented, and make sure the results of any relevant investigations are available (including a sample for blood transfusion)
- You may also need to inform the theatre coordinator.

Bowel preparation for surgery

Bowel preparation	Procedure
No preparation needed	OGD, ERCP, closure (reversal) ileostomy
Phosphate enema (on day of surgery)	Anal fissure, haemorrhoidectomy, EUA, flexible sigmoidoscopy
Full bowel preparation (see below)	Colonoscopy, TEMS, rectoplexy, right hemi-/left hemi-/sigmoid/pancolectomy, anterior resection, AP resection, reversal of Hartmann's procedure

Full bowel preparation

Various preparations are used to empty the bowel, including Picolax®, Fleet Phospho-soda® and Klean-Prep®. These are often given at 12:00 and again at 18:00 the day before surgery. Elderly patients or patients with other co-morbidities should be admitted for bowel preparation and have an intravenous infusion running as soon as the bowel preparation is given to prevent dehydration.

The operating theatre

Theatre design

Operating theatres include an operating area, a scrubbing-up area, a preparation (or prep) room, a sluice and an anaesthetic room. Most theatres have a whiteboard (to document the date, operation and number of swabs used), an X-ray viewing box and an area to write up the operation notes and histopathology form. Above the operating table, there are usually two mobile lights (satellites).

Theatre staff

Each operating theatre has a team of theatre assistants who clean and maintain the theatre. The 'scrub nurse' scrubs for each operation to assist in selecting appropriate instruments, as requested by the surgical team. One other trained nurse and an auxiliary nurse act as 'runners' to fetch equipment for the scrub nurse and to monitor the number of swabs and sutures used (displayed on the whiteboard). An operating departmental assistant (ODA) maintains the anaesthetics equipment and assists the anaesthetist. Each operation is logged into the operating book/computer, with the details of the patient, name of the operating surgeon, patient's consultant and anaesthetist.

Theatre clothing

'Scrubs' should be worn for each operating list and should be changed between lists, or between cases if they become dirty or potentially infected with MRSA. Most hospitals insist on the use of masks or caps, although the benefits are controversial; masks are always worn in orthopaedic, spinal and neuro theatres. Theatre shoes are essential for safety purposes and you will not be allowed to enter without them. Theatre scrubs and shoes should not be worn outsides of theatres unless in an emergency.

Scrubbing up

Scrubbing up is an art and a key part of minimising infection risk to the patient. Ask a theatre nurse to show you how to do it correctly.

- Prior to scrubbing up, remove any jewellery and make sure you put your mask on
- Open a gown pack and drop a pair of sterile gloves on top
- When scrubbing up for the first patient, scrub under your nails using a brush with chlorhexidine/iodine. Wash hands for a further 4–5min
- Unravel your gown, making sure that it does not touch the floor
- Touching its inner aspects only, put it on with the end of the sleeves covering your hands
- Put on your gloves. Do not touch the outside of your gloves with your bare hands
- For high-risk operations (eg Caesarian, HIV +ve) double glove and protect your eyes with a visor or safety spectacles
- Wait for an assistant to tie your scrub gown from behind
- If your hand becomes non-sterile, change your glove. If your gown becomes non-sterile you need to rescrub, change your gown and gloves

Theatre etiquette

- Check the correct patient is undergoing the correct operation on the correct side (match the consent form to the patient's wristband)
- If you are scrubbed up:
    - make sure the light handle has a sterile cover before touching it if you are asked to adjust the light
    - do not pick up instruments which fall to the ground
    - if you are handed an instrument/cable by someone who is not scrubbed, check that you can touch it before accepting it
- In operations involving the abdomen and the perineum, if you are asked to move from the perineal operating site to the abdomen you need to rescrub. This is not necessary when swapping from the abdomen to the perineal site
- If you sustain a needle-stick injury, leave the operation and report to occupational health (p34)
- Always eat/drink before going to an operating list.

Watching an operation

Make sure you can see; get a stool or stand at the patient's head if the anaesthetist allows you to. Some theatres have a mirror or camera attached to the overhead light, which can be adjusted to show the operation. Although you are not actively participating in the operation, use the time to learn surgical techniques – hand ties look easier than they actually are! If you can't follow what's going on, ask (either at the operation or later). As the operation finishes, fill in any histology forms or TTOs if appropriate. Check histology samples are labelled accurately.

Some commonly used instruments in theatre

- ***Dissecting forceps*** used to handle tissue during dissection and suturing. May be toothed or non-toothed, serrated or non-serrated. Examples include De Bakey forceps
- ***Tissue forceps*** used to hold static tissue whilst dissecting around it. They are hinged in the middle with a ratchet lock on the handle. Examples include Allis and Babcock forceps
- ***Haemostatic (artery) forceps*** usually lightweight with spring handles and a delicate tip used to identify and hold bleeding points or vascular pedicles. Examples include Mosquito forceps, Spencer Wells, Kocher's forceps
- ***Abdominal retractors*** much loved by junior doctors nationally! Examples include Langenbeck, Morris and Deaver retractors
- ***Operating scissors*** may be used to separate and dissect tissue or cut through scar tissue. May be straight/curved with round or bevelled blades. Examples include Mayo scissors
- ***Needle-holders*** are designed to hold needles securely with a locking mechanism at the handle. They can be straight or curved with long handles. Examples include Mayo or De Bakey's needle-holders
- ***Needles*** may be cutting (triangular in cross-section) for skin or tendon sutures or round-bodied (oval/round in cross-section) for gut and vascular anastomoses. They can be straight or curved

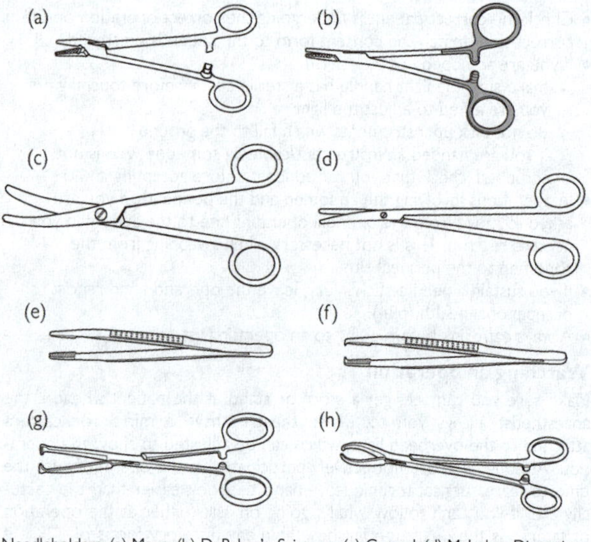

Needleholders: (a) Mayo; (b) DeBakey's. Scissors: (c) Curved; (d) McIndoe. Dissecting forceps: (e) non-toothed; (f) toothed. Tissue forceps: (g) Allis; (h) Littlewoods.

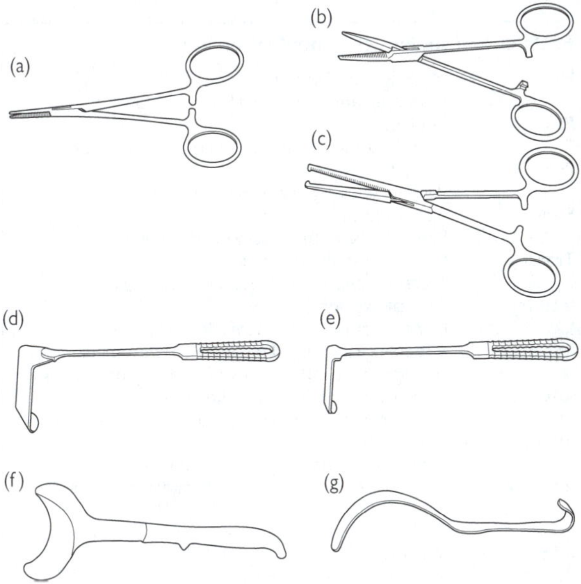

Haemostatic forceps: (a) Mosquito halstead; (b) Spencer Wells; (c) Kocher's artery forceps. Retractors: (d) Langenbeck; (e) Morris; (f) Doyen; (g) Deaver.

Prefixes and suffixes commonly used in surgery

Hemi-	Meaning half of something Hemicolectomy – excising half the colon
Pan-	Total/every Pancolectomy – complete removal of the colon
Per-	Going through a structure Percutaneous – going through the skin
Peri-	Near or around a structure Perianal – Near the anus/around the anus
Trans-	Going across a structure Transoesophageal – across the oesophagus
-ectomy	Surgical excision Nephrectomy – removal of a kidney
-gram	A radiological image often using contrast medium Angiogram – contrast study of an artery or arteries
-oscope	A device for looking inside the body Sigmoidoscope – device for looking into the bowel
-otomy	Cutting something open Craniotomy – opening the cranium (skull)
-ostomy	An artifical opening between two cavities or to the outside Colostomy – opening of the colon to the skin
-olith	Stone-like Faecolith – solid, stone-like stool
-plasty	Reconstruction of a structure Myringoplasty – repair of the tympanic membrane

Hints and tips for budding surgeons

- At the end of each operation, get the scrub nurse to go through each of the instruments on the operating trolley, so you get to know the names and functions of each piece of equipment
- Ask for old sutures to practice suturing and knots

If the case is a day case, write up the patient's TTOs in theatre because the rest of the team is available to check if there are any specific post-operative instructions.

Post-op care

As well as seeing patients pre-operatively, you should review them after the operation, before you go home. This means you can review and discharge day cases with your team, as well as make sure the in-patients are stable after the operation.

Discharging day cases **this may be done by nursing staff**

Before sending day surgery patients home, you should make sure they are alert, have eaten and had fluids without vomiting, are mobilising without fainting and have adequate pain relief. Inspect the operation site and check their observations. Go through the operation procedure and findings with the patient.

Organise appropriate follow-up care and clarify if they need dressing changes, suture removal dates and where this can be done (GP surgery, A+E or ward). If the patient develops any post-operative temperatures, pain or bleeding, they should contact their GP or come to A+E in the first instance.

Common questions about discharge

- Tell the patient if their sutures are dissolvable or if they need to come back to have them taken out (give dates)
- Patients can shower and commence driving again 48h after minor surgery (as long they can perform an emergency stop; see p35)
- Advise patients not to fly for 6wk following major surgery

In-patient post-op care

Post-op patients are at risk of complications associated with the operation, either directly (eg haemorrhage) or indirectly (eg PE, MI).

When reviewing post-operative patients, document the number of days since the operation and the operation they underwent (eg 2d post left mastectomy). Ask about pain, ability to eat and drink, nausea/vomiting, urinary output and colour, bowel movements/flatus and mobilisation. Examine the wound site, chest, abdomen, legs, drains, stoma bags, IV cannulae and catheter bag. Check the drain entry site, the amount drained and the colour of any fluid being drained. Look at the observations for pyrexia, pulse rate, BP, RR and fluid balance (ie NG tube output, urinary output, drains). Review the drug chart for analgesia, antibiotics and fluids. Check post-operative Hb and transfuse if necessary (p276).

Involve other members of the multidisciplinary team if necessary, eg stoma nurse, pain team, physiotherapists, social worker.

Post-operative problems

Low urine output (see p266) urine output <0.5ml/kg/h in adults

Ask about input, drugs, duration of oliguria, thirst, pain, colour of urine, catheter patency

Look for BP, pulse rate, fluid input/output, palpable bladder, signs of hypovolaemia (p262)

Management Flush/replace catheter, U+E, fluid challenge, rarely need to consider furosemide, discuss with your seniors early

Hypotension (see p149)

Ask about pre-op BP, fluid input, epidural, drugs

Look for repeat BP, pulse rate, fluid input/urine output, temperature; is the patient alert, cold, clammy? Check cap refill, signs of hypovolaemia/sepsis, wounds, drain, abdomen, any signs of active bleeding

Management 15min obs, monitor hourly urine output (catheterise bladder). Lie the patient flat, elevate the legs and give oxygen. Get IV access, consider colloid (eg 500ml Gelofusine® stat). Send bloods for FBC and crossmatch (blood cultures if you suspect sepsis). Apply pressure to any obvious bleeding points. Call for senior review early.

Shortness of breath/↓O_2 sats (see p165)

Ask about chronic lung/CVS disease, previous PE, chest pain, ankle swelling, new onset cough

Look for BP, pulse rate, temp, pallor, lungs (consolidation, crackles, air entry), signs of fluid overload, leg oedema/calf swelling

Management Sit up and give O_2. FBC, ABG, CXR, ECG. Consider 0.9% saline nebs, antibiotics and regular chest physiotherapy. If you suspect a PE (p169) call for senior help and specialist advice (medical reg on-call).

Pyrexia Temp >37.5°C, investigate if this persists/increases after the first 24h post-op; refer to p248

Ask about cough/SOB, wound, dysuria/frequency, abdo pain, diarrhoea

Look for BP, pulse rate, temp, wound, catheter, IV cannulae, chest, abdomen

Management MSU, CSU, FBC, U+E, CRP, blood cultures, CXR, abdominal USS or CT, echo if new onset murmur

Abdominal wound breakdown: consider dehiscence and infection

	Ask about	Examine	Management
Dehiscence	Pink serous discharge, haematoma, bowel protrusion	Separation of wound edges	Call for senior help. Cover the bowel with a large sterile swab soaked in 0.9% saline. Check analgesia and fluid replacement
Infection	Pyrexia, pain, erythema, exudate from wound site	Tenderness, odorous discharge, swelling	Wound swab, broad-spectrum antibiotics initially

Post-op confusion, see page 229. **Nausea and vomiting**, see page 206.

Stomas

Colostomy usually in age >50yr

Common locations	LIF or right hypochondrium
Features	May be permanent or temporary; mucosa sutured directly to skin
Output	Soft/solid stool; intermittently passed
Indications	Colorectal cancer, diverticular disease, trauma, radiation enteritis, bowel ischaemia, obstruction, Crohn's disease

Ileostomy usually in age 20–50yr

Common locations	RIF
Features	Usually permanent; bowel mucosa sutured to form a 'spout' to avoid skin contact with bowel contents which are irritating (not flush with skin)
Output	Liquid stool (may be bile-stained); passed continuously
Indications	GI tract cancer, inflammatory bowel disease, trauma, radiation enteritis, bowel ischaemia, obstruction

Urostomy usually in age >20yr

Sometimes referred to as a nephrostomy when originating in the renal pelvis

Common locations	Left or right flank, lower anterior abdominal wall
Features	A ureteric catheter may be protruding from the skin into the stoma
Output	Clear urine passed continuously
Indications	Renal tract cancer, urinary tract obstruction, hydronephrosis, urinary fistulae, spinal column disorders

Common complications

- Electrolyte/fluid imbalance
- Ischaemia/necrosis shortly after
- Obstruction/prolapse/parastomal hernia
- Skin erosion/infection
- Psychosocial implications

It is important to refer patients who are likely to need stomas to the stoma care nurse prior to the operation. Patients with stomas also need to alter their diet to avoid excess flatulence or overly watery stool, so should also be referred to the dietician.

Minor surgical presentations

Lumps

Ask about location, size (is it growing?), speed and duration of onset, associated pain, number of lesions, character (eg is it reducible/pulsatile), infection/erythema, vomiting, trauma, systemic symptoms (eg weight loss)

Look for site, size, shape, consistency, colour, tenderness, temperature, surface (is there a punctum?), edge, pulsatility, mobility, fluctuance, transillumination, auscultation, local lymphadenopathy

Common skin lumps

Diagnosis	Characteristics
Lipoma	Soft swelling of fatty tissue with a well-defined edge; may be multiple
Sebaceous cyst	Fluid-filled cavity lined by epithelium; punctum present; fixed to the skin; may become infected
Ganglion	Swelling around joints and tendons; deep to the skin – usually lined by fibrous tissue
Papilloma	Benign epidermal tumour; may be related to human papilloma virus; may be sessile/pedunculated
Seborrhoeic wart	Benign dark brown lesion on trunk, face and limbs
Basal cell carcinoma	Raised nodule with a pearly edge; may develop a raised rolled edge; usually on face with local invasion
Squamous cell carcinoma	Ulcerated lesion with hard raised edges; on the face or in venous leg ulcers (Marjolin's ulcer); locally destructive
Lymphadenopathy	Localised well-defined rubbery masses, deep to the skin; may be uni/bilateral, isolated/multiple, ±tender (often infective cause if tender)

Hernias

Definition abnormal protrusion of a viscus through its covering

Think about lymphadenopathy, lipoma, aneurysm, undescended testes, saphenovarix, psoas abscess

Ask about site, pain, duration, size, is it reducible/pulsatile? *Risk factors* chronic cough, constipation, heavy lifting, previous abdominal surgery, ascites, obesity, age

Look for examine the patient standing up, asking about pain before palpating; ask the patient to reduce the hernia themselves, check external genitalia and examine the other side

Investigations diagnosis usually based on history and clinical findings; consider ultrasound, herniography, MRI

Management *conservative* weight loss, truss, high-fibre diet, stop smoking, treat lung disease *surgery* day surgery, open approach, laparoscopic repair for bilateral/recurrent herniae. For strangulated hernias see opposite.

Strangulated hernia – Surgical emergency

Presentation fixed irreducible painful lump in hernial orifice, ± abdominal swelling, nausea, vomiting, constipation
Examination tender, red, hot, may have bowel sounds/abdominal distension, peritonism
Investigations *blds* FBC, U+E, glucose, amylase, CRP, G+S *AXR* (exclude bowel obstruction) *erect CXR* (exclude bowel perforation)
Management NBM, analgesia (eg morphine 5mg/1h IV with cyclizine 50mg/8h IV), IV access and fluids (0.9% saline 1l/4h), call for senior review, book theatre

Scrotal swelling *see figure below*

Think about testicular torsion, epididymo-orchitis, hydrocele, femoral hernia, indirect inguinal hernia, saphena varix, lymphadenopathy, aneurysm, ectopic testis, skin lumps, psoas abscess, testicular tumour.

Testicular torsion is a surgical emergency
Ask about location, duration, size and growth, colour, uni/bilateral, pain
Look for Can you get above it? If yes, is it cystic, separate from testis, unilateral, reducible, pulsatile, fluctuant, tender, red, hot? Is it transilluminable?
Investigations *blds* FBC, U+E, LFT, Ca^{2+}, αFP, β-HCG, CRP; urethral swab for M,C+S *imaging* USS
Management treat the cause. If you suspect testicular torsion (young, recent trauma, unilateral severe pain, short history):

- keep NBM, give analgesia IV/IM and inform your seniors
- IV access for fluids; take bloods for FBC, U+E, G+S where indicated
- emergency surgical exploration is required; call theatres and put the patient on the emergency list (p423)

Differential diagnosis of a scrotal lump (OHCM6 p512)

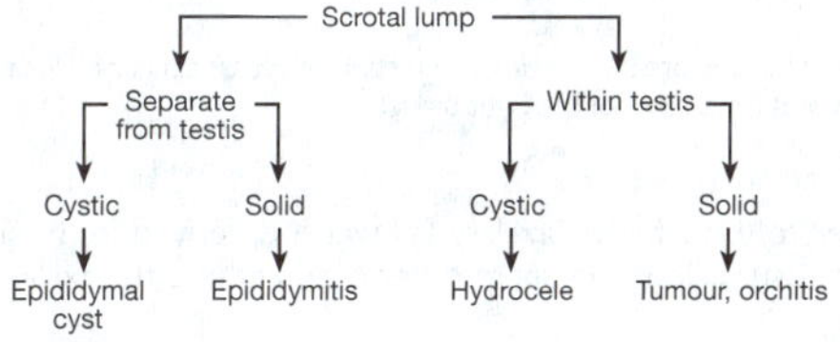

Breast lumps

Breast lumps involve a 'triple assessment' approach:

- clinical examination
- imaging (2 view X-ray mammography or USS)
- histology/cytological analysis

Think about fibroadenomas, fibrocystic change, breast abscess, cancer
Ask about age, size, pain, nipple discharge/bleeding, skin changes (eg eczema), previous breast lumps *FH* breast or gynaecological cancer *hormone use* HRT, COC *obstetric hx* parity, age at first completed pregnancy, menarche, breast-feeding
Look for examine both breasts *inspection* asymmetry, scars, skin changes, nipple discharge/inversion, skin tethering, erythema, oedema *palpation* all four quadrants (see below), axillary tail, assess any palpable masses *lymphadenopathy* axilla, cervical, supraclavicular *other* liver, percuss spine
Investigation *ultrasound* (age <35yr) or *mammography* (oblique and craniocaudal) *fine-needle aspiration* for cytology or *trucut biopsy* if histology shows malignancy, request staging CT, bone scan
Management *Blds* FBC, G+S *surgery* wide local excision/mastectomy, ±axillary dissection/lymph node sampling, involve breast nurse and physiotherapist post-operatively. Consider adjuvant chemotherapy depending on oestrogen receptor status and nodal involvement.

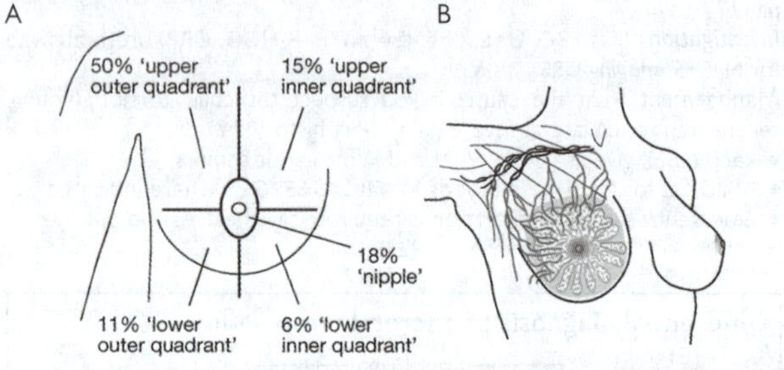

(A) Quadrants of the breast showing proportion of breast cancer by location
(B) Glands and lymphatics of the right breast

Remember to examine the axillary tail which is derived from muscle and other soft tissues along the upper outer quadrant into the axilla.

Trauma and orthopaedics (T+O)

The trauma and orthopaedic beds make up a significant number of all beds in most hospitals. Orthopaedics refers to non-traumatic bone and soft tissue disease (most often congenital, degenerative or malignant) and trauma, as its name suggests, consists of patients with acquired injuries to bone and soft tissues, commonly fractures and dislocations.

Patients with bone and soft tissue problems vary greatly in age and social background, from the child with congenital hip abnormalities, through the young man with osteosarcoma to the 100yr old with a fractured neck of femur.

Orthopaedic surgeons in most large hospitals usually have a sub-speciality interest, eg hips or hands, and therefore your patients may well represent just a small sample of all orthopaedics patients. This makes ward work easier as you will have a limited range of tests and investigations to request, though make sure you get sufficient exposure to the whole range of patients and their management on general T+O takes.

Orthopaedic history

History taking in orthopaedics is like that in other specialities; it is important to make sure you and the patient are comfortable that you have sufficient time and are not going to get disturbed unnecessarily. Most orthopaedic patients are initially seen in out-patients, but will still need pre-operative clerking on admission to hospital (p420) so use this opportunity to practise orthopaedic history taking.

Presenting complaint Enquire what problems it poses the patient (often pain or limitation of function), the duration and change over time of symptoms, together with exacerbating and relieving factors. What limitations on activities of daily living (ADLs) does it cause? What treatments have they tried and have these had any effects?

The trauma history (ATLS is outlined on p312)

History taking for trauma patients is like that in other specialities; it is important to make sure you and the patient are comfortable (adequately analgesed) and that you have sufficient time. Most trauma patients are initially seen in A+E, but still need clerking on admission to the ward. Ensure the patient has sufficient analgesia and remember excess morphine may impair they ability to recall a history.

Presenting complaint Enquire about the patient's injuries and the cause for the injury; a drop-attack resulting in a fracture may suggest an underlying cardiac pathology, whereas a high-velocity car accident should alert you to occult injuries to the head, chest or abdomen that the patient may be unaware of. The mechanism of injury will also suggest likely pathology; fall on the outstretched hand often causes a Colles' fracture, whereas fall onto the dorsum on the hand causes a Smith's fracture. Very elderly and frail patients may not be able to offer much history so use family members or carers to fill in the gaps. With suspected fractures and soft tissue injuries always ask about neurological symptoms which may indicate nerve or vascular damage.

Investigations in trauma and orthopaedics

Plain radiographs are the commonest form of imaging bones and fractures. Always obtain a minimum of two views, ideally at 90° to each other to help localise the lesion in space (most commonly an AP and a lateral film). If looking for a fracture, view the joint above and below the fracture to exclude a dislocation. Most radiographers will mark the film with a red sticker or other marker if they notice an abnormality. CXR p508, AXR p510, C-spine p312.

Blood tests such as baseline U+E and FBC are often undertaken for most trauma and some elective patients; other investigations such as clotting, LFT, CRP/ESR, G+S (or crossmatch) should be requested upon need. Blood cultures must always be sent if osteomyelitis is suspected.

Fluoroscopy uses 'real-time' X-rays to view bones and fractures and allows manipulation of these to be watched on a monitor. Often used in theatre to check alignment during and after fixation of fractures.

CT and MRI are becoming more frequently used to diagnose and monitor treatment. CT is very good at looking at bone, whereas MRI is often more useful for looking at the soft tissues (with a few exceptions).

Ultrasound shows effusions of most joints clearly and will reveal some architecture of the articular surface. Also useful if free fluid is suspected in the pelvis (which may indicate pelvic fracture).

Joint aspiration is often undertaken to establish the cause of a swollen joint or to identify pathogen in septic arthritis (p297). Can be used to examine fluid for crystals in crystal arthropathy.

Arthroscopy ±washout is often undertaken in day-case and allows direct visualisation of the inside of a joint (commonly knee, ankle, wrist) to help confirm a diagnosis and to wash out an effusion or loose body. Many knee procedures can now be undertaken by arthroscopy alone such as cruciate ligament repair and meniscal surgery.

DXA/DEXA scan (dual energy X-ray absorptiometry) is used to assess bone mineral density, which deteriorates with age and in osteoporosis.

Other investigations will depend upon clinical need and include microbiological cultures, histological examination of tissue from biopsy and following excision, electrophysiological studies of nerve transmission and muscle response and radio-isotope uptake studies.

The pelvic radiograph

Confirm patient details and date of film.
Does the film include a good view of both hip joints?
Check inner bony ring and obturator foramina to identify any break in the cortices.
Is the symphysis pubis abnormally wide or asymmetrical?
Are the sacro-iliac joints equal and visible?
Are the contours of the acetabulum smooth and the same on both sides?
Follow the outline of each femur checking for breaks in the cortex.
Check remaining bones individually for breaks in the cortex (ilium, ischium, pubis).

Hip (OHCS6 p628)

Presenting symptoms pain, decreased range of movement (ROM), limitation of activities of daily living (eg walking, rising from seated position)

Past medical and drug history previous episodes or surgery (prosthesis), arthritis, trauma/infections to the joint, problems as a child, steroid therapy (predisposes to osteoporosis), medical reason for falls

Inspection Look for leg shortening or internal rotation (hip dislocation) or external rotation (fractured neck of femur). Examine skin over joint for signs of surgical scars, sinuses, cellulitis or bruising.

Palpation Feel for boney landmarks (greater trochanter, anterior superior iliac crest), are these at similar level on either side? Palpate joint as it is moved to feel for crepitus, clicks etc.

Supine Active (allow patient to demonstrate their ROM) and passive movements (ask the patient to relax and move the joint yourself); flexion, abduction and adduction, internal and external rotation. Check for fixed flexion deformity by placing hand in lumbar lordosis and checking the hips can extend to allow the popliteal fossa to touch the couch.

Prone Active and passive movement to check hip extension.

Stressing is not generally undertaken for the hip.

Gait Trendelenburg gait, uses stick on side opposite to diseased hip.

Other joints Examine the knee and lower spine/sacroiliac joints.

Common pathology in the hip – children

- ***Congenital dislocation*** 1% incidence, can be normal at birth
- ***Tubercular arthritis*** 2–5yr and elderly, common in developing world
- ***Perthes' disease*** osteochondritis of femoral head, commonly 4–7yr
- ***Slipped femoral epiphysis*** usually 10–16yr, often obese children

Common pathology in the hip – adults

Osteoarthritis Often degenerative disease (p416), but can be precipitated by trauma and inflammation, resulting predominantly in pain and limitation of function. Joint replacement (both ball and socket) commonly undertaken which lasts up to 20yr before needing revision/replacement.

Fractured neck of femur (NOF) is a common fracture in the elderly following a simple fall. Classically shortened, externally rotated leg. Confirm with AP and lateral hip X-ray. Often treated by hemi-arthroplasty (replacing femoral head and neck and not the socket) or with dynamic hip screw (DHS). Can be undertaken with spinal anaesthesia so even frailest of patients can undergo surgery; poor prognosis without surgery.

Hip dislocation is commoner in people with prosthetic hips. Can occur in non-prosthetic hips in trauma with a force being applied from the knee up a femur through a flexed hip, eg high-speed car crash.

Referred pain is common between the hip and knee, which is why both should be examined during a new consultation.

Knee (OHCS6 p634)

Presenting symptoms hip/knee pain, decreased range of movement (ROM), locking, clicking, giving way, limitation of activities of daily living (eg walking, climbing stairs)

Past medical and drug history previous episodes or surgery (prosthesis), arthritis, trauma/infections to the joint, problems as a child

Inspection Look for swelling, erythema and the position that the knee is held in by the patient. Is there any varus (bow-legs) or valgus (knock-knees) deformity? Examine the skin over joint for signs of surgical scars, sinuses or cellulitis. Is there any wasting of the thigh muscles compared to the other side (especially vastus medialis)?

Palpation Feel for temperature, boney landmarks (head of fibula, medial and lateral joint lines, patella). Is there an effusion (if large infra-patella sulci will be bulging outwards with a positive patella tap, if small try milking fluid down from thigh and stroking fluid from one side to the other). Palpate joint as it is moved to feel for crepitus, clicks etc.

Supine Active (allow patient to demonstrate their ROM) and passive movements (ask the patient to relax and move the joint yourself), flexion, extension.

Prone Examine the popliteal fossa for cysts and popliteal aneurysms.

Stressing Flex knee to 90°, sit on the patient's foot so the foot is immobilised and perform anterior and posterior draw tests to check for anterior and posterior cruciate ligament integrity, respectively. Holding the knee at about 30° flexion, fix the thigh with your left hand on inner aspect and stress the knee with a valgus strain (force applied over lower leg to mimic bow-legs) and then a varus strain (force applied over lower leg to mimic knock-knees) to check for medial and lateral collateral integrity.

Gait Limp or using walking aids. Gives way on mobilising or patient cautious or in pain.

Common pathology in the knee

Osteoarthritis Often degenerative disease (p416), but can be precipitated by trauma and inflammation, resulting predominantly in pain and limitation of function (rest pain in severe disease). Joint replacement commonly undertaken which lasts 15yr before needing revision.

Acutely swollen knee Common after trauma/sporting injury. Often haemarthrosis (OHCS6 p710), though can be an non-haemorrhagic effusion. Consider septic arthritis (p297).

Locked knee A true locked knee is held in a fixed position, usually by a loose body trapped in the joint. Some knees have a limited ROM due to a loose body which can also be referred to as a locked knee.

Patella problems True dislocation of the patella laterally is uncommon, but very painful (p305). Bursitis is common around the knee joint in people who spend a lot of time kneeling (OHCS6 p638).

Ankle and foot (OHCS6 p640)

Presenting symptoms ankle pain, decreased range of movement or unable to weight-bear, swelling

Past medical and drug history previous episodes or surgery (internal fixation), arthritis, trauma/infections to the joint, problems as a child, steroid therapy (predisposes to osteoporosis)

Inspection Look for swelling, erythema and the position that the foot is held in by the patient, if there is marked deviation of foot in trauma consider fracture-dislocation and summon senior help immediately as requires immediate reduction before undertaking X-rays due to risk of neurovascular compromise to the foot (p305).

Palpation Feel for temperature, boney landmarks (medial and lateral malleolus, tibiotalar joint) for crepitus or pain; always feel the proximal fibula head in ankle injury to exclude its fracture (Maisonneuve fracture). For Ottawa ankle rules see p305. Is there any swelling, if so is it soft tissue or an effusion in the joint. Palpate joint as it is moved to feel for crepitus, clicks etc. Check for foot pulses, cap refill and sensation.

Movement Active (allow patient to demonstrate their ROM) and passive movements (ask the patient to relax and move the joints yourself); flexion (plantarflexion) and extension (dorsiflexion) across the tibiotalar (ankle) joint.

Stressing is not generally undertaken for the ankle.

Gait Is the patient able to weight-bear (able to walk two paces unaided)?

Other joints Examine the knee and foot.

Foot

Presenting symptoms foot pain, unable to weight-bear, swelling

Past medical and drug history previous episodes or surgery (internal fixation), arthritis, trauma/infections to the foot, DM, problems as a child, steroid therapy (predispose to osteoporosis and immunocompromise)

Inspection Look for swelling, erythema and the position that the foot is held in by the patient; are the toes all in a normal alignment?

Palpation Feel for temperature and along each metatarsal and adjacent phalanx, assessing for pain or crepitus. Palpate forefoot bones (navicular, cuboid and medial, intermediate and lateral cuneiform bones). Check for foot pulses, cap refill and sensation.

Movement Active (allow patient to demonstrate their ROM) and passive movements (ask the patient to relax and move the joints yourself); flexion (plantarflexion) and extension (dorsiflexion) across the tibiotalar (ankle) joint, degree of internal and external rotation about talonavicular joint, flexion and extension over the MTPJ and IPJ.

Stressing is not generally undertaken for the foot.

Gait Is the patient able to weight-bear (able to walk two paces unaided)?

Other joints Examine the ankle.

Shoulder (glenohumeral joint) (OHCS6 p610)

Presenting symptoms pain in the shoulder or neck at rest or on movement, reduced range of movement (sometimes 'frozen' in one position)

Past medical and drug history previous episodes or surgery, arthritis, spondylitis, trauma/infections to the joint, problems as a child, steroid therapy (predisposes to osteoporosis)

Inspection Look for swelling, erythema, abnormal bony prominences and the position that the arm and shoulder are held in by the patient; look at the joint from the front, side and back. Examine the skin over joint and clavicle for signs of surgical scars, sinuses, cellulitis, swelling or deformity. Is there any wasting of the muscles around the shoulder girdle compared to the other side (deltoid, supra-spinatus, infra-spinatus)?

Palpation Feel for temp and bony landmarks (acromioclavicular joint, clavicle and spine of scapula). Check the cervical and upper thoracic vertebrae for tenderness. Feel the joint as it is moved for crepitus, clicks.

Movement Active (allow patient to demonstrate their ROM) and passive movements (ask the patient to relax and move the joint yourself); abduction, adduction, internal and external rotation, flexion and extension. Easing the arm through a painful arc (on abduction) should be undertaken carefully and passively.

Stressing *Impingement test*: arm held at 90° abduction and internally rotated, if pain detected positive test. *Scarf test:* left hand placed over right shoulder, and vice versa, if pain detected positive test (acromioclavicular joint pathology).

Other joints Examine the neck and scapulae.

Common pathology of the shoulder

Dislocation is usually recurrent and due to anatomical instability from either congenital or traumatic causes. Anterior dislocation is most common, and can usually be reduced without need for a general anaesthetic (OHAEM2 p434).

Rotator cuff injury often results from supraspinatus tendon damage. Partial tears cause a painful arc, and complete tears prevent normal abduction between 45° and 90°, though passive abduction can be achieved. Pain typically at shoulder tip.

Painful arc syndrome occurs between 45° and 160° and can result from supraspinatus tendinopathy, calcifying tendinopathy and acromioclavicular pathology (commonly osteoarthritis). Passive movement through the painful arc often allows a pain-free arc at the extreme of abduction or flexion (in whichever plane the arc is painful).

Osteoarthritis of the shoulder is much less common than of the knee or hip (presumably because loads across the glenohumeral joint are less). Like hips and knees the joint can be replaced.

Frozen shoulder seldom results in a completely immobile shoulder; commonly presents with pain and reduce external rotation, making combing the hair hard. Cause unknown.

Elbow and wrist (OHCS6 p614)

Elbow

Presenting symptoms elbow pain, forearm pain, decreased range of movement (ROM), locking, clicking

Past medical and drug history previous episodes or surgery, arthritis, trauma/infections to the joint, problems as a child, steroid therapy (predisposes to osteoporosis)

Inspection look for swelling, erythema

Palpation Feel for temperature and bony landmarks (medial and lateral epicondyles, olecranon). Pain over lateral epicondyle suggests 'tennis elbow' and over the medial epicondyle 'golfer's elbow'.

Movement Active (allow patient to demonstrate their ROM) and passive movements (ask the patient to relax and move the joint yourself); flexion and extension, pronation and supination.

Stressing is not generally undertaken for the elbow.

Other joints Examine the shoulder and wrist.

Wrist (OHCS6 p616)

Presenting symptoms wrist pain, forearm pain, decreased range of movement (ROM)

Past medical and drug history previous episodes or surgery, arthritis, trauma/infections to the joint, problems as a child, steroid therapy (predispose to osteoporosis)

Inspection Look for dinner fork deformity (Colles' fracture), break to the skin (open fracture) or features of rheumatoid disease (p416).

Palpation Feel for temperature, boney landmarks (styloid process of radius, head and styloid process of ulna) and for scaphoid in the base of the anatomical snuff-box.

Movement Active (allow patient to demonstrate their ROM) and passive movements (ask the patient to relax and move the joint yourself); flexion, extension, radial and ulna deviation, circumduction of the wrist relies on all four movements, pronation and supination.

Stressing is not generally undertaken for the wrist.

Other joints Examine the forearm and elbow.

Common pathology of the wrist

Traumatic	Non-traumatic
Fractured wrist (Colles' (p304) + Smith's)	De Quervain's tenosynovitis
Scaphoid fracture (p304)	Ganglia
Fractured radial + ulna styloid processes	Rheumatoid arthritis (p416)
Lunate dislocation	Rickets (in children)
	Carpal tunnel (p220)

Hand (OHCS6 p616)

Presenting symptoms hand/finger pain, decreased range of movement (ROM), limitation of activities of daily living (holding drinking cup, doing up buttons, writing etc)

Past medical and drug history previous episodes or surgery, arthritis, trauma/infections to the joints, problems as a child, steroid therapy (predisposes to osteoporosis)

Inspection Look for erythema, swelling, breaks to the skin, features of rheumatoid disease, muscles wasting, pitting of the nails.

Palpation Feel for temperature and along each metacarpal and adjacent phalanx, assessing for pain or crepitus.

Movement Active (allow patient to demonstrate their ROM by making a fist and opening hand fully) and passive movements (ask the patient to relax and move the joints yourself); flexion and extension of all MTPJ, PIPJ and DIPJ, abduction and adduction of all MTPJ and opposition and circumduction of the thumb MTPJ. Ask patient to hold a pencil and write, pick up a mug, undo a button on a shirt or blouse, demonstrate pincer grip and then ask them to oppose thumb and little finger and assess strength of this union.

Stressing of the collateral ligaments of the digits is undertaken following trauma and dislocation to establish joint stability. Extensor and flexor (profundus and superficialis) tendon function should be assessed in penetrating or lacerating trauma to the hand to identify tendon injury.

Other joints Examine the wrist and examine for rheumatoid nodules or psoriatic rash at the elbows.

Common orthopaedic pathology of the hand

Dupuytren's disease results from pathology of the palmar fascia of the hand, causing a puckering of the skin and eventual fixed flexion of little and ring fingers (most commonly), though others can be involved. Most commonly familial. Release can be undertaken surgically, though recurrence is a problem.

Trigger finger results when a nodule on the flexor digitorium profundus tendon catches on the tendon sheath, preventing full digital extension, though the nodule can often slip under the sheath with help. Treated with steroid injections, or surgical laying open part of the tendon sheath.

Rheumatoid hands

In severe disease small joints of the hand can be fused (arthrodesed) or replaced

- Symmetrical small joint polyarthritis (DIPJ usually spared)
- Ulna deviation of fingers
- Palmar subluxation of MTPJ
- Z-deformity of thumb
- Swan neck deformity (flexion DIPJ, extension PIPJ)
- Boutonnière deformity (flexion PIPJ, extension DIPJ)
- Wasting of the small muscles of the hand

Osteoarthritis (OHCS6 p668, p416)
This is a disease of synovial joints which results in degeneration of the cartilage lining the articular surfaces. Patients complain of joint pain, initially on exertion but eventually at rest. The joints are seldom red and inflamed though may become deformed and have ↓ROM. *Commonly* the knees and hips are affected, though spine, shoulder and wrists/hands are often involved. *Classical radiological features* consist of loss of joint space, subchondral sclerosis, bone cysts and osteophyte formation. *Treatment* relies on minimising pain and disability with analgesia and encouragement to lose weight and undertake regular gentle exercise. Joint replacement or fusion should be considered if pain is interrupting sleep or function is greatly affected. Role of joint washout unclear.

Causes of OA • trauma • foreign bodies • destructive arthritis (eg psoriasis) • neuropathic • gout • following septic arthritis • Paget's disease • idiopathic

Osteoporosis (OHCS6 p676, p344)
This is a reduction in the bone mineral density, resulting in increased susceptibility to fractures. *Patients* are often unaware of osteoporosis. *Commonly* the vertebrae are involved (crush fractures) together with the wrists and neck of femur (common fractures in the elderly). *DXA scanning* can be undertaken to assess bone density, though this often is performed after a fracture has occurred. *Treatment* relies on preventing further deterioration of bone density and encouraging remineralisation with calcium, vitamin D and bisphosphonates (inhibit bone mobilisation).

Causes of osteoporosis • genetic • inflammatory disease • dietary deficiency • early menopause • steroids • alcoholism • anorexia nervosa • thyrotoxicosis

Osteomyelitis (OHCS6 p644, p296)
Infection of bone in the absence of trauma or orthopaedic surgery is now rare in the developed world. *Risk factors* include surgical prosthesis, open fractures, penetrating injuries, DM or other forms of immunosupression. *Patients* complain of tenderness and warmth at site and often a draining sinus can be identified on the skin. Inflammatory markers are usually raised and plain radiographs can be normal for up to 6wk, but eventually show hazy bone cortex, loss of bone density and subperiosteal thickening. *Treatment* relies on aggressive antibiotic therapy, draining of abscess cavity within bone and thorough bone toilet in theatre.

Musculoskeletal tumours (OHCS6 p646)
Primary tumours of bone are uncommon and usually present with pain, swelling or following a pathological fracture. Primary tumours of breast, bronchus, prostate, kidney and thyroid, however, commonly metastasise to bone. Malignant soft-tissue tumours are also rare and require urgent oncology input.

Bone and joint surgery (OHCS6 p654)

Elective orthopaedics includes a large proportion of joint replacement/revision surgery. Hips and knees are the most common, though shoulders, finger, wrist and elbow joints are also undertaken.

Hip replacement is undertaken when pain from hip disease is great or the patient's function is severely impaired. Replacement is most commonly due to OA, followed by RA. Prosthetic implants can consist of just the femoral head component (hemi-arthroplasty) or femoral head and replacement of the acetabulum (total hip replacement). Prosthetic joints often last for ~20yr, after which time they can become loose and need revising (removing and new prosthetic joint sited). The operation is often undertaken using a regional anaesthetic (eg spinal) so patients with chronic disease who may not be suitable for a general anaesthetic can be considered for surgery.

Knee replacement is undertaken when pain from the knee is great or the patient's function is severely impaired. Replacement is most commonly due to OA, followed by RA. Knee prostheses are most often 'total' with both articular surfaces are replaced. Like hips, the operation is often undertaken using a regional anaesthetic so patients with chronic disease who may not be suitable for a general anaesthetic can be considered for surgery.

Prosthetic joint infection is disastrous. Strict precautions are taken in theatre to prevent microbes contaminating the operation site and antibiotics are given before and after the procedure. Infected joints commonly have to be taken out and infection and inflammation allowed to settle before a new prosthesis can be inserted.

Trauma surgery is the most commonly performed surgery in most hospitals. Operative management of many fractures which were once treated by non-operative means allows patients to be discharged earlier and have shorter time in plaster of Paris (or equivalent).

Fractured neck of femur surgery commonly uses a screw (or several screws) to unite the shaft of the femur to the existing femoral head which sits in the acetabulum. Occasionally the blood supply to the femoral head is compromised (intracapsular fractures) and either a hemi-arthroplasty or less frequently a total hip replacement is undertaken.

Open reduction and internal fixation (ORIF) surgery is used acutely to treat many fractures of long bones, namely the ankle (and rest of the tibia and fibula), wrist (and rest of the radius and ulna), metacarpals, humerus and mandible (jaw).

Manipulation under anaesthetic (MUA) is often required to obtain an adequate alignment of a fracture and permit the best possible healing and restoration of function. This is particularly true for fractures of long bones in children and in fractures of wrists in adults where internal fixation is not required. Patients are given a short general anaesthetic in theatre and the joint is manipulated under direct vision using fluoroscopy (real-time X-rays) viewed on a monitor. Immobilisation is achieved with plaster of Paris or equivalent material.

Urology

It is important to consider urological disease in patients presenting with abdominal pain, urinary symptoms or haematuria. You may need to liaise with nephrologists and occasionally gynaecologists.

Urological symptoms

- ***Pain*** *renal* constant ache in the back/loin *ureter* colicky pain in the back/loin *bladder and urethra* dysuria, suprapubic pain
- ***Bladder/urethral obstruction*** poor flow/stream, urgency, intermittency, nocturia, incomplete emptying, frequency
- ***Infection*** dysuria (start, end, throughout stream), painful haematuria, suprapubic pain, urgency, frequency, pyuria
- ***Urine quantity*** polyuria, oliguria, anuria *colour* red, pink, brown, ask which phase of urination it occurs in, ie start (urethral), end (bladder) or throughout (bladder/above); if haematuria, make sure the blood is not from the rectum/vagina *air* suggests a fistula (pneumaturia)
- ***Urinary incontinence*** *stress* (associated with ↑intra-abdominal pressure eg coughing, lifting) *urge* (bladder overactivity), ask about risk factors (multiple childbirths, infections, obesity, drugs) and check it is not overflow incontinence

Look for palpable or tender kidneys by balloting, distended bladder (may be palpable and/or percussable), abnormality of the external genitalia, abnormal PV examination (mass/tenderness), prostatic hypertrophy or tumours on PR, swollen ankles

Obs always check for hypertension

Urine analysis see p504

Urodynamic studies see next page

Radiology

Kidneys, ureter and bladder X-ray (KUB) detects 90% of renal stones. The kidneys usually lie at the level of L1/2 (right generally slightly lower than the left) with the ureters passing down the tips of the transverse processes to the inferior edge of the sacroiliac joints, before turning medially into the bladder.

Intravenous pyelography (IVP)/Intravenous urography (IVU) contrast medium is injected IV and serial plain X-rays are taken at intervals to observe the progress of contrast through the kidneys down into the bladder. It is used to detect filling defects (stones, tumours, stenosis), distortion and dilatation (think of distal obstruction). A plain KUB film is used as a control.

Transrectal USS and biopsy to investigate prostate disease.

Abdominal USS will detect small/enlarged kidneys, hydronephrosis, large tumours and cysts of the urinary tract; good investigation for haematuria

Renal Doppler USS may highlight renal artery stenosis (↓flow)

MRI/CT to image the urinary tract and kidneys; often used to stage urinary tract malignancy, investigate stone disease and in trauma

Commonly performed urological procedures/operations

Extracorporeal shockwave lithotripsy (ESWL)	Non-invasive technique using ultrasound to shatter renal/ urinary tract stones *in situ*, which are then passed out in the urine.
Transurethral resection of prostate (TURP)	Prostate is resected from around the bladder neck via a cutting device attached to a cystoscope. No cuts to the skin, so wound infection and post-op pain reduced, though UTI rate is high.
Cystoscopy	Either a flexible or rigid cystoscope is passed through the external urinary meatus, via the urethra into the bladder, under local or general anaesthesia. Ureteric catheter can be passed into the ureters via the ureteric orifices and allows retrograde ureterography to be undertaken.
Ureteroscopy	Undertaken at cystoscopy (see above). Useful emergency investigation for stone disease.

Investigations of the lower urinary tract

Urinary flow rate	Flow rate during micturition is recorded. Peak flow rate of <15ml/s suggests bladder outflow obstruction (BOO) or detrusor failure.
Urodynamics	A specialised catheter is sited into the bladder and another into the rectum. Pressure in both the bladder and rectum (a reflection of intra-abdominal pressure) is recorded during bladder filling and during micturition. Subtraction of one from the other allows true intravesicular (bladder) pressure to be determined to establish detrusor function.

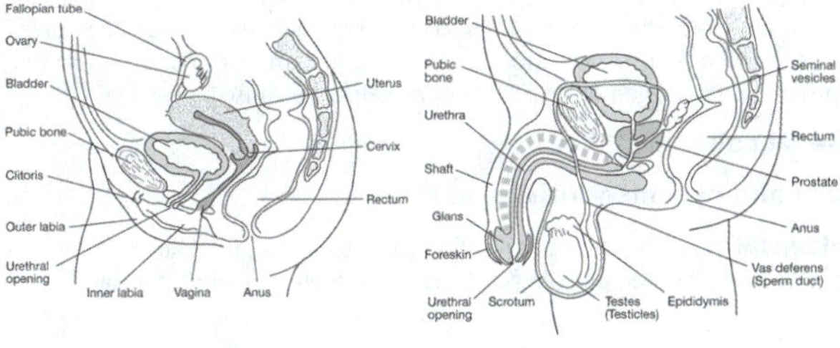

Anatomy of the female (left) and male (right) urogenital systems

Urology presentations

Acute urinary retention

This requires urgent treatment and is very painful. Likely to be painless in patients with spinal injuries or multiple sclerosis.

Ask about suprapubic pain (±sudden onset), anuria, hesitancy, dribbling, poor stream, fluid intake, recent operation, symptoms of coexisting medical disease (DM, MS, spinal cord disease), drugs (anticholinergics, antidepressants, alcohol), concurrent constipation, pre-existing urinary symptoms

Look for agitated patient unable to stay still, palpable distended bladder extending above the symphysis pubis, dull to percussion, enlarged prostate on PR, PV mass in women

Differentials *causes of urinary retention* bladder outflow obstruction (enlarged prostrate, bladder neck pathology, urethral strictures), drugs (anticholinergics, antidepressants), alcohol, constipation or other pelvic mass (especially in ♀) *causes of anuria* acute renal failure, AAA involving renal arteries *causes of abdominal pain* AAA, renal colic, UTI, testicular torsion.

Management:

- Catheterise (p482) – if urethral catheterisation is difficult consider suprapubic catheter (seek senior help)
- Record the volume of urine voided and re-examine abdomen
- Monitor BP and pulse rate. IV fluids if >1.5l drained from bladder
- Urine M,C+S, Hb, U+E, PSA falsely elevated in acute retention
- If isolated episode of retention allow home when passing urine freely without a catheter. Otherwise consider indwelling catheter and trial without catheter (TWOC) in 7–14d after commencing α-blockers (eg alfuzosin). Most patients will require flow rate studies and follow-up

Complications acute renal failure, chronic obstruction, UTI, urethral trauma following bladder catheterisation

Chronic urinary retention

This usually has an insiduous, painless onset with symptoms of bladder outflow obstruction. High pressure retention requires long-term catheterisation of the bladder or TURP to prevent renal damage by back pressure. Low pressure retention often results from dysfunctional bladder muscle and management relies on addressing the cause.

Renal colic see p188

UTI and pyelonephritis see p249

Haematuria the causes and approach to haematuria are shown on p269. There is often a urological cause, eg infection, stones, tumours.

Urogenital tumours

Kidney – renal cell cancer

Typically an adenocarcinoma most often identified incidentally, but can present with haematuria. If no metastases, partial/radical nephrectomy has a 5yr survival of 70%.

Bladder cancer

Usually transitional cell cancers (TCC) presenting with haematuria; distant metastases are rare. Risk factors include smoking or contact with dyes. Important to rule out invasive gynaecological cancer in women or rectal cancer in men. Investigation and treatment may be by cystoscopy (if superficial lesion); cystectomy and urostomy (see p451) may be required for a high-grade tumour or if the tumour extends past epithelial basement membrane. Chemotherapy/radiotherapy may be required

- ***Carcinoma in situ (CIS)*** Pre-malignant condition commonly presenting with dysuria and frequency. May be resectable via cystoscopy or treated with chemotherapy.

Prostate cancer

Usually presents in men aged >60yr, with obstructive urinary symptoms, though age of presentation is falling due to PSA testing, PR may reveal an irregular, craggy mass though this is often a late-stage finding; more commonly the gland is firm, has a nodule or feels normal. Diagnosed and monitored by serum PSA and transrectal USS and biopsy. Management includes 'watch and wait', radiotherapy, radical prostatectomy and hormone therapy (eg goserelin) to suppress testosterone.

Testicular cancer

Most common cancer in men aged 20–34yr. The main risk factor is an undescended testes. Presentation is usually with a painless testicular lump, usually investigated with USS. The two most common types of testicular cancer and their management are outlined below. All patients must have a CXR and tumour markers measured.

Features of seminoma and teratoma testicular tumours

Features	Seminoma	Teratoma
Age	30–40yr	<30yr
Type	Solid	Solid/cystic
Growth	Slow	Fast
Tumour markers	Nil	β-HCG, αFP, LDH
Treatment	Inguinal orchidectomy, radiotherapy	Inguinal orchidectomy, ±chemotherapy
Survival	98% at 5yr	Depends on stage/differentiation

Chapter 9

Procedures

Practical procedures

In experienced hands procedures seem easy and highly rewarding, but this takes practice. Learning new procedures can make you feel frustrated, embarrassed and guilty about inflicting pain. It often doesn't feel great for the patient either but you need to practise to get better.

The saying 'see one, do one, teach one' is an outdated and potentially dangerous attitude. When you are learning a new procedure, especially if it is your first time, ask one of your seniors to take you through it and supervise you. Try to get as much practical experience as you can so that you can work more efficiently and teach others. If the patient is under another team, always check with that team's doctors before you perform the procedure.

Before starting Always introduce yourself and obtain informed consent (verbal or written, p94) before carrying out the procedure. Explain what the procedure involves, how it will feel and why it is necessary in clear, simple language and ask if they have any questions. Mentally prepare yourself by thinking through each step of the procedure and use this process to check you haven't forgotten any equipment.

The procedure As you perform the procedure take your time, plan ahead and be confident in your actions so that you are successful first time. Procedures often become harder with each repeated attempt. Make sure you and the patient are comfortable and in the right position. Ask for an assistant if you need one – especially useful if you have forgotten anything.

If things go well At the end of the procedure clean up (to stay loved by the nurses) and always dispose of your own sharps. Check the patient is alert, comfortable and well; adopt a level of self-satisfaction appropriate to the number of attempts you took.

If things go wrong Ask for help early. Stay calm and reassure the patient while you wait. See p96 if there is a serious problem.

Improving Make sure you get feedback and hints from supervisors so that next time you can do it better. Reflect on your efforts, think about what you did well, what you could do differently and how you would teach someone else doing the procedure. If you have any tips to share please email the address at the front on pvii.

Things to remember when preparing a procedures trolley

- Gloves ±sterile
- Needles (various sizes)
- 0.9% saline
- Antiseptic solution
- Syringes
- Local anaesthetic
- Plenty of swabs – you can never have too many
- Dressings and tape
- Specimen pots/bottles
- Galipots (kidney dishes)
- Sharps bin

Taking blood (venepuncture)

Indications diagnosis, monitoring physiological state, therapeutic drug monitoring

Contraindications *absolute* patient refusal, AV fistula

Consent verbal; explain why a blood sample is required

Site usually the antecubital fossa but any vein can be used (eg hands, arms, feet, legs and groin (femoral stab p459)); never use a limb with an AV fistula (dialysis) or an IV infusion distal to the site

Equipment non-sterile gloves, tourniquet, alcohol swab, needles (green or blue), 5–20ml syringe, cotton/gauze, tape, sharps bin, appropriate blood bottles (see p460)

Checks patient comfortable, vein exposed, accessible and not pulsing, cotton wool to hand, no IV fluids going into the arm

Patient position *upper limb* sit the patient upright, with arm extended and below the heart *lower limb* lie patient flat on their back

Procedure Wash hands and wear non-sterile gloves. Assess both arms and select an appropriate vein. Tighten the tourniquet proximally and palpate along the course of the vein to assess its direction and depth. Swab the skin and hold the vein steady with your non-dominant hand. Warn the patient and advance the needle into the vein at 20° to the skin; look for 'flashback' of blood and hold your position and draw the blood into the syringe. Unclip the tourniquet and apply pressure to the puncture site with cotton wool as you withdraw the needle. Press (or ask the patient to press) on the cotton wool for 2min (longer if bleeding) then tape it in place. Dispose of the needle into the sharps bin. Fill the blood tubes, label them and complete the accompanying request forms.

Confirmation blood flows freely into the syringe

Complications pain, bleeding, haematoma, infection/cellulitis, failure

Safety steady the patient's arm on a pillow to reduce movement and risk of needle-stick injury, dispose of needles into a sharps bin immediately, do not resheath them.

Alternatives
- Blood samples can be taken from cannulas when they are first inserted. It is sometimes possible to take blood at a later date; dispose of the first 5ml and interpret the results with caution
- Vacutainers allow blood to be drawn straight into the blood bottles to reduce the risk of a needle-stick injury, they are good for straight forward veins but can collapse small veins through strong suction.
- For fine veins use a small needle (eg blue) or 'butterfly' (p458) but beware of haemolysis causing artificially ↑K^+
- If you are unable to obtain blood from the upper limb look at the veins in the leg/foot; if you still cannot find veins consider a femoral stab

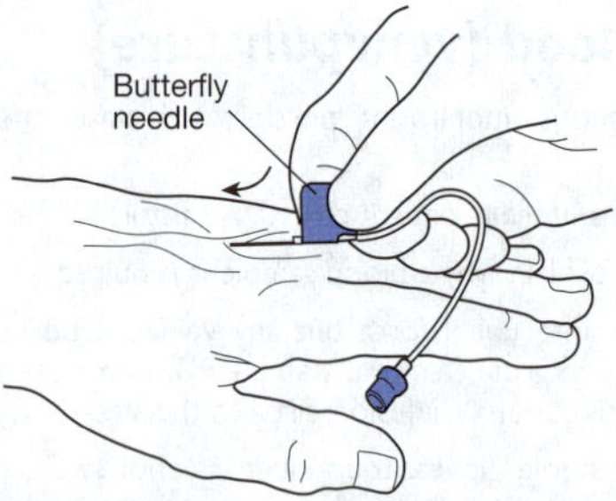

Taking blood using a butterfly needle

Hints and tips

- In patients with poor veins spend a long time finding a suitable vein rather than stabbing blindly.
- In children use topical local anaesthetic, see p390.
- In adults choose veins by palpation with the tourniquet on rather than their appearance; a bouncy vein is usually easy to take blood from.
- Tie the tourniquet tightly and ask the patient to clench their fist repeatedly with their arm below their heart; tap the vein to make it more prominent.
- Before starting, pull the syringe plunger a small distance (<1mm) back to make it move more freely once inside the vein.
- It is best to use a green needle for U+E samples to prevent haemolysis and a ↑K^+; extract blood slowly and gently with blue needles.
- Pull the skin and vein taut to prevent movement away from the needle, especially in older patients.
- Going through the skin is the most painful bit, once under the skin you can take several attempts to manoeuvre the needle into the vein.
- If the syringe is filling slowly/intermittently try slightly less pressure.
- If you can only obtain a small sample consider using paediatric tubes; see the minimum blood requirements on p460.
- Never force blood into blood tubes, the results are spectacular, messy and embarrassing. Consider pulling the top off or withdrawing air.

Procedure for taking blood cultures

Indicated by a repeated/persistent temp >37°C or one-off ≥38°C
Taking antibiotics is a relative **contraindication**
If **bacterial endocarditis** is suspected take 3 sets (6 bottles) from 3 separate veins
Procedure as for normal blood taking except:

- Wear sterile gloves (strict aseptic technique for deep veins)
- A set of blood cultures is two bottles (aerobic and anaerobic)
- After using the alcohol swab do not touch the vein again
- Once the blood has been obtained replace the used needle with a fresh one
- Flip off the culture bottle lids, insert the needle and fill each bottle with 5–10ml

Blood cultures can be stored at room temperature overnight.

Femoral stab

- You do not need a tourniquet for a femoral stab
- Lie the patient flat and expose their groin fully
- Feel for the femoral pulse and choose the side where it is most prominent
- Clean the area with a sterile swab
- With your fingers over the artery insert a green needle vertically 1cm medially
- Pull back on the syringe as you advance; stop moving as soon as you get flashback
- If you get bright red, pulsatile flashback make sure you press firmly for 5min after withdrawing the needle as this is an arterial stab
- Once you have obtained a blood sample, exert pressure over the area for 2min and dress it with a plaster once bleeding has subsided

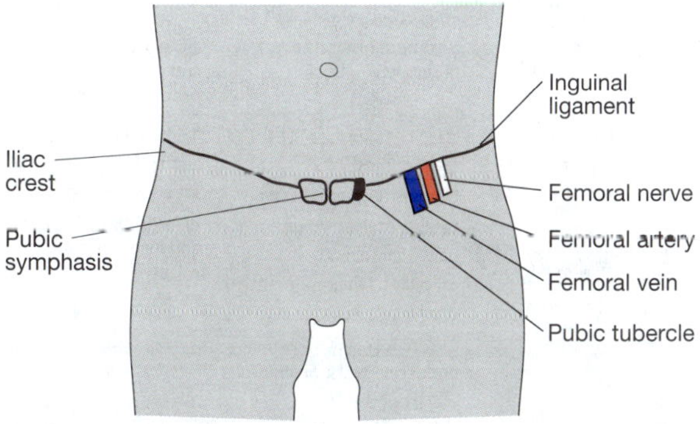

Anatomy of the femoral region

Blood tubes

Use this page as a guide to which bottle is used for each test and to make sure the sample is suitable. Fill in the lab contact numbers, colour of blood bottles and specific blood tests used in your hospital.

Blood tubes

Colour	Contents	Tests	Special instructions
	EDTA	FBC, reticulocytes, HbA_{1C}, sickle screen, Hb electrophoresis, malaria screen	1ml minimum but aim to fill; gently mix to prevent clotting
	EDTA	ESR	Always fill to the line and gently mix to prevent clotting
	EDTA	Blood transfusion (G+S, crossmath)	4ml minimum; always hand write ≥3 forms of patient identification
	Sodium citrate	D-dimer, APTTr, INR, thrombophilia screen, fibrinogen	3.5ml minimum, always fill to the line and gently mix to prevent clotting
	Glucose separating gel	U+E, LFT, amylase, TFT, CRP, Cl^-, Mg^{2+}, Ca^{2+}, PO_4^{3-}, HCO_3^-, urate, LDH, total protein, digoxin, paracetamol and salicylate, lithium, other drug levels, tumour markers, β-HCG, some endocrine tests, protein electrophoresis	1.5ml minimum but aim to fill; try to use a green needle to prevent haemolysis and inaccurate $\uparrow K^+$ results
	Plain	Some endocrine tests, drug levels, serology	1.5ml minimum but aim to fill
	Fluoride oxalate	*Blood* glucose, lactate, alcohol *CSF* glucose, protein, oligoclonal bands	*Blood* 2ml; mix gently *CSF* 6 drops; mix gently
	Heparin	Some endocrine tests, troponins	Mix gently, may need to be transported on ice
	Aerobic + anaerobic medium	Blood cultures (sterile technique)	5–10ml in each bottle; if insufficient blood use aerobic bottle only

IV cannulation

Indications unwell patients, hypovolaemia/shock, IV fluids/drugs, blood product transfusions, other routes of drug administration not tolerated

Contraindications *absolute* patient refusal, AV fistula

Consent verbal; explain why a cannula is required

Site the forearm and back of the hand on the non-dominant arm are best, but any vein can be used (eg hands, arms, feet, legs), antecubital fossa in an emergency, never use a limb with an AV fistula (dialysis)

Equipment tourniquet, non-sterile gloves, alcohol swab, cannulas (appropriate size, see opposite), cannula dressing, 5ml syringe with saline flush, cotton wool, 5–20ml syringe if blood sample required, sharps bin

Checks patient comfortable, skin is clean and free of infection, vein exposed, accessible and not pulsing, cotton wool ±syringe to hand

Patient position *upper limb* sit the patient upright, with arm extended and below the heart *lower limb* lie patient flat on their back

Procedure Wash hands and wear non-sterile gloves. Assess both arms and select an appropriate vein. Tighten the tourniquet proximally and palpate along the course of the vein to assess its direction and depth. Swab the skin and hold the vein steady with your non-dominant hand. Warn the patient and advance the cannula through the skin at 20° with the bevel facing upwards and proximally. Look for flashback, then advance the cannula and needle a little further before withdrawing the metal needle whilst firmly advancing the plastic cannula. Press with your thumb over the tip of the cannula in the vein.

- ***Taking blood*** If blood leaks out try lifting the arm, if still leaking remove the tourniquet. Attach the syringe, take the blood (easier with gentle pressure) and remove the tourniquet then syringe
- ***Not taking blood*** Remove the tourniquet

Place the cap on the end of the cannula, secure with the adhesive dressing and flush with 2–5ml 0.9% saline through the flip-top cap. Dispose of the needle into a sharps bin.

Confirmation flashback seen, 0.9% saline flush requires minimal pressure and does not form a proximal subcutaneous 'bleb' or hurt

Complications *early* haematoma, tissuing (fluid/drugs enter subcutaneous tissues), local damage, air embolism *late* thrombophlebitis, cellulitis

Safety never reinsert the metal needle into the plastic cannula once you have fully removed it as this increases the risk of needle-stick injuries and bits of the plastic cannula may shear off and embolise, steady the patient's arm on a pillow to reduce movement and risk of needle-stick injury, dispose of needles into a sharps bin immediately

Alternatives central venous cannulation (p476), alternative route of drug administration (PO/IM/SC/PR)

Hints and tips

- See comments under blood taking
- Start distally in a limb and work your way proximally if you fail to cannulate initially
- Veins are easier to cannulate at the junction of two veins
- Try to avoid cannulas over a joint as these are uncomfortable and more likely to tissue
- If you go through the wall of the vein, withdraw a small distance until flashback recurs and try to advance the plastic cannula
- In confused patients cover the cannula with a crêpe bandage and tape the IV line to their skin to minimise auto-extraction and further cannulation practice

Size and function of different cannulae

Colour	Size	Flow rate (ml/min)	Use
Blue	22G	31	Small fragile veins
Pink	20G	55	IV drugs and fluids ±blood
Green	18G	90	Blood, fluids, drugs
White	17G	135	Blood, fluids, drugs
Grey	16G	170	Rapid blood, fluids, drugs
Brown	14G	265	Emergency situations

Cannula care

- Inspect cannula daily, looking for inflammation and replace them every 72h
- If asked to replace them, check the cannula is still necessary
- If blocked, try flushing the line gently with 0.9% saline and check it isn't kinked
- Remove the cannula if the surrounding skin is red, swollen or tender
- GTN patches can prolong the life of a drip site, but are expensive

Arterial blood gas (ABG)

Indications assessment of hypoxia, CO_2 retention, acutely ill patients

Contraindications *absolute* patient refusal *radial* AV fistula, poor/absent collateral circulation, bony fractures *femoral* femoral artery graft *relative* abnormal blood coagulation

Consent verbal; explain why the test is required

Site radial artery (usual), femoral artery, brachial artery (last resort)

Equipment non-sterile gloves, alcohol swab, heparin-filled syringe and cap, needle (blue for radial, green for femoral), gauze/cotton ball, tape, sharps bin

Checks Note the concentration of O_2 the patient is on and their temperature. Locate the nearest ABG analysis machine. *Radial ABG* check ulnar circulation adequacy by squeezing the hand into a fist, occluding the radial and ulnar arteries in the wrist, holding for 10s then opening the hand and releasing the pressure on the ulnar artery only; looking for reperfusion of the whole hand (Allen's test)

Patient position *upper limb* sit the patient upright, arm and wrist extended, put a sick bowl under the wrist to hold the position *femoral ABG* lie patient flat on their back with their groin exposed and curtains shut

Procedure Wash hands and wear non-sterile gloves. Attach needle to syringe and expel the heparin (if present). Palpate both radial pulses and select the better side. Roll your finger back and forth over the artery to assess its width and course. Do not use a tourniquet. Place a finger on the radial pulse, hold the syringe like a pen with the bevel facing upwards and proximally. Warn the patient and insert the syringe at 45° to the skin, aiming for the centre of the artery against the direction of blood flow. Once you hit the artery the blood should pulse into the syringe (best method of assessing whether arterial or venous). If not reassess the positions of the pulse and needle by feeling for the needle tip as you gently press the syringe upwards. Once you have about 0.5ml of blood apply gentle pressure to the puncture site with cotton wool and withdraw the needle. Press firmly for at least 3min (do not let the patient do this). Remove the needle using a sharps bin and put the cap on the syringe. Label the syringe with the patient's details, O_2 concentration and temp and take it to the ABG machine.

Confirmations *during procedure* pulsatile, bright red blood fills the syringe automatically *post-procedure* blood O_2 saturation is the same as that measured with a sats probe

Complications bleeding, haematoma, arterial damage and peripheral ischaemia, pain, infection, local tendon/nerve damage

Safety steady the patient's arm on a pillow to reduce movement and risk of needle-stick injury, dispose of needles into a sharps container immediately, do not resheath them

Alternatives

- ***Femoral blood gas*** Similar to femoral stab (p459) but aim for the femoral pulse (usually 2 fingers width below the inguinal ligament), with the patient lying flat on their back. Insert the green needle at 90° to the skin.
- ***Brachial artery gas*** (if unable to get radial or femoral) Extend the patient's arm and insert needle at 45° into the brachial artery (medial to the biceps tendon, on the inner aspect of the upper forearm).
- ***Arterial cannula*** Used for repeated arterial samples or direct BP measurement (seek senior/specialist advice).

Hints and tips

- Consider applying topical (p390) or intradermal local anaesthetic (bleb of 1% lidocaine over the artery using an orange needle).
- If no blood is seen reposition the needle without withdrawing it completely from the skin; ask the patient to dorsiflex the wrist fully.
- You may miss the artery and hit the bone (painful); if this happens gently withdraw the needle to just under the skin, reposition the needle in line with the pulse and try again, taking your time.
- A&E, ITU, HDU, neonatal and labour wards often have ABG machines, if you cannot process the ABG immediately put it in a fridge or on ice.
- Expel air bubbles from the syringe before presenting the sample to the analysis machine.

Interpretation see *p506*

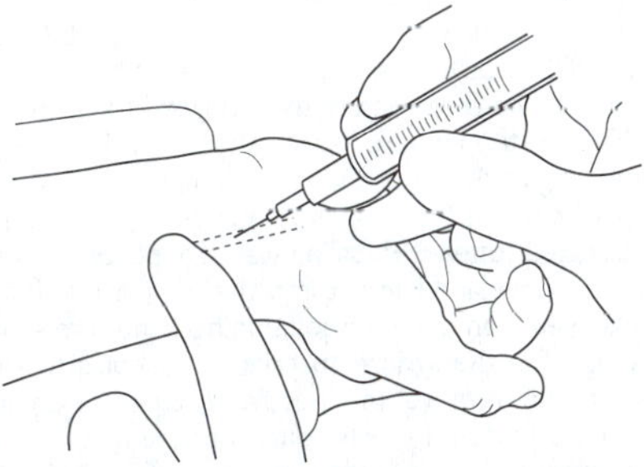

Obtaining an arterial blood sample from the right radial artery

IV injections (intravenous)

Blood transfusions	p276	Heparin infusion	p290
Insulin sliding scale	p235	GTN infusion	p170
IV fluids	p263	Morphine injection	p283

Indications rapid or direct drug administration, steady plasma concentration from infusion, only route of administration available or tolerated

Contraindications *absolute* patient refusal, drug allergy

Consent verbal; explain what fluid/drug/blood you are injecting and why

Site via a cannula (see p462) or central line (p476)

Equipment IV fluid/drug/blood, IV cannula *in situ*, syringe, green needle, giving set (tube connecting the bag to the cannula), 0.9% saline flush

Checks patient's name and DoB (ask patient or check ID band), dose and infusion rate prescribed, batch number and expiry date, allergies (ask patient, check allergy bands or drug chart), cannula is sited appropriately and flushing, some drugs need therapeutic monitoring (p569)

- If you are unfamiliar with an IV drug look it up in the *BNF* before giving
- Always follow the *BNF* and drug instructions

Patient position sitting up with the cannula exposed

Procedure Flush the cannula to make sure it is working then:

- ***IV infusion*** Hang the bag on a drip stand and puncture the port on the bag of fluids with the sharp plastic end of the giving set. Open the valve and run the fluid through into a sink (or kidney bowl) to remove air bubbles. Connect the other end of the giving set to the horizontal cannula porthole (not the coloured top). Alter the drip speed and tape a loop of the tubing to the patient's arm to limit traction on the cannula
- ***Drawing up IV drugs*** If the drug is in powder form reconstitute with solvent as directed (often 0.9% saline/water; appendix 6 of *BNF*). Draw solvent into a syringe and inject it into the drug vial with a green 21G needle. Shake well then draw the solution back into the syringe
- ***Giving IV drugs*** Tap the syringe to bring air bubbles to the top then expel any air and remove the needle. Attach the syringe to the coloured cannula port and slowly administer the medication according to the drug manufacturer's instructions or the *BNF*. Flush with 5ml 0.9% saline

Confirmation infusion running/IV drug successfully administered, assess the patient and monitor the pulse, BP and RR to ensure there is no acute reaction, remember to write the time given and sign the drug chart

Complications anaphylaxis (p156), drug overdose (p310), local irritation/thrombophlebitis, leakage of drug from tissued cannula, haematoma

Safety If multiple infusions are set up check they can be given through the same cannula. If not, insert a second cannula or give the drugs at different times. Stay on the ward for at least 5min after giving IV drugs in case of an acute reaction.

Alternatives Consider other routes of administration (PO, IM, SC, PR, SL, IN). As a last resort IV fluids (0.9% saline ±KCl) can be given very slowly SC (no faster than 1l over 16h). Never give glucose-containing fluids SC due to infection risk. Blood transfusions (p276) can only be given IV. You may need a central line (p476) for some IV infusions/drugs.

Hints and tips

- Flush the cannula, especially after giving irritant drugs
- If you are unsure of infusion rates, consult the *BNF*
- Some medications must be given at a constant rate using a syringe driver (eg heparin, magnesium, GTN, opiates)
- Keep IV infusions above the level of the patient's heart to prevent blood loss
- Keep syringe drivers below the level of the patient's heart to prevent drug siphoning
- Most nurses can administer IV infusions or drugs though some IV injections must be given by a doctor; there is usually good reason for this – find out what it is before giving the injection

SC/IM injections

Indications only route of administration available or tolerated

Contraindications *absolute* patient refusal, drug allergy, bleeding disorder or ↓platelets

Consent verbal; explain why you are giving the drug

Site

- SC upper arm (tricep/deltoid), anterior abdominal wall, anterior thigh
- IM shoulder (deltoid), lateral thigh, superior lateral quadrant of the buttocks (to avoid the sciatic nerve)

Equipment non-sterile gloves, alcohol swab, drug, syringe, green (21G) and blue (23G) or orange (25G) needle, cotton wool

Checks patient's name and DoB (ask patient or check ID band), dose and strength prescribed, batch number and expiry date, allergies (ask patient, check allergy bands or drug chart)

Patient position so that target site is exposed and accessible

Procedure Wash hands and wear non-sterile gloves. Draw up the medication into a syringe using a green needle and expel any air bubbles:

- *SC* Attach an orange needle to the syringe and clean the area for injection with an alcohol swab. Raise the skin and subcutaneous tissue between your fingers by pinching it and insert the needle at 45° into the skin. Pull the syringe back slightly to check you are not in a blood vessel. Inject the medication slowly, watching the patient as you do so, then withdraw the needle and hold cotton wool over the site
- *IM* Attach a blue needle to the syringe and clean the area for injection with an alcohol swab. Insert the needle vertically into the skin and pull back slightly to check you are not in a blood vessel. Inject the medication slowly, watching the patient as you do so, then withdraw the needle and hold cotton wool over the site

Confirmation drug successfully administered, assess the patient and monitor the pulse, BP and RR to ensure there is no acute reaction, remember to write the time given and sign the drug chart

Complications anaphylaxis (p156), drug overdose (p310), local swelling, pain and bruising, bleeding, accidental IV injection

Safety Stay on the ward for at least 5min after giving drugs in case of an acute reaction. Dispose of sharps in a sharps bin.

Alternatives Consider other routes (PO, IV, PR, SL, IN) or alternative drugs (see *BNF*).

Hints and tips

- Use a larger needle in obese patients
- If blood is aspirated, withdraw and repeat the procedure in a different area with a clean needle
- Rotate injection sites to limit local reactions
- Most nurses can give IM/SC injections and are more experienced at it

Drugs commonly given SC and IM routes

Subcutaneous
- Insulin
- Low molecular weight heparin
- Diamorphine

Intramuscular
- Metoclopramide
- Cyclizine
- Tramadol/pethidine
- Chlorpheniramine
- Haloperidol

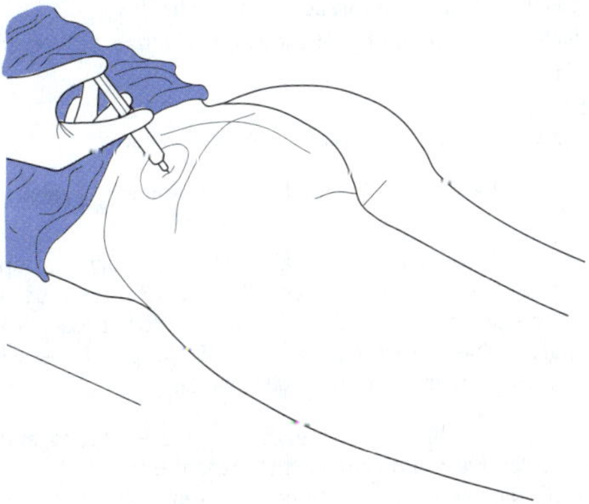

Safe area for IM injection in the buttock

ECGs and cardiac monitors

Indications
- *ECG* chest/back/abdo pain or suspicion of cardiac ischaemia, unexplained shortness of breath, ↓GCS, ↑K^+, arrhythmias, pre-op
- ***Cardiac monitoring*** peri- and post-cardiorespiratory arrest, peri- and post-MI, ↑K^+, arrhythmias, cardioversion, administration of certain drugs, administration of anaesthesia

Contraindications *absolute* patient refusal *relative* patient contaminated with toxic substance or other risk to operator

Consent verbal; explain why the ECG/monitoring is required

Site anterior chest wall and limbs

Equipment ECG/cardiac monitor, adhesive electrodes

Checks sufficient ECG paper, paper moving at 25mm/s, power supply

Patient position sitting at 45° for ECG

Procedure
- *ECG* apply adhesive electrodes and connect as follows:

Limb leads: red right shoulder **yellow** left shoulder **green** left foot **black** right foot

Chest leads: V1 (red) right sternal edge, 4th intercostal space **V2** (yellow) left sternal edge, 4th intercostal space **V3** (green) between V2 and V4 **V4** (brown) mid-clavicular line, 5th intercostal space **V5** (black) anterior-axillary line, horizontal with V4 **V6** (purple) mid-axillary line horizontal with V4 (see diagram on next page).

  Turn the ECG machine on once the leads are applied and ask the patient to relax back and remain still; press the record button (usually has an ECG picture or the number '12'). Once the machine has captured enough data it should print. Common error messages include 'lead disconnection' or 'no paper'; both are self-explanatory
- Cardiac monitoring apply the leads as follows: red right shoulder; yellow left shoulder and green/black over the apex beat or spleen. The machine will show the trace of lead 'II' on a standard 12-lead ECG. Other views can also be obtained with three leads (OHCC2 p108)

Confirmation adequate ECG printout or trace on cardiac monitor

Complications skin reaction to adhesive electrodes (rare).

Safety caution with electricity and wet/bloody environments

Alternatives request help from the ECG technician or nursing staff, posterior leads are used for posterior MIs, the position of leads continues round the chest from V6; connect V1 to V4, V2 to V5 and so on

Hints and tips Adhesive electrodes do not stick well to hairy skin, so you may need to shave a small patch where the electrode is needed. If the patient is sweaty try cleaning the skin with an alcohol wipe first. In desperation use a pen to hold single leads in place. The limb leads can be placed on the ankles and wrists or over the hips and shoulders; both are recognised, although comparing ECGs taken by different methods can be hard. Consider a chaperone for female patients.

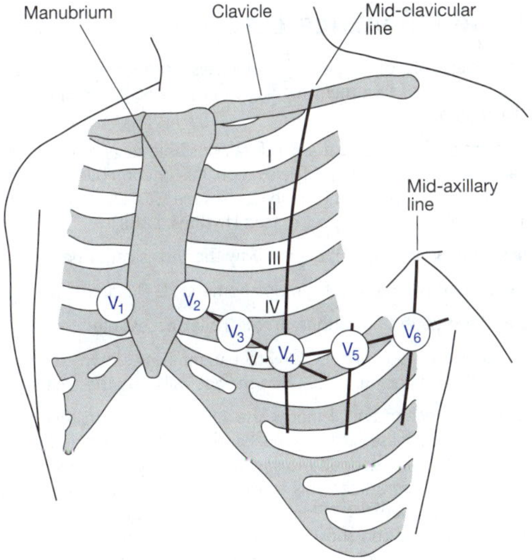

Position of chest leads for 12-lead ECG

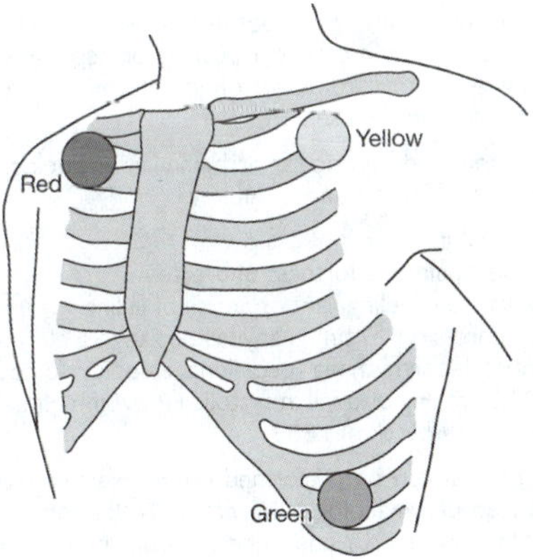

Position of three leads for cardiac monitoring

Exercise tolerance test

Indications diagnosis of suspected IHD, assess cardiac fitness, prognosis post-MI, evaluation of treatment (eg angioplasty, CABG), assessing exercise-induced arrhythmias

Contraindications *absolute* patient refusal, unstable angina *relative* severe aortic stenosis, recent (<5d) ST elevation MI, uncontrolled arrhythmia, ↑BP or heart failure, physical inability (eg severe COPD, stroke, arthritis), β-blockade, inability to interpret (paced rhythms, LBBB)

Consent verbal/written (p94); explain why the test is required

Equipment treadmill, ECG, sphygmomanometer, GTN, arrest trolley

Checks exclude contraindications, arrest trolley accessible

Patient position record first ECG with patient lying down, second with patient standing up and serial ECGs as patient walks on the treadmill

Procedure The technician connects the BP cuff and ECG leads to the patient with a specialised harness; a baseline BP is recorded. The test commences with the treadmill moving slowly then gradually speeding up whilst increasing the gradient; this is pre-programmed and most hospitals use the Bruce protocol (OHCM6 p106). BP is recorded every 3–5min. Real-time ECGs are often shown on a monitor where changes to the ST segment can be observed. The test is complete once the patient reaches ≥90% of their maximal heart rate (220 – age in years) or they complete the protocol (30min). The test is often stopped early (see below). BP and ECG measurement continues for a further 10–15min as the patient rests.

Confirmation Deciding if the test is positive or not is difficult, since stopping early (see below) could be either positive or negative depending on the ECG tracing. A senior cardiologist often determines the result. If the test is stopped early consult a senior.

Complications atrial and ventricular arrhythmias (including VF and VT), syncope, shortness of breath, angina, MI

Safety Stop the test if:
- patient has chest pain or shortness of breath
- patient is exhausted, feeling faint or at risk of falling
- ST segment depression >2mm in any lead or any ST elevation
- atrial or ventricular arrhythmia (occasional ectopics do not count)
- systolic BP ≥230mmHg or a fall in systolic BP ≥20mmHg
- development of AV block or LBBB

Alternatives The test can be performed on an exercise bicycle, an arm bicycle or induced pharmacologically with an IV β-agonist. Stress echocardiography (OHCM6 p110) and nuclear cardiography (OHCM6 p112) can also be used to assess cardiac disease.

Hints and tips Most hospitals have specific protocols for exercise testing. The technician is usually much more experienced than the junior doctor and if they suggest stopping a test it is worthwhile doing so.

Cardioversion and defibrillation

Indications *emergency* VF, VT, fast AF (new onset or haemodynamically unstable), SVT if other treatments have failed (p139) or patient haemodynamically unstable *elective* AF

Contraindications *absolute* patient refusal *relative* wet or bloody environment (moisture and electricity don't mix)

Consent verbal/common law in an emergency, otherwise verbal/written (p94)

Site one electrode to the right of the upper sternum below the clavicle, and the other level with the 5th left intercostal space in the anterior axillary line (see diagrams A+B opposite). In refractory VF/VT consider shocking in the anterior/posterior position (diagram C).

Equipment defibrillator with paddles and gel-pads or hands-free electrodes, arrest trolley, ECG machine

Checks Defibrillator working and battery charged; gel-pads and resuscitation drugs available, at least one assistant, patient's cardiac rhythm requires cardioversion. In elective cases (OHAM2 p894) check the patient is starved and adequately anticoagulated with good IV access.

Patient position supine; left lateral position for AP cardioversion

Procedure

- ***Emergency*** Follow BLS (p121) and ALS(p123)/APLS algorithms. Attach gel-pads or hands-free electrodes. Set defibrillator to required energy, make sure no one is in contact with the patient or bed and the O_2 is removed. **Give a clear verbal warning to stand clear**. Shock. Repeat in accordance with ALS/APLS algorithm. After third shock replace electrodes into defibrillator and continue with the algorithm.
- ***Elective*** Ensure the anaesthetist is available and inform the nursing staff. Apply gel-pads or hands-free electrodes before the patient is anaesthetised. Once asleep set the defibrillator to 'synchronised shock' (OHCM6 p754) and shock in accordance to ALS/APLS algorithms, checking that no one is in contact with the patient/bed and that O_2 is removed. **Give a clear verbal warning to stand clear**. Shock.

Confirmation restoration of sinus rhythm for elective cases or a cardiac output in the emergency situation; perform 12-lead ECG

Complications life-threatening arrhythmias, thromboembolism, aspiration, local burning to skin, risks to user and bystanders

Safety users of the manual defibrillator must have passed an ALS or ILS course; caution with electricity and wet/bloody environments

Alternatives Automated external defibrillators (AEDs) are becoming widespread and require no rhythm recognition by the user. Two hands-free electrodes are applied to the patient and the AED determines if a shock is advisable or not; if a shock is advisable the operator just presses the 'shock' button when the AED tells them to. AEDs should not be used for elective cardioversions.

Hints and tips Always defibrillate safely; if in doubt contact your resuscitation officer for some extra training.

(A) (B)

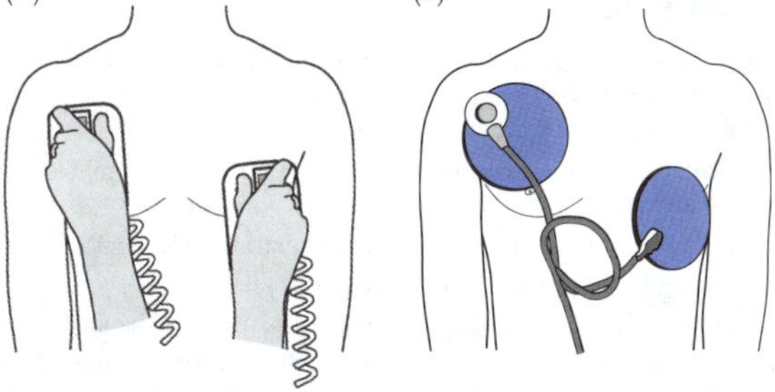

(A) Position of manual defibrillator paddles. Make sure gel-pads are placed on the skin underneath the paddles as these reduce the impedence and limit skin burns. ***(B) Position of hands-free adhesive defibrillation electrodes.*** The electrodes for most hands-free systems indicate where they should be placed: over the right shoulder and over the left side of the chest.

(C)

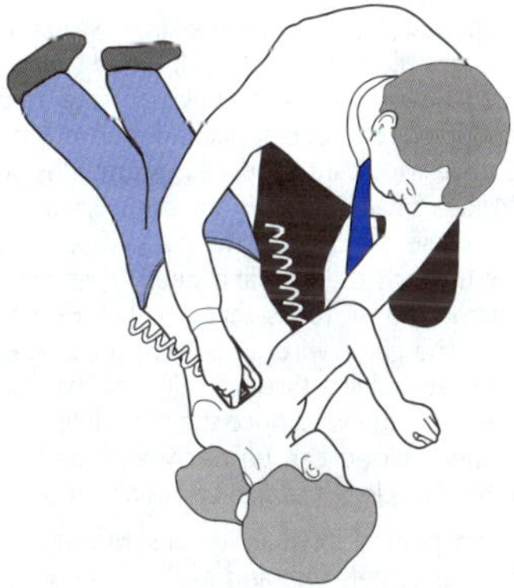

(C) Position of either manual paddles or hands-free electrodes in the anterior/posterior position. The anterior site is to the left of the lower sternal border and the posterior position is just inferior to the left scapula.

Central lines

Indications monitoring fluid balance, pulmonary artery catheterisation (Swann-Ganz catheters), temporary pacing wires, drug administration, parenteral feeding, permits blood sampling

Contraindications *absolute* patient refusal *relative* infection at site, bleeding diathesis/anticoagulation, shock

Consent verbal/written (p94); explain why the central line is required

Site internal jugular, subclavian or femoral vein

Equipment 5ml/10ml syringes, blue (23G) and green (21G) needles, non-absorbable suture, Seldinger central line kit (introducing needle, 5ml syringe, guide-wire, dilator, small blade, central line with 2–5 lumens and bungs), 1% lidocaine, sterile gloves, dressing pack, sterile drapes, ±portable ultrasound

Patient position flat on their back with their head down for internal jugular and subclavian cannulation; flat on their back with head up for femoral cannulation – helps fill the vein

Procedure Using aseptic technique, clean and drape the area. Identify landmarks (see opposite) and anaesthetise skin and deep layers with 10ml lidocaine. Whilst anaesthetic takes effect, flush all lumens of the central line and cap all except the green one. Attach 5ml syringe, insert the introducer needle through skin and towards vein, aspirating whilst advancing. Once dark red blood is aspirated freely into the syringe, stop advancing. Remove syringe whilst holding needle firmly in place. If blood spurts out in a pulsatile fashion it is likely to be an arterial cannulation (see opposite). Advance guide-wire though lumen of needle (should occur without resistance). Once most of the guide-wire is inserted, remove needle, but always holding onto guide-wire. Make a small incision in the skin adjacent to the guide-wire with the blade; thread the dilator over the guide-wire and gently but firmly advance the dilator through the skin and deep layers, rotating to ease its passage. Stop once half the dilator is through skin. Remove dilator, whilst always holding on to the guide-wire. Pass the central line over the guide-wire and advance the central line through skin, holding onto the guide-wire at all times. Remove the guide-wire once the central line is inserted and cap the open lumen. Check blood can be easily aspirated from each lumen. Suture the line to the skin, clean the skin and apply clear sterile dressing.

Confirmation blood aspirated from all lumens, blood O_2 sats < finger O_2 sats, CXR to locate the catheter tip and exclude pneumothorax

Complications arterial cannulation, bleeding, pneumothorax (subclavian >internal jugular), failure to identify vein, air embolism, infection

Safety Never perform this procedure for the first time on your own.

Hints and tips Make sure you and the patient are both comfortable before you start. Use sufficient LA and consider premedicating the patient with good PO/IV analgesia 30min before the procedure. A SonoSite® (ultrasound) shows the vascular anatomy very clearly.

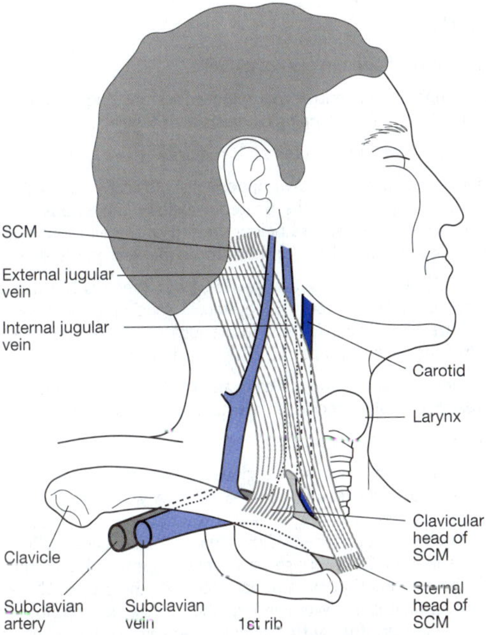

(A) Anatomy of the major vessels in the neck The right internal jugular is the commonest site for central cannulation and has fewer complications than subclavian cannulation; femoral cannulation has a higher rate of infection and is used less frequently. The right internal jugular lies deep to sternocleidomastoid muscle (SCM) and appears between the two heads, just above the clavicle, lateral to the carotid.

Accidental arterial cannulation

Signs of arterial cannulation

- Bright red blood, rather than dark red
- Pulsatile blood, rather than constant low flow
- High O_2 sats (>95%) of blood compared with finger O_2 saturation
- If the right carotid artery is cannulated the central line will cross the midline on the CXR

What to do if the artery is cannulated

- Identify arterial cannulation
- Remove all lines and press firmly over site for 10min
- Seek senior help

You can reattempt on the same side or the other side; if you don't feel confident, ask your seniors for assistance.

Pleural tap

Indications diagnosis of effusion, symptomatic relief

Contraindications *absolute* patient refusal *relative* local infection, contralateral pneumothorax/effusion, bleeding diathesis/anticoagulation

Consent verbal; explain why the pleural tap is required

Site simplest and safest sites are shown opposite (A), directly below the inferior angle of the scapula or in the posterior-axillary line; choose an intercostal space two or three spaces below the top of the effusion; if in doubt request an ultrasound and ask for a site to be marked on the skin

Equipment 5, 10, 20, 50ml syringes, orange (25G) and green (21G) needles, ±intravenous cannula (14–16G), 3-way tap, 3 specimen containers and fluoride oxalate blood tube (p460), sterile jug/bowel, 1% lidocaine, sterile gloves, dressing pack, antiseptic cleaning solution

Checks confirm side of the effusion clinically and on CXR; lay equipment out on clean treatment trolley; recruit an assistant to pass you things

Patient position see diagram A opposite

Procedure Wash hands and wear sterile gloves. Clean area thoroughly with Betadine® or chlorhexidine. Infiltrate 2–5ml of LA with orange needle into subcutaneous and then deeper layers towards pleura, avoiding neurovascular bundles (C opposite). Allow 2min to take effect. Using either a green needle on a 20ml syringe or a cannula, gently advance the needle through the anaesthetised area directly towards the pleura. Once in the pleural space, fluid is easily drawn into the syringe or a flashback will be seen in the cannula; if using the cannula then remove the needle, leaving the plastic component in place, and attach a syringe. Aspirate volume required and divide into specimen containers. If performing a therapeutic procedure use the cannula and attach a 3-way tap with a 50ml syringe; withdraw and dispose of fluid into a jug. Once complete withdraw needle/cannula and apply plaster to skin.

Confirmation pleural fluid aspirated, always get a CXR (pneumothorax and reassess the level of the effusion if a therapeutic procedure)

Complications pneumothorax, haemothorax, pain, bleeding, damage to intercostal nerve, local or intrapleural infection

Safety Never perform this procedure for the first time on your own; take care not to allow air into the chest.

Alternatives retry in a different rib space; radiology might perform a diagnostic tap under ultrasound guidance; chest drain for large effusions

Hints and tips Make sure you and the patient are both comfortable before you start; try to anaesthetise and insert the needle 100% vertically.

Aspiration of pneumothorax Tension pneumothorax is a medical emergency and requires immediate treatment (p171). Aspiration of 'simple' pneumothoraces can also be performed (OHAM2 p238).

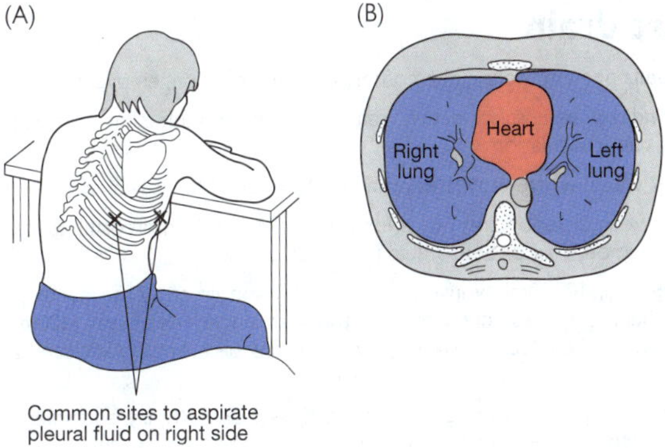

(A) Position of the patient for aspiration of pleural fluid. Get the patient to lean forwards over a table or the back of a chair to open up the rib spaces and prevent excessive movement. ***(B) Position of the normal heart within the thorax at level of T6/T7 vertebra.*** Posterior and lateral approaches for pleural aspiration with standard green (21G) needle or IV cannula are highly unlikely to puncture the heart, even on the left side of the chest.

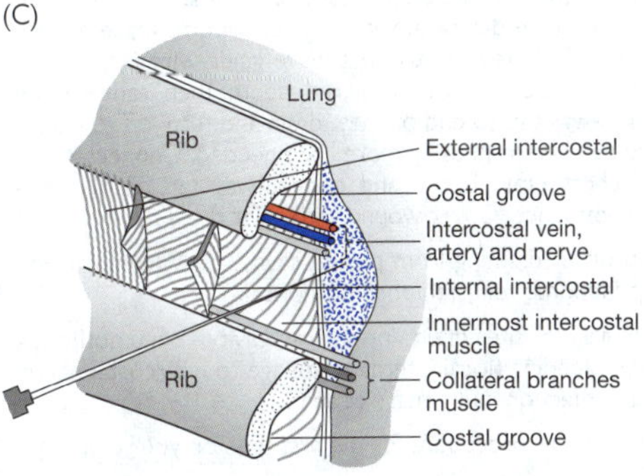

(C) Safe pleural aspiration approach to avoid neurovascular bundles. The main bundle sits just posterior to the inferior rib edge, though collateral branches are located adjacent to the superior border. The safe approach is to advance the needle above a rib, but not right against its superior edge.

Chest drain

Indications pneumothorax, haemothorax, pleural effusion, empyema

Contraindications *absolute* patient refusal *relative* local infection, bleeding diathesis/anticoagulation

Consent verbal/written (p94); explain why the pleural tap is required

Site between anterior and posterior axillary lines, 5th intercostal space for a pneumothorax or below fluid level in an effusion

Equipment 5, 10, 20ml syringes, orange (25G) and green (21G) needles, suture, Seldinger chest drain pack, bottle with under-water seal (400ml sterile water), 1% lidocaine, sterile gloves, dressing pack, antiseptic cleaning solution

Checks confirm side of the effusion clinically and on CXR; lay equipment out on clean treatment trolley; recruit an assistant to pass you things

Patient position hunched forwards over a table (A) or reclining back with their arm behind the head (B); choose according to comfort

Procedure Wash hands and wear sterile gloves. Clean area thoroughly with Betadine® or chlorhexidine. Infiltrate 5ml of LA with orange then green needle into subcutaneous and then deeper layers towards pleura, avoiding neurovascular bundles (see C, p479). Allow 2min to take effect. Attach Seldinger needle onto the syringe and advance through the area of infiltration as for a pleural tap (p478). Once needle tip is inside the pleural space, remove the syringe and pass the guide-wire through the needle. Never let go of the guide-wire. Withdraw the needle fully leaving half the guide-wire in chest. Make a small incision with scalpel alongside the guide-wire and pass the dilator along the guide-wire to make a track to the pleural space. Withdraw dilator, but leave guide-wire *in situ*. Pass chest drain over the guide-wire to required depth then remove the guide-wire. Attach 3-way tap to end of chest drain and turn 'off to chest'. Suture chest drain to chest wall using more LA if needed. Connect 3-way tap to tubing of chest drain bottle and open 3-way tap. Fluid drainage/bubbling will commence. Cover wound with clear dressings.

Confirmation fluid or air draining from pleural cavity, CXR (confirmation of position and reduction of effusion/pneumothorax)

Complications failure to site drain in pleural cavity, pneumothorax, haemothorax, pain, bleeding (local/internal), damage to intercostal nerve, local or intrapleural infection, pulmonary oedema

Safety Never perform this procedure for the first time on your own.

Alternatives Radiology might insert a Seldinger chest drain under ultrasound, but these block easily if the fluid is too viscous. Traditional/blunt/surgical chest tubes can also be used (OHAM2 p920, OHCM6 p750).

Hints and tips Make sure both you and the patient are comfortable before you start; use sufficient LA and consider premedicating the patient with good PO/IV analgesia 30min before the procedure.

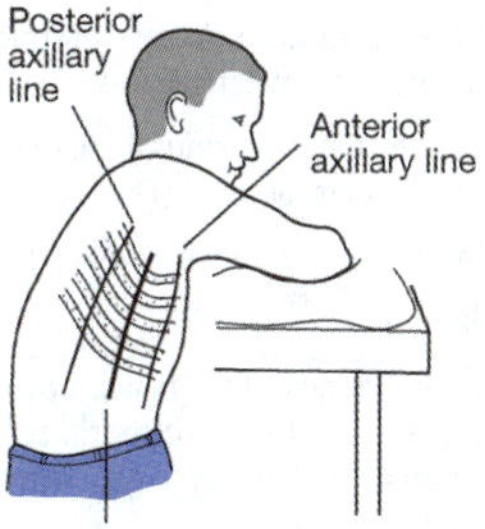

(A) Position of the patient for chest drain insertion. Ask the patient to lean forwards over a table or the back of a chair, since this opens up the rib spaces and prevents them from moving too much.

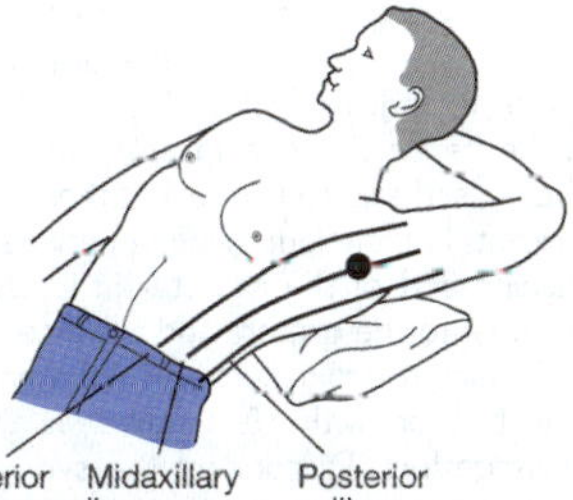

(B) Alternative position of the patient for chest drain insertion. Position the patient at about 45° with their arm above and behind the head, exposing the axilla.

Removing a chest drain

- Leave the drain unclamped
- Remove dressings from skin
- Clean skin with Betadine® or chlorhexidine
- Remove all sutures
- Gently but firmly remove drain as patient exhales, occlude wound
- Re-suture mattress sutures around drain site (p494)
- Apply sterile dressing. Sutures should stay in for 5d.
- CXR not specifically required following removal of chest drain

Urinary catheterisation

Indications monitor urine output, urinary retention, incapacitation (eg ↓GCS), incontinence, urological investigations

Contraindications *absolute* patient refusal *relative* suspected urethral injury, urethral strictures/fistulas, active UTI

Consent verbal; explain why a catheter is required

Site via urethra into bladder

Equipment catheter pack (kidney dish, bowl, cotton balls, sterile towel and gloves), Foley catheter (10–16F), antiseptic solution, gauze, 10ml 1% lidocaine/lubricant gel in pre-filled syringe, 10ml saline-filled syringe, catheter bag

Checks no latex allergy/UTIs, correct sex catheter

Patient position lying on back, genitalia exposed (legs apart in women)

Procedure Wash hands and wear sterile gloves. Prepare the equipment, using aseptic technique. Pour antiseptic solution into the sterile bowl.

Male Create a hole in the centre of the towel and drape it over the patient's pelvis, exposing the penis through the hole. Hold the penis with some gauze in your non-dominant hand. Retract the foreskin and clean the penis with antiseptic – work from the urethral meatus outwards. Hold the penis upright and instil 10ml lubricant/lidocaine gel into the meatus. Occlude the penile tip to help push the gel along the urethra. Allow 1min for the anaesthetic to take effect then lubricate the tip of the catheter with lubricant. Put the kidney bowl between the patient's thighs and place the draining end of the catheter in it. Using your clean hand insert the catheter tip into the urethra and advance. Continue to advance once urine starts draining to make sure the catheter balloon is within the bladder. Inflate the balloon with 10ml saline via the side port. Stop if there is pain or discomfort. Disconnect the syringe and pull back the catheter until you feel resistance. Attach a draining tube and bag to the free end of the catheter. Clean and redress the patient. Remember to replace the foreskin at the end of the procedure.

Female Drape the sterile towel between the patient's thighs. Separate labial folds with your non-dominant hand and clean with antiseptic solution from the urethra outwards. The urethra is between the vagina and clitoris. Continue as for a male patient.

Confirmation urine drains freely, no pain on inflating balloon

Complications pain, infection, local trauma, strictures (long-term), retention on removing catheter

Safety never force the catheter or fill the balloon under force

Alternatives suprapubic catheter – seek senior advice

Hints and tips

- Double glove on your dominant hand and remove the top glove once you have finished cleaning the genitalia so that you remain sterile when handling the catheter.
- Avoid touching the lubricant gel with the hand holding the catheter as this makes the catheter slippery and difficult to grip and insert.
- Try not to touch the catheter; it usually comes in a plastic cover which can be shuffled down or torn away as you insert it into the urethra.
- If you feel resistance at the prostatic urethra hold the penis vertically and try to advance the catheter.
- The urethra is 4–7cm in women so urine should be seen after 8cm; the male urethra is much longer (20cm) so the catheter must be inserted further.
- If no urine appears check the catheter is in the correct place and advanced far enough; flush the catheter with saline to make sure it is not blocked with lubricant gel.
- Urine samples can be taken from a catheter (CSU).

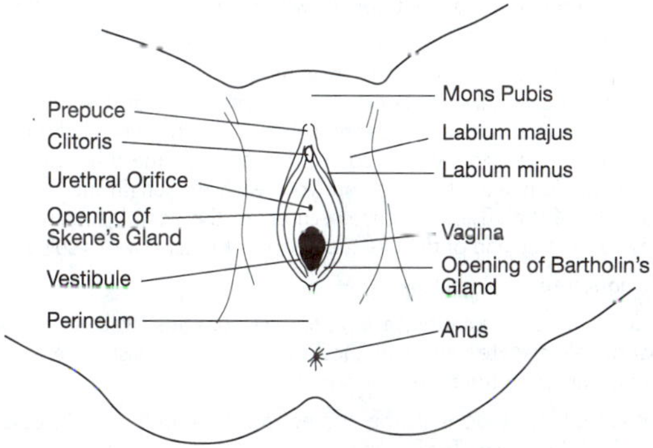

Anatomy of the female genitalia for catheterisation

Nasogastric tubes (NG tubes)

Indications stomach emptying eg bowel obstruction (wide-bore or Ryle's tube), nutrition (fine bore)

Contraindications *absolute* basal skull fracture, facial trauma, patient refusal *relative* infection

Consent verbal; explain why a NG tube is required and warn the patient about initial discomfort (which does improve)

Site inserted into the stomach via a nostril

Equipment non-sterile gloves, NG tube, lubricant jelly, glass of water, adhesive tape, drainage bag and bowl (or spigot)

Checks Make sure the patient is alert, with no history of head injury. Use an appropriate sized tube (10 (small) to 16 (large)). Gauge the length of tube to insert by measuring the distance from the nostril to the angle of the jaw and from the angle of the jaw to the lower edge of the ribs.

Patient position Sit the patient upright with their head against a pillow.

Procedure Wash hands and wear non-sterile gloves. Ask the patient to take a sip of water and hold it in their mouth. Cover the tip of the NG tube with lubricant jelly and insert into the patient's nostril. Aim the tube directly backwards, ***not*** up. Once the patient feels the tube at the back of the throat ask them to swallow so you can advance the tube down their oesophagus. Continue advancing until you reach the length measured earlier (usually ~40cm). Tape the tube securely to the nostril. Attach a drainage bag to the free end of the NG tube or plug the tube with a spigot.

Confirmation see table below

Complications pain/irritation, aspiration, oesophagitis, tracheal/duodenal intubation, electrolyte depletion, local tissue necrosis, gastric perforation, tube may curl up in the mouth or pharynx

Safety Check the tube is in the correct position with a CXR, essential before the tube is used for feeding.

Alternatives If you cannot insert the tube via one nostril, try the other nostril or consider passing it orally; see next page for other options.

Hints and tips Use a chilled NG tube as these are less flexible.

Methods of confirming NG tube placement

Chest X-ray	Essential before a fine-bore feeding tube is used and highly recommended for a wide-bore tube. Check the tip of NG tube is visible below the diaphragm and not in the bronchial tree
NG aspiration	Aspirate fluid and test pH (stomach content is usually acidic). This does not confirm the NG tube is in the stomach
Air injection	Listen for air over the stomach as 20–50ml of air is injected. This does not confirm the NG tube is in the stomach

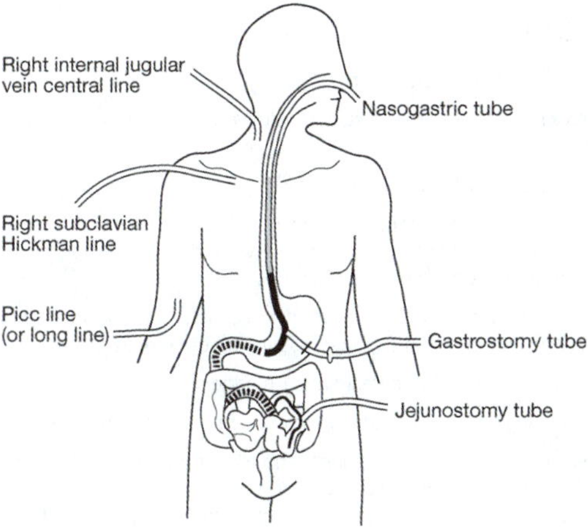

Methods of enteral and parenteral feeding

Enteral feeding – using the gut (excluding intake by mouth)

Types	Nasogastric, nasoduodenal, nasojejunal tubes Gastrostomy (sited endoscopically, surgically or radiologically) Jejunostomy (sited endoscopically, surgically or radiologically)
Uses	If the gut is functional, best to feed a patient via their gut
Risks	Complications of insertion (sitting in bronchial tree, vomiting) Aspiration following reflux or regurgitation

Parenteral feeding – not using the gut

Types	Central line (internal jugular, subclavian, Hickman, femoral) Peripheral long-line (Picc line) Peripheral cannula (can be used for short term but not advisable)
Uses	Means of providing nutrition when the gut is non-functional Should not be used for <7d as risks likely to outweigh benefits
Risks	Complications of line insertion (bleeding, pneumothorax) Sepsis from line Thrombosis and risk of embolism Metabolic imbalance (electrolyte abnormalities)

Laboratory monitoring of nutritional support

Consult local policy, but monitor U+E, LFT, Ca^{2+}, Mg^{2+}, Zn^{2+}, Iron, FBC

Ascitic tap

Indications diagnosis from ascitic fluid

Contraindications *absolute* patient refusal *relative* abnormal coagulation, local infection

Consent verbal; explain why a tap is required

Site left/right iliac fossa, horizontal to the umbilicus, but lateral to the mid-inguinal point (see diagram opposite). Avoid the suprapubic area with the bladder and inferior epigastric arteries

Equipment sterile gloves, antiseptic solution in a bowl, 10ml 1% lidocaine, swabs, green (21G) needle, 20ml syringe, sterile adhesive dressing

Checks INR – seek advice if abnormal empty bladder

Patient position lying flat on their bed, tilt the bed slightly to one side

Procedure Percuss the abdomen to assess the location and extent of the ascites. Wash hands and wear sterile gloves. Using aseptic technique clean the target area. Infiltrate around the area with 1% lidocaine initially into subcutaneous, then deeper layers towards the peritoneum. Allow 2min, then insert a green needle with a 20ml syringe vertically into the skin. Advance whilst aspirating until fluid flashback is seen (usually straw-coloured; may be bloodstained). Obtain 20ml fluid, then remove the needle and apply a sterile adhesive dressing.

- *Send fluid for* FBC, bacteriology (M,C+S, ±ZN stain/TB culture), biochemistry (protein, glucose, LDH, amylase), cytology

Confirmation fluid aspirated from abdominal cavity

Complications pain, bleeding (local or perforated viscus), perforated bowel/bladder, infection (skin or peritonitis), fluid leakage from wound

Safety do not have repeated attempts, if unsuccessful contact a senior

Alternatives therapeutic paracentesis (see box opposite)

Hints and tips Avoid sites close to old surgical scars to avoid going through adhesions; in obese patients use a bigger needle. Afterwards lie the patient with the puncture site upwards to minimise fluid leakage.

Diagnosis of ascites

	Transudate ascites	Exudate ascites
Total protein	<30g/l	>30g/l
Aetiology	• Cirrhosis • Nephrotic syndrome • CCF	• Infection (>250 white cells/mm^3) • Pancreatic cause • Malignancy • Budd–Chiari syndrome

Therapeutic paracentesis (OHAM2 p926)

Ascites may need to be drained for symptomatic relief, to reduce infection risk and prevent respiratory compromise. Drainage should take place over <6h to reduce the risk of infection. Up to 6l can be drained in this time so long as 100ml salt-poor albumin IV is given for every 1.5l ascitic fluid drained to prevent hypotension. The patient's FBC, U+E, LFT and INR should be checked after the procedure.

A Seldinger paracentesis set is used for paracentesis. The procedure is similar to an ascitic tap except that a guide-wire is inserted through the needle followed by the drain over the guide-wire. The drain must be removed within 6h.

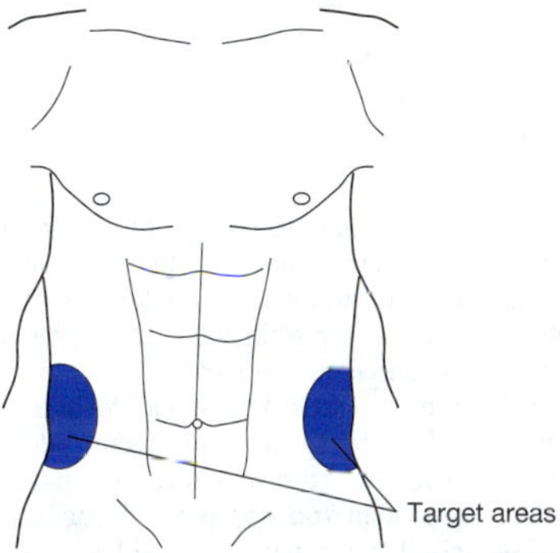

Target areas for ascitic tap at the level of the umbilicus, 3–4cm lateral to the mid-inguinal line

Lumbar puncture (LP)

Indications suspected meningitis, encephalitis, sub-arachnoid haemorrhage, investigation of other neurological conditions

Contraindications *absolute* patient refusal, raised intracranial pressure (see p212, check CT), infection at the site, cardiorespiratory compromise (treat first, including antibiotics) *relative* bleeding diathesis/anticoagulation, spinal deformity

Consent verbal; explain why the lumbar puncture is required

Site Draw a line between the iliac crests and feel for a gap in the spine where the line crosses it, this is L3/L4. Ask the patient if this feels like the middle of their back. The cord ends at L1/L2, mark the spaces using arrows away from the spine so they are not cleaned off.

Equipment 2ml syringe, orange (25G) needle, 4ml 1% lidocaine, antiseptic, gauze, lumbar puncture pack, sterile gloves, 3 specimen pots (labelled 1, 2, 3), fluoride oxalate blood tube (p460)

Checks Check the pots are numbered and the assistant knows this

Patient position Lying on their side on the edge of the bed with their back exposed, legs curled up and neck flexed (fetal position). Their body should be 90° to the floor.

Procedure Wash hands and wear sterile gloves. Clean area thoroughly with betadine or chlorhexadine. Infiltrate subcutaneously with 2–3ml of 1% lidocaine and 25G needle. Allow 2min to take effect during which you should assemble the manometer (thin tube, check the numbers match up). Insert spinal needle between the spinous processes with the bevel facing up and aim for the umbilicus. You should feel resistance from the supraspinous ligaments then the ligamentum flavum and dura followed by a lack of resistance as you enter the sub-arachnoid space. Withdraw the stylet and look for clear fluid (do not panic if you see blood, this is probably a spinal vessel), if there is no CSF pull back 2–3cm and realign. If the patient feels pain shooting down their leg you are hitting a nerve root so head more towards the midline. Once CSF is seen attach the manometer and measure pressure (7–20cm is normal). Use the three-way tap to drain the manometer fluid into the three specimen pots (10 drops in each) and the fluoride tube (six drops). Withdraw the entire needle and cover the wound with a sterile plaster. Take a blood sample in a fluoride (grey/yellow) tube and send for glucose levels. Advise the patient to lie flat for 1h and ask the nurses to check neurological obs and BP.

Confirmation CSF fluid seen

Complications headache post procedure (30%, worse sitting up, occurs within 24h and lasts 3–4d, p213), infection, trauma to nerve roots

Safety never perform this procedure for the first time on your own

Alternatives can be performed under X-ray guidance though this is rare; there is no equivalent, consider asking a senior to help

Hints and tips Position is everything; explain exactly what you want the patient to do, make sure their back is straight and their legs are tightly curled up. If you are having difficulty finding the midline ask the patient if it feels to the left, right or middle. Make sure the needle is horizontal.

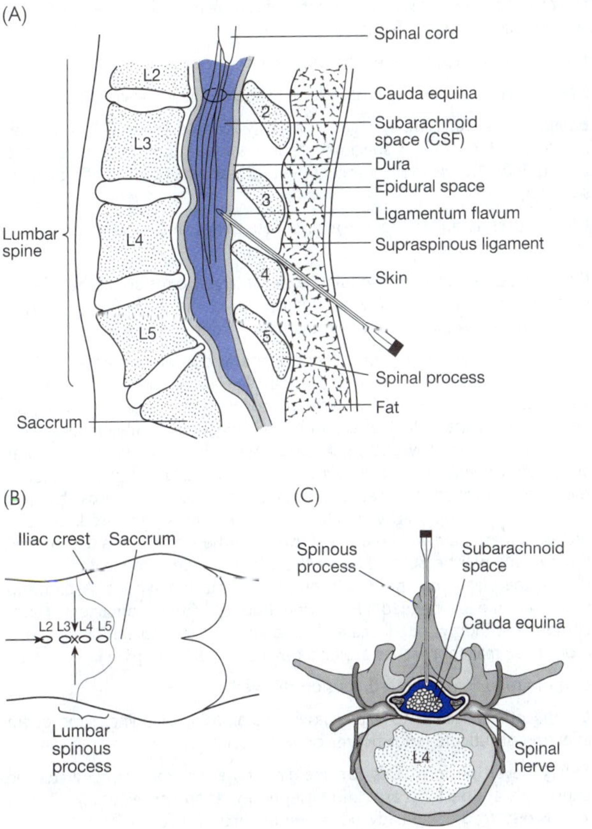

(A) Anatomy of a lumbar puncture
(B) Position and surface anatomy for a lumbar puncture
(C) Cross-section of the spine during a lumbar puncture

Joint aspiration and injection

Indications *diagnostic* look for blood/crystals/pus *therapeutic* steroid injection, drain tense/septic effusion or haemarthrosis

Contraindications *absolute* patient refusal *relative* bleeding diathesis/anticoagulation, local infection

Consent verbal; explain why the procedure is needed

Site any synovial joint (eg wrist, elbow, shoulder, knee, ankle, 1st MTPJ)

Equipment 2, 10, 20ml syringes, orange (25G) and green (21G) needles ±IVcannula (16–18G), 3 specimen containers and fluoride oxalate blood tube (p460), 1% lidocaine, sterile gloves, dressing pack, antiseptic cleaning solution

Checks recruit an assistant to pass you things, make sure aspiration/injection is required

Patient position Depends on joint; easier if larger joints are slightly flexed such as the knee and elbow as this opens up the joint. Position larger joints over a few pillows to make the patient more comfortable.

Procedure for aspirating knee Identify lateral border of patella and the depression posterior to it over the joint line (B opposite). Wash hands and wear sterile gloves. Clean area thoroughly with Betadine® or chlorhexidine. Infiltrate 2–5ml of LA with 25G needle into subcutaneous and then deeper layers towards joint space. Allow 2min to take effect. Either attach 21G needle to a 10ml syringe or a 16G cannula; gentle advance the needle through the area of LA infiltration directly towards the joint space. A slight 'pop' might be felt as the synovium is punctured. Once in the joint space fluid will be easily drawn into the syringe, or a flashback in the cannula will be seen; if using the cannula then remove the needle, leaving the plastic component in place, and attach a syringe. Aspirate as much volume as needed and divide into specimen containers. Once complete withdraw needle/cannula and apply plaster to skin. Medial and more proximal approaches are also described (OHAM2 p946).

Confirmation fluid aspirated, tension relieved

Complications failure to tap synovial fluid, pain, bleeding, subsequent infection of subcutaneous tissues or within joint

Safety never perform this for the first time on your own, watch an expert; always perform aspiration aseptically, as an iatrogenically infected joint is disastrous; avoid advancing needle through infected skin

Alternatives seek help from orthopaedic surgeon/rheumatologist; some radiologists will perform this under ultrasound guidance

Hints and tips Thick viscous effusions are difficult to draw up through small needles, so use a larger needle or cannula. Always speak to the relevant laboratory beforehand and enquire what volume and in which container they need their sample.

Joint injection

Steroid injections are used for a number of inflammatory disorders, but should be performed by an expert. If there is doubt whether a joint is infected or not, then steroids must not be injected into that joint (OHCS6 p656).

Synovial fluid in health and disease

Aspiration of synovial fluid is used primarily to look for infectious or crystal (gout and pseudogout) arthropathies.

	Appearance	Viscosity	WBC/ml	Neutrophils
Normal	Clear, colourless	High	<200	<25%
Noninflammatory[1]	Clear, straw	High	<5000	<25%
Haemorrhagic[2]	Bloody, xanthochromic	Variable	<10,000	<50%
Acute inflammatory[3]	Turbid, yellow	Decreased		
• Acute gout			~14,000	~80%
• Rheumatic fever			~18,000	~50%
• Rheumatoid arthritis			~16,000	~65%
Septic	Turbid, yellow	Decreased		
• TB			~24,000	~70%
• Gonorrhoeal			~14,000	~60%
• Septic (non-gonococcal)[4]			~65,000	~95%

1 eg degenerative joint disease, trauma.
2 eg tumour, haemophilia, trauma.
3 Includes eg Reiter's, pseudogout, SLE etc.
4 Includes staphs, streps, Lyme, and *Pseudomonas* (eg post-op).

For inflammatory causes of arthritis: Synovial fluid WBC >2000/ml is 84% sensitive (84% specific); synovial fluid neutrophil count >75% is 75% sensitive (92% specific). ►NB: not all labs are equally skillful.

(A) Synovial fluid analysis together with the history and examination findings should allow a diagnosis to be reached

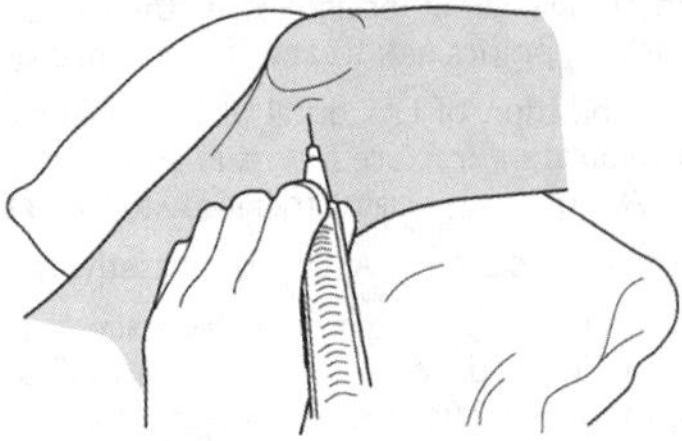

(B) Aspirating a knee joint. Rest the flexed knee on a pillow

Local anaesthetic (LA)

Local anaesthetics (LAs) should not be used without knowledge of their side-effects, toxic doses and properties. A basic understanding about this drug class is essential as it will improve the patient's outcome.

Indications suturing, wound cleaning, FB removal, cannulation, cardiac arrhythmias, minor and major surgery (cataracts/hip replacement); topical preparations for cannulation, catheterisation, corneal anaesthesia

Types of block A *field block* is infiltration of LA into the tissue around a wound; this numbs small cutaneous nerves. In a *peripheral nerve block* a specific nerve is anaesthetised (eg digital, median) with subsequent dermatomal anaesthesia. A *spinal anaesthetic* blocks motor and sensory nerves below the level at which it is injected (often L3/L4). For full descriptions see OHCS6 p776.

Which LA to use Most wards will stock lidocaine (formerly lignocaine); 1% lidocaine solutions are usually sufficient. Other LAs are more likely to be used in the operating theatre or A+E. Different LAs vary in their speed of onset and duration of action. The table opposite shows the basic properties of common LAs.

LAs with epinephrine (adrenaline) The vasoconstricting action of epinephrine prevents the LA from being rapidly redistributed by the circulation, prolonging its action at the injection site and allowing a larger dose to be administered. It is especially useful for scalp and facial anaesthesia. LAs with epinephrine must **never** be used near end arteries, (fingers, toes, penis, nose, ears) as this may lead to ischaemia/gangrene.

LA toxicity This usually occurs when serum concentrations peak (45–60min after use). The symptoms and signs of toxicity are shown opposite. The toxic dose of LAs represents the maximum dose that should be injected into the tissues.

Management of LA toxicity If suspected, stop any further injection or infusion of LA, check ABC and give O_2; midazolam 1–4mg increases the convulsion threshold and may prevent seizures; consider:

- ***Intubation*** if conscious level falls or seizures are resistant to conventional therapy (p215)
- ***CPR*** if there are signs of cardiovascular collapse (p122)

Allergy to LAs This is rare and much more likely with the ester group of LAs (cocaine, tetracaine, amethocaine) than the amide group of LAs (lidocaine, bupivacaine, prilocaine); treat as for anaphylaxis (p156).

Bier's block An IV injection of LAs distal to a double-cuffed tourniquet, often used to manipulate a fractured wrist in an awake patient (OHCS6 p700). IV use of LA requires specialist training with close supervision.

Alternatives Entenox®, sedation ±LA, general anaesthesia ±LA

Hints and tips LAs sting as they are injected; lidocaine is less painful if it is diluted, warmed and injected slowly. LAs are 'activated' by alkaline conditions and so are much less effective when injected into inflamed/infected tissues which have a lower pH.

Commonly used local anaesthetics and their properties

Local anaesthetic	Onset	Duration	Toxic dose
Bupivacaine (Marcaine®)	Medium	Long	2mg/kg
Levobupivicaine	Medium	Long	2mg/kg (data lacking)
Lidocaine	Fast	Medium	3mg/kg
Lidocaine (with epinephrine)	Fast	Medium	7mg/kg
Prilocaine	Fast	Medium	6mg/kg

To calculate the concentration of a solution of LA, multiply the percentage solution by 10 to give the concentration in mg/ml

% solution	mg/ml	% solution	mg/ml
0.25%	2.5mg/ml	1%	10mg/ml
0.5%	5mg/ml	2%	20mg/ml
0.75%	7.5mg/ml	4%	40mg/ml

Maximum dose of lidocaine without epinephrine per body weight (volume in brackets represents ml of 1% lidocaine solution)

Weight (kg)	Maximum dose	Weight (kg)	Maximum dose
50	150mg (15ml)	75	225mg (22.5ml)
55	165mg (16.5ml)	80	240mg (24ml)
60	180mg (18ml)	85	255mg (25.5ml)
65	195mg (19.5ml)	90	270mg (27ml)
70	210mg (21ml)	95	285mg (28.5ml)

Symptoms and signs of systemic local anaesthetic toxicity

Mild toxicity	• Tingling around the mouth • Metallic taste • Tinnitus • Visual disturbance • Slurred speech
Moderate toxicity	• Altered consciousness • Convulsions • Coma
Potentially fatal toxicity	• Respiratory arrest • Cardiac arrhythmias • Cardiovascular collapse

Suturing

Indications The two main indications for skin suturing are:
- wound closure
- keeping drains in place.

Contraindications *absolute* patient refusal, foreign body embedded in the wound, wound infection

Consent verbal (in A+E), written (elective surgery)

Site appropriate to wound/drain site

Checks tetanus status (p307), no infection or foreign bodies, no neurovascular deficit requiring referral, no damage to the underlying structures; if in doubt ask for senior opinion

Patient position patient lying in a comfortable position which exposes the wound site

Equipment sterile drape, sterile gloves, sterile water, 10ml syringe, green (21G) needle, orange (25G) needle, local anaesthetic, appropriate suture material, suture pack (toothed forceps, needle-holder, scissors, gauze)

Anaesthetic Prepare the sterile pack on the trolley with sterile gloves and antiseptic solution in the receiver. Wash hands and wear sterile gloves. With a 10ml syringe, draw up LA using a green needle. Change to an orange needle for infiltration. Clean the skin with antiseptic solution and use the sterile drape to expose the area for suturing only, producing a sterile field. Warn the patient before infiltrating the skin with LA. Draw back before injecting to check you are not injecting into a blood vessel, infiltrate superficially. Allow 2min for the LA to work. During this time prepare your suture material and hold it with the needle facing upwards in the needle-holder. Before starting to suture, ensure the skin is numb.

Suturing Starting at the middle of the wound, pick up the skin edge with tooth forceps and pass the needle perpendicularly through the skin 5mm from the wound edge and into the wound just under the dermis. Grasp the needle point and pull it through gently. Hold the other skin edge with toothed forceps and again pass the needle through the skin, this time through the dermis first, up to the surface. Aim to come out 5mm from the wound edge. Pull most of the suture through then grasp both ends of the suture, tighten and appose the skin edge so the edges evert slightly but without tension. Hold the free end of the suture with the needle-holding forceps and make 3 knots around the forceps (anticlockwise, clockwise, anticlockwise). Make sure you 'lock' each knot by pulling the knot initially in the direction of the wound and then perpendicular to it. Cut the ends of the knot about 1cm long. The knots should lie to the side of the wound not on top of it. Repeat the procedure with sutures 5–10mm apart, depending on the area being sutured. When you have finished clean the wound gently and apply a dry dressing. Tell the patient when the sutures need to be removed (see table opposite).

Confirmation stitches apposing wound edges but not under tension

Complications infection, poor healing, hypertrophic/keloid scarring

Safety Avoid handling the suture needle with your fingers; use the needle-holder. When you do not need the needle keep it in a 'guarded' position – held in the needle-holder forceps, with the point towards the forceps.

Alternatives steristrip and glue (p306); staples have a lower infection rate, but can cause prominent hypertrophic scarring and require staple removers to take them out (may need to attend ward)

Hints and tips

- Make sure you and the patient are in a comfortable position with good lighting before you start.
- Use toothed forceps on skin.
- Local anaesthetic can be dangerous, see p492; epinephrine helps haemostasis, but should not be used on extremities.
- Avoid nylon for securing lines or drains as this is often uncomfortable for the patient.
- Consult a senior if the edges need a lot of tension to meet; may need deep sutures on sub-cut sutures.
- See p306 for treatment of wounds in A+E.
- Don't hesitate to get senior help; if the sutures do not look right the patient will have the scar for life.
- Patients often judge their operation by the scar.

Suture size and suggested dates for removal of sutures (ROS)

Location	Absorbable?	Suture size	ROS at day
Face and neck	No	6/0	3–4
Lips/mouth/tongue	Yes	6/0 vicryl	N/A
Chest/abdomen	No	3/0	7–10
Limbs	No	4/0	5–7

Types of suture material

Non-absorbable sutures	Absorbable sutures
Nylon (ethylon)	Vicryl
Prolene	PDS
Silk	Monocryl

Wound care advice for patients

- Keep the wound area clean and dry for at least 48h
- Come in if signs of infection at the wound site develop, ie redness, swelling, tenderness
- Unless the patient has a scalp/face wound, avoid heavy lifting for at least 6wk
- Drive when you can perform an emergency stop (see p35)

Chapter 10

Interpreting results

Full blood count (FBC)

There are three main components – red cells (haemoglobin or Hb), white cells (leukocytes or WCC) and platelets (plts). Remember these components represent the three cell lines from bone marrow.

Main FBC abnormalities		
Anaemia	↓ Hb	p272
Acute blood loss	FBC initially normal	p274
Infection/inflammation	↑ WCC, ↑ plts	p248
Haematological malignancies	↑↑ WCC	p348
Bone marrow disorders	Persistent change in ≥1 cell line	p348

Hb – red bloods cells (♂ 13–18g/dl: ♀ 11.5–16g/dl)

- ↓*Hb* Anaemia, classified according to MCV, see p272 for causes, investigations and management
- ↑*Hb* Dehydration (p267), secondary polycythaemia eg heart/lung disease, polycythaemia rubra vera (p348). Consider prophylactic LMWH (p289) due to the increased thrombosis risk

Reticulocytes ($50–100 \times 10^9$/l or 0.5–2.5%) These are immature red cells released from bone marrow in response to haemolysis or blood loss (response detectable after a few hours, not acutely). They are also raised secondary to inflammation and infection.

WCC – white blood cells ($4–11 \times 10^9$/l)

Causes of abnormal WCC

Cell		Causes
Neutrophils ($2.0–7.5 \times 10^9$/l)	↑	Bacterial infection, inflammation, acute illness, myeloid leukaemia
	↓	Viral infection, sepsis, drugs (chemotherapy, steroids, carbimazole), splenomegaly, bone marrow failure, ↓B_{12} or folate, autoimmune disease
Lymphocytes ($1.3–3.5 \times 10^9$/l)	↑	Viral infection, inflammation, lymphocytic leukaemia
	↓	Steroids, chemotherapy, HIV, autoimmune disease, bone marrow failure
Eosinophils ($0.04–0.44 \times 10^9$/l)	↑	Parasitic/fungal infection, asthma, atopy, lymphoma
	↓	Rarely pathological

Plts – platelets ($150–400 \times 10^9$/l)

Causes of abnormal plts

↑	Inflammation, infection, acute illness, recovery from splenectomy, essential thrombocytosis, polycythaemia rubra vera
↓	Heparin (5% of patients), idiopathic thrombopaenic pupura (ITP), chronic alcoholism, bone marrow failure, DIC, viral infections, splenomegaly

Clotting

Clotting is often measured before procedures and operations if there is suspicion of an abnormality (eg jaundice). It is also measured to allow correct dosing of warfarin and heparin.

Causes of abnormal clotting

Test		Causes
INR (0.8–1.2)	↑	Warfarin, liver disease, DIC, deficiency of factors II, V, VII or X, heparin
	↓	Rarely pathological
APTTr (0.8–1.2)	↑	Heparin, haemophilia A+B, von Willebrand disease, DIC, deficiency of factors II, V, VII, IX, X, XI or XII, liver disease, warfarin
	↓	Rarely pathological
INR and APTTr	↑	DIC, liver disease, warfarin

Cardiac markers

The types of cardiac markers measured differ between hospitals, however most will measure creatine kinase (CK) and a troponin (either I or T). These tests are used to diagnose myocardial infarction and acute coronary syndromes, especially to distinguish from stable angina.

Causes of abnormal cardiac markers

Test		Causes
CK (25–195u/l)	↑	MI, rhabdomyolysis (muscle break down – check renal function), exercise, recent surgery, hypothyroidism
	↓	Rarely pathological
Troponin	↑	MI (only raised after 6–12h), small rise may be seen with CRF, PE, septicaemia
CK and troponin	↑	MI

Inflammatory response

Acute or chronic inflammation can affect a wide range of blood results, including:

- ↑ ESR
- ↑ CRP
- ↑ Ferritin
- ↑ Plts
- ↑ WCC
- ↓ Albumin

A very high ESR (>100mm/h) should raise suspicions of giant cell arteritis (p213) or myeloma (p245).

Urea and electrolytes (U+E)

These are measured to assess renal function and the concentration of the two main electrolytes in the blood.

Main urea and electrolyte abnormalities

Dehydration	↑urea, ±↑Cr	p267
Acute renal failure	↑K^+, ↑↑urea, ↑Cr	p268
Chronic renal failure	↑urea, ↑↑Cr, ↓Hb	p269
Upper GI bleed	↑↑urea, others normal	p175
Addison's disease	↓Na^+, ↑K^+, ↑urea, ↑Cr	p240

Urea and creatinine

Urea and creatinine (Cr) are metabolic waste products excreted by the kidney. An increase in either measure suggests a degree of renal dysfunction. If both urea and creatinine are raised the patient has renal failure. Check previous U+E results to distinguish between chronic and acute renal failure. Acute renal failure is an emergency, see p268.

Causes of abnormal urea and creatinine

Test		Causes
Urea (2.5–6.7mmol/l)	↑	Dehydration, excess protein intake eg upper GI bleed, acute illness
	↓	Rarely pathological, can be caused by a lack of protein eg alcoholism, anorexia, liver failure, starvation
Creatinine (Cr) (70–150μmol/l)	↑	Renal failure, may be acute, chronic or acute on chronic, muscle injury
	↓	Rarely pathological
Urea and creatinine	↑	Renal failure, check K^+ and ECG

Sodium and potassium

Numerous diseases can affect electrolyte levels, these are discussed in the section on electrolyte imbalance. Small changes in potassium can induce fatal arrhythmias in the heart so abnormal potassium levels should be treated as an emergency (p242).

Abnormal sodium and potassium

Electrolyte		Causes
Na^+ – Sodium	↑	See p243
(135–145mmol/l)	↓	See p244
K^+ – Potassium	↑	Urgent ECG, inform senior, see p242
(3.5–5.3mmol/l)	↓	Urgent ECG, inform senior, see p242

Liver function tests (LFT) and amylase

These are measured to detect jaundice, liver disease, biliary disease and pancreatitis. Liver dysfunction may affect clotting, particularly INR.

Main liver function abnormalities

Pre-hepatic jaundice	↑bilirubin (unconjugated), ↓Hb, ↑reticulocytes	p196
Hepatic jaundice	↑bilirubin (mixed), ↑ALT/AST, ↑γGT	p191
Cholestatic jaundice	↑bilirubin (conjugated), ↑ALP	p196
Hepatocellular damage	↑↑AST/ALT, ↑γGT, ↑ALP	p191
Liver failure	↑bilirubin, ↑INR, ↓albumin	p192
Alcoholism	↑γGT, ↑MCV, ↓plts	p24
Pancreatitis	↑↑amylase, ↓Ca^{2+}, ↑glucose, ↑↑CRP	p198

Liver function tests

See p196 for the investigation and management of jaundice and liver disease.

Causes of abnormal liver function tests

Test		Causes
ALT (or AST) (3–35u/l)	↑	Liver disease/damage, biliary disease, alcohol, muscle damage, MI, pancreatitis
	↓	Rarely pathological, consider ↓vitamin B6
ALP (40–120u/l)	↑	Biliary disease/damage, liver disease, alcohol, bone disease (especially Paget's), pregnancy
	↓	Rarely pathological
γGT (10–55u/l)	↑	Biliary or liver disease, alcohol
	↓	Rarely pathological
Bilirubin (3–17μmol/l)	↑	Jaundice (p196 – haemolysis, liver disease, obstruction), Gilbert's syndrome
	↓	Rarely pathological
Albumin (35–50g/l)	↑	Dehydration
	↓	Inflammation, cirrhosis, malnutrition, pregnancy

Amylase

Causes of abnormal amylase

Test		Cause
Amylase (0–180u/dl)	↑	Acute or chronic pancreatitis, abdominal disease (eg perforation), burns, anorexia, salivary adenitis, renal disease
	↑↑	Acute pancreatitis (eg 3x upper limit of normal)

Calcium and phosphate

Calcium and phosphate are electrolytes predominantly stored in bones. Blood levels are affected by many diseases including parathyroid and bone abnormalities.

Main calcium and phosphate abnormalities

Bone metastases	↑Ca^{2+}	p245
Hypoparathyroidism	↓Ca^{2+}, ↑PO_4^{3-}, ↓PTH	p246
Hyperparathyroidism	↑Ca^{2+}, ↓PO_4^{3-}, ↑ALP, ↑PTH	p245
Myeloma	↑Ca^{2+}, ↑urea, ↑Cr, ↓Hb, ↑ESR	p245
Paget's	↑↑ALP, ↔Ca^{2+}, ↔PO_4^{3-}	

Causes of abnormal calcium and phosphate

Test		Causes
Ca^{2+} – Calcium (2.12–2.65mmol/l)	↑	See p245
	↓	See p246
PO_4^{3-} – Phosphate (0.8–1.25mmol/l)	↑	Chronic renal failure, ↓PTH, myeloma, excess vitamin D, rhabdomyolysis, cell lysis (eg post chemo), acidosis
	↓	Malabsorption/malnutrition, alcohol, ↑PTH, burns, alkalosis, post DKA treatment

Effects of parathyroid hormone disease on blood tests

Disease	Ca^{2+}	PO_4^{3-}	PTH
Primary hyperparathyroidism	↑	↓	↑
Secondary hyperparathyroidism	↓	↓	↑
Tertiary hyperparathyroidism	↑	↓	↑
Hypoparathyroidism	↓	↑	↓

CSF

What to do with the samples

Hold the specimen pots up to the light, CSF should be crystal clear and colourless. Cloudy CSF suggests bacterial infection. Red CSF suggests blood, bottle 3 may be less red than bottle 1 suggesting a bloody tap (hit a spinal vessel). Yellow (xanthochromic) suggests a recent sub-arachnoid. Send the samples to the following places:

- ***Bottles 1 and 3*** microbiology for M,C+S, consider asking for viral culture/PCR if encephalitis is suspected
- ***Bottle 2 and fluoride tube*** biochemistry for protein, glucose, request xanthochromia if sub-arachnoid suspected
- ***Blood in fluoride tube*** biochemistry for paired serum glucose

There are many other tests available, however you should only need these if specifically requested by a senior.

Microscopy

Red cells (0 per mm^3) these are raised from a bloody tap (more in 1 than 3) or from a sub-arachnoid haemorrhage (same in 1 and 3), however the two can only be distinguished reliably by measuring for xanthochromia (sub-arachnoid only). High levels of blood cells will disrupt the measurement of WBC and protein. The following calculations may help:

- True CSF WBC = CSF WBC – (bld WBC x CSF RBC ÷ bld RBC)
- True CSF protein = CSF protein – (RBC ÷ 100)

White cells (<4 per mm^3) raised levels in infection or 48h post sub-arachnoid, levels tend to be higher in bacterial meningitis. The main type of white cell suggests the infectious agent:

- *Neutrophils/Polymorphs* (0 per mm^3) bacterial infection
- *Lymphocytes/Mononuclear* (<4 per mm^3) viral infection or TB

	Bacterial	TB	Viral	MS
Appearance	Cloudy	Clear	Clear	Clear
White cells	5–2000	5–500	5–1000	5–50
Type of cell	Neutrophils	Lymphocytes	Lymphocytes	Lymphocytes
Glucose	Very low	<50% plasma	>70% plasma	>70% plasma
Protein	>1	>1	0.5–0.9	0.5–0.9

Biochemistry

Protein (<0.4g/l) Levels >1.0g/l are usually only seen in bacterial or TB meningitis. Less dramatic rises can occur in all types of meningitis and also multiple sclerosis or Guillain-Barré.

Glucose (>2.2mmol/l or >70% plasma) Reduced in meningitis, especially bacterial meningitis.

Xanthochromia is a yellowing of the CSF caused by the breakdown of blood; it is present following a sub-arachnoid haemorrhage.

Urine tests

Urine samples should be 'mid-stream' (MSU) to limit contamination, alternatively they can be taken from a catheter (CSU).

Dipstick

UTIs can be asymptomatic and urinary symptoms (dysuria, frequency, urgency) can be present without a UTI. This table gives the chance of a positive urine culture from dipstick readings. Dipsticks are not sensitive:

	Leuks +ve	Leuks –ve
Nitrites +ve	>95%	90%
Nitrites –ve	70%	<20%

Nitrites are produced by Gram negative bacteria (eg *E. coli*) and suggest urinary tract infection (UTI).

Leukocytes (white cells) are raised from inflammation of the kidneys and urinary tract, most commonly UTIs, but also stones, trauma, neoplasia, infection of related structures (eg prostate, appendix) and renal disease.

Blood Dipsticks detect haemoglobin and may distinguish this from blood cells. Send the urine for microscopy if either are seen. A positive dipstick with no red cells on microscopy suggests myoglobinuria or haemoglobinuria. See p269 for the causes of haematuria.

Protein Dipsticks detect albumin which should not be present in urine. If protein is persistently positive then a 24h collection should be tested. Bence–Jones protein (seen in myeloma) is not detected by dipsticks.

Glucose should not be present in urine but is common with ↑age; its presence suggests, but cannot diagnose or exclude, diabetes (see p236).

Ketones are raised in diabetic ketoacidosis (along with glucose). They can also be raised after fasting, low carbohydrate diets and acute illness.

pH Normal range 4.5–8; urine pH can be affected by systemic acidosis and alkalosis. Acid pH suggests systemic acidosis and vice versa.

Specific gravity A rough guide to the concentration of urine. The normal range is 1.005–1.030; increased in hypovolaemia, heart failure, proteinuria and glycosuria; reduced in acute tubular necrosis and diabetes insipidus.

β-HCG A separate urine dipstick can be used to test for pregnancy; it should be positive within 12d of conception. It is important to test all women of reproductive age to exclude pregnancy as a cause of their symptoms and before harmful medications or investigations (eg X-ray).

Microscopy

A mid-stream urine (MSU) or catheter specimen of urine (CSU) should be sent for microscopy if there are nitrites, leukocytes, blood or protein on the dipstick or if there is clinical suspicion of a UTI. In children a clean catch or suprapubic aspirate is used (p390).

White cells >10/mm^3 is abnormal; same causes as leukocytes on dipstick.

Bacteria may be seen on simple microscopy and this is highly suggestive of a UTI; Gram staining may help identify the pathogen. The sample needs to be cultured for complete identification.

Red cells >2/mm^3 is abnormal; see p269 for management of haematuria

Casts Hyaline and fine granular casts are not significant; dense granular, red cell and epithelial casts suggest renal disease; white cell casts are found with pyelonephritis.

Culture and sensitivity

Samples sent for microscopy are routinely cultured over 48h. The culture is said to be positive if >100,000 organisms/ml are present. The sample is recultured in different mediums to determine the bacteria present and its sensitivity to antibiotics. A mixed culture (more than one organism present) suggests the sample is contaminated. Urine culture is not 100% sensitive or specific – it can often be wrong and require repeating.

Biochemistry

Sodium concentration This is a useful test in acute renal failure. A low urine sodium (<20mmol/l) suggests hypoperfusion, eg hypovolaemia, while a raised concentration (>40mmol/l) suggests acute tubular necrosis. It is also used in the assessment of hyponatraemia (p244).

Urine osmolality This is a measure of the concentration of the urine; the normal range is 500–800mosmol/kg. It is used in the investigation of renal disease and diagnosis of diabetes insipidus (p241). In acute renal failure it can distinguish between prerenal failure (>500mosmol/kg) and acute tubular necrosis (<350mosmol/kg).

24h urine protein Total protein and microalbumin can be measured, total protein is the more common test; microalbumin is used to detect developing renal failure in diabetics and a value of >30mg/24h is abnormal. Urine creatinine should also be measured to determine GFR.

24h Protein	Significance
<150mg	Normal
150mg–3g	Proteinuria, probably renal if >2g p269
>3g	Nephrotic syndrome p269

Creatinine clearance The excretion of creatinine per minute can be calculated from a 24h urine collection and this gives an estimation of the glomerular filtration rate (GFR).

Catecholamines/VMA If a phaeochromocytoma is suspected a 24h urine sample is analysed for free catecholamines (eg adrenaline) or their metabolites (eg vanillylmandelic acid, VMA).

Toxicology Urine can be screened for a wide range of recreational and medical drugs. In practice the results often take several days.

Arterial blood gases (ABG)

Arterial blood gas (ABG) analysis calculates PaO_2, $PaCO_2$ and HCO_3^- in a heparinised specimen (can also be undertaken on venous or capillary blood or on fluid aspirated from the chest or abdomen), as well as the pH, O_2 saturation, base excess, anion gap and on some machines concentrations of Na^+, K^+, Ca^{2+}, Cl^- and lactate. For advice on how to perform an ABG see p464.

Normal ranges (patient breathing room air)

pH	7.35–7.45
PaO_2	10.5–13.5kPa
$PaCO_2$	4.5–6.0kPa

HCO_3^-	22–28mmol/l
Base excess (BE)	−2 to +2
O_2 saturation	95–100%

NB Note that a normal pO_2 in a patient on a high concentration of O_2 is very worrying.

First look at the pH:
- pH <7.35 = acidaemia
- pH 7.35 to 7.45 = normal pH
- pH >7.45 = alkalaemia

Next look at the $PaCO_2$ and bicarbonate (HCO_3^-):

Types of acidaemia

	↓ HCO_3^-	↔ HCO_3^-	↑ HCO_3^-
↓$PaCO_2$	Metabolic acidosis	×	×
↔$PaCO_2$	Mixed acidosis	×	×
↑$PaCO_2$	Mixed acidosis	Acute respiratory acidosis	Chronic respiratory acidosis

Types of alkalaemia

	↓ HCO_3^-	↔ HCO_3^-	↑ HCO_3^-
↓$PaCO_2$	Chronic respiratory alkalosis	Acute respiratory alkalosis	Mixed alkalosis
↔$PaCO_2$	×	×	Mixed alkalosis
↑$PaCO_2$	×	×	Metabolic alkalosis

× – incompatible

Base excess

This is the amount of 'base' needed to restore pH to the normal range
- Base excess >+2, patient has excess base present (ie alkalosis)
- Base excess <−2, patient has insufficient base present (ie acidosis)

Causes of acid-base disturbance

	Acidosis	Alkalosis
Metabolic	Shock DKA Renal/liver failure Drug overdose (eg TCA) Renal tubular acidosis Lactate (p154) Refer to 'anion gap' below	Vomiting Diarrhoea Hypokalaemia
Respiratory	Severe asthma/COPD Severe pneumonia Severe pulmonary oedema Myasthenia gravis Drugs (eg sedatives, opiates) Chest trauma/scoliosis Obesity	Hypoxaemia Cranial lesions (eg stroke) Anxiety/hyperventilation

If all else fails calculate the anion gap or speak to a biochemist

If the differentials for an acid-base disturbance are still unclear then calculate the anion gap which should answer any remaining problems (see below); alternatively ask a senior or speak directly to the clinical biochemist in the laboratory.

The anion gap

This is calculated by $([Na^+] + [K^+]) - ([Cl^-] + [HCO_3^-])$
Normal value is 10–18mmol/l
It helps to distinguish the different causes of a metabolic acidosis:

- **Raised anion gap**
  - Lactic acidosis (p148 shock, sepsis/infection)
  - Urate (renal failure)
  - Ketones (DKA, alcohol, starvation)
  - Drugs/toxins (salicylates, biguanides, ethylene glycol, methanol)
- **Normal anion gap**
  - Renal tubular acidosis
  - Diarrhoea
  - Drugs (acetazolamide)
  - Addison's disease
  - Pancreatic fistula
  - Ammonium chloride ingestion

Chest X-ray (CXR)

The main patterns of acute disease are:
- ***Pneumonia*** asymmetrical shadowing (consolidation), blunting of angles, blurring of heart and diaphragm borders, air bronchograms
- ***Pulmonary oedema*** enlarged heart, symmetrical hazy/reticular shadowing, blunted costophrenic angles or pleural effusions, indistinct hilar vessels, enlarged upper lobe vessels, Kerley B lines, distinct septa
- ***Pleural effusion*** featureless white area at the base with loss of costophrenic angle ±meniscus (upper surface sloping up to the chest wall)
- ***Asthma/COPD*** hyperinflated, flattened diaphragm, barrel chested
- ***Pneumothorax*** line of separated pleura with peripheries lacking lung markings – may be large and deviating mediastinum (eg tension)

Adequacy of a CXR – interpret cautiously unless the following are normal

• **Rotation** medial clavicles should be the same distance from the vertebral bodies on each side; the spinous processes should be in the middle of the vertebral bodies • **Penetration** intervertebral discs should be visible behind the heart and the lung fields should have markings • **Inspiration** ≥7 posterior ribs should be visible

Develop a routine so you spot all the abnormalities:
- ***Lung outline***
  - Blunting/loss of costophrenic and cardiophrenic angles
  - Indistinct heart border, lung border or diaphragm edges
  - Pneumothorax – this is best seen by rotating the CXR 90°
  - Kerley B lines – 1–2cm horizontal lines at the edges
  - Pleural plaques/thickening: does the edge look whiter in some areas?
- ***Lung fields***
  - *Colour* too dark suggests pneumothorax, emphysema or high penetration, while white shadowing suggests pulmonary oedema, pneumonia, effusion or over-penetration. Describe shadowing as nodular (lumpy), reticular (fine lines eg pulmonary oedema) or alveolar (fluffy eg consolidation)
  - *Vascular markings* the upper lobe vessels should be thinner than lower lobe ones
  - *Cavities* ie dark circles, consider bronchiectasis, bullae or abscesses (may have a air/fluid level)
  - *Localised white lesions* eg carcinoma
- ***Lung size*** There should be 8 posterior ribs (see diagram opposite), ≥10 hyperinflated, ≤6 poor inspiratory effort. For anterior ribs the numbers are two lower, ie ≥8, 6, ≤4
- ***Diaphragm***
  - Is there a pneumoperitoneum (perforated bowel), thin black line under the diaphragm
  - Is the right side slightly higher than the left? If not consider excess chest or abdomen pressure
  - Are the domes convex? Flat suggests hyperexpansion

- ***Mediastinum***
  - This should be <8cm wide at the aortic arch, wider suggests swelling eg aortic dissection or lymphadenopathy
  - The heart should be <50% the width of the chest on a PA (non-portable) film, larger suggests cardiomegaly
  - Is there collapse or consolidation behind the heart?
- ***Trachea*** Should be central and uncompressed
- ***Hila*** These should have a concave shape with distinct vessels
- ***Bones*** Look at the spine, clavicles, scapulae, shoulder and ribs. Look for fractures, osteolytic and osteosclerotic lesions. Is the spine straight?
- ***Soft tissues*** Surgical emphysema (pneumothorax), breast lesions

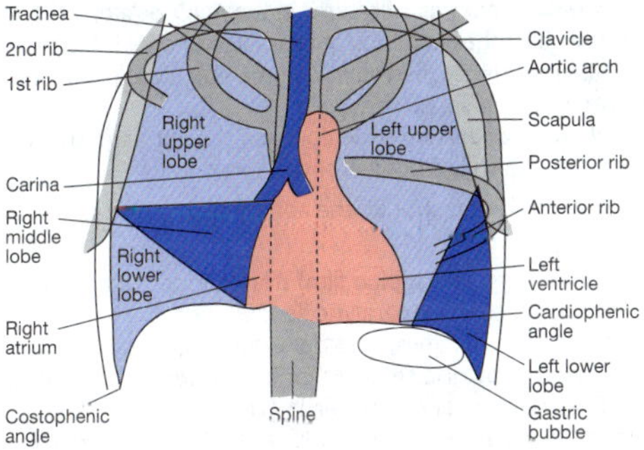

Major features on a AP CXR

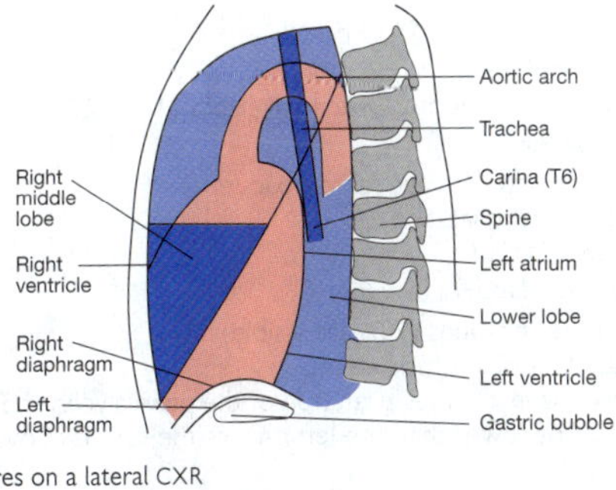

Major features on a lateral CXR

Central lines (p476) Check for pneumothorax and haemothorax; note the position of the end of the line, it should be in the right atrium.

Feeding NG tubes (p484) The end of the tube should be seen below the diaphragm; if not advance the tube 5cm and repeat CXR.

Chest drains (p480) The end should be inside the chest wall without touching the opposing wall, ideally angled downwards for effusions and up for pneumothoraces. Note the size of pneumothorax or effusion.

Abdomen X-ray (AXR)

The main patterns of acute disease are:

- ***Bowel perforation*** free gas seen on lateral decubitus abdominal film or erect CXR underneath the diaphragm
- ***Dilated*** loops of small bowel >2.5cm or large bowel >6cm (see table opposite)
- ***Sigmoid volvulus*** grossly dilated loop of bowel ('coffee bean' shaped)
- ***Constipation*** faecal loading in the large bowel, often starting from the rectum
- ***Pyloric stenosis*** dilated stomach proximally, stricture at pylorus
- ***Gallstones/renal stones*** calcifications in the RUQ or along the urinary tract; 10% of gallstones and 90% of renal stones are visible on AXR
- ***Chronic pancreatitis*** calcified specks in the epigastric/pancreatic area
- ***Chronic renal failure*** small kidneys
- ***Abdominal aortic aneurysm*** wide aorta on the left hand side of the spine; may see a calcified outline of the aortic walls

Develop a routine so you spot all the abnormalities:

Bowel pathology

- *Bowel gas* (best seen in a supine film) dilated loops of bowel due to mechanical obstruction or paralytic ileus
- *Fluid levels* obstruction, ileus, gastroenteritis
- *Stomach* dilated in pyloric stenosis; look for linitis plastica ('leather bottle stomach') in advanced stomach cancer
- *Gas outside the lumen* bowel perforation (look for air under the diaphragm on erect CXR or lateral decubitus AXR)

Liver Look for:

- Calcification
- Cysts/abscess cavities
- Irregular opacities associated with malignancy (1° or 2°)

Biliary tree Look for:

- Gallstones (NB only 10% are radio-opaque)
- Common bile duct dilatation
- Is there a stent *in situ*?

Urinary tract and bladder Look for:

- Renal and ureteric stones (90% are visible)
- Urinary catheters or ureteric stents
- Size of the kidneys, obvious dilatation of the pelvicalyces; the right kidney should be lower than the left one, as the liver is above it

Pelvis

- *Uterus/ovaries* foreign bodies (eg IUCD, ring pessary), fibroids, cysts
- *Prostate* size, calcification

Bones

- *Lytic lesions (pale)* think bronchial/breast/renal carcinoma, myeloma
- *Sclerotic lesions* think prostate/breast carcinoma, Paget's disease
- *Fusion of the vertebrae/sacroiliac joints, curving of the spine* degenerative disease, scoliosis, ankylosing spondylosis

Other soft tissues

- *Psoas muscle* if absent, think of a retroperitoneal mass or haematoma
- Is there any ascites?

Hints and tips

- AXRs are daunting to interpret initially, so it's important to keep in mind what you are trying to confirm/exclude on it
- Stand back and approach things in a systematic manner
- Take the findings on AXR together with the clinical picture and discuss what management is necessary with the rest of your team

Large bowel vs small bowel obstruction

	Small intestine	Large intestine
Number of loops	Lots	Few
Distribution of loops	Central	Peripheral
Diameter of loops	>2.5cm	>6cm
Haustrae[1]	No	Yes
Valvulae conniventes[2]	Yes	No
Faeces present	Nil	Yes

1 Haustrae folds which do not completely cross the bowel lumen wall.
2 Valvulae conniventes folds which do completely cross the bowel lumen wall.

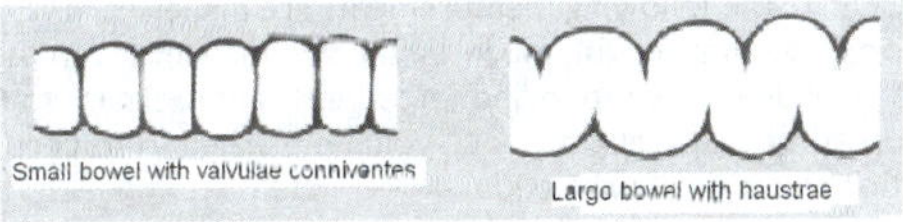

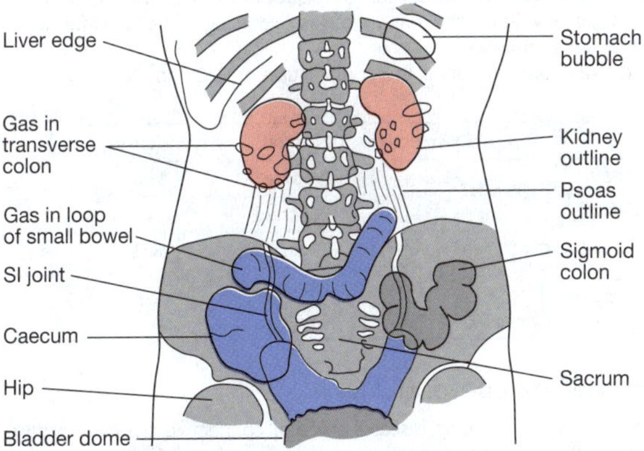

Main features of the abdominal X-ray

Respiratory function tests

Peak expiratory flow rate (PEFR)

Indications Used for the diagnosis, monitoring (eg daily diary/obs) and severity assessment of obstructive lung disease (asthma and COPD).

Method Reset the tab and fit a clean mouthpiece. Ask the patient to stand up and hold it in their hand (not covering the scale), breathe in deeply and blow as hard and fast as they can (with encouragement), they do not need to exhale maximally. Use the best reading of three attempts.

PEFR[1]	>80%	80–50%	33–50%	<33%
Asthma severity	Normal	Mild–moderate	Severe	Life-threatening

1 Compared with best or predicted (see chart on opposite page)

Spirometry

Indication diagnosis and monitoring of respiratory disease

Before testing Leave out morning inhalers or nebulisers (unless severely ill) to allow reversibility assessment.

Method Usually performed by trained technicians in a respiratory function laboratory. The patient must inhale as deeply as they can then exhale as fast and as long as they can manage. This is difficult enough without COPD. The following measurements are made:

- **FEV_1** Forced expiratory volume in 1s, the volume exhaled in the first second after deep inspiration and forced expiration, similar to PEFR
- **FVC** Forced vital capacity, the total volume exhaled from deep inspiration to maximal exhalation

Beyond spirometry respiratory function laboratories can also measure:

- **RV** Residual volume, the volume of gas remaining in the lung after a maximum expiration
- **TLC** Total lung capacity is the combination of FVC and RV

	Obstructive	**Normal**	**Restrictive**
FEV_1	↓↓	Predicted	↓
FVC	↓	Predicted	↓↓
FEV1/FVC	<75%	75–80%	>80%
RV	↑	Predicted	↓
TLC	↑	Predicted	↓

Obstructive asthma, COPD, emphysema

Restrictive interstitial lung disease, sarcoid, connective tissue disorders, neuromuscular disease (including myasthenia gravis and Guillain–Barré)

Other spirometry measurements

Reversibility Asthma (a reversible obstruction) is diagnosed if there is >200–400ml improvement in PEFR or FEV_1 with bronchodilators. Asthma can coexist with COPD (non-reversible obstruction).

Gas transfer, also called *transfer factor*; is measured using carbon monoxide. It is reduced in emphysema, acute asthma, anaemia and interstitial lung disease and increased with chronic asthma, left heart failure, polycythaemia and exercise.

Flow volume loops Graphical representations of the results with volume on the X-axis and flow rate on the Y-axis. Exhalation is above the line and inhalation below the line. There are four main patterns:

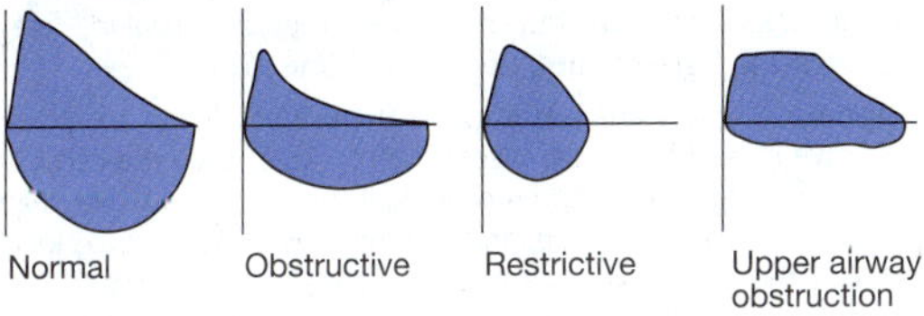

Upper airway obstruction lesion occluding the bronchi, trachea or larynx associated with stridor, see p378.

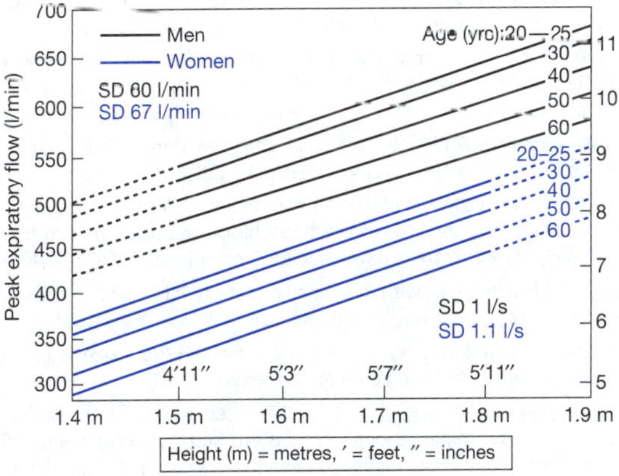

Normal peak expiratory flow values

Electrocardiogram (ECG)

Examine all ECGs in a systematic manner to avoid missing the basics.

Check patient details, date and time of ECG, speed of paper (25mm/s)

Rate At 25mm/s each large square represents 0.2s and each small square 0.04s. To calculate rate divide 300 by the number of large squares between one R wave and the next R wave (see box opposite).

Rhythm *Sinus rhythm* each QRS has a P wave before it. *Atrial fibrillation* no P wave and the QRS complexes are irregularly irregular. *Atrial flutter* the baseline is described as saw-tooth and the QRS are often regularly spaced. *Ventricular rhythm* QRS is wide (>0.12s or >3 small squares) and has no association with P waves. *Nodal rhythm* P wave may be absent or part of the QRS complex, but rhythm is regular. *Regularly irregular* rhythms suggest a degree of heart block (OHCM6 p96).

Axis Imagine the limb leads are a clock. If the complexes are predominantly positive in lead I (R wave bigger than S wave) then the cardiac axis must lie between 12 o'clock and 6 o'clock; if the S wave is larger than the R wave then the reverse is true, and the axis lies between 6 o'clock and 12 o'clock. If the complexes are predominantly positive in aVF (R wave bigger than S wave) then the cardiac axis must also lie between 3 o'clock and 9 o'clock; again the reverse is true if the S wave is greater than the R wave. The overlap suggests the axis is between 3 o'clock and 6 o'clock. The true axis is at right angles to the lead position which is isoelectric, where the height of the R wave and S wave are equal (OHCM6 p94). Normal cardiac axis is between –30° (2 o'clock) and +90° (6 o'clock), where 0° is 3 o'clock; see OHCM6 p95 for causes of axis deviation.

P wave Absent in AF, atrial flutter and sinoatrial block. Bifid P wave suggests left atrial hypertrophy. Peaked P waves are seen in right atrial hypertrophy (pulmonary hypertension) and transiently in $\downarrow K^+$.

PR interval Normally 0.12–0.2s (3–5 small squares). Longer in heart block (OHCM6 p96) and shorter in WPW (OHCM6 p128).

QRS complex Normally <0.12s (<3 small squares). Wider QRS implies ventricular rhythm, either 3rd degree heart block or bundle branch block (OHCM6 p98). Paced rhythms have wide QRS complexes (OHCM6 p134).

ST segment Usually level with baseline; elevation >1mm or depression >0.5mm suggests infarction (p130) or ischaemia (p131) respectively.

T wave Inversion (pointing down) in leads I, II or V4–V6 suggests ischaemia. Often peaked in $\uparrow K^+$ and acute MI, flattened in $\downarrow K^+$.

Other components of the ECG The QT interval is often calculated by modern ECG machines, though can be worked out manually (p140). A U wave (positive in most leads) follows the T wave and precedes the P wave and if present can imply $\downarrow K^+$ though can be a normal finding.

Hints and tips Being able to read an ECG systematically is much more important than a spot ECG diagnosis. The common ECG abnormalities which should not be missed are: AF, MI or ischaemia, LBBB/RBBB, 3rd degree heart block, ventricular tachycardia and ventricular fibrillation.

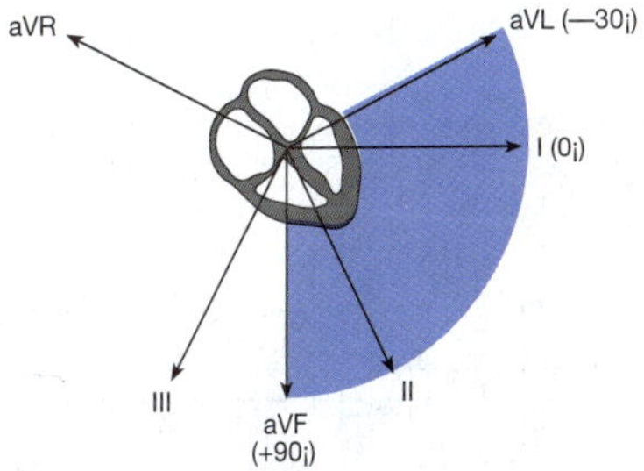

(A) Normal cardiac axis (shaded area) and view each limb lead represents

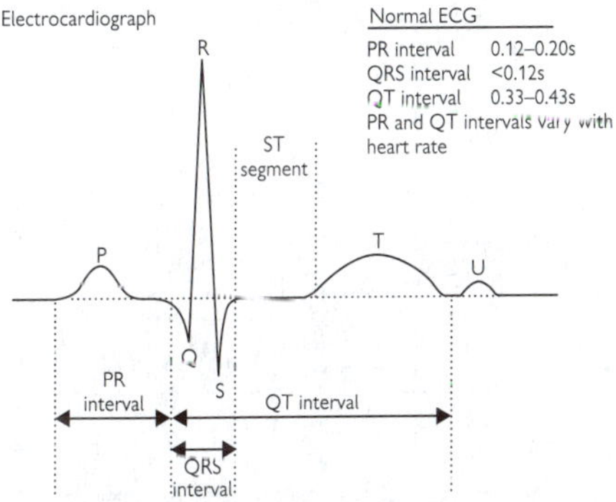

(B) The normal ECG and its various complexes and intervals.

To calculate heart rate divide 300 by the number of large squares between adjacent R waves

Number of large squares between adjacent R waves	Heart rate (beats per minute)
1	300
2	150
3	100
4	75
5	60
6	50
7	43
8	38
9	33
10	30

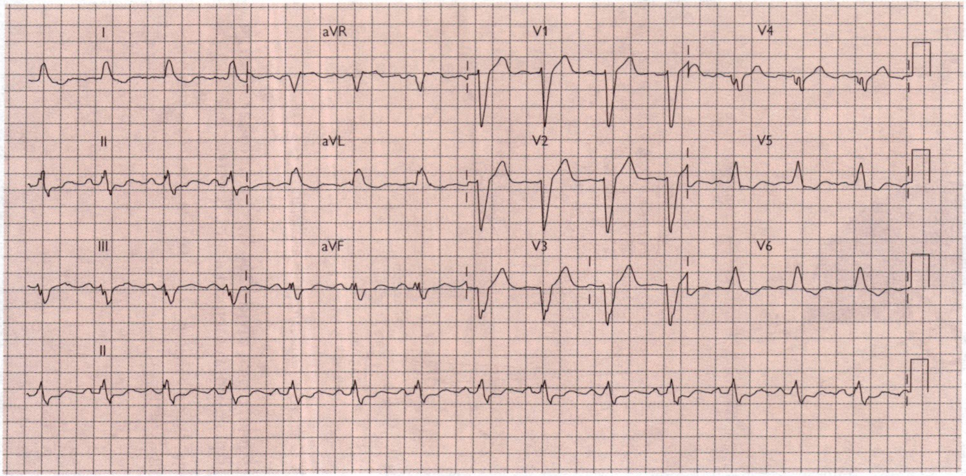

(A) **Left bundle branch block:** Note W pattern in V1 and M pattern in V5/V6, also no Q wave in V5/V6 and inverted T wave in I and aVL. Remember 'William Marrow'.

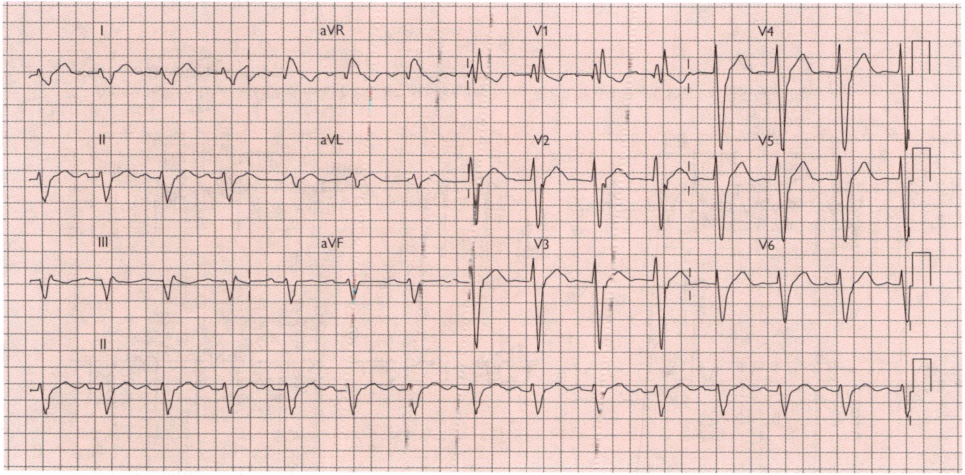

(B) **Right bundle branch block:** Note M pattern (RSR') in V1, W pattern in V5/V6 and inverted T wave in V1. Remember 'William Marrow'.

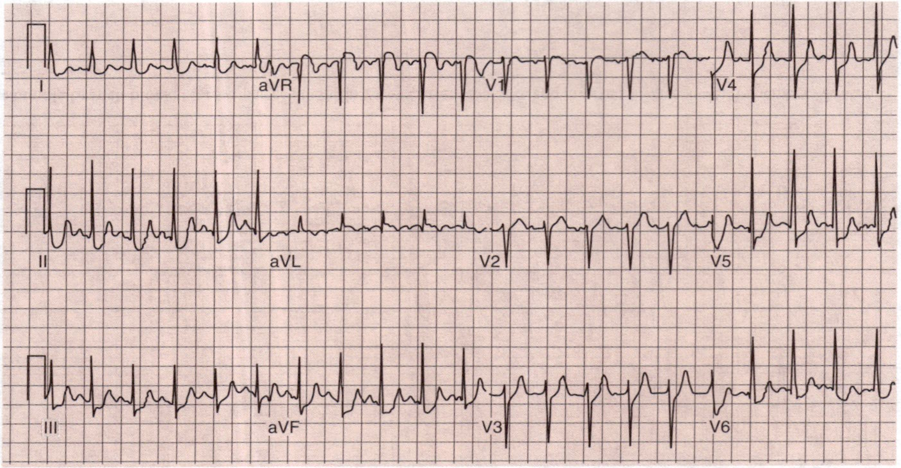

(C) **Acute infero-lateral ischaemia:** Note ST depression in leads I, II, II aVF and V3 to V6, also wave inversion in AVR (normal variant) and aVL.

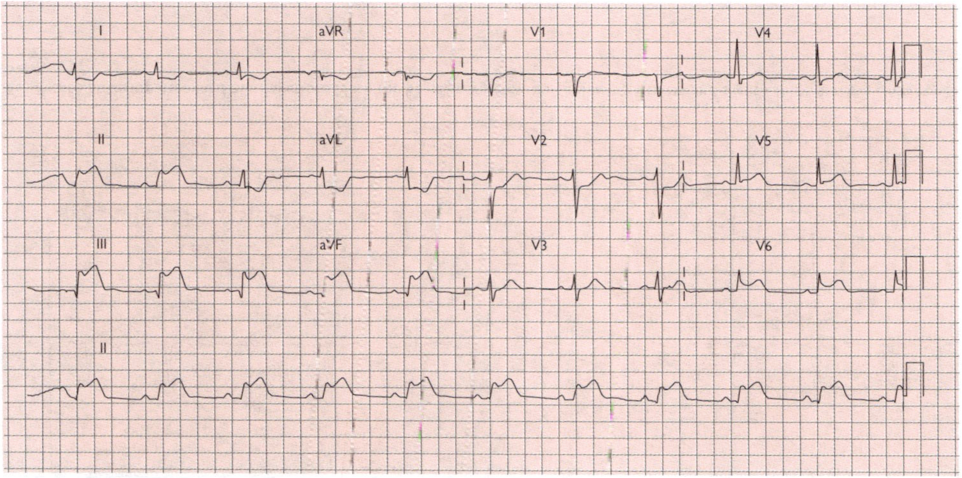

(D) **Acute infero-lateral myocardial infarction:** Note ST elevation in leads II, III and aVF (inferior leads) and also in V5 and V6 (lateral leads). The ST depression in I and aVL are reciprocal changes and often seen with large infarcts.

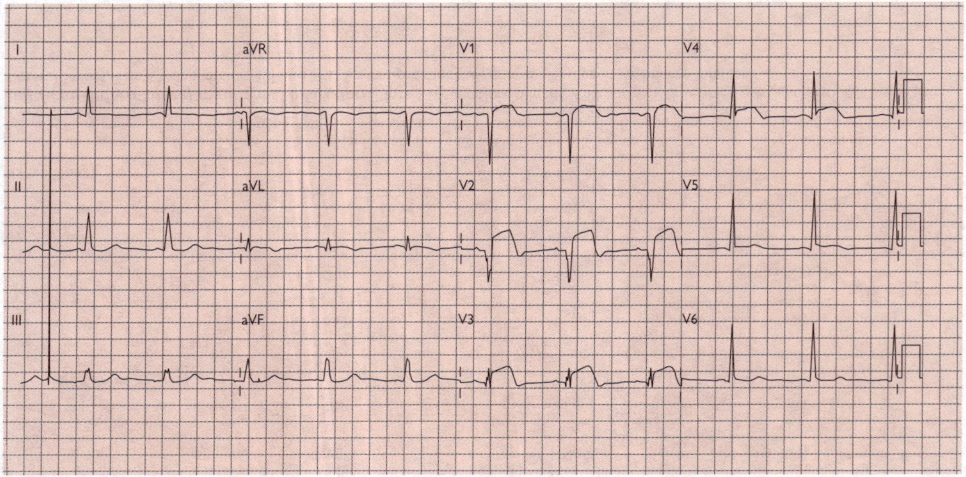

(E) **Acute anterior myocardial infarction:** Note the ST segment elevation in leads V1 to V4 and slightly in V5 and the evolving Q wave.

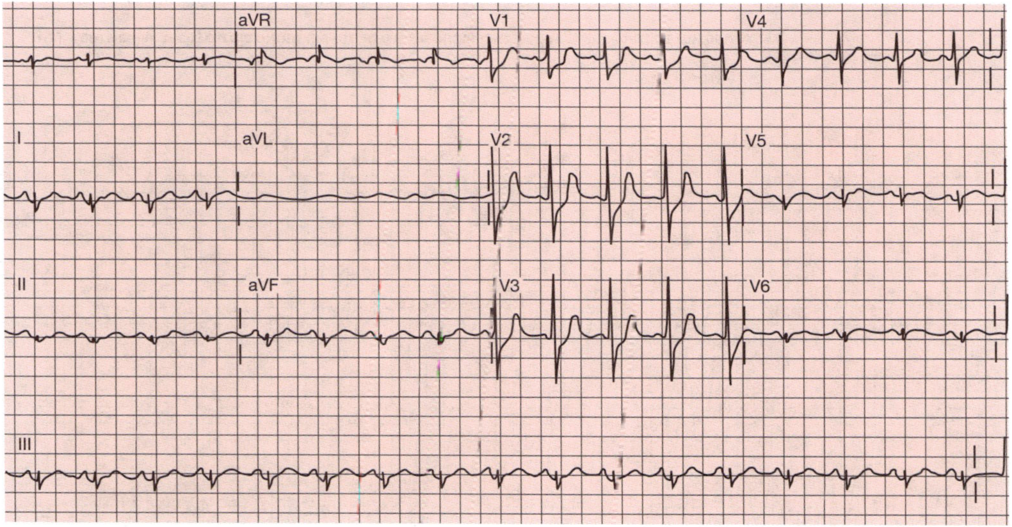

(F) **Acute postero-lateral infarct:** Note dominant R wave and ST depression in V1/V2 and ST elevation in V5/V6.

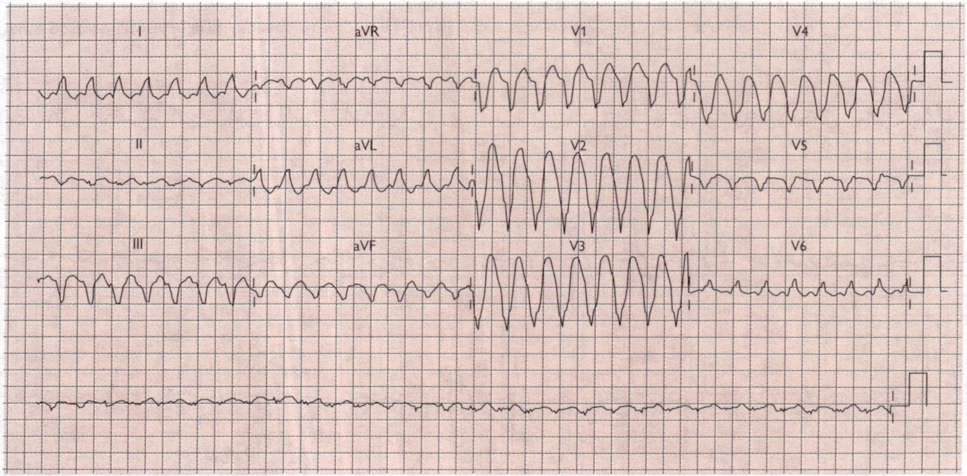

(G) **Ventricular tachycardia:** Note the broad nature of the QRS and regular repeating rhythm.

Appendices

Useful numbers and websites

Medical organisations

General Medical Council (GMC)
- 08453 578001 www.gmc-uk.org
- Registration issues 08453 573456

British Medical Association (BMA)
- 020 7387 4499 www.bma.org.uk

Medical Defence Union (MDU)
- 0800 716 376 www.the-mdu.com
- **24h help 0800 716 646**

Medical Protection Society (MPS)
- 08457 187 187 www.medicalprotection.org
- **24h help 0845 605 4000**

Medical Doctors' and Dentists' Defence Union of Scotland (MDDUS)
- 0141 221 5858 www.mddus.com
- **24h help 0141 221 5858**

Counselling lines

BMA Counselling Service
- 08459 200169

National Counselling Service for Sick Doctors
- 0870 241 0535 www.ncssd.org.uk

Doctors' Support Network (mental Illness)
- 0870 321 0642 www.dsn.org.uk

Sick Doctor's Trust (alcohol and drug addiction)
- 0870 444 5163 www.sick-doctors-trust.co.uk

Financial organisations

Medical Sickness
- 0800 358 6060 www.medical-sickness.co.uk

BMA Services
- 0800 358 0014 www.bmas.co.uk

MLP Private Finance
- 0207 423 6350 www.mlp-plc.co.uk

Other

Gay and Lesbian Association of Doctors and Dentists (GLADD)
- 0870 765 5606 www.gladd.org.uk

Medical Research Council (MRC)
- 020 7636 5422 www.mrc.ac.uk

Medical Women's Federation
- 020 7387 7765 www.medicalwomensfederation.co.uk

Médecins Sans Frontières (MSF)
- 020 7404 6600 www.msf.org

Voluntary Services Overseas
- 020 8780 7500 www.vso.org.uk

Wellcome Trust
- 020 7611 8888 www.wellcome.ac.uk

Royal College of

Anaesthetists	020 7813 1900	www.rcoa.ac.uk
General Practitioners	020 7581 3232	www.rcgp.org.uk
Obstetricians & Gynaecologists	020 7772 6200	www.rcog.org.uk
Ophthalmologists	020 7935 0702	www.rcophth.ac.uk
Paediatrics & Child Health	020 7307 5600	www.rcpch.ac.uk
Pathologists	020 7451 6700	www.rcpath.org
Physicians	020 7935 1174	www.rcplondon.ac.uk
Physicians of Edinburgh	0131 225 7324	www.rcpe.ac.uk
Physicians of Ireland	00 353 1 661 6677	www.rcpi.ie
Physicians & Surgeons of Glasgow	0141 221 6072	www.rcpsglasg.ac.uk
Psychiatrists	020 7235 2351	www.rcpsych.ac.uk
Radiologists	020 7636 4432	www.rcr.ac.uk
Surgeons of Edinburgh	0131 527 1600	www.rcsed.ac.uk
Surgeons of England	020 7405 3474	www.rcseng.ac.uk
Surgeons of Ireland	00 353 1 402 2100	www.rcsi.ie

A selection of medical websites

For doctors	For patients
www.emedicine.com	www.netdoctor.co.uk
www.nelh.nhs.uk (NHS library)	www.patient.co.uk
www.bmjpg.com (BMJ publishing)	www.macmillan.org.uk (cancer)
www.vh.org (virtual hospital)	www.medlineplus.gov (USA based)
www.bnf.org	health.allrefer.com (USA based)

A selection of locum agencies

NHS Professionals	0845 606 0345	www.nhsprofessionals.nhs.uk
JCJ	0800 590 979	www.jcj.co.uk
Quality Locums	0800 043 7318	www.qualitylocums.com
Medacs	0800 037 5050	www.medacs.com
Nationwide Locum Service[1]	0845 650 7018	www.nlsandumrweb.co.uk

1 specifically for overseas doctors.

Height conversion

Metres (m) to inches (inch), multiply by 39.37 (12 inches to the foot)
Inches to meters, multiply by 0.0254

m	inch	feet	inch
1.36	53.5	4	5.5
1.37	54	4	6
1.38	54.5	4	6.5
1.40	55	4	7
1.41	55.5	4	7.5
1.42	56	4	8
1.43	56.5	4	8.5
1.45	57	4	9
1.46	57.5	4	9.5
1.47	58	4	10
1.48	58.5	4	10.5
1.50	59	4	11
1.51	59.5	4	11.5
1.52	60	5	0
1.54	60.5	5	0.5
1.55	61	5	1
1.56	61.5	5	1.5
1.57	62	5	2
1.59	62.5	5	2.5
1.60	63	5	3
1.61	63.5	5	3.5
1.62	64	5	4
1.64	64.5	5	4.5
1.65	65	5	5
1.66	65.5	5	5.5

m	inch	feet	inch
1.67	66	5	6
1.69	66.5	5	6.5
1.70	67	5	7
1.71	67.5	5	7.5
1.73	68	5	8
1.74	68.5	5	8.5
1.75	69	5	9
1.76	69.5	5	9.5
1.78	70	5	10
1.79	70.5	5	10.5
1.80	71	5	11
1.81	71.5	5	11.5
1.83	72	6	0
1.84	72.5	6	0.5
1.85	73	6	1
1.87	73.5	6	1.5
1.88	74	6	2
1.89	74.5	6	2.5
1.90	75	6	3
1.92	75.5	6	3.5
1.93	76	6	4
1.94	76.5	6	4.5
1.95	77	6	5
1.97	77.5	6	5.5
1.98	78	6	6

Temperature

Degrees Fahrenheit (°F) to Degrees Centigrade (Celsius °C)

$$°C = (°F - 32) \times 0.56$$

Degrees Centigrade (Celsius °C) to Degrees Fahrenheit (°F)

$$°F = (C \times 1.8) + 32$$

Pressure

Millimetres of mercury (mmHg) to kilopascals (kPa)

$$kPa = mmHg \times 0.113$$

Kilopascals (kPa) to millimetres of mercury (mmHg)

$$mmHg = kPa \times 7.519$$

Weight conversion

kg to pounds (lbs), multiply by 2.2046 (14lb to the stone; 16oz per lb)
Pounds to kg, multiply by 0.4536

kg	St	lbs	kg	St	lbs	kg	St	lbs
1	0	2.2	43	6	11	85	13	5
2	0	4.4	44	6	13	86	13	8
3	0	6.6	45	7	1	87	13	10
4	0	8.8	46	7	3	88	13	12
5	0	11	47	7	6	89	14	0
6	0	13	48	7	8	90	14	2
7	1	1	49	7	10	91	14	5
8	1	4	50	7	12	92	14	7
9	1	6	51	8	0	93	14	9
10	1	8	52	8	3	94	14	11
11	1	10	53	8	5	95	14	13
12	1	12	54	8	7	96	15	2
13	2	1	55	8	9	97	15	4
14	2	3	56	8	11	98	15	6
15	2	5	57	9	0	99	15	8
16	2	7	58	9	2	100	15	10
17	2	9	59	9	4	101	15	13
18	2	12	60	9	6	102	16	1
19	3	0	61	9	8	103	16	3
20	3	2	62	9	11	104	16	5
21	3	4	63	9	13	105	16	7
22	3	7	64	10	1	106	16	10
23	3	9	65	10	3	107	16	12
24	3	11	66	10	6	108	17	0
25	3	13	67	10	8	109	17	2
26	4	1	68	10	10	110	17	5
27	4	4	69	10	12	111	17	7
28	4	6	70	11	0	112	17	9
29	4	8	71	11	3	113	17	11
30	4	10	72	11	5	114	17	13
31	4	12	73	11	7	115	18	2
32	5	1	74	11	9	116	18	4
33	5	3	75	11	11	117	18	6
34	5	5	76	12	0	118	18	8
35	5	7	77	12	2	119	18	10
36	5	9	78	12	4	120	18	13
37	5	12	79	12	6	125	19	10
38	6	0	80	12	8	130	20	7
39	6	2	81	12	11	135	21	4
40	6	4	82	12	13	140	22	1
41	6	6	83	13	1	145	22	12
42	6	9	84	13	3	150	23	9

Body mass index (BMI)

BMI calculation

BMI = weight (kg)/height^2 (m^2)

eg: 77kg, 1.83m
77/(1.83 x 1.83) = 23 (normal)

BMI	Weight status
<18.5	Underweight
18.5–24.9	Normal
25.0–29.9	Overweight
>30	Obese
>40	Morbidly obese

Body mass index chart for adults

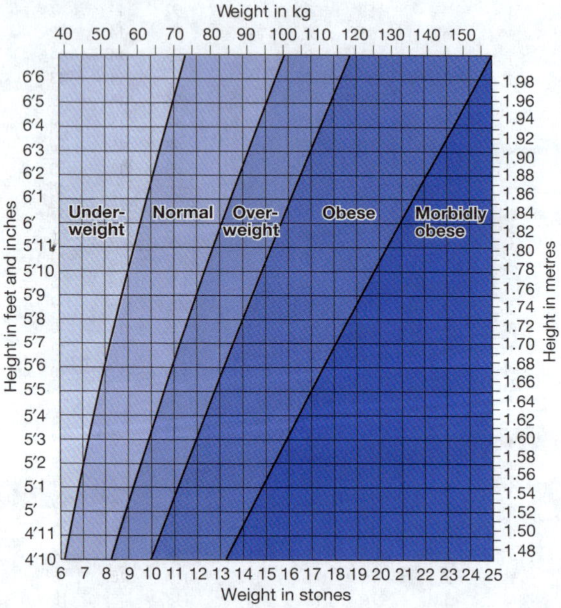

Plotting weight against height estimates BMI

Interesting cases

Note down any interesting or unusual cases which could be used for a teaching or a Grand Round case presentation.

Hospital number	
Details	

Hospital number	
Details	

Hospital number	
Details	

Hospital number	
Details	

Telephone numbers 1

Hospital:	Telephone:	
	Extension	Bleep
Consultants		
Consultant Secretary		
Registrars		
SHOs		
PRHOs		
Ward		
On-call registrar		
On-call SHO		
On-call PRHO		
Haematology		
Blood bank		
Clinical chemistry		
Microbiology		
Radiology		
ITU		
Porters		
Pharmacy		

Your firm's timetable

Time	Monday	Tuesday	Wednesday	Thursday	Friday

Telephone numbers 2

Hospital:	Telephone:	
	Extension	Bleep
Consultants		
Consultant Secretary		
Registrars		
SHOs		
PRHOs		
Ward		
On-call registrar		
On-call SHO		
On-call PRHO		
Haematology		
Blood bank		
Clinical chemistry		
Microbiology		
Radiology		
ITU		
Porters		
Pharmacy		

Your firm's timetable

Time	Monday	Tuesday	Wednesday	Thursday	Friday

Telephone numbers 3

Hospital:	Telephone:	
	Extension	Bleep
Consultants		
Consultant Secretary		
Registrars		
SHOs		
PRHOs		
Ward		
On-call registrar		
On-call SHO		
On-call PRHO		
Haematology		
Blood bank		
Clinical chemistry		
Microbiology		
Radiology		
ITU		
Porters		
Pharmacy		

Your firm's timetable

Time	Monday	Tuesday	Wednesday	Thursday	Friday

Index

Notes: Index entries appear in their full form; a list of abbreviations appears on pp. xi–xxii. **Bold** type indicates main references.

B

D

F

G

H

J